CONGESTIVE HEART FAILURE

Logic gives man what he needs
Magic gives man what he wants
Care that heals is magic

CONGESTIVE HEART FAILURE

WITHDRAWN

Edited by

CYDNEY R. MICHAELSON, R.N., M.N., C.C.R.N.

Cardiovascular Clinical Specialist,
Health Care Consultant and Educator,
Santa Barbara, California

with 170 illustrations

The C. V. Mosby Company

ST. LOUIS   TORONTO   1983

MOSBY

A TRADITION OF PUBLISHING EXCELLENCE

Editor: **Barbara E. Norwitz**
Assistant editor: **Bess Arends**
Manuscript editors: **Jennifer Collins, Gayle May**
Book design: **Jeanne Bush**
Cover design: **Suzanne Oberholtzer**
Production: **Linda R. Stalnaker, Judy England**

Printed in the United States of America

The C.V. Mosby Company
11830 Westline Industrial Drive, St. Louis, Missouri 63146

Library of Congress Cataloging in Publication Data

Main entry under title:

Congestive heart failure.

Includes index.
1. Congestive heart failure. I. Michaelson,
Cydney R. [DNLM: 1. Critical care—Nursing texts.
2. Heart failure, Congestive—Nursing. WY 152.5 C749]
RC685.C53C64   1983   616.1′29   83-8300
ISBN 0-8016-3443-1

AC/VH/VH 9 8 7 6 5 4 3 2 1   01/B/085

Contributors

DANIEL S. BERMAN, M.D., F.A.C.C.

Division of Cardiology,
Department of Medicine,
Department of Nuclear Medicine,
Cedars-Sinai Medical Center,
U.C.L.A. School of Medicine,
Los Angeles, California

MADELEINE DISTASO BRUNING, R.N., B.S.N., M.A.

Assistant Director of Nursing,
Cedars-Sinai Medical Center,
Los Angeles, California

MAGDA BUNOY, R.N., B.S.

Critical Care Clinical Instructor,
Department of Nursing Education,
Cedars-Sinai Medical Center,
Los Angeles, California

LORA E. BURKE, R.N., M.N.

Cardiovascular Clinical Specialist,
Collaborative Practitioner,
Los Angeles, California

MARY M. CANNOBIO, R.N., M.N.

Assistant Clinical Professor,
School of Nursing,
University of California, Los Angeles,
Los Angeles, California

JANE FREIN, R.N., M.N., C.C.R.N.

Cardiac Rehabilitation Coordinator,
French Hospital,
San Luis Obispo, California

ANNA GAWLINSKI, R.N., M.S.N., C.C.R.N.

Cardiovascular Clinical Nurse Specialist,
U.C.L.A. Center for the Health Sciences,
Los Angeles, California

MAUREEN HARVEY, R.N., M.P.H., C.C.R.N.

Consultants in Critical Care,
Pasadena, California

LESLIE FLICKINGER KERN, R.N., M.N.

Clinical Nurse Specialist,
Department Nursing Service;
Assistant Clinical Professor, School of Nursing,
U.C.L.A. Center for Health Sciences,
Los Angeles, California

KATHRYN M. LEWIS, R.N., B.S.N., M.Ed., C.C.R.N.

Critical Care Clinical Services,
Good Samaritan Medical Center,
Phoenix, Arizona

CYDNEY R. MICHAELSON, R.N., M.N., C.C.R.N.

Cardiovascular Clinical Specialist,
Health Care Consultant and Educator,
Santa Barbara, California

LINDA S. PURA, R.N., B.A., C.C.R.N.

Coordinator,
Blood Donor and Apheresis Center,
Cedars-Sinai Medical Center,
Los Angeles, California

CARMELA RIZZUTO, R.N., M.S.

Consultant, Continuing Professional Education,
Santa Barbara, California

CONCHITA S. SAM, R.N., M.N.

Clinical Specialist Critical Care Education,
Cedars-Sinai Medical Center,
Los Angeles, California

JANET UZANE SCHNEIDERMAN, R.N., M.N.

Assistant Clinical Professor of Nursing,
California State University,
Los Angeles, California

PREDIMAN K. SHAH, M.D., F.A.C.C.

Department of Medicine,
Cedars-Sinai Medical Center,
School of Medicine,
University of California, Los Angeles,
Los Angeles, California

CHARLEEN A. STREBEL, R.N., C.C.R.N., C.N.R.N.

Critical Care Instructor,
Santa Barbara Cottage Hospital,
Santa Barbara, California

NANCY PANTALEO STÜDER, R.N., M.S.

Research Associate,
Division of Nuclear Medicine,
Cedars-Sinai Medical Center,
Los Angeles, California

LISA M. TAORMINA-PAPLANUS, R.N., B.S.N., C.C.R.N.

Critical Care Instructor,
Santa Barbara Cottage Hospital,
Santa Barbara, California

Foreword

This monograph, *Congestive Heart Failure*, edited by Cydney R. Michaelson, represents yet another milestone in the maturation of the role of the non-physician health care specialist in the management of cardiac patients. With the regrettable decline of the nurse-midwife and the limited growth of the nurse anesthetist, it was the development of cardiac care units in the early 1960s that underscored a fundamental truth—acute treatment had to be provided by qualified personnel in immediate attendance. This fact was the initial impetus for the development of the coronary care system, which focused on the pivotal role of appropriately trained cardiac care unit nurses. It is difficult for the current graduate to recognize that 20 years ago cardiac resuscitation, hemodynamic monitoring, and electrical defibrillation were either in their infancy or restricted in their application to qualified licensed physicians. In actuality and predictably, the nurse readily accepted these new responsibilities and the application of such techniques in the management of the cardiac patient. These developments parallel the required expertise in management of ventilation and in the broad field of critical care medicine and critical care nursing.

With the emergence of critical care as a specialty in its own right, the role of non-physician health personnel in general and critical care nurses in particular is rapidly becoming clear. The principle that management of critically ill patients at a distance is unsatisfactory is generally accepted, and additional responsibilities are appropriately given to nurses and physician assistants who are available on a regular and predictable basis at the bedside. The management of the postsurgical patient, trauma and shock, acute pulmonary insufficiency, and a wide variety of other medical ills in addition to cardiovascular disease characterize the critical care field. Familiarity with hemodynamic monitoring, respiratory gas exchange, ventilation, acid-base balance, and a wide variety of other matters basic to the pathophysiology of disease is now required. An understanding of monitoring devices, the intra-aortic balloon, and ventilators themselves is necessary. Familiarity with the actions and complications of a vast array of powerful pharmacological agents is required on a day-to-day basis. Critical care personnel spend almost all of their professional time in direct contact with seriously ill patients, and they have greater opportunity for gathering experience in this field than the majority of practicing physicians. While physician supervision and direction are essential in the management of the critically ill patient, effective care can be delivered only by a highly informed, well-trained, and disciplined cadre of nursing personnel.

Congestive Heart Failure bears striking resemblance to many texts designed primarily for a physician audience. This reflects the fact that the same basic information is as fundamental to the role of the critical care nurse and physician assistant as it is to the physician. It further underscores the mutually supportive and participative role of all personnel engaged in the management of such patients. In addition to the basic knowledge of pathophysiology, it contains updated and detailed specific recommendations that are practical in nature and intended to allow for the effective performance of such duties. Non-physician critical care or cardiology specialists will find this book essential to effective performance in the future in their accepted role of rendering care to the sick in the most meaningful and positive manner.

H.J.C. Swan, M.D., Ph.D.

Director, Cardiology,
Cedars-Sinai Medical Center
Los Angeles, California

Preface

Congestive heart failure is a clinical syndrome that precipitates generalized organ dysfunction. It results from myriad causes and is the terminal event of most disease. It is a syndrome that has been the object of extensive research and intensive treatment, yet it still prevails as a leading cause of death. The complexity and prevalence of heart failure require diligent study and comprehensive knowledge in order to fully appreciate its biopsychosocial complexities. This book presents a comprehensive clinical approach to care of patients with congestive heart failure. Prior knowledge of cardiovascular anatomy and physiology, nursing theory, physical assessment, and pharmacology has been assumed to permit a more sophisticated approach to each topic. Emphasis is on multidisciplinary care. This monograph is intended for use by nursing, medical, and paramedical clinicians in critical care, acute care, and outpatient facilities. For this reason, some chapters focus on care of the critically ill and others deal with care of the chronically ill.

As editor, I have endeavored to structure a book that presents material in a logical, consistent manner. There is some duplication of major physiological principles and pathophysiological alterations to eliminate elaborate cross referencing. This allows the reader to use selected chapters as complete references. Major illustrations and diluent charts are prominently set off on a single page for the reader's convenience. Several chapters contain health care plans, which will aid clinicians in application of principles and health care considerations that are intended to direct and clarify the clinician's role in caring for individuals who have heart failure.

Congestive Heart Failure is divided into four sections. Part I, "Physiology and Pathophysiology," includes three chapters. Chapter 1 describes each component of the cardiovascular system in terms of its anatomical, physiological, and functional relationships. It provides a review of major physiological principles to help the reader retrieve information essential to understanding pathophysiology, underlying causes, clinical indicators, and intervention rationale for treating congestive heart failure. Chapter 2 is a comprehensive presentation of the pathophysiology of heart failure. It provides a conceptual framework for understanding the origin of clinical indicators and the rationale for therapeutic intervention. Chapter 3 presents a review of underlying causes and precipitating factors of heart failure. It includes an overview of adult congenital heart disease, valvular dysfunction, and systemic disorders that may precipitate cardiac decompensation.

Part II, "Patient Assessment," presents four chapters that address the major diagnostic components essential to accurately assess individuals in congestive heart failure. Chapter 4 reviews physical assessment principles and delivers a detailed presentation of the physical assessment process as it relates to individuals in heart failure. It clearly describes the major subjective and objective findings that characterize the syndrome.

Chapter 5 discusses noninvasive cardiological investigations that assist in the diagnosis and management of heart failure. These include echocardiography, chest roentgenography, electrocardiography, and laboratory analysis. The chapter addresses the role of selected pulmonary function tests used to evaluate heart failure and provides instructional information for the patient relating to potential health problems that may result from the performance of these studies.

Chapter 6 presents the clinical application of radionuclide angiography in congestive heart failure. The main objective of this chapter is to familiarize health care clinicians with the nuclear noninvasive diagnostic tests available to assess the condition and to evaluate the treatment of individuals with congestive heart failure.

Chapter 7 deals with bedside hemodynamic monitoring. It is the intent of this chapter to provide relevant information to critical care personnel that will enable them to accurately interpret hemodynamic data as they relate to hemodynamic alterations of heart failure. The chapter also addresses the predictive value of such data and the relationship of this information to the selection and alteration of therapy.

Part III, ''Patient Intervention,'' contains six chapters that address major interventions used to treat heart failure. Emphasis is on rationale and indications for use rather than on methodology and techniques. Chapter 8 is a comprehensive presentation of the major intervention for heart failure, namely pharmacological therapeutics. It addresses the prescriptives for use and action of inotropic agents, vasodilators, and diuretics in the setting of both acute and chronic heart failure. It contains excellent drug tables and diluent charts, which may be particularly useful in critical care settings.

Chapter 9 emphasizes the significance of arterial blood gas interpretation on accurate assessment and treatment of heart failure. It speaks to oxygen therapy, modes of delivery and ventilation, and the attendant cardiovascular effects. The effects of oxygen toxicity and the management of mechanically ventilated patients are also discussed.

Chapter 10 addresses the use of mechanical devices to support the failing heart. It presents an overview of intra-aortic balloon counterpulsation, left ventricular assist devices, abdominal left ventricular assist devices, and the total artificial heart. There is an illustration of the Jarvik-7 heart with an accompanying explanation of its mechanics. The physiological principles of mechanical devices and mechanics of operation are presented, as well as the role of critical care clinicians during the preinsertion, insertion, maintenance, and weaning phases of therapy. Complications and major health problems are addressed individually, and the chapter concludes with a case study and health care plan.

Chapter 11 discusses the physiological basis for sodium-restricted diets in the treatment of heart failure. It presents the major objective of dietary restrictions, identifies foods high and low in sodium and potassium, and describes the nurse clinician's role in using and evaluating diet therapy.

In chronic heart failure, rehabilitation focuses on modifying the patient's behavior in order to increase performance within the restrictions of the illness. Chapter 12 focuses on the education component of rehabilitation. It identifies the essential teaching principles and techniques, important assessment data, scope of content, evaluation criteria, and available resources and material.

The purpose of Chapter 13 is to attend to the psychological problems experienced by those with chronic congestive heart failure. There is little in the literature that deals specifically with the problems caused by chronic progressive heart failure. Much is written about the psychological problems arising from response to an acute myocardial infarction and to heart surgery. This chapter outlines the disease trajectory and provides a theoretical framework for assessment of and intervention in selected patient problems. These include change in life-style, loss of physical integrity, change in role function, and interdependence. Special attention is given to the grieving process and to the problem of facing death.

Part IV, ''Special Health Care Considerations,'' contains one chapter dealing with surgical treatment of underlying heart disease and another presenting the health care problems of infants and children with congestive heart failure.

Chapter 14 gives an overview of major surgical procedures performed to correct heart disease that may precipitate heart failure. The procedures and techniques required to perform coronary artery bypass grafts, aortic and mitral valve replacement, and heart transplantation are presented. They are accompanied by a comprehensive discussion of nursing care as it relates to patient management during the preoperative, intensive care, postintensive care, and discharge phases of recovery. Emphasis is placed on the biopsychosocial problems that may complicate recovery and appropriate interventions. A case study and a health care plan are presented to demonstrate application of major concepts addressed in the chapter.

Chapter 15 reviews the major cardiac congenital anomalies and accompanying clinical indicators that may precipitate heart failure in infants and children. It delineates the diagnostic studies used on a pediatric population and relates the psychological implications of these tests to children. The chapter discusses the effect of the disease process on the child's developmental status and presents the major psychological implications of heart disease and congestive heart failure on the parent-child-family interaction. A case study and health care plan demonstrate application of the major concepts set forth in the chapter.

A work such as this represents a concerted effort of many talented and dedicated individuals. I wish to extend my sincere appreciation to the contributors for sharing their professional expertise that has so endowed this book. I am indebted to Elizabeth Geffers for her recommendation at the onset of this project and to Pamela Swearingen for her confidence in my editorial ability. It has been a pleasure to work with the support of Bess Arends, Barbara Norwitz, and Peggy Fagen at The C.V. Mosby Company. I wish to thank Jorge Rameriz and May Cheney for their superb illustrations, which are a most important part of this monograph, and Cyndy Kelly for her secretarial skills, which expedited manuscript preparation.

I am personally indebted to Connie Rizzuto for her endless support, helpful advice, and constructive criticism during the development of this monograph and to my family, Jay, Jonathan, Jeremy, and Jenny, for their enduring patience and support.

To the readers, I invite you to partake of this work with the hope that it will aid in delivering expert, efficient professional health care.

Cydney R. Michaelson

Contents

PART I

PHYSIOLOGY AND PATHOPHYSIOLOGY

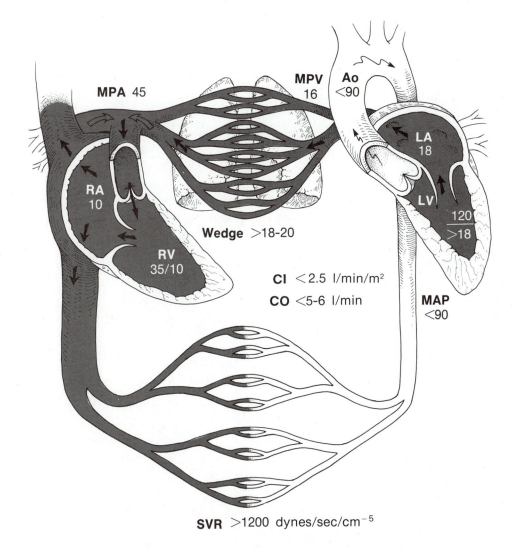

Clinical congestive heart failure

CHAPTER 1

Review of functional cardiovascular anatomy and physiology

KATHRYN M. LEWIS

Observation and evaluation of body functions through the use of multiple physical assessments, diagnostic tests, and monitoring devices has made it mandatory to possess a working knowledge of cardiovascular anatomy and physiology. These concepts are key components of the integrated comprehensive knowledge base required by the skilled professional health practitioner. Furthermore, they are essential to the decision-making process involved in providing the mechanical, pharmacological, and electrical interventions that are vital to providing safe and consistent care for the patient with heart failure.

The art and science of nursing and the technical advances in medicine have provided greater insight into the physiological function of the cardiovascular system. Although much research was done in chapter preparation, the reader would be well advised to remain updated by constant review and study of texts and current periodicals.

Every effort has been taken to develop and present material in a practical manner. The purpose of this chapter is to describe each component of the cardiovascular system in terms of its anatomical, physiological, and functional relationships within the body. An additional goal is to provide clinicians with a basic review of normal cardiovascular function so that they are able to recognize abnormality, evaluate implications, and provide appropriate interventions.

The cardiovascular system is composed of the heart, vessels, and blood. This system has two main functions: the delivery of oxygen and vital nutrients to the tissues and the removal of carbon dioxide and other waste products. Each component of the cardiovascular system will be described in detail to give insight into its ability to perform unique and vital functions.

CARDIAC ANATOMY
Location

The heart, a muscular organ that pumps blood throughout the circulatory system, is located in the center of the chest within the mediastinum between the lungs (Fig. 1-1). One third of the heart lies to the right of the midline, and two thirds of the heart lie to the left of the midline. The heart is superior to the diaphragm, with the apex located to the left of the central portion of the diaphragm. The base of the heart is located superiorly, posteriorly, and to the right of the midline at about the level of the second intercostal space. The heart is protected anteriorly by the sternum and the rib cage and posteriorly by the vertebral column and the rib cage.

Chambers

The heart consists of four chambers. The two upper compartments are thin, low-pressure chambers called the right and left atria. Each atrium has an appendage or pouch called an auricle that increases the surface area of each atrium. The atria are separated by a wall called the interatrial septum. The two lower compartments are thick-walled, high-pressure chambers called the right

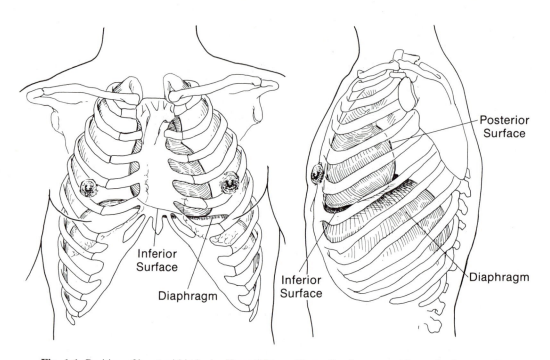

Fig. 1-1. Position of heart within body. Heart is located in mediastinum, superior to diaphragm with bulk of left ventricle to left side and posterior.

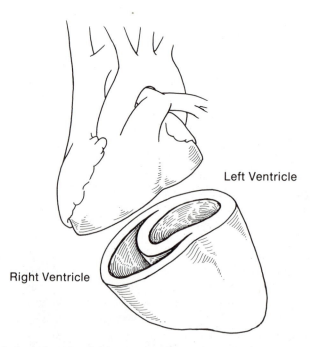

Fig. 1-2. Anatomical relationship of right ventricle illustrating globular shape of left ventricle and half-moon shape of right ventricle as it drapes around left ventricle. (Adapted from Guyton, A.C.: Basic human physiology, Philadelphia, 1977, W.B. Saunders Co.)

and left ventricles. They are separated by the thick interventricular septum.

The right ventricle, which is larger than the left ventricle, is shaped like a half-moon and wraps over the left ventricle (Fig. 1-2). The right ventricle pumps blood at 25 to 32 mm Hg pressure into the lungs for oxygenation and for release of carbon dioxide. The left atrium receives oxygenated blood from the lungs. The blood then passes into the left ventricle, which pumps it at 120 mm Hg pressure into the arterial system.[12]

Walls

The muscular walls of the atria and ventricles are separated by connective tisues that form the atrioventricular (AV) ring. This band of tissues is referred to as the cardiac skeleton because it serves as the origin for ventricular muscles. Externally the anterior and posterior interventricular sulci contain the coronary blood vessels and a variable amount of fat. The layers of the muscles of the ventricles are developed so that the muscle mass of the right ventricle is considerably less than that of the left ventricle. This is the result of the difference in pressures between the muscular chambers. Although each ventricle pumps essentially the same amount of blood, the major difference in structure reflects the difference in function (Fig. 1-3).

Layers of the heart wall. The wall of the heart is divided into three layers: the inner layer called the *endocardium,* the middle layer or *myocardium,* and the outer layer or *epicardium* (Fig. 1-4).

Endocardium. The endocardium is a thin layer of endothelial tissue that lines the inside of the myocardium, and is permeated by tiny blood vessels and bundles of smooth muscle. The endocardium is the inner lining of the heart and covers the valves of the heart and the chordae tendineae, the tendons that hold cardiac valves open. The endocardium is also continuous with the inner lining of the great vessels.

Myocardium. Structurally the myocardium is described as a latticework of long, faintly striated, fiber-like cells that divide, recombine, and divide again. They are separated by extensions and modifications of the plasma membrane called intercalated disks. These myocardial fibers are so tightly intertwined that when a muscle cell propagates an impulse, the potential spreads from cell to cell as a result of the low electrical resistant interconnections at the intercalated disks. This creates a system referred to as a functional syncytium (Fig. 1-5). The syncytial nature of cardiac muscle accounts for its unique response to stimulation. An impulse originating from a single cell can trigger an action potential to travel over the entire muscle mass. This is referred to as the "all-or-nothing principle."

There are two independently functional cardiac syncytia: the atrial syncytium and the ventricular syncytium. They are separated by the fibrous band surrounding the AV valvular rings. An impulse from a single atrial cell can cause the action potential to travel over the entire atrial muscle mass. Concurrently, an impulse arising in a single ventricular cell can cause an action potential to travel over the entire ventricular muscle mass, allowing the chambers to beat independently. However, impulses normally travel from the atria to the ventricles through special conductive tissue in the AV junction, resulting in coordinated function of these chambers.

The ultrastructure of the myocardium differs from skeletal muscle in that myocardial muscle has more mitochondria crowded between contractile filaments, and it contains more myoglobin than skeletal muscle.[11] Myoglobin is a conjugated protein that contains iron porphyrin prosthetic groups similar to hemoglobin. It is found in the sarcoplasm of cardiac muscle and is most abundant in ventricular muscle where the strong repetitive contractions require oxidative metabolism. Myoglobin is limited in its ability to store oxygen and primarily facilitates transport of oxygen from the cell membranes to the mitochondria for tissue oxygenation. For this reason myocardial tissue is unable to tolerate an oxygen deficit.

Epicardium. The epicardium is the thin trans-

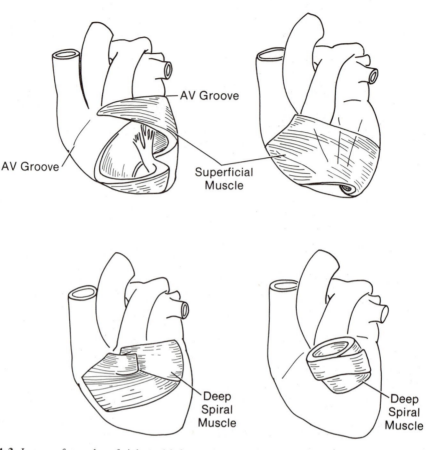

Fig. 1-3. Layers of muscles of right and left ventricles. Two groups of fibers surround outside of both ventricles and their origin in atrioventricular (AV) groove. Deep spiral muscle *(lower left)* also has its origin in AV groove and encircles both ventricles. Deep spiral muscle *(lower right)* is specific to left ventricle. (Adapted from Folkow, B., and Neil, E.: Circulation, New York, 1977, Oxford University Press.)

parent outer layer of the heart wall. It is continuous with the visceral pericardium.

Pericardial sac

The heart is enclosed in a serous pericardial cavity within the mediastinum. This sac is composed of two layers, the parietal and the visceral pericardium. The outer parietal layer is a fibrous pericardium that is attached to the large blood vessels that enter and leave the heart, to the diaphragm, and to the inner sternal wall of the thorax. The fibrous pericardium anchors the heart within the mediasti-

num and allows it to complete its unique gyrations without being intimated by or imposing on adjacent thoracic structures.

The inner layer of the parietal pericardium is composed of serous tissue and is continuous with the visceral pericardium, which directly overlies the heart and encloses the great vessels. The visceral pericardium is also called the epicardium (Fig. 1-4).

Between the smooth moist surfaces of the parietal and visceral pericardium (epicardium) is a potential space known as the pericardial cavity. It con-

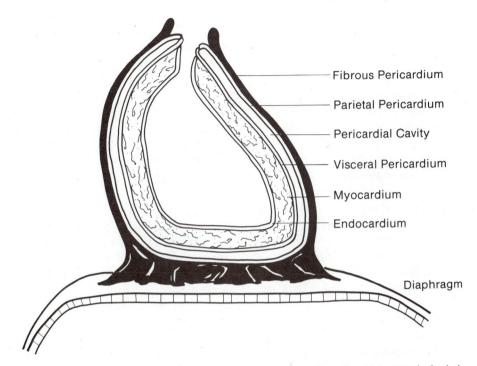

- Fibrous Pericardium
- Parietal Pericardium
- Pericardial Cavity
- Visceral Pericardium
- Myocardium
- Endocardium
- Diaphragm

Fig. 1-4. Schematic representation of layers of heart and pericardium showing anatomical relationship between pericardial layers, cardiac tissue, and diaphragm. (Adapted from Walls of the heart and pericardium, plate 49. In Kapit, W., Elson, L.M.: The anatomy coloring book. Copyright © 1977 by Wynn Kapit and Lawrence M. Elson. By permission of Harper & Row, Publishers, Inc.)

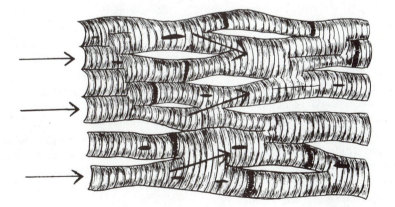

Fig. 1-5. Anatomical representation of functional syncytial structure of cardiac muscle. Because of interconnections of muscle fibers, an electrical current spreads rapidly from cell to cell. (Adapted from Guyton, A.C.: Basic human physiology, Philadelphia, 1977, W.B. Saunders Co.)

tains a minute amount of lubricating fluid that allows the heart to move freely within the sac. It is in this potential space that fluid may accumulate, hampering cardiac function.

Valves

The forward flow of blood through the heart is controlled by a series of one-way valves that prevent back flow within the heart chambers. The valve between the left atrium and the left ventricle has two cusps and is called the mitral valve (Fig. 1-6). The valve between the right atrium and right ventricle is called the tricuspid valve; this valve has three cusps. The AV valves are connected by the chordae tendineae to the muscular extensions of the myocardium called the papillary muscles. The papillary muscles and their chords keep valve cusps pointing in the direction of blood flow. The contraction of the papillary muscles helps to prevent the valves from swinging too far up into the atria during ventricular contraction (Fig. 1-7).

Semilunar valves are situated between the ventricles and the large vessels and are so named because of their half-moon shapes. These valves prevent the back flow of blood into the ventricles. The pulmonary semilunar valve lies between the right ventricle and the pulmonary artery, a vessel carrying unoxygenated blood to the lungs. The aortic semilunar valve is situated between the left ventricle and the aorta, a vessel carrying blood to the systemic circulation.

There are no valves between the returning venous circulation and the atria; therefore the atria must always accept blood returning to them. This accounts for the venous neck distention as seen in right-sided heart problems and the pulmonary congestion seen with left-sided heart problems.

The opening and closing of valves are a result of changes in pressure within the cardiac chambers. Whenever inlet pressures are higher than outlet pressures, the valves open. When outlet pressures are higher than inlet pressures, the valves close. When the ventricles begin to contract, the mitral and tricuspid valves close in response to rising ventricular pressure. When ventricular pressure is

greater than outflow pressure in the arteries, the semilunar valves open, and blood is pumped into the pulmonic and systemic circulations.

Once contraction is complete the ventricles relax and pressure within them falls below that of the outflow tracts, resulting in closure of the semilunar valves. Ventricular muscle then relaxes. AV valves open when ventricular pressure drops below atrial pressure, allowing blood to fill the ventricles.

Coronary blood supply

Like other organ systems the heart has its own blood supply (Fig. 1-8). However, unlike other organ systems coronary artery perfusion is affected by the cardiac cycle. The right and left sides of the heart receive oxygenated blood from the coronary arteries, yet the time during which optimal perfusion occurs differs.[8] The right ventricular myocardium receives a continuous flow of oxygenated blood from the coronary circulation throughout the cardiac cycle. This occurs because the right ventricle generates lower systolic pressure. The left ventricular myocardium receives oxygenated coronary blood flow only during the diastolic phase of the cardiac cycle, because the left ventricle exerts systolic pressure equal or greater than aortic pressure. As a result, intramyocardial tension and pressure hamper blood flow within the myocardium, particularly to the subendocardial layers.

The coronary arteries have their origin behind the cusps of the aorta. The left coronary artery divides into the anterior descending branch and the left circumflex branch. The anterior descending branch supplies arterioles to the left and right ventricles; the circumflex branch supplies arterioles to the left atrium and left ventricle. There are very few anastomoses between the coronary arteries, but many exist between the arterioles. This allows for the development of collateral arteriolar circulation should obstruction occur in one of the main branches of the coronaries.

The coronary arteries are also responsible for blood supply to the electrical conduction system. In 60% of individuals, the right coronary artery is responsible for the blood supply to the sinus node,

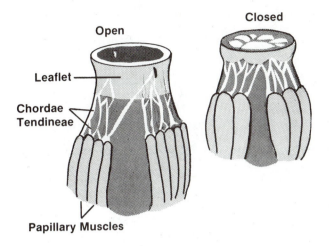

Fig. 1-6. Mitral valve. Cusps are shut in ventricular systole to prevent backflow of blood. Papillary muscles and their chordae tendineae keep valve cusps pointing in direction of blood flow during ventricle diastole. (Adapted from Huszar, R.J.: Emergency cardiac care, Bowie, Md., 1974, Robert J. Brady Co.)

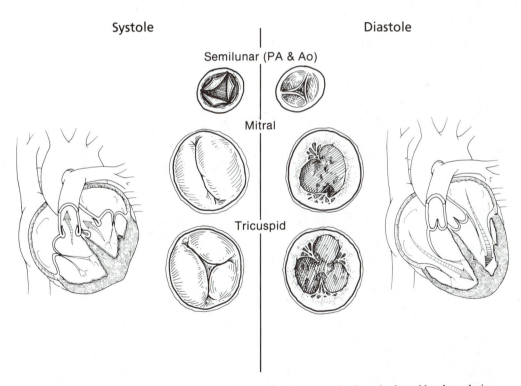

Fig. 1-7. Schematic representation of position of semilunar, mitral, and tricuspid valves during systole and diastole.

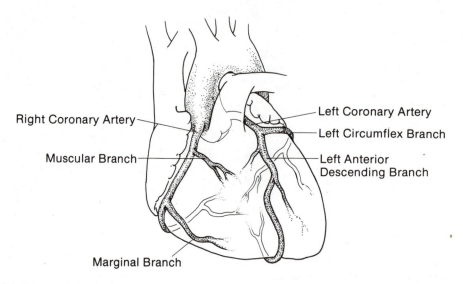

Fig. 1-8. Right and left coronary arteries exit from ascending aorta and cross ventricular muscle mass.

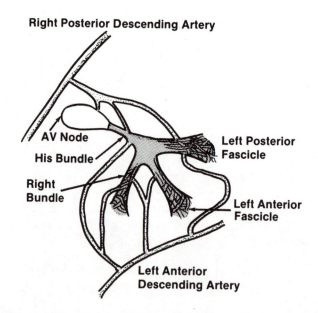

Fig. 1-9. Schematic representation of coronary blood supply to myocardial electrical conduction system. Dual blood supply from right coronary artery and from left anterior descending branch of left coronary perfuse the AV junction and fascicles of bundle branches. Note supply to fascicles of left; this may account for protection to conduction in event of right coronary heart disease. (Adapted from Hindman, M., and Wagner, G.: Bundle branch block during myocardial infarction. In Primary cardiology, New York, December 1980, PW Communications, Inc.)

the major pacemaker of the heart. The left circumflex branch supplies the sinus node in the remaining 40% of individuals.

In about 90% of individuals, the posterior descending branch of the right coronary artery perfuses the electrical conduction system at the AV junction. In the remaining 10% dual blood supply from the right posterior descending branch of the right coronary artery and the anterior descending branch of the left coronary artery perfuse the conduction system, supplying the ventricular myocardium (Fig. 1-9).[4]

As blood is perfused through the coronary circulation system, oxygen and nutrients are delivered to myocardial tissue substrate and carbon dioxide and metabolic waste products are removed. The deoxygenated blood is collected by smaller cardiac veins that empty into the great cardiac vein, coronary sinus, and finally the right atrium. The venous blood from the anterior aspect of the heart empties into the great cardiac vein, and the venous blood from the posterior aspect is drained into the middle cardiac vein. The remaining blood empties directly into the right ventricle by way of the small thebesian veins.

VASCULAR SYSTEM
Great vessels

There are three major venous systems within the body: the first is the superior vena caval system, which receives blood from the subclavian and jugular veins, originating from the head, neck, and upper extremities; the second is the inferior vena caval system, which receives blood from the lower extremities by way of the iliac veins and from the liver, spleen, and other gastrointestinal organs by way of the portal circulation; the third are the cardiac veins, which open into the right atrium, allowing venous return from the heart's coronary blood supply.

Venous blood draining into the right atrium is pumped into the right ventricle and out the pulmonary trunk. The pulmonary trunk divides into the right and left pulmonary arteries, and each branch carries blood to its respective lung for release of carbon dioxide and assimilation of oxygen. Blood is then returned to the left heart by way of four pulmonary veins that deliver oxygenated blood into the left atrium. Blood is then squeezed into the left ventricle, which pumps it into the ascending aorta.

The aorta is the largest of the arterial vessels. It leaves the heart from the left ventricle and is divided into three major anatomical sections: the ascending aorta, the aortic arch, and the descending aorta. The descending aorta is further divided into the thoracic and abdominal sections. This vessel is the major conduit of arterial blood to all organ systems except the lungs.

Structure of vessel walls. All blood vessels have a common wall structure, yet they differ in size and in purpose. The three anatomical layers of the vascular system are: (1) the tunica intima, (2) the tunica media, and (3) the tunica adventitia or externa (Fig. 1-10).

The tunica intima is an extension of the heart's own inner lining, the endocardium. It is composed of a thin layer of simple squamous epithelium that comes into direct contact with circulating blood. Thickening of the tunica intima, such as occurs with lipid-related lesions, impedes blood flow in affected vessels and damages the organ systems they supply. Also, plaque formation on the endothelium causes a roughened surface susceptible to clot formation. The tunica intima also has a thin layer of areolar connective tissue overlying the endothelium and an outer layer of elastic tissue called the internal elastic membrane.

The tunica media, or middle layer, is the thickest layer of the vessel wall. It contains elastic fibers and smooth muscles that give strength and recoil to blood vessels. This structure is responsive to the dilating and constricting effects of volume, pressure, hormones, and specific medications. An external elastic membrane separates the tunica media from the tunica adventitia.

The tunica adventitia (or externa) is composed of loose connective tissue, elastic and collagen fibers, smooth muscle fibers, and fibrous tissue that help vessels maintain anatomical configuration

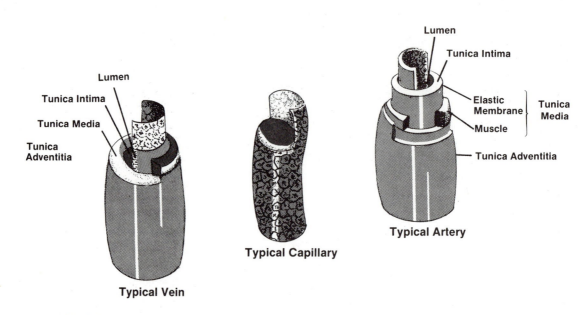

Fig. 1-10. Schematic representation of structure of artery, capillary, and vein, illustrating difference in size and wall structure. (Adapted from Huszar, R.J.: Emergency cardiac care, Bowie, Md., 1974, Robert J. Brady Co.)

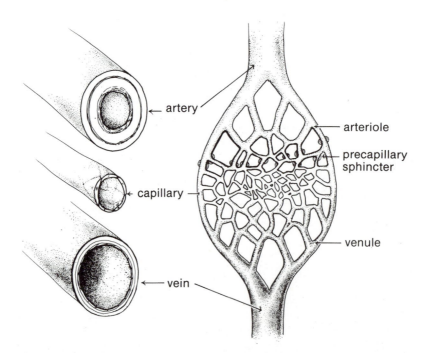

Fig. 1-11. Anatomical relationship of artery, arteriole, capillary bed, venule, and vein. Note precapillary sphincter—ring of smooth muscle that controls amount of blood entering capillary circulation.

in the face of high intravascular pressures.

The anatomical layers of the vascular system contain their own blood vessels. The cells lining the endothelium are supplied directly by blood flow through the vessels; cells of the media and adventitia are supplied by tiny vessels known as the vasa vasorum, or vessels of vessels.

The cavity within a blood vessel is referred to as the lumen. The size of vessel lumina varies and is dependent on the location and the function of the vessels. The radius of the lumen is the primary controlling factor of circulation. For example, the smaller the radius of a vessel, the more resistance there is to blood flow; the larger the radius of a vessel, the less resistance there is to blood flow. Regulation of the size of the radius is controlled by the central nervous system vasomotor center, the autonomic nervous system, hormones, enzymes, and local vasoactive metabolic substances. A pathophysiological process such as atherosclerosis may also affect lumina of vessels; however, the process is usually obstructive rather than vasoactive.[5]

Arteries. Arteries are thicker and stronger than the other vessels in the body. This is necessary because of the elevated pressure within the arterial system. Arteries are composed of a thick middle layer, the tunica media, which provides arteries with two important functional properties: elasticity and contractility.

When the ventricles of the heart contract and eject blood into the arteries, the elastic property of the arteries allows them to expand to receive the volume. As the ventricles relax, the elastic recoil of the arteries propels the blood into the circulatory system.

Arterioles are small arteries that deliver blood to the capillaries. They have fewer elastic fibers as compared to arteries and they become progressively smaller in size as they approach the capillaries. They are subject to constriction and elastic recoil, and they are the primary structure controlling the amount of blood entering the capillary bed.

Capillaries. Capillaries are microscopic vessels measuring approximately 7 to 8 μm in diameter.

The exact value of capillary pressure is not known, but normal mean capillary pressure is estimated at about 17 mm Hg.[12] The term "capillary bed" refers to the sum of all the capillary networks. Capillaries have no tunica media or adventitia and are composed of a single layer of endothelial cells that are permeated with minute passageways called pores. These pores are responsible for the passage of water and the many dissolved nutrients from the lumen of the capillary into the interstitial spaces and back again. Blood does not flow at a continuous rate through the capillaries. At a point where blood enters the capillary, there is a ring of smooth muscle called the precapillary sphincter, which relaxes and contracts and thus controls the amount and force of blood entering the capillary bed (Fig. 1-11). This phenomenon of capillary blood flow is called vasomotion; it is directly related to the amount of oxygen in tissues and circulating blood. When oxygen concentration in blood and/or in tissues is very low, the rate and duration of blood flow increase to meet tissue metabolic demand.

Capillary dynamics—Starling forces. The two main processes that occur across the capillary walls are diffusion and filtration/absorption. These are controlled by a balance of forces across the capillary membrane that include four principal pressures. The two pressures for inward flow are interstitial fluid pressure and interstitial fluid colloid osmotic pressure. The two pressures responsible for movement of fluid outward through the capillary membranes are capillary pressure and plasma colloid osmotic pressure. These factors are better depicted in the following diagram:

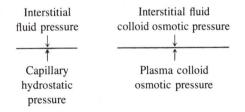

Capillary hydrostatic pressure. Hydrostatic pressure is the pressure resulting from the weight of water at rest inside a system. Capillary hydrostatic pressure is the force exerted by blood inside the capillary bed. Pressure at the arterial end of a true capillary averages 35 mm Hg and 15 mm Hg at the venous end.[19] However, these pressures are variable depending on the activity of the arterioles and venules. For example, when arterioles are closed, capillary pressure falls to values close to venous pressure. When arterioles are dilated, pressures may rise to values as high as 50 mm Hg. The exact value of capillary hydrostatic pressure is not known, but normal mean pressure is estimated at 17 mm Hg.

Plasma colloid osmotic pressure. The colloid osmotic pressure of normal human plasma averages about 25 to 28 mm Hg pressure, and it is directly related to the amounts of the plasma proteins, albumin, globulin, and fibrinogen.[12] There is almost twice as much albumin in plasma as globulin and each gram of albumin exerts about twice the osmotic pressure of 1 g of globulin. Fibrinogen accounts for a very small fraction of pressure. Therefore about 70% of the total colloid osmotic pressure of the plasma results from the albumin fraction, and about 30% results from the amounts of globulin and fibrinogen.

Interstitial fluid pressure. Interstitial fluid pressure averages less than atmospheric pressure. This negativity accounts for the suction of fluid out of the capillary.

Interstitial fluid colloid osmotic pressure. The average colloid osmotic pressure of interstitial fluid is about 5 mm Hg. This is because small amounts of plasma proteins do leak into interstitial spaces. The average protein concentration of the interstitial fluid is a fraction, less than one fourth, of that in plasma, and it is equivalent to 2 g in 100 ml of blood.[12]

Effective filtration pressure. Effective filtration pressure (PEff) is the difference between the two forces that move fluid out of the intravascular space and the two forces that push fluid into the intravascular space. Effective filtration pressure at the arterial end of a capillary is about 8 mm Hg and is about −8 mm Hg at the venous end of a capillary.[10] Because of this difference, fluid tends

to be filtered out of the capillary at the arterial end and reabsorbed at the venous end.

The low pressure at the venous end of the capillary bed changes the balance of Starling forces and accounts for reabsorption of fluid into the capillary. This change in pressure accounts for about 90% of the reabsorption of fluid that had filtered out at the arterial end.

An abnormal increase in net filtration pressure causes a disruption of the fluid balance between the interstitial fluid compartment and the intravascular fluid compartment. This results in tissue edema. There are two primary causes of edema: the first is hypertension or an increase in blood hydrostatic pressure; the second is inflammation. Inflammation causes capillaries to become more permeable to plasma proteins, thereby changing the balance of oncotic forces. When this occurs, plasma proteins increase interstitial osmotic pressure and fluid accumulates in tissues, causing edema.

Diffusion. While filtration is the net movement of fluid out of the capillaries at the arterial end, diffusion occurs in both directions. The diffusion of water and water-soluble substances back and forth across the capillary membrane is about 80 times greater than the rate at which plasma flows through the capillaries.

There is a slight difference between the forces at the capillary membranes, which favors more filtration of fluid into interstitial spaces. This increased filtration is balanced by the return of fluid to circulation by the lymphatics. The lymphatic fluid is reabsorbed into the circulation from the venous system.

Veins. Venules are the small vessels that are contiguous with the capillaries and ultimately form veins, as illustrated in Fig. 1-11. Venules closest to capillaries consist of tunica interna made up of endothelial cells and tunica adventitia made of connective tissue. As the venules merge into veins, they develop a tunica media characteristic of veins.

While veins consist of the same three layers found in arteries, there are three characteristics that account for functional differences. These are: less elastic tissue and smooth muscle, more fibrous tissue, and the presence of valves.

The lesser amount of elastic tissue and smooth muscle allows for the greater distensibility of veins. This permits the veins to adapt to variations in blood flow. A large amount of blood can be added to the venous system before veins become distended to the point where venous pressure rises. For this reason, veins are referred to as capacitance vessels. The fibrous tissue surrounding these vessels in the lower extremities helps maintain anatomical configuration in the face of elevated hydrostatic pressures resulting from gravitational force. Valves are also present in the extremity vessels to prevent the back flow of blood. An insufficiency in venous valves, particularly in the lower extremities, can result in progressive loss of vessel elasticity, vessel distention, and pressure overload of the affected vein. Veins close to the surface are most vulnerable since they are not surrounded by supportive skeletal muscle.

Blood and blood components

Blood volume is approximately 7% of total body weight. Almost one half of the blood is composed of circulating cells. The other half is plasma, which is an isotonic solution in which sodium and chloride are the major electrolytes. Plasma is part of the extracellular fluid and is considered the transport medium for carbohydrates, amino acids, and proteins.

A breakdown of blood components is illustrated in Fig. 1-12. Blood is primarily plasma that contains a suspension of red cells, white cells, and platelets. Red cells constitute about 45% of the blood. The percentage of red blood cells is measured as hematocrit. The principal function of red cells is the transport of hemoglobin, which has the unique ability to bind and release oxygen. Hematocrit and hemoglobin concentrations are measured quantitatively and reflect the red cell concentrations found in a sample of blood drawn from an individual.

White blood cells make up about 1% of the circulating blood volume and are classified into two major categories, polymorphonuclear leukocytes (PMNs) and mononuclear leukocytes.[12] PMNs are the body's first line of defense against bacterial infections. This subgroup contains the following granulocytes: neutrophils, eosinophils, and basophils. Mononuclear leukocytes contain lymphocytes and monocytes. The lymphocytes are formed in the lymph nodes, thymus, and spleen, and they play a key role in immunity. The monocytes are formed in the bone marrow and by their phagocytic action on bacteria function similar to neutrophils. In conjunction with lymphocytes, they may also kill tumor cells.

Platelets are small bodies 2 to 4 mm in diameter containing a variety of chemicals and enzymes active in the process of inflammation and the coagulation of blood. Platelets are the agents that initiate clot formation. When blood vessel walls are injured or tissue is damaged and exposed to air, platelets change shape and collect at the site of injury by adhering to exposed collagen. This aggregation forms a temporary hemostatic plug and is the first step in a complex clotting mechanism. The hemostatic plug is converted into a definitive clot by fibrin. The mechanism responsible for fibrin formation involves a series of complex "cascade" reactions. Discussion of this is beyond the scope of this book. There also exists within the blood a fibrinolytic system that limits clot formation. The active component is plasminogen or fibrinolysin. This enzyme causes clot degradation as healing occurs.

Plasma proteins contribute to cardiovascular function by maintaining blood volume, blood viscosity, and osmotic pressure. These proteins comprise 8% of the plasma and consist of albumin, globulin, and fibrinogen fractions. Since the capillary walls are essentially impermeable to them, they exert an oncotic pressure of 25 to 28 mm Hg. Plasma proteins are also responsible for 15% of the buffering capacity of the blood. Circulating antibodies in the globulin fraction of plasma proteins are synthesized in the plasma cells, and the albumin fraction and fibrinogen are synthesized in the liver.

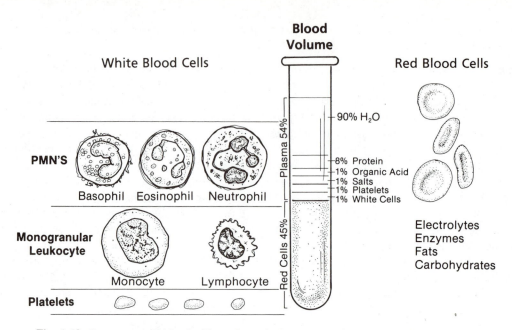

Blood Volume

White Blood Cells

Red Blood Cells

PMN'S

Basophil   Eosinophil   Neutrophil

Monogranular Leukocyte

Monocyte   Lymphocyte

Platelets

Plasma 54%

— 90% H_2O

8% Protein
1% Organic Acid
1% Salts
1% Platelets
1% White Cells

Red Cells 45%

Electrolytes
Enzymes
Fats
Carbohydrates

Fig. 1-12. Components of blood with mathematical analysis of volume and cellular contents.

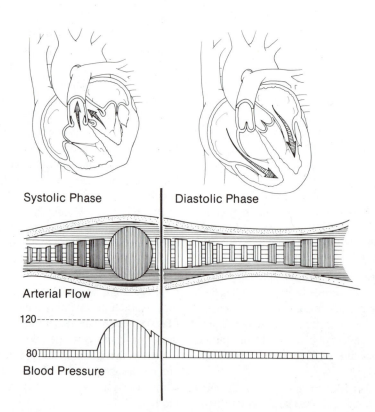

Systolic Phase   Diastolic Phase

Arterial Flow

120 - - - - - - - - - - - - - - - - -

80

Blood Pressure

Fig. 1-13. Systolic and diastolic phases of cardiac cycle with relationship to arterial blood flow and pressure. (Adapted from Huszar, R.J.: Emergency cardiac care, Bowie, Md., 1974, Robert J. Brady Co.)

Lymphatic circulation

The lymphatic system circulates 2 to 4 L of fluid in 24 hours. This fluid originates primarily in the interstitial fluid compartment where fluid efflux normally exceeds fluid influx across the capillary membrane.

Lymph moves as the result of skeletal muscle contraction, negative intrathoracic pressure, and the suction effect of high-velocity blood flow in the veins. A significant amount of protein enters this system from the interstitial fluid in the liver, intestines, and other tissues. This is because of the permeability of the lymphatics to large molecules. These proteins and the interstitial fluid are returned to the venous side of circulation where lymphatic channels terminate. The amount of protein returned to the circulation by the lymphatics per day equals 25% to 50% of the total plasma protein. Consequently, changes in lymphatic function resulting from obstruction and elevated venous pressure will significantly affect interstitial fluid volume and capillary dynamics.

CARDIAC CYCLE

The cardiac cycle is the coordinated activity of the heart that results in circulation of blood throughout the cardiovascular system. It is comprised of two phases: contraction (systole) and relaxation (diastole) (Fig. 1-13).

The lapse time from the beginning of one beat of the heart to the next includes systole, a period of atrial and ventricular muscular contraction when blood is propelled forward, and diastole, a period of muscle relaxation, when the heart's cavities are refilled with blood. The cardiac cycle is less than 0.80 second from the onset of atrial excitation to the completion of ventricular excitation and onset of ventricular relaxation. During a complete cardiac cycle, the atria are in systole 0.10 second and in diastole 0.70 second, and the ventricles are in systole 0.30 second and in diastole 0.50 second.[17,18]

Ventricular diastole

During the first third of the ventricular relaxation phase of diastole, the atria are also in diastole. During this time the AV valves are open and approximately 75% of ventricular filling occurs. During the middle third of diastole only a small amount of blood flows into the ventricles, and during the latter third phase of ventricular diastole the atria contract, contributing an additional 30% of blood volume to the circulation.[1] (See the boxed material below.)

At the end of ventricular diastole, just before ventricular systole, the pressures within the chambers of the heart are similar. The atrial and ventricular pressures as well as the communicating pulmonary pressures are summarized in Fig. 1-14. Note the equivalent diastolic pressures in the pulmonary artery, left atrium, and left ventricle. The

---

**THE THREE PHASES OF EACH OF THE TWO COMPONENTS
OF THE CARDIAC CYCLE**

Ventricular contraction	= Systole	= Isolation phase Rapid ejection phase Reduced ejection phase	=	Atrial filling
Ventricular relaxation	= Diastole	= Isovolumic relaxation phase Rapid ventricular filling Reduced ventricular filling	=	Atrial contraction

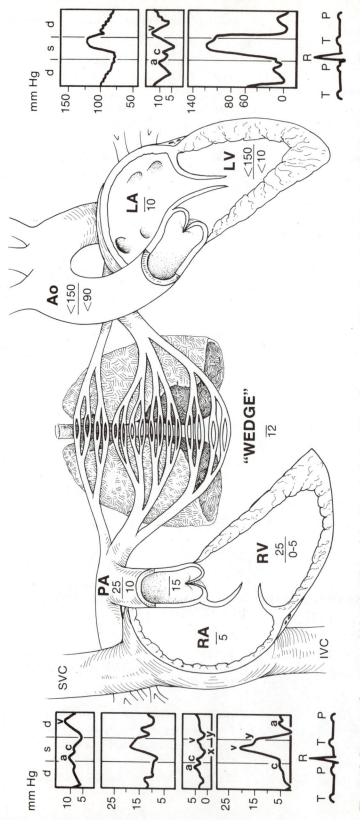

Fig. 1-14. Summary of pressures within atria and ventricles. Note similarity of diastolic pressures within communicating chambers of pulmonary artery, left atrium, and left ventricle. During diastolic phase of contraction this pressure may be transmitted to pulmonary capillary bed and may be measured using flow-directed balloon-tipped catheter.

recognition of the continuity of this pressure system helps one to understand why left venericular function can be indirectly observed by monitoring pulmonary artery diastolic pressure.[2,6,10]

Ventricular systole

Once the ventricles are filled, pressures rise abruptly, causing the AV valves to close. Within hundredths of seconds, the ventricles accumulate pressures needed to force open aortic and pulmonic valves. During this phase, known as isometric or isovolumic contraction, there is no shortening of muscle fibers and no ejection of blood. There is only an increase in muscle tension and a build-up of pressures within the system. Intraventricular pressures finally elevate to a point when contraction and ejection of blood takes place. Aortic and pulmonic valves are forced open, and blood is pumped out of the ventricular chambers. This is called the ejection phase. During the period of rapid ventricular ejection, almost one half of the ventricular volume is pumped into the aorta, and the remaining blood is ejected shortly thereafter. Finally, at the end of systole, the ventricles suddenly begin to relax and elevated pressures in the pulmonary artery and the aorta allow blood to flow backward, closing the aortic and pulmonic valves. The ventricular muscle mass continues to relax, dropping intraventricular pressures to their original levels during diastole, and the cardiac cycle begins again.

Heart sounds

The four heart sounds, referred to as S_1, S_2, S_3, and S_4, are thought to be produced by the contraction and relaxation of the muscles of the heart, and they are associated with the closure of the valves of the heart. Two of the heart sounds, S_1 and S_2, are heard normally, and S_3 and S_4 are considered abnormal unless proved otherwise.

S_1 is the first heart sound and corresponds to the onset of ventricular contraction. It is associated with the closure of mitral and tricuspid valves, which sends sound waves through each respective ventricle.

The mitral valve closes a fraction of a second before the tricuspid. Occasionally, the timing is such that it is possible to hear the splitting of the first sound. This is a very staccato sound that is then followed by the second heart sound.

The second heart sound, S_2, occurs at the end of ventricular contraction and corresponds with the onset of ventricular diastole. When aortic and pulmonic pressures are elevated, blood flows backward closing the aortic and pulmonic valves. Sounds from the valve closures are transmitted along the respective great vessels. The second heart sound may also be heard as a split sound. The disparity in closing time between the aortic and pulmonic valve is greater during inspiration since during this phase more blood flows into the right heart, which will delay ventricular contraction. Subsequent pulmonic valve closure will also be delayed. Split S_2 sounds also have a very staccato quality.

The third heart sound, S_3, occurs early in diastole, a fraction of a second after the second heart sound. At this time, during the period of rapid ventricular filling, vibrations are produced by the rapid inflow of blood and are transmitted by the ventricular muscle. In older adults, the presence of the third heart sound denotes altered cardiac function; however, it is considered normal in healthy children and young adults. S_3 is a rather rhythmic sound in comparison to the staccato sounds of split S_1 and S_2.

The fourth heart sound, S_4, occurs during ventricular diastole after atrial contraction immediately preceding S_1. In certain pathological conditions such as congestive heart failure, a ventricle may be dilated with decreased compliance. This is accompanied by elevated end-diastolic pressure, and such pressure increases the resistance of the ventricle to filling. S_4 is rhythmic and is heard over the apical area.

Normal electrical cardiac conduction

The heart has an intrinsic regulating system called the conduction system. The components of the conduction system are the sinus node, the interatrial tract, the AV junctional tissue, the bundle of His, and the His-Purkinje system (Fig. 1-15).

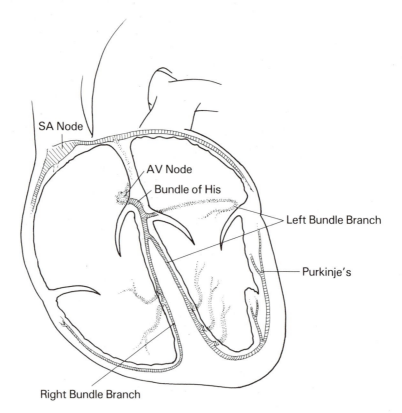

Fig. 1-15. Graphic representation of position of cardiac conduction system within myocardium.

The conduction system is composed of specialized muscle tissue that generates and distributes the electrical impulses that stimulate the cardiac muscle fibers to contract. Normal cardiac rhythms result from the spontaneous excitation of cells in the sinoatrial node.

The sinus node is located near the junction of the superior vena cava and the right atrium just beneath the atrial epicardial surface. It varies considerably in size. It is about 15 mm long, 5 to 7 mm wide, and 1 to 2 mm thick. The shape of the sinus node is described as being a distorted elliptical structure that can range between 10 and 20 mm in length and 3 and 5 mm at its widest part. Since it is less than 1 mm beneath the epicardial surface, it is vulnerable to disease (Fig. 1-16).[7]

The cells of the sinus node are arranged in a very fine pattern within a framework of dense collagen tissue. There are a number of stellate cells found in the central portion of the node. These are believed to be the source of pacemaking activity. Once an electrical impulse is initiated by the sinus node, the impulse spreads out over both atria causing them to contract. At the same time, this impulse depolarizes the AV node.

The AV node is located in the right atrium medial and anterior to the opening of the coronary sinus and directly above the attachment of the tricuspid valve. It is described as a flattened structure that varies in size and usually measures 5 to 6 mm in length and 2 to 3 mm in width at its widest surface (Fig. 1-17).[4,7] The cells of the AV node connect freely with one another, forming a dense

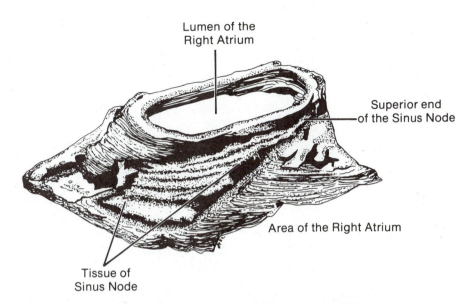

Fig. 1-16. Location and shape of sinus node within right atrium. It is inferior to superior vena cava. (Adapted from Ritota, M., and Mangiola, S.: Cardiac arrhythmias, Philadelphia, 1974, J.B. Lippincott Co.)

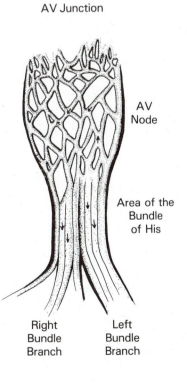

Fig. 1-17. Schematic representation of AV junction, demonstrating entrance fibers into AV node, orientation of AV node to bundle of His, and entrance fibers into intraventricular septum.

network. Near the distal end of the node, the cells become organized in a parallel fashion before entering into the bundle of His. Delayed transmission of electrical impulse from the atria to the ventricles occurs in the AV node to allow further filling of the right and left ventricle before ventricular electrical stimulation. In the AV junction, the fibers at the crest of the AV node are considerably thinner than fibers lower within the AV node. This anatomical arrangement is probably a mechanism to delay impulses.

The AV junction has two functions. One is to conduct impulses at a specific rate of speed. The second is to form impulses that are now thought to originate only in the lower areas of the AV junction in the region of the bundle of His rather than in the AV node itself.

During normal electrical conduction, impulses reach the crest of the AV node and enter the thin fibers that temporarily slow conduction. The impulses then pass through the AV bundle and enter the bundle branches more or less simultaneously. If the tissues at the bundle of His are not activated, they are capable of reaching their own threshold potential and of initiating and propagating an impulse.

After transmission through the AV node, the impulse is normally transmitted into the ventricular conduction network. The bundle of His is a continuation of the AV node and divides into two major branches called the right and left bundle branches. The right bundle branch, or fascicle, is a very slender group of fibers running along the right side of the interventricular septum; it reaches the base of the right ventricle where it divides into a network supplying the right ventricular myocardium. For this reason, it is said that the endocardial septum of the right ventricle is most electrically sensitive.[14,18] This is a condition that probably supports successful electrical pacing, and may explain sensitivity and ventricular ectopy that occurs with pulmonary catheter insertion.

The left bundle branch runs along the left side of the interventricular septum and divides into an anterosuperior fascicle and an inferoposterior fascicle. The anterior division is a relatively long and thin pathway that reaches the base of the anterior capillary muscle. It supplies the anterosuperior part of the left ventricle. The posterior division is a relatively short, but thick, structure passing to the base of the posterior capillary muscle. It supplies the inferoposterior aspect of the left ventricle.

The right bundle branch and both the anterior and the posterior fascicles of the left bundle branch divide into a complex network of fibers called the Purkinje fibers. They are distributed throughout the ventricular myocardium. The fibers are more abundant in the subendocardial layers, are longer than common myocardial fibers, and are believed to lack nervous supply.

The entire electrical conduction system is very complex and lies just under the endocardial surface of the heart. This accounts for the susceptibility of the conduction system to disease and/or lack of blood supply.[13]

The events of myocardial electrical conduction are depicted on the electrocardiograph as specific wave forms (Fig. 1-18).

ELECTROPHYSIOLOGICAL PROPERTIES OF THE HEART

The electrophysiological properties of cardiac cells have four major characteristics: (1) automaticity, (2) excitability, (3) conductivity, and (4) contractility.

Automaticity

Automaticity is the property of self-excitation and the maintenance of rhythmic activity. The myocardial cells possessing this property are called pacemaker cells. Under normal circumstances, the pacemaker cells have the highest degree of rhythmicity and the most rapid discharge of impulse. These pacemaker cells are located in the sinus node, the primary focus for pacing the heart. There are pacemaker cells with a lesser degree of automaticity and a slower inherent or natural discharge present in the atria, the AV junctional tissues, and the ventricles.

The more peripheral the site of the pacemaking cells, the slower their rhythmicity and inherent dis-

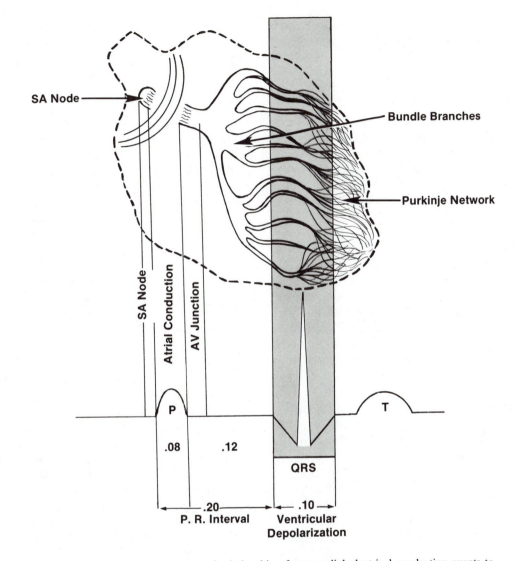

Fig. 1-18. Schematic representation of relationship of myocardial electrical conduction events to electrocardiogram. (From Marriott, H.J.: Workshop in electrocardiography, Tarpon Springs, Fl., 1980, Tampa Tracings, slide 7, p. 5.)

charge rate. The sinus node usually controls the heart rate because its more rapid impulses spread to the atria, the AV junction, and the ventricles, overriding the slower impulses of the other pacemaking foci. An ectopic pacemaker located in the atria, in the AV junction, or within the ventricles must discharge impulses faster than the most rapid pacemaker in order to usurp control.

Excitability

Excitability is the cellular responsiveness to a natural or artificial stimulus. Both pacer and nonpacemaker myocardial cells have this property. The degree of excitability varies during the phases of the cardiac cycle, but the response of the myocardial cell to a given stimulus at a particular moment is either maximal or not present at all. Excitability exists because of an ionic imbalance across the membranes to the cells. The degree of negativity within the cells is an important factor determining excitability.

Conductivity

Conductivity is a property that allows the myocardial cell to propagate an impulse to its neighboring cell. An impulse of adequate strength originating in any area of the heart during the resting period can cause a wave of excitation that is then propagated to the whole of the heart muscle.

Conduction velocity

Conduction velocity is the speed at which the propagation of an impulse occurs from cell to cell. Conduction velocity will vary in different cardiac muscles and is dependent on cellular ionic balance. It is the fastest in Purkinje fibers and can reach almost 4000 mm/sec.[4,18] Conduction between the atria and ventricles normally occurs in a forward fashion, but it can occur in a retrograde manner.

Contractility

Contractility is the ability of the muscle fibers to shorten when electrically stimulated. It is discussed later in the chapter under "Physiology of Cardiac Contraction."

Refractory period of myocardial cells

The term "refractory" describes the ability with which a cell is able to reject an impulse. The refractory period of cardiac cells is divided into the absolute refractory period and the relative refractory period. During cellular excitation, the myocardial cells are rendered unresponsive to any stimulus, regardless of its strength. This is called the absolute refractory period of that cell and extends from Phase 0 in rapid depolarization to about −60 mV in repolarization.

A relative refractory period will follow, during which some of the cells are capable of responding to a stimulus stronger than normal. During this time the impulse will be conducted, but the conduction velocity will be slow. The duration of the refractory period is influenced by heart rate. For example, when heart rate is increased, the refractory periods are shorter.

The term "supernormal" applies to a phase during the last part of repolarization just before the cell returns to its resting potential. A weak stimulus from inside or outside the myocardium can evoke an action potential at this time.

Various drugs can affect the refractory periods of the myocardial cells by altering the level of the threshold potential or the duration of the action potential. Conditions causing ischemia and hypoxia can also alter membrane responsiveness.

Resting potential

During the resting state, a negative and steady potential gradient is present inside a nonpacer cell. This gradient is termed the "resting potential." When an impulse propagates across the cell membrane, the inside of the cell rapidly becomes positive in relation to extracellular fluid. A phase of recovery or repolarization follows, and the potential again becomes negative. Repolarization is initially rapid, then slow, and then rapid again.

The phase of rapid depolarization is called Phase 0. Phase 1 is the phase of early rapid repolarization, Phase 2 the plateau, and Phase 3 is the phase of rapid repolarization. The resting potential that follows is called Phase 4 (Fig. 1-19, *A*).

During the resting state, or Phase 4, of repolarization, the potential gradient inside the pacemaker cell is unsteady and negative. As soon as repolarization from the preceding excitation is completed, the action potential will show a spontaneous slope that slowly reaches the threshold level. At this point, rapid depolarization takes place and the action potential is transmitted through adjacent fibers and cells. The slow slope of the resting state is called spontaneous (diastolic) depolarization and represents the mechanism normally responsible for rhythmic and autonomic activation of cells.

Action potential

During the resting period of the cardiac cycle, the myocardial cells maintain a negative potential

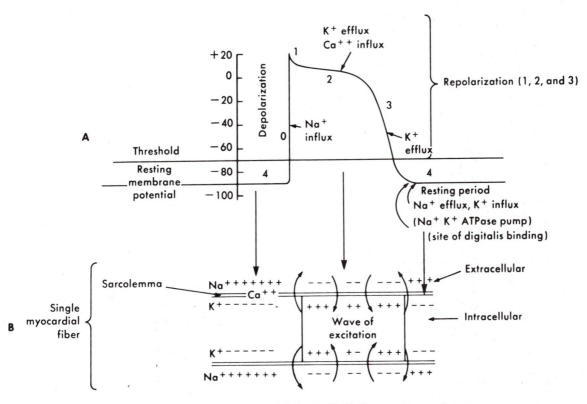

Fig. 1-19. **A,** Action potential of single myocardial fiber (cell). **B,** Ionic exchanges that occur across cell membrane of single myocardial fiber during action potential. (From Hahn, A.B., Barkin, R.L., and Oestreich, S.J.K.: Pharmacology in nursing, ed. 15, St. Louis, 1982, The C.V. Mosby Co.)

of about −90 mV in atrial and ventricular muscle and about −50 mV in the sinus node and the AV junctional tissue. This negative potential is the result of specific concentrations of intracellular and extracellular ions. Ions concerned with the electrical activity are primarily sodium, potassium, and calcium.

Normally, the greatest concentration of sodium is extracellular and of potassium is intracellular. Because of these differences, the inside of the cell is negative in relation to the outside. In the process of depolarization, the negative intracellular charge rapidly diminishes and becomes positive, creating an action potential (Fig. 1-19, *B*).

Phase 0 is the result of an influx of sodium into the cell. When the intracellular concentration of the sodium ion is sufficient to change the resting membrane potential to about −65 mV, a self-sustained wave of complete depolarization occurs. The influx of sodium is a passive process that does not require energy use. Once the critical level of the threshold potential is reached, the cell membrane increases its permeability to sodium, and this intense inward movement completes Phase 0.

In the sinus node and in the AV junction, the fast channels for sodium are thought to be absent. Instead, slow inward channels for sodium and calcium predominate. This peculiarity is an important concept to remember when discussing certain antiarrhythmic drugs.[14,23]

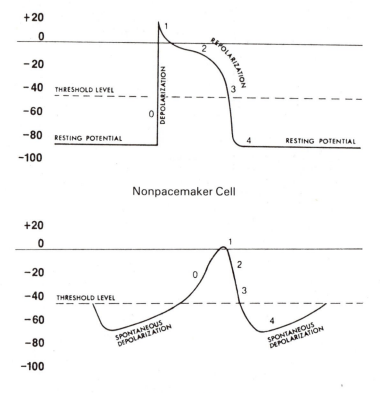

Fig. 1-20. Schematic representation of action potential of pacemaker and nonpacemaker cells. (Adapted from Ritota, M., and Mangiola, S.: Cardiac arrhythmias, Philadelphia, 1974, J.B. Lippincott Co.)

Phase 1 is the initial phase of repolarization. During this phase there is a rapid influx of the negative chloride ion as well as an inactivation of the inward sodium current. During Phase 2, the decreasing outward potassium currents balance a similarly timed slow inward calcium current so that membrane voltage remains almost constant and a plateau effect is achieved. This allows a more sustained myocardial contraction while the membrane is maintained in a depolarized state. It also allows contraction to be completed before another can be activated. Both the potential of the plateau phase and the magnitude of the slow inward calcium current depend on extracellular calcium concentration. Ischemia and hypoxia alter

intracellular calcium concentration; they can also modify the processes responsible for the slow inward current. This may shorten the plateau phase, thus decreasing the time available for myocardial contraction.

The major portion of repolarization is accomplished during Phase 3 and results mainly from passive efflux of potassium outside of the cell. The slow calcium current is inactivated at this time. As the membrane potential rapidly returns to the resting state, the action potential terminates for ventricular and atrial cells. The cell membrane is returned to its original −90 mV at the end of repolarization. During Phase 4, the ionic pumps move sodium to the outside of the cell and move potassium to the inside of the cell to reestablish resting potential.

Automatic and working cells

The rate of diastolic depolarization in Phase 4 is different for pacemaker (automatic) and nonpacemaker (working) cells. Cells having pacemaker activity do not remain at a resting state and instead begin a slow diastolic depolarization caused by a decreased potassium efflux and increased sodium influx. This event causes threshold to be reached sooner than in nonpacemaker cells. Fig. 1-20 describes the slope of depolarization in pacemaker cells and the difference in potential.

Automatic cells undergo depolarization without any outside stimulus and are located in the sinus node, in the orifice of the coronary sinus, at the junction of the AV node, and throughout the His-Purkinje system. Under normal circumstances, the working cells of the atrial and ventricular myocardial system do not possess the quality of inherent automaticity.

The automatic cells of the sinus node possess the steepest slope of Phase 4 depolarization. The other automatic ·cells do not reach their threshold as rapidly as the sinus node, which undergoes spontaneous depolarization at about 60 to 100 times/minute in the adult. For this reason, it is regarded as the dominant pacemaker of the heart. Lower pacemakers such as the AV junction reach inherent threshold potential at a rate of 40 to 60 times/minute and the cells in the His-Purkinje system reach inherent threshold potential at 20 to 40 times/minute. If a normally dominant pacemaker fails to reach threshold potential fast enough to maintain control, the pacemaker with the most rapid inherent rate will assume control. For example, should the rate of the sinus node discharge less than 40 times/minute, or fail to activate atrial tissue, the AV junction pacemaker will reach threshold potential and depolarize at a rate of 40 to 60 times/minute. In doing so, it becomes the dominant pacemaker. Normally the AV junction pacemaker cells are considered protective in nature and do not compete with sinus activity.

PHYSIOLOGY OF CARDIAC CONTRACTION

The mechanical response of myocardial cells to electrical depolarization is called contractility. Contractility is the myocardial cellular response to a flow of ions across cellular membranes.

The myocardium consists of long strands of myocardial cells. Each cell is made up of a nucleus and longitudinal myofibrils. Multiple parallel fibrils are cross-banded into a series of units. The sarcomere is composed of two sets of filaments that are elongated, polymerized, protein molecules. These filaments are responsible for contraction. They are composed of thin filaments called actin filaments and thick filaments called myosin filaments. The ends of the thin actin filaments insert into Z bands, which are structures that join the sarcomere longitudinally. Fig. 1-21 illustrates these structures.

Within the sarcomere, the individual actin and myosin filaments maintain a constant length. Each actin filament has a number of receptor sites. To promote movement, cross-bridges are formed between the globular extensions of myosin and the receptors on the actin filaments. Each cross-bridge undergoes a conformational change that pulls the two filaments toward each other, sliding the thin actin filament over the thick myosin filament. This reduces the length of the sarcomere and results in muscle contraction.[15]

The globular ends of the myosin molecule contain a hydrolyzing enzyme that acts on the high-energy substrate, adenosine triphosphate (ATP), to facilitate the formation of the cross-bridges between actin and myosin. The contraction would occur continuously and result in rigor if it were not for regulation by two other protein complexes. These regulating proteins are called tropomyosin and troponin and are also integral parts of the actin complex. Troponin and tropomyosin control contraction by inhibiting cross-binding sites on the actin filament. This causes myofibril relaxation. The presence of troponin and tropomyosin is essential to normal cellular contraction and relaxation.[16]

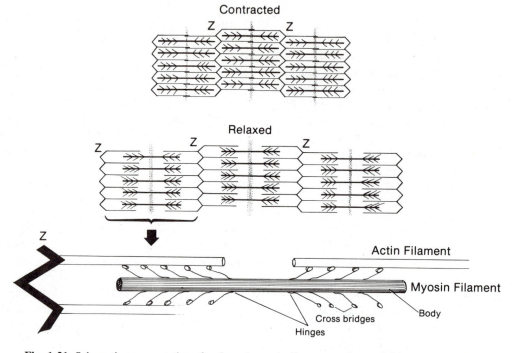

Fig. 1-21. Schematic representation of actin and myosin filaments and cross bridges responsible for conformational change that shortens myocardial muscle fibers resulting in cardiac contraction. (Adapted from Guyton, A.C.: Basic human physiology, Philadelphia, 1977, W.B. Saunders Co.)

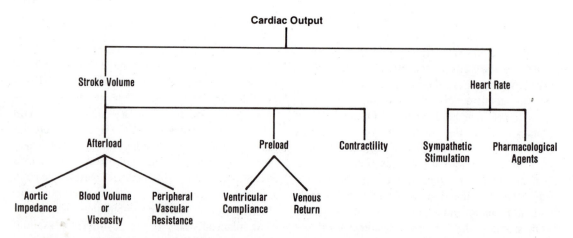

Fig. 1-22. Determinants of cardiac output. Factors influencing cardiac output include changes in heart rate and stroke volume. Stroke volume, in turn, is affected by afterload and preload.

Role of calcium

In the presence of calcium ions, the inhibitory effect of troponin and tropomyosin on the actin filament is itself suppressed. Troponin has an extremely high affinity for calcium. When calcium ions combine with troponin, the troponin molecule undergoes a conformational change that is thought to uncover the active sites on the actin filament, allowing cross-bridges to form and contraction to occur. The exact mechanism of the creation of the cross-bridges is still unknown.

Contraction can be augmented by increasing the amount of calcium at the cross-bridge by several mechanisms. First the external source of calcium can be increased, thereby increasing the amount of available extracellular calcium. When this occurs, more calcium will diffuse into the cell so more will be available at the contractile sites. This is a temporary, short-lived effect.

A second method is to increase the permeability of the cell membrane to calcium. Catecholamines may increase cellular permeability by activating enzymes that open the calcium channels. Circulating catecholamines are normally present in conditions of stress or can be introduced into the system by administration of sympathomimetic agents.

A third method is to increase the amount of intracellular sodium, which would then interchange with extracellular calcium. This interchange functions as a revolving mechanism whereby excess sodium leaves a cell and calcium enters in the same proportion. This mechanism may be stimulated by digitalis. Digitalis inhibits the sodium-potassium pump so more sodium remains in the cell. Intracellular sodium is then available for exchange with extracellular calcium. The net result is the increase of free intracellular calcium to support myocardial contractility.

After the muscle has contracted, calcium must be removed from troponin to allow myocardial relaxation. This takes place by an energy-consuming process that causes the cross-bridges to separate so that the sarcomeres relax. During this time, free calcium is removed from the cell by the sarcoplasmic reticulum and is bound to the cell membrane and extruded into the extracellular space.

DETERMINANTS OF CARDIAC PERFORMANCE

Cardiac output, the quantity of blood pumped from the left ventricle to the aorta, is calculated from the product of heart rate and stroke volume. Normal cardiac output in the adult male at rest is about 5.5 L/minute and tends to decrease with age.[12]

Stroke volume

Stroke volume is the amount of blood ejected by a ventricle during each systolic contraction. In a resting adult, stroke volume is about 70 cc. Factors that increase heart rate or stroke volume tend to increase cardiac output; factors that decrease heart rate or stroke volume tend to decrease cardiac output. For example, if stroke volume falls below normal, the heart rate will increase in an effort to compensate. Fig. 1-22 illustrates the functional relationship of the determinants of cardiac output.

Stroke volume is determined by the force of ventricular contraction. The more forcefully the cardiac fibers contract, the more blood they are able to eject. Within limits, contraction is most efficient when muscle fibers are optimally stretched. The heart always acts to accept blood returning to it, so the important determining factor is right atrial pressure generated by the entry of blood into the heart. For example, during increased activity, large amounts of blood return to the heart. This causes increased diastolic filling pressures, which in turn stretch the muscle fibers of the ventricles. The increased length of these muscle fibers activates more cross-bridges at a cellular level and consequently intensifies the force of ventricular contraction. Thus the increased volume of venous return is handled by an increased cardiac output through a more forceful contraction. This phenomenon by which the length of cardiac muscle fiber determines the force of contraction is referred to as "Starling's law of the

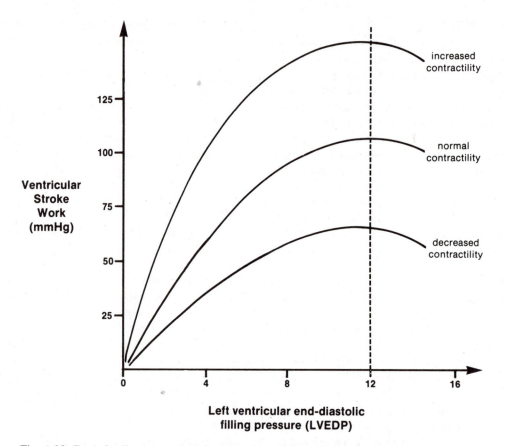

Fig. 1-23. Frank-Starling curve. As left ventricular end-diastolic volume increases, so does ventricular stroke work, or contractility. When left ventricular end-diastolic filling pressure exceeds a maximal point, stroke work, contractility, and cardiac output diminish.

heart'' and is illustrated in Fig. 1-23.

The maximal percentage of the cardiac output that can increase above normal in response to stress is referred to as the cardiac reserve. During strenuous exercise, the cardiac output can be increased 3 to 4 times normal. With a progressive increase in exercises and given a healthy myocardium, cardiac reserve can increase 5 to 6 times normal. Although cardiac reserve depends on many factors, it is influenced most by conditions affecting contractility. These include ischemic heart disease, valvular disorders, and myocardial necrosis.

Preload

Stroke volume depends on three factors, the first being preload. Preload is the volume of blood in the ventricles at the end of diastole, immediately before the onset of ventricular contraction. This volume is indirectly measured by left ventricular end-diastolic filling pressure. According to Starling's law, in the normal heart, as left ventricular end-diastolic filling pressure increases, the ventricles should respond with a more vigorous contraction, increasing stroke volume and cardiac output to meet increased demand. However, if stroke volume is not sufficient, there is an increase in the amount of blood remaining in the ventricle. During diastole, the blood entering the ventricles adds to the blood remaining and leads to an increase in left ventricular end-diastolic filling pressures.

An increase in left ventricular filling pressure will result in an increase in left atrial pressure, which is transmitted to the pulmonary venous circulation and from there into the pulmonary capillary system. When pulmonary capillary pressure increases to a critical degree, fluid may transudate from the pulmonary capillaries into the alveoli. This accounts for the presence of basilar rales and the adventitious sounds heard during chest auscultation in patients with heart failure.

Compliance is another determinant of left ventricular filling pressure. Compliance refers to the stiffness of the ventricles, or their distensibility. Fibrosis, hypertrophy, and scar tissue from myocardial disease may contribute to a reduced compliance, which will result in an elevated left ventricular filling pressure.

Right ventricular filling pressures also affect left ventricular function. The interrelationships between right ventricular filling pressure and cardiac output is such that when venous pressures and right ventricular filling pressures increase, cardiac output will increase (according to Starling's law).[5] Blood will be moved into the systemic arterial tree, ventricular diastolic pressure will decrease, and equilibrium will be maintained.

If left ventricular contractility is diminished and right ventricular pressures continue to rise, the high right ventricular pressure will cause blood to back up into the peripheral venous system. This accounts for the systemic circulatory congestion that occurs in heart failure.

Afterload

Another determinant of stroke volume is afterload, or the resistance against which the ventricles must pump. When applied to the intact ventricle, afterload may be defined as the tension, force, or stress in the ventricular wall after the onset of muscle shortening.[12,20] Afterload is related to aortic impedance, peripheral vascular resistance, and blood viscosity. One type of mechanical impedance is a narrowing of the aortic opening caused by stenosis of the aortic valve. This narrowing causes a resistance to the ejection of blood from the left ventricle. Aortic regurgitation or backflow of blood into the ventricle also causes an increase in heart work.

Peripheral vascular resistance refers to the resistance to blood flow by the force of friction between blood and the walls of the blood vessels. It is related to the diameter of arterioles. Slight changes in the radius of a blood vessel cause tremendous changes in its ability to conduct blood flow. Conduction of blood within a vessel increases in proportion to the fourth power of its diameter. Poiseuille's law states that the quantity of blood that will flow through a vessel in a given period of time is:

$$Q = \frac{\pi P r^4}{8nl}$$

Where Q = blood flow, r = radius, l = length, P = pressure difference, and n = blood viscosity.

Note that the equation demonstrates that the rate of blood flow is directly proportional to the fourth power of the radius of the vessel.[3] This relationship demonstrates that the radius of the blood vessel has the greatest influence in determining the rate of blood flow through a vessel. Consequently, as the vessels constrict the impedance to flow is increased. It follows that peripheral vascular resistance becomes a direct influence on the afterload. Both arterial blood pressure and peripheral vascular resistance are clinical indices of cardiac afterload.

Afterload increases the work of the heart by its effect on myocardial muscle tension. As afterload increases, the myocardial fibers must be able to shorten against this load for the ventricle to effectively eject blood. This requires an increase in the isometric component of muscle contraction. During this phase, muscle length remains the same, but the muscle tension increases greatly, causing a marked elevation in myocardial energy requirements and oxygen consumption.

Increased afterload and preload also trigger a change in ventricular geometry. Laplace's law (P = T/R) states that pressure developed by a level of wall tension in a hollow organ is inversely proportional to the radius of the chamber.[20] Muscle tension (T) necessary to maintain a level of pressure (P) is increased when the radius (R) of the vessel or chamber is increased. As the hollow organ dilates, wall tension increases to maintain pressure and flow. In order to maintain pressure and eject blood into the aorta, tension in an enlarged heart must be greater than tension in a normal heart. This means a dilated heart with large end-diastolic volume must develop more wall tension than a normal-sized heart. To adapt to this demand, the ventricles increase in muscle mass by replication of myofibrils and mitochondria. This process is called ventricular hypertrophy, and it occurs in two forms, concentric and eccentric hypertrophy, depending on the nature of the load.

Blood volume

Normally the amount and viscosity of blood returning to the heart help regulate the stroke volume and affect cardiac output. The normal viscosity of blood results in part from the red cell content and the amount of plasma protein. Conditions increasing viscosity, such as dehydration or an unusually high production of red cells, will cause increased afterload. When there is increased retention of salt and water by the kidneys there will generally be an increase in blood volume. However, if the blood volume is reduced because of disease, dehydration, or excessive bleeding, venous pressure will fall, and venous return to the heart will be inadequate. Consequently, ventricular filling drops and cardiac output is reduced.

Contractility

Inherent myocardial contractility is difficult to precisely define. Physiological measurements are related to maximum velocity of fiber shortening,

and clinical measurements are related to stroke volume and cardiac output. Increased contractility results from sympathoadrenergic stimulation, circulating catecholamines, epinephrine and norepinephrine, or administration of selective pharmacological agents. Depressed contractility may occur secondary to changes in myocardial cellular physiology and loss of functional tissue resulting from disease.

NEUROHUMORAL CONTROL OF THE HEART

The autonomic control of the heart is a result of opposing sympathetic (stimulating) and parasympathetic (inhibitory) influences. Sensory impulses from receptors in different parts of the cardiovascular system act upon these centers so that a balance is achieved.

Within the cerebral medulla is a group of neurons called the cardioacceleratory center. Arising from this center are sympathetic fibers that travel down a tract in the spinal cord and pass outward into the cardiac nerves and the nerves of the sinus node, AV node, junctional tissue, and small portions of the myocardium (Fig. 1-24).[5,12] When this center is stimulated, nerve impulses travel along the sympathetic fibers and cause a release of norepinephrine at the synaptic site. This substance acts on adrenergic receptors to cause an increase in heart rate and contractility. Located in the cerebral medulla is another group of cardioinhibitory neurons that function in opposition to the cardioaccelerator center. In this inhibitory center are the parasympathetic fibers that reach the heart by way of the vagus nerve. These vagal fibers also innervate the sinus node and the AV node. When this center is stimulated, nerve impulses transmitted along the parasympathetic fibers cause the release of acetylcholine at synaptic sites. This substance decreases the heart rate (Fig. 1-25).

Adrenergic receptors

Adrenergic receptor sites are classified as alpha, $beta_1$, and $beta_2$. The nature of response to drug interventions depends on its relative ability to ac-

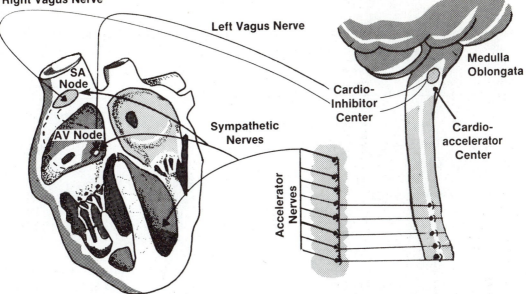

Fig. 1-24. Schematic representation of innervation of specific portions of myocardial conduction system from cardioinhibitor and accelerator centers within medulla of brain. (Adapted from Huszar, R.J.: Emergency cardiac care, Bowie, Md., 1974, Robert J. Brady Co.)

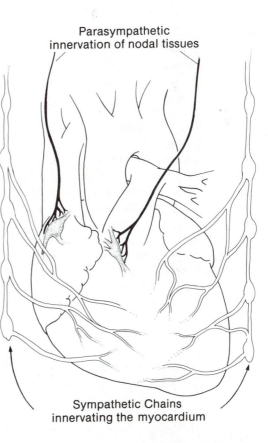

Fig. 1-25. Autonomic nervous system innervation of nodal tissue and myocardium by parasympathetic vagus nerve fibers and sympathetic chains.

Table 1-1. Responses of effector organs to sympathetic activation by catecholamines or sympathomimetic drugs

Effector organ	Adrenergic receptor	Predominant physiological or pharmacological effects	Predominant response observed
Heart			
Sinoatrial node	Beta$_1$	↑ Rate	↑ Heart rate
Conduction tissues	Beta$_1$	↑ Conduction velocity	↑ Heart rate
Myocardium	Beta$_1$	↑ Contraction	↑ Force of contraction
Arteries and arterioles			
Renal, abdominal viscera	Alpha	Vasoconstriction	↓ Local blood flow ↑ Systemic blood pressure
Subcutaneous	Alpha	Vasoconstriction	↓ Local blood flow
Skeletal muscle	Beta$_2$	Vasodilation	↑ Local blood flow ↓ Systemic blood pressure
Veins	Alpha	Vasoconstriction	↑ Venous return ↑ Cardiac output
Kidney	Beta$_2$	↑ Renin secretion	↑ Sodium reabsorption ↑ Blood pressure

Adapted from Gerald, M.C., and O'Bannon, F.V.: Nursing Pharmacology and Therapeutics, © 1981, pp. 40, 46. Reprinted by permission of Prentice-Hall, Inc., Englewood Cliffs, N.J.

tivate one or more of these receptor sites and on the relative distribution of these sites within a given organ or tissue. Table 1-1 summarizes the responses of effector organs to sympathetic activation.[9]

Receptor sites are described and categorized in terms designating their response to sympathetic stimulation. Alpha-adrenergic receptors are sites along the autonomic nervous pathways where excitatory responses occur when adrenergic agents, such as epinephrine and norepinephrine, are released. There are alpha-adrenergic receptors in peripheral vascular beds and in the gastrointestinal tract. Stimulation of these alpha receptors has little direct cardiac effect but raises blood pressure by constricting peripheral vascular arterioles. There is also an increase in the sphincter tone in the stomach and the intestines. Alpha-adrenergic blocking agents are substances that interfere with transmission of adrenergic stimuli along the nervous pathways.

Other receptor sites exist along the autonomic nervous pathways. These are the beta-adrenergic receptors, which are only mildly excited by norepinephrine release. There are two types of beta-adrenergic receptors, beta$_1$ and beta$_2$. Beta$_1$ receptors are located in the heart and small intestines. Stimulation of the beta$_1$ receptors causes an increase in conduction velocity over the AV node increase in myocardial contractility, and an increase in conduction velocity over the AV node and the ventricular conduction system. There is also an increase in the automaticity and the rate of discharge at ventricular ectopic foci.

Beta$_2$ receptors are located in bronchial smooth muscle and the peripheral vascular beds. Stimulation of the beta$_2$ receptors results in peripheral vasodilation and relaxation of constricted bronchial muscle.

Pressoreceptors (baroreceptors)

Nerve cells capable of responding to changes in blood pressure are called pressoreceptors or baroreceptors. These receptors affect the heart rate, and they are involved in three complex feedback mechanisms: the carotid sinus reflex, the aortic reflex, and the reflex in the right atrial wall.

The carotid sinus reflex maintains normal blood pressure within the cerebral circulation. The carotid sinus is a small widened portion of the internal carotid artery located just above the point where the carotid artery branches off from the common carotid artery. In the walls of the carotid sinus lie the pressoreceptors or baroreceptors. Any increase in blood pressure will stretch the walls of the carotid sinus, activating the pressoreceptors, which initiate nerve impulses. These impulses then travel over the ninth cranial nerve into the medulla. In the medulla, the impulses stimulate the cardioinhibitory center and inhibit the cardioacceleratory center. Consequently, more parasympathetic impulses pass from the cardioinhibitory center by way of the vagus nerve to the heart. Fewer sympathetic impulses come from the sympathetic center. The result is a decrease in heart rate and force of contraction, which leads to a drop in blood pressure.

Conversely, if blood pressure drops below normal, reflex acceleration of the heart takes place. This occurs because the pressoreceptors in the carotid sinus do not stimulate the cardioinhibitory center, and the cardioacceleratory center is free to dominate. The heart rate and the force of cardiac contraction increase to restore normal blood pressure.

The aortic reflex is initiated by the pressoreceptors or baroreceptors in the walls of the arch of the aorta. When blood volume decreases, the receptors will be stimulated and the reflex response will increase cardiac rate. The reflex in the right atrial wall responds to venous blood pressure. It is initiated by pressoreceptors in the superior and inferior venae cavae and in the right atrium. When venous pressure increases, the pressoreceptors send impulses to the cardioacceleratory center, which in turn increases heart rate.

Chemoreceptors

Receptors that are sensitive to chemical changes in the blood are located in the carotid sinus and in the aorta. They react to a deficiency in oxygen or to an increase in carbon dioxide levels, and they send impulses to the vasomotor center in the medulla. The response is an increase in sympathetic stimulation, which results in peripheral arteriolar vasoconstriction and an increase in blood pressure.

Emotions

Strong emotions such as fear, anxiety, and anger will stimulate the cerebral cortex, which in turn stimulates the vasomotor center to fire sympathetic impulses. Heart rate will increase and peripheral arteriolar vasoconstriction will occur, causing an increase in blood pressure.

In cases of profound depression, when a decrease in carbon dioxide levels associated with hyperventilation occurs, the cardioinhibitory center is stimulated and this results in peripheral arteriolar vasodilation and a concomitant decrease in blood pressure.

Temperature

Increased body temperature will cause the AV node to discharge impulses faster, thereby increasing heart rate. Decreased body temperatures decrease heart rate and contractility.

Electrolytes and hormones

Certain chemicals in the body have an effect on heart rate. For example, epinephrine is produced by the adrenal medulla in response to sympathetic stimulation, and it increases the automaticity of the sinus node, which in turn increases heart rate.

The excess of potassium and extracellular fluids within the heart muscle will cause the heart to become extremely dilated and flaccid and will subsequently depress the heart rate. Large quantities of potassium can also block conduction of electrical impulses from the atria to the ventricles. Elevations of serum potassium concentrations to about 8 mEq/L will usually cause such a profound weakness within the heart that death will ensue.[21] High potassium concentrations in extracellular fluid are believed to cause a decreased negativity within the cell. As the resting membrane potential decreases, Phase 0 of the action potential will be reduced and conduction will be slowed. In addition, elevated potassium levels will interfere with the participation of calcium in muscle contraction.

Hypokalemia, reduced levels of potassium, causes increased automaticity and interference with normal myocardial repolarization. Ectopic beats may also occur.

SYSTEMIC CIRCULATION

Systemic circulation is the largest route through which blood travels to and from the organs of the body. The four divisions of the systemic circulation intimately related to cardiovascular function are the coronary circulation, the hepatoportal circulation, the renal circulation, and the cutaneous circulation.

Coronary circulation

Coronary blood flow is phasic and dependent on aortic blood pressure, blood volume, and oxygen debt. Other determinants include systolic myocardial resistance and increased impedence in hypertrophied muscle.

Coronary blood flow occurs during ventricular diastole when aortic valves are closed. The pressure gradient between the aorta and the coronary sinus allows blood to flow into the coronary vessels. A reduction in aortic pressures in cases of profound hypovolemia can cause retrograde coronary blood flow, resulting in myocardial ischemia.

In an individual at rest, coronary blood flow is about 5% of cardiac output. Coronary blood flow can increase; however, myocardial oxygen extraction remains fixed at an estimated 65% to 70%. The myocardium functions exclusively by aerobic metabolism and cannot support an oxygen debt. Therefore coronary arterial vasodilation is the primary mechanism of compensation that is activated in response to myocardial hypoxia.

Factors that contribute to myocardial oxygen demand include increased heart rate, increased myocardial contractility, and increased muscle fiber tension. Increased muscle tension plays a significant role in cases of hypertrophy and/or chamber enlargement. If a dilated ventricle uses in-

creased tension in order to maintain stroke volumes, high coronary flow rates must be maintained to provide adequate myocardial oxygen supply.

Hepatoportal circulation

The liver receives blood from two origins. About 350 ml/minute is delivered by way of the hepatic artery at systemic arterial pressure, while about 1100 ml/minute, is venous blood received from the capillaries of the gastrointestinal tract and spleen.[12] This venous blood is part of the portal circulation and has a hydrostatic pressure of approximately 8 mm Hg. The total hepatic blood flow is about 1500 ml/minute or 29% of cardiac output, while the normal blood volume within the liver is about 500 ml or 10% of cardiac output.

The liver is a compliant organ and large quantities of blood can be stored in its vascular compartment or mobilized to support central circulation. For example, in an individual in shock, severe vasoconstriction of the gastrointestinal arterioles may reduce portal blood flow, thereby shunting blood to the central ciruclation. This reduction in portal blood flow may be so severe that hepatic necrosis develops. However, when elevated pressure in the right atrium and inferior vena cava is transmitted to the liver, it expands and may pool as much as 1 L of blood in its veins and sinuses. This quality of hepatoportal circulation accounts for the hepatomegaly and hepatojugular reflux associated with heart failure.

Renal circulation

The kidneys receive 20% to 25% of cardiac output. Approximately 90% of this blood is directed to the nearly one million nephrons in the cortex of each kidney. The remaining 10% of blood flow is directed to the inner medullary portion.[8]

Each kidney is supplied by one or more of the renal arteries branching from the abdominal aorta. The renal arteries enter the hilum and divide into the interlobar arteries. The interlobar arteries then extend to the junction of the cortex and the medulla. Here they branch into the arcuate arteries, which arch over the pyramids at right angles to the interlobar arteries. The arcuate arteries become the interlobar arteries, and they are perpendicular to the arcuate arterial system in the renal cortex. The interlobular arteries form the afferent arterioles, which divide in the cortex into the glomerulus, a capillary network. The capillaries rejoin to form the network called the efferent arterioles. Blood leaves the glomerulus by way of the efferent arterioles, which open into a network of peritubular capillaries that surround the convoluted and straight tubules and collecting ducts (Fig. 1-26).

Capillaries surrounding the straight tubules and ducts in the medulla form a series of interconnecting loops called the vasa recta. Veins draining these peritubular networks join the interlobar veins, and the venous blood proceeds to renal veins and finally empties into the inferior vena cava.

Unobstructed blood supply to the kidneys is a critical factor since collateral circulation is inadequate. Obstruction of an artery can result in the loss of the entire segment supplied by that artery.

The circulatory pattern among the functioning units of the kidney, nephrons, and collecting ducts is vital to the preservation of fluid and electrolyte balance. The high perfusion rate to the kidneys reflects the primary function of the kidneys to continuously reconstitute the extracellular fluid. The perfusion rate is thought to be maintained by an autoregulatory mechanism of the kidneys. However, when oxygen supply is inadequate, blood flow to organ tissues with low oxygen extraction such as the kidneys is decreased in favor of tissues

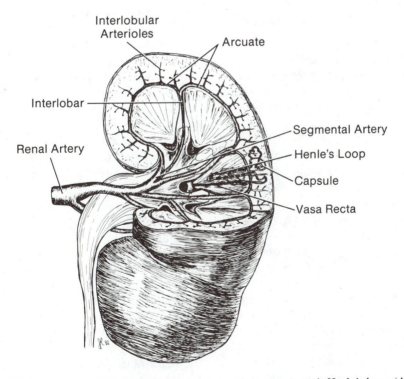

Fig. 1-26. Arterial circulation of kidney showing vasa recta as it surrounds Henle's loop. (Adapted from an original painting by Frank H. Netter, M.D., copyright by CIBA Pharmaceutical Company, Division of CIBA-GEIGY Corporation.)

and organs with higher oxygen extraction, such as the brain and the heart.

Reduction in renal perfusion is accomplished by intrarenal redistribution of blood flow so relatively less blood reaches the renal cortex. The cumulative effects of the intrarenal redistribution are diagramed below.

Decreased renal perfusion

Decreased perfusion
of cortical
nephrons

↓

Increased perfusion
of juxtamedullary
nephrons

↓

Maintenance of
sodium balance

Increased glomerular
vascular resistance

↓

Maintenance of glo-
merular filtration rate

↓

Increased protein concen-
tration

↓

Increased colloid osmotic
pressure

↓

Increased reabsorption
of sodium

Increased reabsorption of sodium causes less fluid to reach distal portions of the nephron. This reduces urine volume and increases urine concentration.

Cutaneous circulation

The rate of blood flow through the skin is about 200 ml/min, or 4% of cardiac output. It is the most variable of any organ system in the body, functions primarily to control body temperature, and is regulated by the autonomic nervous system rather than by local tissue control.[8,12,19]

Cutaneous blood vessels are innervated by sympathetic vasoconstrictor nerve fibers and contain only alpha-adrenergic receptors; therefore they are extremely sensitive to circulating norepinephrine and epinephrine. Because of this, the large capacity of cutaneous vascular beds and their ability to change volume, the skin is an important blood reservoir. The cutaneous circulation responds to the baroreceptor reflex in the following way: increased systemic arterial pressure causes reflex vasodilation, and hypotension produces reflex vasoconstriction. In addition, the extreme sensitivity of skin vessels to circulating catecholamines potentiates the vasoconstrictor response in hypotensive episodes. These characteristics account for the skin pallor, cool temperature, and diaphoresis that occur in cardiocirculatory failure.

Neurohumoral controls

The relationship of flow, pressure, and resistance is a concept important to understanding control of peripheral circulation. To review, flow is the amount of blood passing through the arterial vessels. Resistance is the amount of restriction to that blood flow. Flow and resistance combine to produce pressure in an artery. In a closed system, if blood pressure falls but blood flow remains the same, the peripheral vascular resistance or vasomotor tone must have decreased. Decreased peripheral vascular resistance is caused by vasodilation. Conversely, if blood pressure rises but blood flow remains unchanged, then resistance or vasomotor tone must have increased. Increased resistance is caused by vasoconstriction. This may occur in both the arterial and venous sides of circulation.

The portion of the nervous system that regulates peripheral vascular resistance is the autonomic nervous system. Receptor sites on arterioles are stimulated by autonomic nerve impulses and circulating catecholamines. These receptor sites are grouped into those that respond to adrenalin, commonly referred to as sympathetic-adrenergic receptors, and those that respond to acetylcholine, called cholinergic receptors.

The adrenergic receptors are subdivided into two groups. The first is comprised of alpha-adrenergic receptors that cause arteriolar constriction. The second is comprised of beta-adrenergic receptors that cause arteriolar relaxation. Arteriolar constriction is referred to as vasoconstriction, while arteriolar relaxation is referred to as vasodilation. Constriction of veins is called venoconstriction, while dilation of veins is called venodilation. The response of the peripheral vascular system to these autonomic controls regulates peripheral perfusion, affects organ system function, and provides the rationale for extensive use of pharmacological agents. (See Table 1-2.)

Table 1-2. Comparison of the responses of cardiovascular effector systems to autonomic nerve impulses

Effector system	Sympathetic (adrenergic) nerve impulses	Parasympathetic (cholinergic) nerve impulses
CARDIOVASCULAR SYSTEM		
Heart		
Rate of contraction	Increase	Decrease
Force of contraction	Increase	Decrease
Blood pressure	Increase	Decrease
Blood vessels		
Skin and mucous membranes	Constriction	Dilation
Skeletal muscle	Dilation	Dilation
Coronary	Dilation, constriction	—
Renal	Constriction	—

Adapted from Gerald, M.C., and O'Bannon, F.V.: Nursing Pharmacology and Therapeutics, © 1981, pp. 40, 46. Reprinted by permission of Prentice-Hall, Inc., Engelwood Cliffs, N.J.

Table 1-3. Comparison of approximate values in flow distribution among the various organs at rest and during strenuous exercise

At rest cardiac output 5 L/min	Organ perfused	Exercise cardiac output 25 L/min
13%	Brain	4%
5%	Heart	5%
22%	Liver and gastrointestinal tract	5%
25%	Kidneys	4%
25%	Muscle and skin	80%
10%	Bone and bone marrow	2%

Adapted from Folkow, B., and Neil, E.: Circulation, New York, 1971, Oxford University Press.

Selective redistribution. Organ system perfusion is controlled in part by local tissue autoregulation and a reflex increase in vascular resistance. This causes selective redistribution of blood flow to preserve circulation to organs with the most critical oxygen needs.

Systemic veins contain about 59% of all the blood volume in the circulatory system and are collectively referred to as the blood reservoirs. They store blood that can be quickly mobilized and shunted to organ systems with high oxygen requirements. For example, during exercise when there is increased skeletal muscle activity, the cerebral vasomotor center increases sympathetic impulses to venous reservoirs. The result is venoconstriction in the liver and gut and vasodilation in the skeletal muscles. This allows redistribution of blood from the venous reservoir to muscles to meet increased metabolic demand. A similar mechanism exists in stress, such as depressed cardiac output, when both blood volume and/or pressure decrease.

In this situation, selective vasoconstriction shunts critical blood volume from renal, splanchnic, and cutaneous circulation to vital organs, such as the brain and heart. Consequently, the central circulatory volume is supported by blood reservoirs located in the veins of the abdominal organs and the skin and by diminished perfusion to the kidneys. (See Table 1-3.)

Electrolyte effects

Changes in the normal levels of electrolytes, such as calcium, magnesium, potassium, and sodium, also affect peripheral circulation. As mentioned previously, moderate increases of calcium ion will augment cardiac contractility; however, at high levels it promotes peripheral vasoconstriction and increased afterload as well as interference with the relaxation phase of cardiac contraction.

Elevated levels of extracellular potassium ion concentration affect peripheral circulation by promoting vasodilation by its inhibiting effect on smooth muscle contraction. Elevated levels of magnesium also cause powerful vasodilation. It is postulated that this occurs because magnesium, in combination with potassium, inhibits smooth muscle contraction in an even more profound manner.

High levels of sodium ion concentration cause

vasodilation by its effect on fluid osmolality rather than from a direct effect of the sodium ion on blood vessels. Increased osmolality resulting from other nonvasoactive substances, such as glucose, also promotes arteriolar dilation. However, decreased osmolality will cause vasoconstriction. This may be a response to the effects of solutes on blood viscosity.

Disruption of fluid and electrolyte balance usually occurs secondary to injury or malfunction of an organ or to massive bacterial invasion. The metabolic consequences of fluid and electrolyte imbalances often cause more dangerous circulatory effects than primary organ dysfunction.

PULMONARY CIRCULATION

The amount of blood flowing through the lungs is essentially the same as the amount flowing through the entire systemic circulation. However, the distribution of blood flow within the lungs is a unique characteristic of the pulmonary circulation.

The pulmonary artery is the vessel leading away from the right ventricle to the lungs. It extends about 3 to 4 cm beyond the apex of the right ventricle, and it divides into the right and left main branches to supply blood to the lungs. The pulmonary artery is very thin, with a wall thickness approximately twice that of the vena cava but one-half to one-third less than that of the aorta. The branches supplying lung segments are very short. All the pulmonary arteries and arterioles have much larger diameters than their systemic counterparts. This, along with the very thin distensible structure of these pulmonary vessels, accounts for the large compliance of the pulmonary vascular system. This compliance is almost equal to the compliance of the entire systemic arterial system, and it allows the pulmonary arteries to accommodate all the stroke volume received from the right ventricle. Pulmonary veins, like pulmonary arteries, are very short, and their distensibility is similar to that of systemic venous circulation.

Pressure in the pulmonary artery during systole is approximately equal to the pressure in the right ventricle. At the end of ejection, after the pulmonary valve closes, the pulmonary arterial pressure gradually falls as blood flows into the capillaries of the lungs. The normal systemic pulmonary arterial pressure is about 25 mm Hg; the diastolic pulmonary arterial pressure is about 8 to 10 mm Hg; and the mean pulmonary arterial pressure ranges from 12 to 18 mm Hg[22] (Fig. 1-14).

Blood volume in the lungs

The blood volume in the lungs is approximately 9% of the total blood volume of the circulatory system. In different physiological and pathological settings, the amount of blood within the lungs may vary from as little as 50% to as high as 300% of normal.[22] For instance, if individuals were to forcefully exhale air so that they build up high intrapulmonary pressure, up to 250 ml of blood can be expelled from the pulmonary circulation into the systemic circulation. Other compensatory mechanisms also exist within the pulmonic system. For example, loss of blood from the systemic circulation by hemorrhage can be partly compensated for by pulmonary vasoconstriction, which shifts blood from the lungs to the systemic circulation.

Blood flow in the lungs

Blood flow in the lungs is essentially equal to cardiac output. Under most conditions, the pulmonary vessels act as passive distensible tubes that enlarge with increasing pressure and constrict with decreasing pressure.

In order for blood to be aerated and oxygenated adequately, it should be evenly distributed to all segments of the lungs. During exercise, increased cardiac output delivers a proportional amount of blood to the lungs. Because of the distensibility of pulmonary vessels, arterioles and capillaries expand in all lung segments to accommodate the elevated volume.

The distribution of blood flow in the normal lung is also affected by posture. For example, in the upright position the blood flow within the lungs is decreased in a linear fashion from the bottom to the top. If the body is changed from an upright position to a supine position, the apical flow will increase and the basilar flow will remain un-

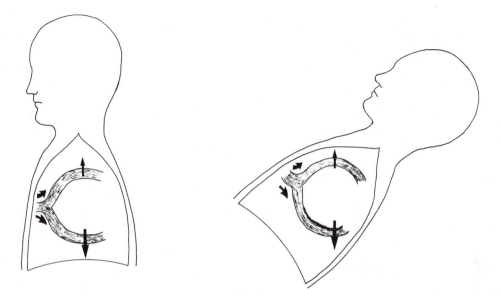

Fig. 1-27. Conceptual relationship of distribution of blood flow affected by posture. In upright position, flow within lungs is decreased from base to apex. If thorax is positioned at 45-degree angle, flow to posterior regions will increase and flow to anterior regions will decrease.

changed, while flow to the posterior regions of the lung will increase and flow to the anterior regions will decrease (Fig. 1-27).

This gravitational force affects pulmonary hydrostatic pressure in the same way it affects systemic pressure. For example, an individual who is sitting in an upright position will display apical pressures 10 mm Hg less than pressures at the level of the heart and will display basilar pressures approximately 8 mm Hg greater than pressures in the upper regions of the lungs.[22]

The effect of gravitational force and regional distribution on blood flow and pulmonary pressures accounts for the difference in the densities in radiographs taken of the chest on individuals in a supine and an upright position. It also provides an explanation for increased adventitial sounds over the lung bases of a sleeping patient or one with depressed cardiac function.

Alveolar oxygen pressures

Alveolar oxygen pressures will autoregulate local pulmonary blood flow. When alveolar oxygen concentration decreases, the adjacent blood vessels slowly constrict, causing a marked increase in the pulmonary vascular resistance. There is no known explanation for this effect, although most authorities believe low oxygen concentration effects the release of some type of vasoconstrictive substance that acts on the pulmonary arterioles.

Low oxygen saturation has an important effect on the pulmonary vascular resistance. It results in redistribution of blood to areas of the lungs that are better aerated, and it provides an automatic control system for distributing blood flow in proportion to the metabolic need for ventilation. Normally, if cardiac output is adequate, blood will circulate through the pulmonary capillaries in about 1 second. Increasing cardiac output shortens the amount of time blood remains in the pulmonary capillaries.

Pulmonary capillary pressure

The pulmonary capillary pressure is the most significant factor that accounts for the difference between pulmonary and systemic capillary dynamics. In the lungs, pulmonary capillary pressure is about 10 mm Hg compared with a mean systemic capillary pressure of about 17 mm Hg.[22] Because of the very low pulmonary capillary pressure, the hydrostatic force tends to favor the movement of fluid out of the capillaries and into the pulmonary interstitial spaces. This pressure is counterbalanced by the colloid osmotic pressure of plasma, which is about 25 to 28 mm Hg. Therefore the elevated osmotic pressure maintains dehydration of the interstitial space in the lungs. There is approximately 6 mm Hg of negative interstitial pressure that pulls the alveolar epithelial membrane toward the capillary membrane, thus squeezing the pulmonary interstitial space to almost nothing. As a result the distance between the air in the alveoli and the blood in the capillaries is minimal, and this facilitates rapid diffusion of gases between pulmonary capillaries and alveoli. The negative interstitial pressures also facilitate movement of fluid from the alveoli through the alveolar membrane into the interstitial spaces and are yet another mechanism that keep the alveoli dry.

During stress, cardiac output increases, as does ventilation, to meet metabolic demand. This is accomplished in two ways: by pulmonary vasodilation to increase the surface area of functional capil-

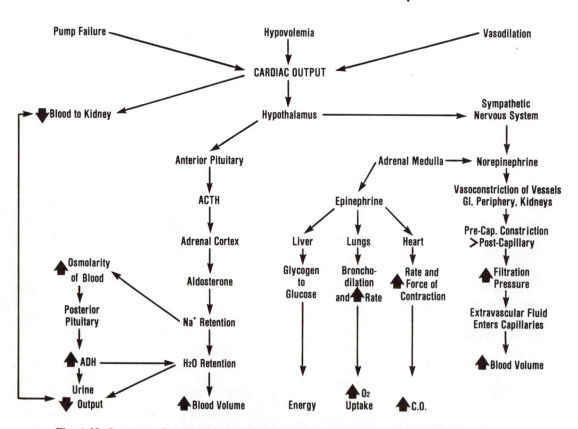

Fig. 1-28. Summary of physiological changes that occur when cardiac output is depressed. Major control mechanisms of cardiovascular system are activated and are diagrammatically presented.

laries and by increasing perfusion of the capillaries. In resting conditions, blood flow is minimal in many of the pulmonary capillaries, particularly those in the apical regions of the lungs. As cardiac output rises, most of these capillaries will open, causing a drop in pulmonary vascular resistance. The ability of the lungs to accommodate this increased blood volume with little or no elevation in vascular pressure conserves energy for the right side of the heart while preventing a significant rise in pulmonary capillary pressure. This adaptive response defends against the development of pulmonary edema.

SUMMARY

Anatomy and physiology of the cardiovascular system are complex topics requiring diligent and intensive study in order to understand their complexities. This system is governed by physical laws; is regulated by autonomic, hormonal, and local controls; and is subject to complex reflex feedback mechanisms (Fig. 1-28). Research continues to identify and explain these complex processes. This chapter has reviewed selected concepts to help the reader retrieve information essential to understanding the pathophysiology, causes, clinical indicators, and rationale for treatment of congestive heart failure.

REFERENCES

1. Aronson, R.: The hemodynamic consequences of cardiac arrhythmias, cardiovascular reviews and reports, New York, 1981, Le Jacq Publishing Co., Inc.
2. Bechimol, A.: Noninvasive techniques in cardiology for the nurse and technician, New York, 1978, John Wiley & Sons, Inc.
3. Berne, R.M., and Levy, M.N.: Cardiovascular physiology, ed. 4, St. Louis, 1981, The C.V. Mosby Co.
4. Conover, M.B.: Understanding electrocardiography, ed. 3, St. Louis, 1980, The C.V. Mosby Co.
5. Criley, J.M., and Ross, R.S.: Cardiovascular physiology, Tarpon Springs, Fla., 1971, Tampa Tracings.
6. Daily, E.K., and Schroder, J.S.: Techniques in bedside hemodynamic monitoring, ed. 2, St. Louis, 1981, The C.V. Mosby Co.
7. Ferrar, M.I.: The heart's primary pacemaker: types of dysfunction, Primary Cardiology **6**:55, 1980.
8. Folkow, B., and Neil, E.: Circulation, New York, 1971, Oxford University Press.
9. Gerald, M.C., and O'Bannon, F.V.: Nursing pharmacology and therapeutics, Englewood Cliffs, N.J., 1981, Prentice-Hall Inc.
10. Gregoratos, G.: Hemodynamic monitoring in the coronary care unit. In Karlinger, J.S., and Gregoratos, G., editors: Coronary care, New York, 1981, Churchill Livingstone Inc.
11. Gross, R.W., and Sobel, B.E.: Biochemical and metabolic aspects of ischemia. In Karlinger, J.S., and Gregoratos, G., editors: Coronary care, New York, 1981, Churchill Livingstone Inc.
12. Guyton, A.C.: Textbook of medical physiology, ed. 6, Philadelphia, 1981, W.B. Saunders Co.
13. Hindman, M.E., and Wagner, G.S.: Bundle branch block during acute myocardial infarction, Primary Cardiol. **12**:73, 1980.
14. Huszar, R.J.: Emergency cardiac care, Bowie, Md., 1974, Robert J. Brady Co.
15. Katz, A.M.: Contractile proteins of the heart, Physiol. Rev. **50**:63, 1970.
16. Langer, G.A.: Heart: excitation-coupling, Annu. Rev. Physiol. **35**:55, 1973.
17. Mangiola, S., and Ritota, M.C.: Cardiac arrhythmias, Philadelphia, 1974, J.B. Lippincott Co.
18. Marriott, H.J.L.: Practical electrocardiography, ed. 6, Baltimore, 1978, The Williams & Wilkins Co.
19. Ross, G.: Essentials of human physiology, Chicago, 1978, Year Book Medical Publishers, Inc.
20. Rushmer, R.F.: Cardiovascular dynamics, ed. 4, Philadelphia, 1976, W.B. Saunders Co.
21. Smith, K., and Brain, E.: Fluids and electrolytes: a conceptual approach, New York, 1980, Churchill Livingstone Inc.
22. West, J.B.: Respiratory physiology, Baltimore, 1979, The Williams & Wilkins Co.
23. Zschoche, D., editor: Mosby's comprehensive review of critical care, ed. 2, St. Louis, 1981, The C.V. Mosby Co.

ADDITIONAL READINGS

Daly, B.J.: Intensive care nursing, Garden City, N.Y., 1980, Medical Examination Publishing Co. Inc.

Guyton, A.C.: Basic human physiology: normal function and mechanism of disease, Philadelphia, 1977, W.B. Saunders Co.

Higgins, C.B., and Batteler A.: Chest radiograph in acute myocardial infarction. In Karliner, J.S., and Gregoratos, G., editors: Coronary care, New York, 1981, Churchill Livingstone Inc.

Phillips, R.E., and Feeney, M.K.: Cardiac rhythms, ed. 2, Philadelphia, 1977, W.B. Saunders Co.

CHAPTER 2

Pathophysiology of heart failure: a conceptual framework for understanding clinical indicators and therapeutic modalities

CYDNEY R. MICHAELSON

Congestive heart failure is a syndrome that was described in ancient literature long before William Harvey discovered the circulation of blood. It is a disorder that bridges the many subspecialties in medicine and nursing. Furthermore, it may afflict individuals at any point during human development and is likely to complicate health maintenance of neonates as well as of octogenarians.

The management of this condition is intimately related to cardiovascular physiology. Consequently, therapeutic modalities are rapidly changing as research uncovers more details of heart and circulatory function. Technological advances in diagnostic and monitoring devices have added yet another complex dimension to the management of this condition.

Current therapeutic intervention requires sophisticated management of pharmacological agents, judicious administration of fluid and electrolytes, vigilant observation of physical manifestations, comprehensive knowledge of circulatory and respiratory support devices, and skilled application of counseling and educational concepts.

To effectively care for individuals suffering from congestive heart failure, professionals in all dimensions of health care from critical care units to community rehabilitation centers must systematically assess and reassess the patient's clinical status and diagnose, intervene, and evaluate response to therapy as delineated by their roles. To

do so with the utmost sophistication requires detailed understanding of the pathophysiology of this syndrome. This chapter contains a comprehensive presentation of the pathophysiological changes characteristic of heart failure and provides the conceptual framework for understanding the origin of clinical indicators and rationale for therapeutic intervention.

Heart failure (HF) is a general term used to describe a pathophysiological state in which abnormal cardiac function results in the failure of the ventricles to pump blood at a volume commensurate with venous return and the metabolic needs of multiple organ systems. It may result from conditions causing abnormal volume overload, abnormal pressure overload, myocardial dysfunction, filling disorders, or increased metabolic demand (Table 2-1).

The basic function of the heart is to transfer blood coming to the ventricles from the low pressure venous system into the higher pressure arterial system. Impaired cardiac function results in failure to empty venous reservoirs and in reduced delivery of blood into the arterial circulation. This causes elevation of systemic and pulmonary venous volume and depression of the volume of blood ejected into the pulmonary artery and aorta. Hemodynamically, these alterations appear as elevated ventricular end-diastolic pressure, elevated systemic and pulmonary venous pressures, and re-

Table 2-1. Conditions causing heart failure

Abnormal volume load	Abnormal pressure load	Myocardial dysfunction	Filling disorders	Increased metabolic demand
Aortic incompetence	Aortic stenosis	Cardiomyopathy	Mitral stenosis	Anemias
Mitral incompetence	Idiopathic hypertrophic subaortic stenosis	Myocarditis	Tricuspid stenosis	Thyrotoxicosis
Tricuspid incompetence	Coarctation of the aorta	Coronary artery disease	Cardiac tamponade	Fever
Overtransfusion	Hypertension	Ischemia Infarction	Restrictive pericarditis	Beriberi
Left-to-right shunts	Primary	Dysrhythmias		Paget's disease
Secondary hypervolemia	Secondary	Toxic disorders		Arteriovenous fistulas
		Presbycardia		

duced cardiac output. Clinical indicators are related to activated compensatory mechanisms, reduced cardiac reserve, accumulation of extracellular fluid, and impaired organ perfusion.

Congestive heart failure (CHF) is a term used to describe a composite of clinical manifestations that result from circulatory congestion. Associated with the development of circulatory congestion is a progressive reduction in the contractile state of the myocardium with a concomitant reduction in the pump function of the heart. Both may cause the same physiological alteration and clinical manifestations. In this book therefore, the term ''congestive heart failure'' and ''heart failure'' will be describing the same conditions.

There are many descriptive terms related to associated indicators of heart failure. However, it is important to remember that these terms refer to the complex interrelationship of physiological adjustments and clinical manifestations of the syndrome. Definition and clarification of these semantics will facilitate communication among professionals caring for these patients.

DEFINITION OF TERMS
Myocardial failure

Myocardial failure is a term used to describe myocardial muscle dysfunction—the inability to develop adequate contractile tension. Damage may result from myocardial ischemia, infarction, cardiomyopathies, and myocarditis. It may also be associated with mechanical restriction to ventricular filling or emptying as seen in valvular disorders, increased aortic impedance, and pericardial restriction. Furthermore, myocardial failure may result from inadequate coronary perfusion secondary to obstruction or from altered cardiac rhythm and conduction sequence. Progressive myocardial failure causes circulatory failure.

Circulatory failure

Circulatory failure is a general term that refers to the inability of the cardiovascular system to perform its basic function of meeting tissue metabolic requirements. It may result from myocardial failure or noncardiac circulatory dysfunction.

Circulation may be impaired by elevated or depressed intravascular blood volume or by altered vascular tone. Some noncardiac conditions that increase blood volume include overtransfusion of blood, blood components, and crystalloids, accumulation of extracellular and intravascular volume caused by renal and gastrointestinal dysfunction, high-dose steroid therapy, and elevated venous return resulting from arteriovenous fistulas. Conditions that reduce blood volume include burn injuries, hemorrhage secondary to trauma, or surgery; others altering vascular tone include bacterial infections, vitamin deficiencies, and severe anemias. Noncardiac circulatory failure may exist independently of myocardial failure; however, if untreated, the heart muscle sustains damage and heart failure ensues.

Right and left ventricular failure

In clinical practice, reference is frequently made to right and left ventricular failure depending on associated clinical indicators (Table 2-2). Right ventricular failure is associated with failure to empty the systemic venous reservoirs causing elevated systemic venous pressure that, in turn, gives rise to the clinical signs of jugular venous distention, hepatomegaly, dependent peripheral edema,

Table 2-2. Clinical indicators of right and left ventricular failure

Left ventricular failure	Right ventricular failure
SUBJECTIVE INDICATORS (behaviors reported by patient)	
Weakness	Weight gain
Fatigue	Transient ankle swelling
Memory loss and	and pigmentation
confusion	Abdominal distention
Breathlessness	Subcostal pain
Cough	Gastric distress
Insomnia	Anorexia, nausea
Anorexia	
Palpitations	
Diaphoresis	
OBJECTIVE INDICATORS (findings observed by clinician)	
Tachycardia	Edema
Decreased S_1	Ascites
S_3 and S_4	Left parasternal lift
Moist rales	Increased jugular venous
Pleural effusion	pressure
Diaphoresis	Hepatomegaly
Pulsus alternans	Neck vein pulsations and
	distention
	Positive hepatojugular
	reflux

and ascites. Left ventricular failure is associated with reduced left ventricular stroke volume and failure to empty the pulmonary venous reservoirs. This causes elevated pulmonary venous pressures and reduced cardiac output that in turn appears clinically as breathlessness, weakness, fatigue, dizziness, confusion, pulmonary congestion, hypotension, and death.

Since the right and the left sides of the heart are separate pumps, theoretically it is possible for one to fail independently of the other; however, the ventricles are arranged in series and blood travels in a circle within the circulation. Consequently, this anatomical relationship results in transmission of circulatory abnormalities from the affected to the unaffected side. Pure unilateral heart failure is rare, and when it does occur, it usually lasts a very brief time before total circulatory involvement occurs. For example, an abrupt increase in right ventricular volume secondary to obstruction by a large pulmonary embolus would markedly elevate systemic venous pressure. This results from accumulation of blood in the venous system behind the failing right ventricle. The embolus would also obstruct blood flow into the pulmonary circulation and to the left side of the heart, thereby altering blood oxygenation, depressing cardiac output, and interfering with arterial circulation and organ perfusion.

Initially when the left side of the heart fails, left ventricular output drops and blood accumulates inside the heart and in the pulmonary circulation behind the failing left ventricle. Consequently, left ventricular end-diastolic filling pressure rises and is transmitted backward across the mitral valve, left atrium, and pulmonary circulation to increase the load against which the right ventricle must work. If pulmonary venous pressure remains elevated, the right ventricle will be unable to sustain forceful contraction against this outflow resistance and will subsequently dilate and fail. This anatomical relationship accounts for left ventricular failure being the most common cause of right ventricular failure.[16,22] Fig. 2-1 is a schematic representation of circulatory alterations in heart failure.

Text continued on p. 51.

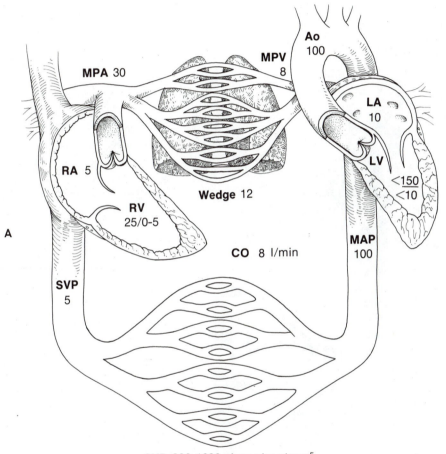

Fig. 2-1. Circulatory alterations in heart failure. Shaded portions of diagrams correspond with affected areas of circulation. **A,** The normal circulation. As blood moves continuously in a circle, outputs of the two ventricles are equal; the normal cardiac output is approximately 8 L/min. Normal mean pressures are approximately 5 mm Hg in systemic veins, 30 mm Hg in pulmonary artery, 8 mm Hg in pulmonary veins, and 100 mm Hg in aorta. (Values adapted from Katz, A.M.: Physiology of the heart, New York, 1977, Raven Press, pp. 398-399.)   *Continued.*

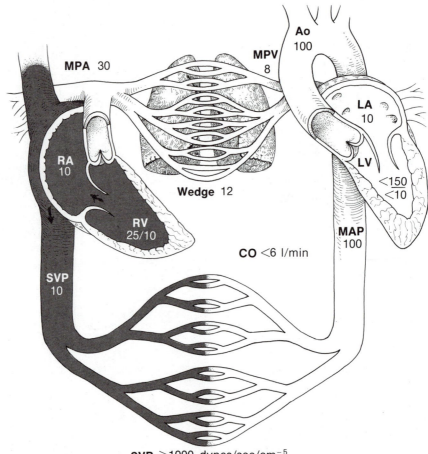

Fig. 2-1, cont'd. B, Right ventricular failure. Impaired pumping by right ventricle causes output of both ventricles to be reduced so that cardiac output falls to 6 L/min. Systemic venous pressure rises to 10 mm Hg because right ventricular end-diastolic pressure is increased, but circulatory reflexes tend to maintain mean pulmonary artery pressure and left ventricular end-diastolic pressure at virtually normal levels.

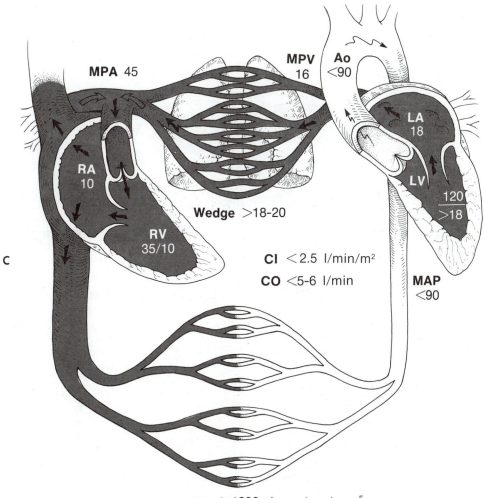

C

Fig. 2-1, cont'd. C, Severe clinical congestive heart failure. This degree of heart failure is caused by impaired pumping of left ventricle. When moderately severe, heart failure is accompanied by fall in cardiac output (e.g., to less than 5 to 6 L/min), significant elevation of pulmonary venous pressure (e.g., 16 mm Hg), pulmonary artery pressure (e.g., 45 mm Hg), and systemic venous pressures (e.g., 10 mm Hg), which occur because of transmission of pressure across pulmonary capillary bed. Drop in cardiac output is reflected by decrease in mean arterial pressure (e.g., less than 90 mm Hg). These patients have clinical symptoms of pulmonary and systemic congestion and decreased peripheral perfusion.   *Continued.*

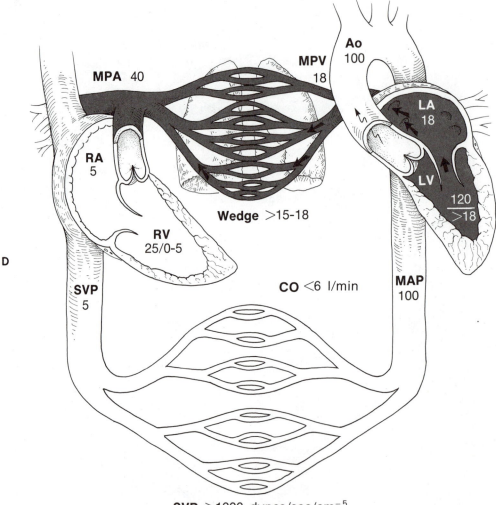

D

Fig. 2-1, cont'd. D, Left ventricular failure. Impaired pumping by left ventricle causes output of both ventricles to be reduced; cardiac output falls to 6 L/min. Pulmonary venous pressures rise to 18 mm Hg because left ventricular end-diastolic volume is increased, but circulatory reflexes tend to maintain mean aortic pressure at virtually normal levels. Elevated pulmonary venous pressure is transmitted through lungs, causing a rise in mean pulmonary artery pressure (e.g., to 40 mm Hg).

Forward and backward failure

Forward and backward failure also refer to a constellation of clinical indicators of circulatory failure. Forward failure, or the low-output theory, relates clinical manifestations to inadequate delivery of blood into the arterial system. Backward failure, or the congestive theory, relates clinical manifestations to a rise in pulmonary and systemic venous pressure that results from failure of the ventricles to empty the veins. When these changes result from myocardial failure, they are accompanied by a drop in cardiac output and some of the clinical features of forward failure.

Because these terms do not describe a complete and accurate picture of congestive heart failure, they are being used less frequently in clinical practice. Fig. 2-2 illustrates the complex interrelationship of the forward and backward effects of right and left heart dysfunction and their relationship to the clinical indicators of congestive heart failure.

Acute and chronic heart failure (Table 2-2)

Generally, the clinical manifestations of acute and chronic congestive heart failure are predicated on the difference in the capacity of the pulmonary and systemic circulations and on how rapidly heart failure develops. Since the capacity and pressure of the pulmonary circulation is significantly less than the systemic circulation, a small imbalance in output between the left and right sides of the heart can result in acute pulmonary congestion. On the other hand, the larger and more distensible systemic circulation is able to adjust to a greater imbalance for a more sustained period of time. Therefore the clinical picture of chronic heart failure generally reflects symptoms of systemic congestion, whereas acute heart failure reflects symptoms of pulmonary congestion and diminished systemic perfusion.

Chronic heart failure is the most common observable syndrome in an outpatient setting and is generally preceded by myocardial failure. It is associated with the pathophysiological alterations of depressed cardiac output, renal conservation of salt and water, and systemic venous congestion. It most frequently appears in patients with a past history of hypertension, coronary artery disease, and/or myocardial infarction. These individuals may exhibit any and all of the following manifestations depending on the extent of cardiac involvement and the effectiveness of therapy:

1. Decreased exercise tolerance
2. Fatigue
3. Exertional dyspnea
4. Weight gain
5. Dependent peripheral edema
6. Jugular venous distention
7. Hepatomegaly
8. Serous effusions

Therapeutic intervention may include administration of digitalis and diuretics, dietary sodium restrictions, and oral vasodilator therapy.

Acute heart failure occurs most frequently from a marked decrease in left ventricular function, secondary to acute myocardial infarction, acute valvular dysfunction, and hypertensive crises. As a consequence, mean pulmonary filling pressure rises because of a shift of blood from the systemic to the pulmonary circulation accompanied by a precipitous drop in cardiac output. These events occur so rapidly that sympathoadrenergic compensation is ineffective, resulting in rapid evolution of pulmonary edema and circulatory collapse. Clinical manifestations include:

1. Marked dyspnea and orthopnea
2. Expectoration of frothy pink-tinged sputum
3. Restlessness
4. Pallor and cyanosis
5. Hypotension
6. Diaphoresis
7. Obtundation and confusion

Acute heart failure may be the initial manifestation of heart disease or may indicate exacerbation of a chronic cardiac condition. In this situation, systemic congestion of chronic heart failure may also be present; however, regardless of the patient's past history, acute heart failure is the condition demanding immediate and vigorous therapeutic intervention.

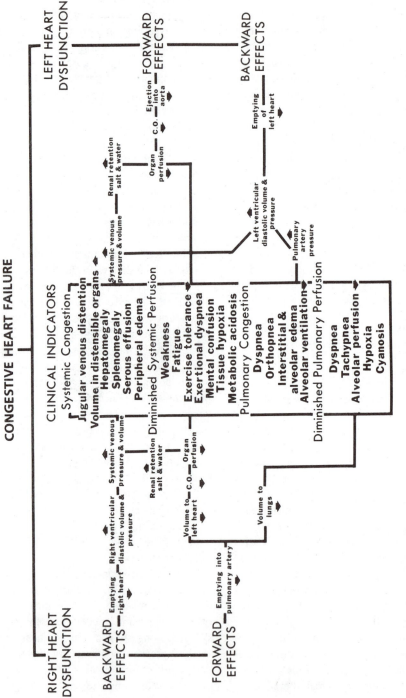
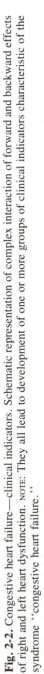

Fig. 2-2. Congestive heart failure—clinical indicators. Schematic representation of complex interaction of forward and backward effects of right and left heart dysfunction. NOTE: They all lead to development of one or more groups of clinical indicators characteristic of the syndrome "congestive heart failure."

High output failure

High output failure is a condition in which cardiac output is markedly elevated before the development of clinical manifestations and remains high afterward.[12] It may be caused by increased metabolic requirements as seen in hyperthyroidism, fever, and pregnancy; or it may be triggered by hyperkinetic conditions such as arteriovenus fistulas, anemia, and beriberi. These conditions are rarely the primary cause of heart failure but rather are the precipitating factors when cardiac function is not sufficient to meet tissue metabolic demands.

Reduced systemic vascular resistance rather than intrinsic cardiac stimulation is characteristic of most conditions that cause chronic high-output states. Decreased vascular resistance augments peripheral circulation and venous return, which in turn increases stroke volume and cardiac output. The clinical findings of a hyperkinetic circulatory state are often the key to assessing high-output heart failure.

The subjective findings include dyspnea on exertion, fatigue, and reports of transient dependent peripheral edema and are difficult to distinguish from heart failure secondary to other disease. The objective findings include tachycardia disproportionate to the degree of heart failure, a hyperdynamic cardiac impulse, and clinical evidence of cardiac enlargement. Further signs of hyperkinetic circulation include pounding peripheral pulses, apical systolic murmur caused by increased stroke volume, and the presence of a third heart sound.

Hemodynamic measurements reveal elevated venous pressure, slightly elevated systolic arterial pressure, a wide pulse pressure, decreased systemic vascular resistance, and elevated cardiac output. The cardiac output of these individuals must be evaluated in light of the hyperkinetic circulatory state. These individuals had a previously elevated cardiac output; therefore as heart failure progresses and ventricular function diminishes, the cardiac output may be depressed relative to its prior level. Consequently when heart failure is severe, cardiac output may appear as normal or at the upper limits of normal compared to mean values. Therefore in conditions of normal cardiac outputs and moderate to severe heart failure, one should think of high output failure and look for the underlying cause.[12]

Intractable and refractory heart failure

Intractable and refractory heart failure, as defined in texts by Hurst and Braunwald, imply persistent heart failure in spite of all known pharmacological, mechanical, and dietary efforts to improve myocardial contractility, control heart rate, and manipulate preload and afterload.[2,14] Affected patient's typically display persistent pulmonary and systemic congestion with a low cardiac output at rest. Depending on their coping mechanisms, they may also exhibit symptoms of denial, anxiety, and depression. It is important to remember that what was intractable a few years ago may not be so today and hopefully, with better intervention, will be less in the future.

MECHANISMS OF COMPENSATION

When the heart is presented with an increased work load, a number of physiological alterations are evoked in an attempt to sustain pump function. The integrity of cardiovascular function depends on the effectiveness of these mechanisms of compensation. They include:

1. Sympathoadrenergic stimulation
2. Cardiac dilation—the Frank-Starling response
3. Myocardial hypertrophy
4. Renal-mediated fluid retention and peripheral vasoconstriction
5. Increased tissue oxygen extraction

As the heart fails, a decrease in cardiac output occurs. This triggers the major circulatory reflexes resulting in maximal stimulation of the sympathoadrenergic system and inhibition of the parasympathetic system. Increased sympathetic stimulation of the beta-adrenergic receptors in the heart cause an elevation in heart rate and contractility that may increase pump function as much as 100%.[13]

Sympathetic effects on the peripheral vascular system increase vascular tone to raise systemic vascular resistance and mean systemic filling pressure, thereby augmenting venous return, preload, and afterload. Increased preload in turn augments cardiac contractility by the Frank-Starling response.

The initial phase of heart failure is followed by a stage in which compensation occurs as a result of partial recovery of the heart and renal conservation of fluid. Renal compensation is triggered by a drop in kidney perfusion that decreases glomerular filtration and activates the renin, angiotensin, and aldosterone hormonal axis. These mechanisms in turn increase peripheral vascular resistance, increase salt and water reabsorption, which augments blood volume, and increase systemic filling pressure and venous return. Enhanced preload, afterload, heart rate, and contractility return cardiac output to normal or near normal levels and adequate circulation is restored. This is described as compensated heart failure and is often accompanied by clinical indicators of elevated blood volume, increased pulmonary venous pressures, and moderately elevated systemic venous pressures.

When the heart has sustained severe damage and when cardiac output is not sufficiently augmented, then the mechanisms of increased vascular tone and salt and water retention may perpetuate feedback mechanisms that lead to degeneration of clinical status. Cardiac output is further impaired, congestive symptoms rapidly progress, and the patient is described as being in decompensated heart failure.

Myocardial hypertrophy is a compensatory mechanism whereby the heart alters its geometrical configuration and increases its muscle mass in response to prolonged stress. It is clinically observable in patients with chronic heart failure. This compensatory mechanism is self-limiting and will interfere with contractility if ventricular work is unaltered.

Increased tissue oxygen extraction is a physiological adjustment that occurs with sustained depressed cardiac output and reduced tissue perfusion. It is manifested by a rightward shift of the oxyhemoglobin dissociation curve (Fig. 9-1). This allows release of more oxygen to meet tissue metabolic demands and clinically is reflected as an increase in the arteriovenous oxygen difference.

All mechanisms of compensation act primarily to restore cardiac output to normal or near normal levels. Sympatho-adrenergic stimulation, with its attendant changes of tachycardia, enhanced myocardial contractility, and redistribution of blood flow, is the primary adjustment to normal stress of exercise and emotion. It also works in concert with the other mechanisms to adjust to the prolonged stress of heart disease.

The extent to which these mechanisms must be employed to sustain cardiac output at a given time in response to stress constitutes cardiac reserve.[13] Individuals with normal cardiac reserve are able to tolerate moderate to heavy exercise without symptoms. Those with very limited cardiac reserve display indications of depressed cardiac output—weakness, fatigue, dizziness, dyspnea, hypotension—even at rest. The New York Heart Association has devised a classification of cardiac status based on cardiac reserve or functional capacity, etiological, anatomical, and physiological diagnosis, and prognosis or responsiveness to therapy.[9] Table 2-3 classifies congestive heart failure as it relates to these categories.

In the remainder of this chapter, reference to mild, moderate, and severe heart failure is based on criteria outlined in Table 2-3.

Sympathoadrenergic stimulation

The most immediately responsive mechanisms of compensation in heart failure result from a reflex increase in sympathoadrenergic stimulation. This represents a major control mechanism to maintain adequate circulation in response to altered cardiac function, exogenous stress, or decreased intravascular volume (Table 2-4).

In heart failure, reflex stimulation of the sympathetic nervous system is triggered by a momentary drop in cardiac output. This depresses arterial pressure, stroke volume, pulse pressure, and cardiac filling, which in turn stimulate baroreceptors, atrial stretch receptors, and myocardial receptor sites to

Table 2-3. Classification of heart failure

Congestive heart failure	Cardiac reserve (functional capacity)	Cardiac status	Prognosis
None	Moderate to heavy activity → no symptoms	Uncompromised	Good
Mild	Moderate or ordinary activities of daily living → dyspnea	Slightly compromised	Good with therapy
Moderate	Mild activities → dyspnea	Moderately compromised	Fair with therapy
Severe	Dyspnea at rest	Severely compromised	Guarded in spite of therapy

Adapted from 8th Edition, *Nomenclature and Criteria for Diagnosis of Diseases of the Heart and Great Vessels,* The Criteria Committee of the New York Heart Association, Little, Brown & Company, 1979.

Table 2-4. Effects of sympathoadrenergic stimulation in heart failure

Heart	Peripheral circulation
↑ Heart rate	↑ Arterial vasoconstriction
↑ Contractility	↑ Venoconstriction
↑ Stroke volume	↑ Systemic vascular resistance
↑ Cardiac output	↑ Redistribution of blood flow
↑ Conduction velocity	↑ Renal vasoconstriction
↑ Myocardial oxygen consumption	

emit afferent nerve impulses to the cardioregulatory centers in the brain. These centers respond by transmitting efferent impulses to sympathetic nerve fibers located in the adrenal medulla, heart, arteries, and veins. These fibers release a neurotransmitter substance, norepinephrine, into the synaptic cleft of adrenergic receptors; in conjunction with elevated levels of circulating catecholamines released by the adrenal medulla, these nerve terminals trigger the following adaptive responses:

1. Increased heart rate and contractility to raise stroke volumes and cardiac output
2. Arterial vasoconstriction to raise blood pressure and distribute peripheral blood flow to vital organs

3. Venoconstriction to shift vascular volume to large veins, thereby augmenting cardiac filling and ventricular performance by the Frank-Starling Response
4. Renal vasoconstriction to stimulate retention of sodium and water to raise effective blood volume

The net effect of sympathoadrenergic stimulation is to increase cardiac output and to effect a redistribution of peripheral blood flow to preserve circulation to vital organs. However, during the course of heart failure, these cardiac and peripheral circulatory adjustments may eventually cause deleterious effects to pump function. Many of the therapeutic interventions used to treat heart failure are predicated on altering or supporting these adjustments.

Cardiac adjustments. There are sympathetic nerve terminals located in all parts of the heart, and upon stimulation, these terminals discharge large stores of myocardial norepinephrine. This substance acts on beta$_1$-receptor mechanisms to increase heart rate by stimulation of the sinoatrial node and by increasing conduction velocity through the atrioventricular junctional tissues. Augmentation of myocardial contractility occurs when beta$_2$ receptors are stimulated in the myocardium.

Research has determined two important factors affecting cardiac response to norepinephrine in heart failure.[19] First, the myocardium becomes hypersensitive and dependent on sustained sympathoadrenergic stimulation and elevated levels of exogenous norepinephrine. This accounts for tachycardia disproportionate to stress and exercise, which is frequently the first sign of compromised cardiac function. Initially, this is a positive adaptive response; however, as the cardiac dysfunction progresses, persistent tachycardia will further stress the heart by increasing myocardial metabolic rate and decreasing coronary artery perfusion, thereby causing an imbalance in the myocardial supply/demand ratio. Second, depletion of endogenous or cardiac stores of norepinephrine interferes with sympathetic augmentation of contractility during stress, which further reduces cardiac reserve.[19]

These findings support the administration of supplemental catecholamines and inotropic agents in selected patients. Furthermore, it provides an explanation for deterioration of cardiac function seen when patients receive agents such as propranolol and reserpine that block the action of catecholamines.

Sustained sympathetic stimulation of the heart may also depress cardiac function in heart failure by elevating myocardial oxygen consumption (see boxed material below). The two determinants of oxygen consumption directly affected by sympathetic stimulation are heart rate and contractility. In the normal heart, increased myocardial oxygen demand is met by coronary artery dilation and increased myocardial oxygen extraction. However, in heart failure, particularly when complicated by coronary artery disease and ventricular hypertrophy, elevated heart rate further compromises coronary circulation by shortening diastolic filling time. This in turn sets up a positive feedback mechanism that further depresses myocardial function. Major therapeutic objectives are directed toward augmenting ventricular performance without increasing heart rate. This is accomplished by administering synthetic sympathomimetic agents such as dobutamine to augment contractility, by using unloading agents to decrease aortic impedance, and by avoiding alpha and beta agonists that markedly elevate heart rate and systemic vascular resistance.

Peripheral circulatory adjustments. Adaptive changes in the peripheral circulation of patients in heart failure also occur because of a generalized increase in sympathoadrenergic stimulation. Vasoconstriction results from sympathetic stimulation of alpha-adrenergic receptors in the arterioles, whereas venoconstriction results from stimulation of a network of sympathetic nerve fibers in the veins. The net effect of these changes coupled with tissue autoregulation results in redistribution of blood flow to preserve circulation to vital organs.

It should be emphasized that peripheral circulatory adjustments in heart failure are the same as those normally occurring with exercise. However, these patients have compromised cardiac function

---

MAJOR DETERMINANTS OF MYOCARDIAL OXYGEN CONSUMPTION

1. Heart rate
2. Contractility
3. Ventricular wall tension
4. Ventricular mass
5. Afterload
6. Activation energy
7. Metabolism resulting from catecholamine levels

so these adaptive changes are more sustained and may ultimately have deleterious effects on pump function (Table 2-5).

The positive effects of vasoconstriction include an increase in blood pressure and a net increase in capillary blood flow to meet tissue metabolic demands. The negative effects result from sustained elevated systemic vascular resistance that increases intramyocardial wall tension and impedes ejection of blood from an already compromised ventricle. This is a prevailing condition in heart failure that elevates afterload on the heart. As such, it provides the rationale for administration of unloading or vasodilator therapy.

The positive effects of venoconstriction accrue from increased resistance in the veins. This augments venous return to the heart, increases cardiac filling or preload, and by the Frank-Starling response results in more efficient cardiac contraction. However, venoconstriction, like other sympathetic adaptive mechanisms, is a nonselective response. It occurs because of reflex feedback mechanisms in response to a drop in blood pressure. Therefore when volume overload causes low-output heart failure, venoconstriction continues to augment diastolic volume and may exacerbate cardiac function by overfilling the ventricles. Therapeutic interventions to alter this response by decreasing preload is accomplished by administration of venodilating drugs such as nitroglycerin and isosorbide dinitrate, diuretics, and mechanical techniques to impede and reduce venous return.

Redistribution of blood flow. This peripheral circulatory adjustment in heart failure follows the same physiological pattern triggered by normal stress such as exercise (Table 2-6). Vasoconstriction in renal, cutaneous, splanchnic, and nonexercising muscle beds supports total vascular resistance at higher levels than normal. This helps maintain adequate arterial pressure essential to achieve high flow rates through the dilated arterioles of exercising muscle, cerebral, and coronary circulation.[18]

When individuals with heart failure are subjected to even minimal exercise, change in regional circulation becomes markedly exaggerated. This results from depressed cardiac function that limits the capacity of the heart to increase cardiac output in response to sympathoadrenergic stimulation. Therefore central circulation is maintained by a marked reduction in blood flow to the kidneys, gut, and skin. When cardiac function is severely limited, redistribution occurs even at rest.

This adaptive response also has both positive and negative effects on cardiocirculatory function. The positive effects result from dilation in the cerebral circulation to support regulatory feedback mechanisms and in the coronary circulation to meet myocardial oxygen demands. The negative effects result from sustained renal and cutaneous vasoconstriction. Renal vasoconstriction impairs blood flow to the kidney. This in turn stimulates several complex responses to produce angiotensin II, a powerful vasoconstrictor agent that elevates afterload and activates renal tubular reabsorption of salt and water. These are also nonselective responses triggered by a drop in arterial pressure and may add to an already elevated hemodynamic burden, thereby hampering cardiac function. Therapeutic intervention includes administration of selective agents to support cardiac contractility and reduce renal vasoconstriction; it also includes administration of agents to decrease afterload by inhibiting or interfering with the synthesis of angiotensin II.[18] Such agents may include oral administration of converting enzyme inhibitor captopril.[8] Other interventions include use of diuretics to decrease intravascular volume and restriction of dietary sodium to diminish fluid retention.

Research has demonstrated that during stress and exercise maximal cutaneous vasoconstriction predominates in patients with heart failure. It is postulated that hypothalamic control in response to increased body temperature is inhibited by strong afferent sympathetic stimulation[27] and may be an operative factor that limits the patient's ability to tolerate thermal stress. Thermal intolerance indirectly adds another burden to the heart because of increased tissue metabolic rate and oxygen demand that results from elevated body temperature.

Table 2-5. Effects of altered peripheral circulation on cardiac function

Adaptive mechanism	Positive effects	Negative effects
Arterial vasoconstriction	↑ Blood pressure ↓ ↑ Perfusion to vital organs ↓ ↑ Oxygen supply	↑ Systemic vascular resistance ↓ ↑ Afterload ↓ ↓ Cardiac function
Venoconstriction	↑ Venous return ↓ ↑ Cardiac filling ↓ ↑ Preload ↓ ↑ Cardiac contractility (by Frank-Starling law)	↑ Excessive venous return ↓ ↑ Excessive cardiac filling ↓ ↓ Depressed cardiac function
Redistribution of blood flow	↑ *Perfusion to heart* ↓ ↑ Myocardial oxygen supply ↓ ↑ Cardiac function ↑ *Perfusion to brain* ↓ Preservation of CNS controls	↓ *Perfusion to kidney* ↓ ↑ Retention of salt ↓ ↑ Retention of water ↓ ↑ Cardiac load ↓ *Perfusion to skin* ↓ ↓ Thermal tolerance ↓ ↑ Body temperature ↓ ↑ Metabolic oxygen requirements ↓ ↑ Cardiac burden

Table 2-6. Changes in regional circulation (percent of cardiac output)

Organ system	Rest (cardiac output 5.5 L/min, cardiac input 3.25 L/m²)	Heavy exercise (cardiac output 25 L/min)
Brain	13-15%	3-4%
Heart	3-4%	3-4%
Lungs	100%	100%
Liver and gastrointestinal tract	20-25%	3-5%
Kidneys	20%	2-4%
Muscle	15-20%	80-85%
Skin*	4%	

Modified from Folkow, B., and Neil, E.: Circulation, New York, 1971, Oxford University Press.
*Blood flow to the skin is increased in moderate exercise to dissipate body heat and decreased in maximal exercise to maintain arterial pressure.

Therapeutic interventions for this problem include educating the patient to avoid extreme temperatures when possible, to decrease activity in hot, humid environments, and to recognize symptoms of thermal intolerance.

Alteration in regional blood flow to exercising muscle coupled with limited cardiac reserve also accounts for decreased exercise tolerance. Unlike normal individuals, who have a moderate increase in blood pressure during exercise, patients with heart failure have little or no increase in pressure. Consequently, they may exhibit exertional hypotension and syncope. Therapeutic objectives include educating these individuals to recognize symptoms of exercise intolerance, to moderate activity to avoid intolerance, and to administer digitalis preparations and vasodilator agents to enhance cardiac function when necessary.

Clinical manifestations of sympathoadrenergic stimulation. The earliest and most easily detectable sign of sympathoadrenergic stimulation in heart failure is an increase in resting heart rate. A more specific finding is an excessive rise in heart rate with minimal exertion that may be precipitated by merely a change of position in bed.

Increased vasoconstriction is reflected by transient elevation of blood pressure, while venoconstriction may contribute to increased jugular venous distention. This may be detected by the presence of hepatojugular reflux and by the prominent pulsation of the deep jugular veins and venous distention above the sternal notch when the patient is elevated approximately 45 degrees.[22] As heart failure progresses and cardiac output drops, renal and cutaneous vasoconstriction becomes markedly pronounced. Depressed kidney perfusion is reflected by oliguria or abnormal renal function tests, whereas depressed cutaneous perfusion is reflected by a decrease in skin and extremity temperature, pallor, and diaphoresis. These manifestations of elevated sympathetic tone add to the constellation of indicators characteristic of severe low-output failure and cardiogenic shock. Congestive manifestations result primarily from elevated pulmonary and systemic venous pressure and will be discussed in detail later in the chapter.

Cardiac dilation—Frank-Starling response

When heart failure develops, diastolic filling increases and ventricular dilation occurs because of one or more of the following:

1. Primary pathological volume overload
2. Secondary increase in venous return resulting from sympathetic stimulation
3. Expansion of blood volume resulting from renal conservation of salt and water

As a consequence of increased diastolic volume, the Frank-Starling response is immediately activated as a mechanism of compensation.

To briefly review, there is a physiological law that states that the greater the heart is filled during diastole, the greater the quantity of blood pumped into the aorta.[13] This is referred to as the Frank-Starling length/tension relationship and relates presystolic myocardial fiber length or preload to the force of ventricular contraction.

In the normally compliant heart, the end-diastolic volume (preload) causes the ventricular muscle fibers to stretch. Increased fiber length results in activation of the force generating cross-bridges of actin and myosin filaments that in turn, give rise to cardiac contraction. Maximal contractile force develops at a myofibrillar length of 2.2 μm.[4] When stretch exceeds this length, cellular abnormalities may occur that decrease the force and velocity of contraction.

The Frank-Starling response is the major mechanism by which the right and left ventricles maintain equal output when their stroke volumes vary. This mechanism of compensation is activated in response to normal stress of exercise, as well as to the pathophysiological stress of heart failure; however, it also has limited capabilities.

When the mechanism is functional, elevated preload causes enhanced cardiac contraction, and the heart is described as functioning on the ascending limb of the Frank-Starling curve (Fig. 2-3). This response may return cardiac output to normal or near normal levels, but at the expense of elevated pulmonary and/or venous pressures. As hemodynamic burden and myocardial dysfunction persist, pump failure progresses, which is reflected by further elevation of end-diastolic volume and

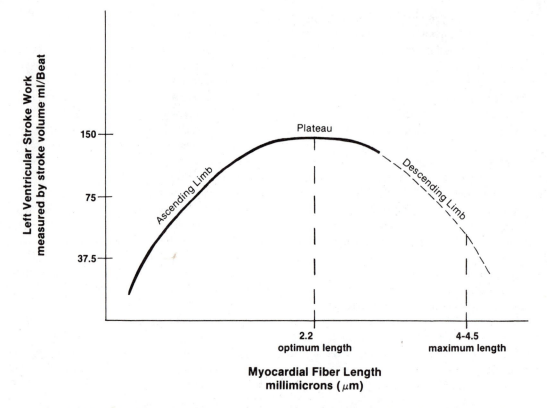

Fig. 2-3. Frank-Starling curve. Schematic representation of theoretical relationship of myocardial fiber length and left ventricular stroke work. The ascending limb illustrates a progressive increase in stroke work corresponding to increase in presystolic myocardial fiber length to optimum stretch of 2.2 μm. Plateau illustrates a stable relationship between fiber length and stroke work; descending limb represents point where fiber length is no longer related to ventricular work. It is uncertain if descending limb can be plotted against preload or excessive stretch or if it results from increased afterload.

ventricular dilation. This in turn may further contribute to depressed ventricular contractility and development of severe congestive symptoms. Therapeutic interventions are directed toward manipulating preload, afterload, heart rate, and contractility in an effort to return ventricular performance to an optimal point on the Frank-Starling curve.

Left ventricular function curve. Clinical application of the Frank-Starling law may be accomplished by analysis of left ventricular function curves. The data provided by these curves are a valuable tool for assessing the clinical status of the patient in heart failure.

A left ventricular function curve uses available hemodynamic parameters to obtain an index of ventricular performance. Cardiac output or cardiac index is used as a measure of ventricular work or contractility; left ventricular end-diastolic pressure or pulmonary wedge pressure is used to measure preload. Fig. 2-4 illustrates several left ventricular function curves and their alteration

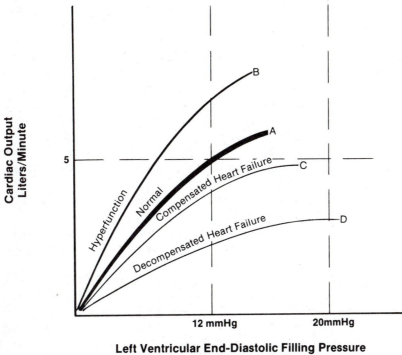

Fig. 2-4. Left ventricular function curves. *Curve A:* represents cardiac output at physiological filling pressures. *Curve B:* represents cardiac hyperfunction caused by sympathoadrenergic stimulation yielding marked increase in cardiac output at physiological filling pressures. *Curve C:* represents compensated heart failure reflecting normal cardiac output with elevated filling pressures. *Curve D:* represents decompensated severe heart failure illustrating a marked decrease in cardiac output in spite of high filling pressures. Shift to left, as occurs when cardiac function moves from curve *B* to *A,* represents increase in ventricular contractility resulting from sympathetic stimulation. Shift to right, as occurs when ventricular function moves from curve *C* to *D,* represents depressed cardiac contractility resulting from hemodynamic burden or intrinsic myocardial dysfunction.

during the course of heart failure.

The normal left ventricle is quite distensible and adapts to increased diastolic volume or preload without significantly increased filling pressure. Generally, optimum contractility occurs at a fiber length of 2.2 μm or 12 to 18 mm Hg.[25] Theoretically, elevation in pressure beyond this limit results in a reduction in ventricular contractility. When the heart is initially stressed, as occurs in acute myocardial infarction, a momentary drop in cardiac output is accompanied by a concomitant rise in sympathoadrenergic stimulation. This elevates heart rate and contractility and is illustrated by a shift to the left of the ventricular function curve. It represents a period of hyperfunction when cardiac output rises with little or no change in filling pressure and may also occur in the syndrome of high-output failure.

As heart failure progresses, the compensatory mechanisms of sympathoadrenergic stimulation, myocardial hypertrophy, and renal conservation of salt and water are activated and result in elevated vascular tone, increased blood volume, and decreased ventricular compliance. These factors cause a shift to the right of the ventricular function curve reflecting a more pronounced increase in filling pressure with no further increase in cardiac performance.

As hemodynamic burden and/or myocardial dysfunction continue to increase, the compensatory mechanisms are no longer effective and cardiac decompensation occurs. Filling pressures continue to rise, ventricular compliance diminishes, and cardiac output drops. These changes are reflected by a further shift to the right of the left ventricular function curve and illustrate a serious reduction in ventricular work. When the curve becomes markedly depressed, it reflects the point at which cardiac performance fails to satisfy tissue metabolic requirements and filling pressures are high enough to cause marked pulmonary and peripheral edema. It is at this level that severe clinical heart failure exists.

Therapeutic interventions are directed toward initiating physiological changes to shift these curves to the right or left. For example, a failing ventricle functioning at curve "C" may be restored to curve "A" by the action of an inotropic agent such as digitalis. Conversely, a compensated ventricle functioning at curve "C" caused by sympathoadrenergic stimulation or elevated preload may be shifted to curve "D" by the action of a depressant drug such as propranolol or by volume depletion resulting from high-dose diuretic therapy. Therefore these ventricular function curves may be used in conjunction with other clinical data to evaluate actual or projected cardiac performance and the effects of clinical therapeutics on heart failure.

Myocardial hypertrophy

Myocardial hypertrophy represents a compensatory response of the heart to sustained hemodynamic burden and may be a clinical finding in both acute and chronic heart failure. The cells of an organ respond to stress by increasing in size (hypertrophy) and in number (hyperplasia). The myocardial cell has the capacity to reproduce by the process of hyperplasia only during embryonic and neonatal development; therefore it adapts to a sustained elevated work load primarily by hypertrophy—increased muscle mass and altered geometrical configuration.

By the process of hypertrophy, increased cardiac work is distributed among a greater number of contractile elements that initially reduces *total* energy requirements and improves pump function. However, this compensatory mechanism is also self-limiting. Each hypertrophied cell requires more energy because of its increased mass and has less inherent contractile force. It is therefore more likely to fail under prolonged stress. For this reason, therapy in heart failure is directed toward reducing hemodynamic burden and decreasing heart size.

The heart increases in size in two distinct structural patterns depending on the nature of stress[24] (Fig. 2-5). *Eccentric hypertrophy* produces a proportional increase in ventricular wall thickness and dilation of the ventricular chamber. It occurs with normal growth and in response to diastolic volume overload. Some conditions causing these geometrical changes include mitral and tricuspid incompetence and/or arteriovenous fistulas. *Concentric hypertrophy* produces an increase in the thickness of the ventricular wall without dilation of the ventricular chamber. It occurs in response to pressure overload and may be caused by aortic stenosis, hypertrophic subaortic stenosis, coarction of the aorta, and hypertension.

Although the exact stimulus of myocardial hypertrophy is unknown, it is postulated that an increase in systolic wall tension associated with elevated pressure or afterload stimulates the synthesis of myocardial cells in parallel, producing concentric hypertrophy, whereas an increase in diastolic tension resulting from elevated volume or preload stimulates the elongation or synthesis of myocardial cells in series, producing eccentric hypertrophy. Regardless of the type of hypertrophy, this mechanism of compensation is effective when the alterations in ventricular mass and geometry are sufficient to decrease the stress on the ventricle and still maintain functional contractility.

Types	Concentric	Eccentric
	Pressure Load 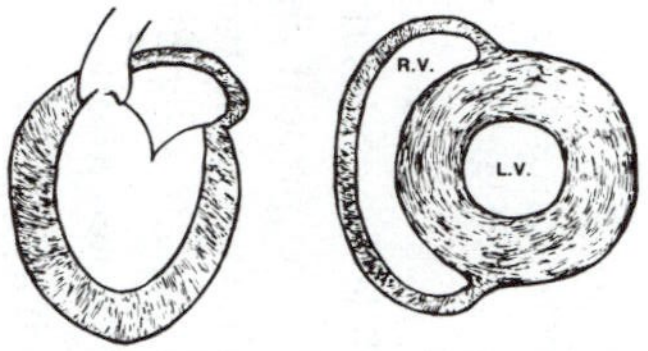	Volume Load 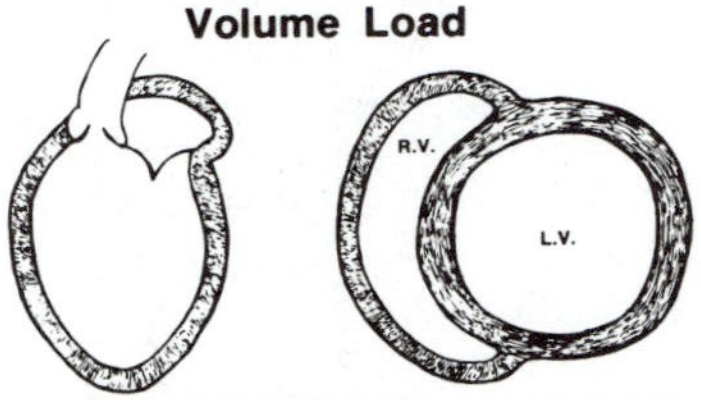
Anatomical Changes		
Structural Changes	Increase in ventricular wall thickness. Little or no change in chamber size.	Proportional increase in ventricular wall thickness and chamber size.
Causes	Elevated afterload Elevated peripheral vascular resistance Outflow obstructions	Elevated preload Regurgitant valvular disorders Arteriovenous fistulas Hypervolemia
Cellular Response	Duplication of cells in parallel	Duplication of cells in series
Cardiac Effects	Decreased ventricular compliance Moderate increase in heart size Marked increase in heart mass	Net decrease in ventricular compliance Marked increase in heart size Moderate increase in heart mass Decrease in rate and force of contractions

Fig. 2-5. Left ventricular hypertrophy. Summary table and anatomical representation of structural and physiological changes of ventricular hypertrophy. (Adapted from Rushmer, R.F.: Cardiovascular dynamics, ed. 4, Philadelphia, 1976, W.B. Saunders Co. p. 538.)

Effects of hypertrophy on ventricular performance. Hypertrophy alters cardiac function by its effect on ventricular compliance and on the rate and force of ventricular contraction. The patient with concentric hypertrophy is likely to develop a less compliant or distensible ventricle. This occurs because of the increased wall thickness. As a result, the ventricle requires a higher diastolic filling pressure to provide normal filling of the heart. On the other hand, the patient with eccentric hypertrophy may have an increased end-diastolic volume with normal filling pressure. This results from chamber enlargement and may reflect a net increase in ventricular compliance. These alterations in compliance then limit the vaue of end-diastolic filling pressures as an index of left ventricular performance.[20] It is therefore vital for clinicians to recognize the effect of hypertrophy on ventricular compliance and to evaluate left ventricular performance in light of this factor.

The chamber dilation that accompanies eccentric hypertrophy causes an alteration in the length/tension relationship of myocardial fiber shortening. This is reflected by an increase in the isometric tension required by the myocardial fibers to develop a given pressure inside a dilated ventricle (law of Laplace). Because of the elevated isometric requirement, it takes longer to develop the required force to elicit rapid fiber shortening characteristic of strong cardiac contraction. Therefore chamber dilation alters the physical properties of fiber shortening, causing a slower and less efficient rate of cardiac contraction that in turn is reflected by a decrease in stroke volume and cardiac output.[20] Furthermore, elevated intramyocardial wall tension increases cellular metabolism and myocardial oxygen requirements. These physiological alterations provide the rationale for directing therapeutic interventions toward decreasing heart size and myocardial oxygen requirements and increasing coronary artery perfusion. They also provide a partial explanation for the operative factors causing intrinsic depressed myocardial contractility characteristic of severe heart failure with associated myocardial hypertrophy.

Clinical recognition of cardiac hypertrophy. *Physical findings* of ventricular hypertrophy occur to some extent in most patients with heart failure. However, according to Burchell, ventricular hypertrophy is difficult to recognize using traditional bedside assessment methods until it is well developed, and it is most discernible when accompanied by chamber enlargement.[6]

Most physical findings result from an increase in ventricular muscle mass and a decrease in compliance. The classic physical sign of left ventricular hypertrophy is a left ventricular heave, palpated at the apex of the heart.[21] The heave is a localized sustained systolic outward motion of left ventricular contraction and is characterized by an apical lift rather than retraction. Frequently, this impulse is only felt during the expiratory respiratory phase with the patient lying in the left lateral decubitus position. The diagnosis is also made when the point of maximal impulse is displaced downward and to the left.

Auscultation of a hypertrophied failing heart may reveal a third heart sound (S_3) or ventricular gallop. This occurs during the rapid filling phase of diastole as a result of sudden deceleration of blood as it meets resistance from a noncompliant ventricle. An audible fourth heart sound (S_4) or atrial gallop may also be present and is also related to decreased ventricular compliance. It occurs most commonly when left ventricular hypertrophy is secondary to elevated afterload or is accompanied by left atrial hypertrophy associated with mitral stenosis.

Right ventricular hypertrophy may be diagnosed by palpation of a right ventricular heave perceived over the lower central chest. It is frequently accompanied by a right-sided S_3 and sometimes with an atrial gallop (S_4), especially if compliance is markedly reduced. Some conditions that cause these physical alterations associated with right ventricular failure include mitral stenosis with left atrial hypertrophy and pulmonary hypertension, pulmonary valvular disorders, and cor pulmonale.

Radiological findings are a primary aid in the diagnosis of ventricular hypertrophy. This method is particularly helpful in detecting sudden changes in heart size associated with acute volume overload and dilation of the ventricle. Generally, dilation of the ventricle is reflected by diffuse enlargement of the cardiac shadow. When precipitated by acute heart failure, it is often accompanied by signs of pulmonary congestion (Fig. 2-6).

Enlargement of the left ventricle caused by increased wall thickness is indicated in the postero-anterior (PA) view by displacement of the apex of heart downward and to the left. The left ventricular shadow may extend below the diaphragm and may be visualized within the gas bubble of the stomach[11] (Fig. 2-7).

Early enlargement of the right ventricle may appear on the PA view and is visible as an increase in the transverse diameter of the cardiac shadow when compared with serial readings.[11] Later stages of right ventricular hypertrophy usually reflect right-sided enlargement of the cardiac shadow and may be associated with clinical indicators of systemic venous congestion characteristic of chronic heart failure.

Electrocardiogram findings may reveal several changes indicative of a stressed hypertrophied heart. It is postulated that biochemical mechanisms of heart failure may cause defects in calcium release and calcium binding by the mitochondria and sarcoplasmic reticulum affecting the excitation-coupling mechanism.[20] There also occur defects in the activity of membrane transport of sodium, potassium, and ATPase causing accelerated and aberrant electrical conduction.[20] These alterations in cellular function, as well as the anatomical alterations resulting from increased ventricular mass, appear on the electrocardiogram as changes in voltage, QRS duration, alteration in conduction, ST-T wave changes, and axis deviation[6] (Fig. 2-8). The more specific ECG changes are discussed in Chapter 5.

Renal compensation

Renal function plays a key role in the pathogenesis of congestive heart failure. When the heart fails, several hemodynamic and neurohumoral adjustments occur to stimulate renal conservation of sodium and water and renal-mediated peripheral vasoconstriction. These regulatory functions are compensatory in early heart failure; however, by their nonselective feedback response they continue to augment preload and afterload to the point where ventricular performance may become severely impaired. The key components of altered renal function include intrarenal hemodynamic changes, neurohumoral control, and alteration in nephron function.

To briefly review, sodium is the chief extracellular cation and chloride and bicarbonate are the principal anions. These constitute the major osmotic forces in this fluid compartment. Normally there is no significant extrarenal sodium loss from the body. Consequently, sodium balance is maintained by matching urinary excretion to dietary sodium intake. Sodium excreted in the urine is the difference between that filtered at the glomerulus and that reabsorbed throughout the nephron.

Sodium reabsorption occurs at different rates within the nephron and is altered by effective arterial blood volume and glomerular filtration rate (GFR) (Fig. 2-9). Effective arterial blood volume is an unmeasurable quantity affected by cardiac ejection, the capacity and compliance of arteries and arterioles, and peripheral run-off.[7] In congestive heart failure, cardiac ejection is impaired, sympathetic vasoconstriction reduces vascular capacity and compliance, and consequently the effective arterial blood volume and renal perfusion are significantly reduced. A drop in renal perfusion pressure changes intrarenal blood flow and stimulates the juxtaglomerular apparatus to activate the renin-angiotensin-aldosterone (RAA) humoral axis. This in turn alters peripheral circulation by increasing vasomotor tone, alters nephron function by decreasing renal perfusion pressure, and alters fluid balance by increasing the rate of sodium reabsorption in the proximal and distal tubules.

These physiological changes progress in proportion to the degree of cardiac dysfunction. In mild heart failure, renal compensation occurs as a negative feedback mechanism. By conserving fluid, it

Text continued on p. 70.

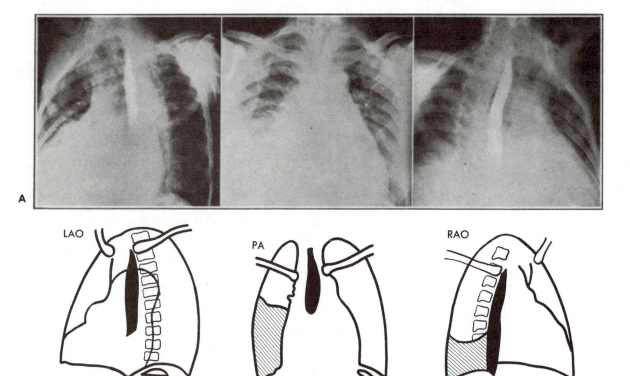

Fig. 2-6. Chest radiogram showing left ventricular dilation. **A,** Generalized dilation of heart from congestive heart failure. Edges of cardiac silhouette are not sharp because of dilation. Notice right pleural effusion in PA and RAO views. (From Goldberger, E.: Textbook of clinical cardiology, St. Louis, 1982, The C.V. Mosby Co., p. 285.)

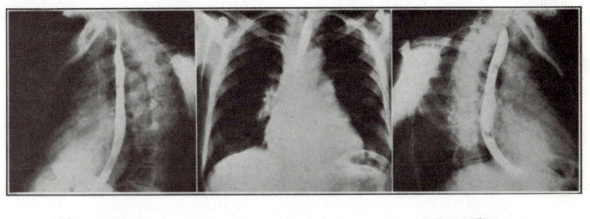

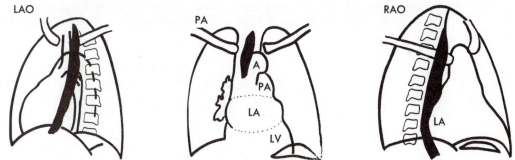

Fig. 2-6, cont'd. B, Same patient 3 months later. Size of heart has decreased greatly and outlines of individual cardiac chambers are now visible. Enlargement of right ventricle and left atrium and dilation of pulmonary trunk are present. Patient has rheumatic mitral stenosis.

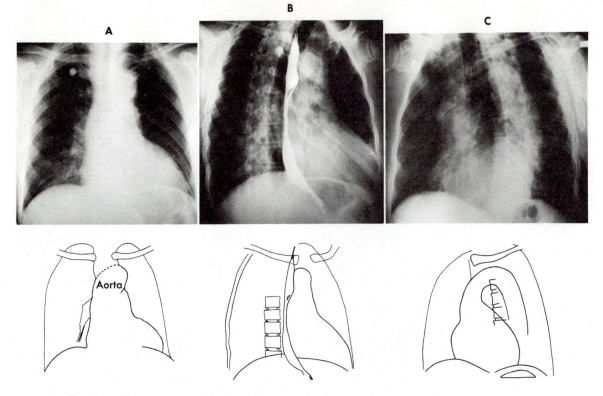

Fig. 2-7. Chest radiogram showing left ventricular hypertrophy. Left ventricular hypertrophy, dilation, and tortuosity of aorta in 47-year-old male with severe hypertension. **A,** PA view. **B,** RAO view. **C,** LAO view. (From Goldberger, E.: Textbook of clinical cardiology, St. Louis, 1982, The C.V. Mosby Co., p. 282.)

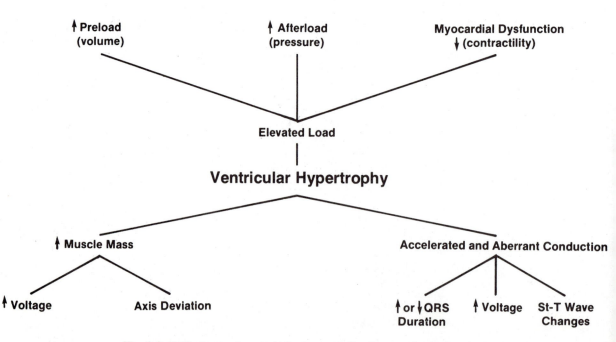

Fig. 2-8. ECG changes in ventricular hypertrophy. See text for explanation.

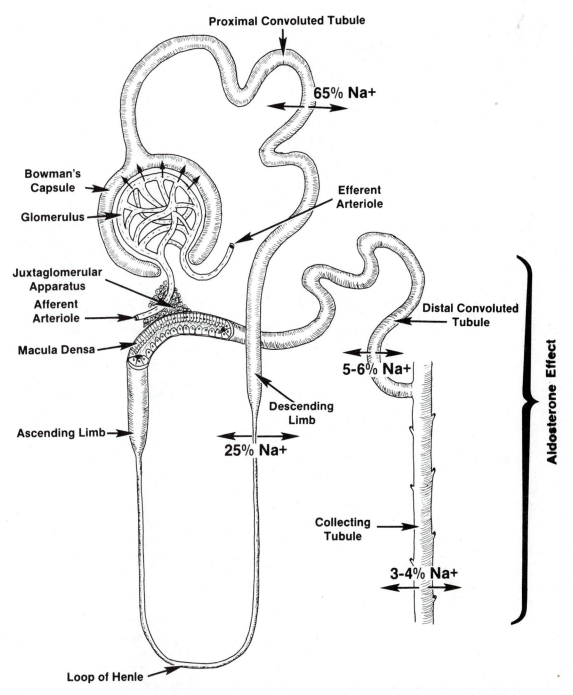

Fig. 2-9. Nephron-sites of sodium and water reabsorption. Schematic representation of a nephron with sites of sodium and water reabsorption. Proximal tubule is primary site of sodium reabsorption and water regulation; distal tubule and collecting ducts are secondary sites of sodium reabsorption and water regulation. In heart failure aldosterone effect on distal tubule enhances sodium and water retention, ultimately leading to cardiac edema.

augments blood volume and diastolic filling pressure and helps to return cardiac output to normal or near-normal levels. However, as heart failure progresses, these mechanisms are unable to restore normal renal perfusion pressure, hence they continue to operate by increasing preload by volume retention and afterload by peripheral vasoconstriction (Fig. 2-12). By this positive feedback mechanism, hemodynamic burden is elevated and ventricular performance becomes more compromised, resulting in the evolution of cardiac edema.

Edema formation in heart failure (Fig. 2-10)
Early mild heart failure—renal hemodynamics. During the phase of early mild heart failure, a drop in renal perfusion pressure results primarily from decreased cardiac output and sympathoadrenergic stimulation that shunts peripheral blood flow away from the kidneys and toward critical organs such as the brain and heart. In response the kidneys, through a process of autoregulation, reduce the amount of sodium and water excreted in the urine. Renal retention of salt and water increases plasma and interstitial fluid volume. This compensatory mechanism may produce a new steady state, where arterial perfusion pressure is restored to normal but is accompanied by elevated venous pressure and an expanded interstitial fluid space.

The mechanisms that account for fluid retention during this phase of heart failure are thought to be mediated by efferent renal arteriolar vasoconstriction and redistribution of intrarenal blood flow. Both of these hemodynamic factors enhance proximal tubular reabsorption of sodium and water within the nephron.[3]

Individuals with mild heart failure usually have normal glomerular filtration rate despite reduced renal blood flow. This occurs because vasoconstriction of the efferent arterioles lowers hydrostatic pressure in the peritubular capillaries so that the fraction of plasma filtered at the glomerular membrane is increased in spite of decreased renal plasma flow. Because the delivery rate of protein-free plasma to the proximal tubules is enhanced, the concentration of proteins in the peritubular capillary plasma is elevated. It follows that de-

creased hydrostatic pressure in the proximal tubule and increased osmotic pressure in the peritubular capillaries favor movement of salt and water from the proximal tubules back into the renal capillaries and circulatory system.

The second hemodynamic factor thought to facilitate proximal tubular reabsorption of sodium results from redistribution of intrarenal blood flow. Studies with inert gas suggest that blood flow is decreased to the outer renal cortex and is increased to the juxtamedullary regions of the kidney.[26] The outer cortical nephrons have shorter loops of Henle and less capacity for reabsorption than the longer juxtamedullary nephrons. Therefore preferential shunting of blood to nephrons with a greater capacity of sodium reabsorption facilitates renal conservation of fluid.

It is important to remember that redistribution of intrarenal blood flow is mediated by both sympathoadrenergic stimulation and renin secretion, and as a function of these processes it may be a contributing factor to inappropriate fluid retention occurring in moderate and advanced heart failure.

Moderate heart failure—renin-angiotensin-aldosterone effects. During this phase the effects of renal hemodynamics is potentiated by the activation of the RAA humoral axis. This is the most important humoral system involved in renal compensation and pathogenesis of cardiac edema. It may be mobilized within hours after the onset of heart failure by the following effects on the kidney[8]:

1. Reduced perfusion pressure
2. Reduced intravascular volume
3. Sympathoadrenergic stimulation of the juxtaglomerular cells
4. Reduced sodium load to the macula densa

In response to these stimuli, renin is secreted by the juxtaglomerular cells that surround the afferent renal arterioles as they enter the glomerulus (Fig. 2-9). In the plasma renin acts on the liver substrate, angiotensinogen, to produce angiotensin I. During a single pass through the lungs, angiotensin I is transformed by a converting enzyme to angiotensin II. This substance is a potent vasoconstrictor

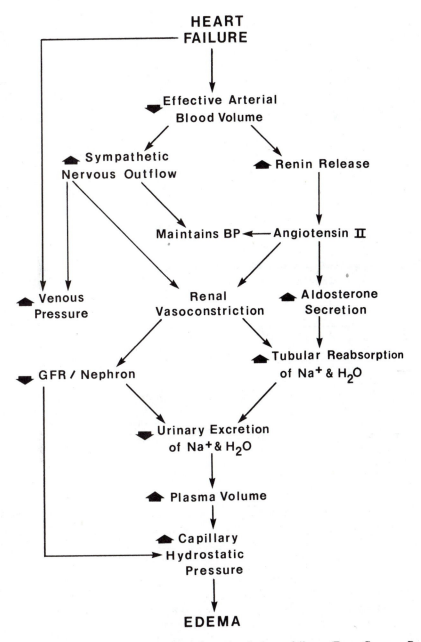

Fig. 2-10. Postulated mechanisms of edema formation in heart failure. (From Cannon, P.: The kidney in heart failure. Reprinted by permission of the N. Engl. J. Med. **296**[1]32, Jan. 6, 1977.)

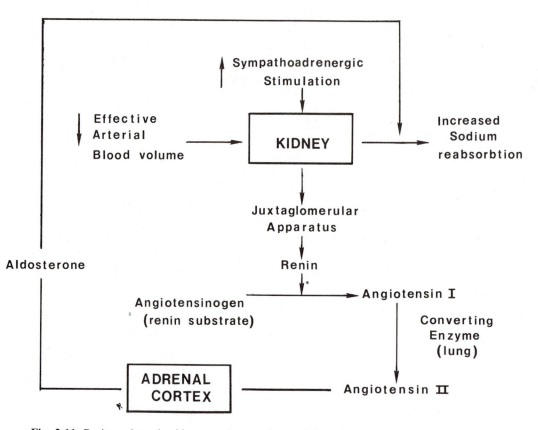

Fig. 2-11. Renin-angiotensin-aldosterone hormonal axis. Schematic summary of activation of the renin-angiotensin-aldosterone hormonal axis by sympathoadrenergic stimulation and low effective arterial blood volume. (Adapted by permission of Augus, Z.S., and Goldberg, M.: Renal function in congestive heart failure. In Levine, H.J., editor: Clinical cardiovascular physiology, New York, 1976, Grune & Stratton, Inc.)

and is the principal stimulus for adrenal secretion of aldosterone (Fig. 2-11). Furthermore, as a regulatory feedback mechanism, it inhibits renin secretion by direct action on the juxtaglomerular cells.[10]

Aldosterone affects the distal tubule of the nephron to promote active reabsorption of sodium and chloride. As sodium and water conservation expands extracellular fluid volume, renal perfusion pressure rises and the stimulus for aldosterone release is inhibited.

In moderate heart failure, renal hemodynamics and the RAA system increase both proximal and distal tubular reabsorption of sodium and water, and the kidneys are unable to excrete any increase in sodium load. Because of the retained fluid and depressed cardiac action, venous capillary hydrostatic pressure increases, promoting transudation of fluid into the interstitial spaces. This is the process thought to contribute to cardiac edema.

Moderate chronic heart failure is also characterized by sustained hypersecretion of renin by the kidney. This may have a dual effect on the pathogenesis of heart failure. Heightened RAA activity potentiates sympathetic vasomotor tone to produce a marked increase in peripheral vascular resistance. This may raise effective arterial pressure, but it also increases a major determinant of left ventricular afterload, thereby altering pump function.

Renin hypersecretion also stimulates production of high levels of aldosterone even when circulating blood volume is adequate. This, coupled with decreased degradation of aldosterone by the liver, results in marked hyperaldosteronism that, in turn, supports inappropriate fluid retention in heart failure. In this manner, a positive feedback cycle is established where depressed cardiac function and low effective arterial blood volume activate the RAA and sympathoadrenergic systems. This results in elevated preload and afterload that, in turn, increases hemodynamic burden, causing further depression of myocardial function (Fig. 2-12).

Research on the effects of RAA humoral axis in hypertension has lead to the development of several new therapeutic agents called converting enzyme inhibitors. These substances inhibit the production of angiotensin II and by this action may serve as vasodilating agents. They are currently being analyzed for their unloading effects in the treatment of chronic congestive heart failure.

Advanced heart failure. In advanced congestive heart failure, all compensatory efforts by the kidney are unsuccessful in restoring effective arterial blood volume; consequently, renal perfusion pressure remains depressed. This factor, coupled with intense renal vasoconstriction and hypersecretion of RAA, precipitates several changes in kidney function that promote further edema formation, electrolyte, and biochemical disorders.

Intense renal vasoconstriction reduces blood flow in both the afferent and the efferent renal arterioles, causing a marked reduction in the GFR. A depressed GFR decreases the ability of the kidney to eliminate end-products of metabolism and to handle any elevation in sodium or fluid load. As a result, the following clinical signs may occur: (1) blood urea nitrogen concentration rises, indicating the presence of prerenal azotemia; (2) urine becomes dilute and the volume is depressed to oliguric levels; (3) a small increase in sodium inges-

tion leads to severe volume overload; and (4) the kidney becomes refractory to diuretic therapy because agents do not reach the site of action in the nephron.[1]

In advanced heart failure there is evidence of increased secretion of antidiuretic hormones. This may account for the inability of some patients to secrete a water load. Although this is not considered a significant factor influencing cardiac edema formation, it is thought to play a role in dilutional hyponatremia frequently seen in these patients.[1]

Other operative factors in edema formation may include the effect of natriuretic hormones and kidney prostaglandins on fluid retention. Normal individuals escape the sodium-retaining action of aldosterone, whereas this escape phenomenon does not occur in patients with heart failure. There is experimental evidence of a natriuretic hormone that promotes sodium and water excretion; however, its chemical nature and site of action have not yet been identified.[7,26] It has been postulated that the absence of this hormone in subjects with congestive heart failure may be a factor contributing to severe fluid retention and edema formation.

The kidneys synthesize local hormones, prostaglandins F_2 and $F_2\alpha$ in the interstitial and collecting ducts of the renal medulla. They are released into the renal interstitial fluid and venous blood and are metabolized in the liver and lungs. Their precise role in sodium retention of congestive heart failure is unclear; however, research studies inhibiting prostaglandins with indomethacin have increased sodium excretion, leading to the conclusion that prostaglandins may indeed play a role in sodium reabsorption in the kidneys. Although this assumption has not yet been validated, it presents yet another area to be researched as a possible contributing factor to cardiac edema.[17]

Clinical recognition of cardiac edema. Cardiac edema, a cardinal sign of congestive heart failure, develops relatively late in the syndrome, appearing a number of days after the onset of the precipitating event. It is most commonly associated with chronic heart failure where it may

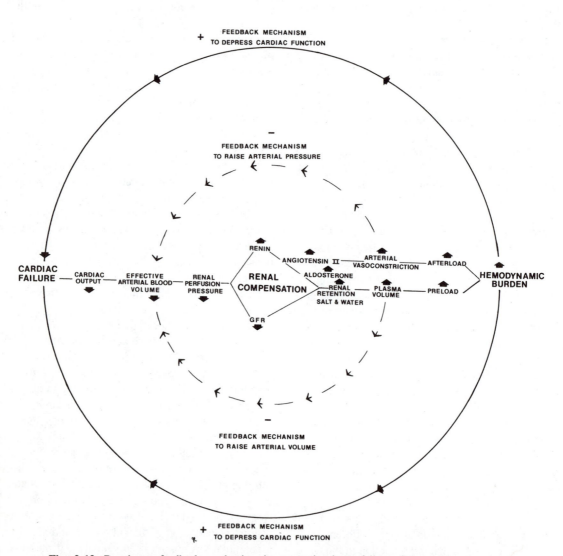

Fig. 2-12. Regulatory feedback mechanism in congestive heart failure. Schematic summary of compensatory mechanisms that trigger negative feedback response to increase cardiac performance (indicated by broken line and arrows). Heavy line indicates positive feedback response in which renal and sympathetic compensatory mechanisms are activated, causing increase in vascular resistance (afterload) and vascular volume and venous return (preload). Increase in preload and afterload adds to hemodynamic burden and results in further reduction of ventricular performance with concomitant increase in cardiac failure.

appear in conjunction with elevated venous pressure, jugular venous distention, and hepatomegaly. However, it is important to remember that cardiac edema may also occur when left ventricular function is depressed and systemic venous pressures are normal or only slightly elevated. This occurs when individuals with low cardiac output have compensated by expanding the extracellular fluid volume enough to produce peripheral edema, but with minimal change in systemic venous pressure.[3] Since cardiac edema does not always correlate with elevated venous pressure, it is necessary to assess it in light of the total clinical picture in order to make an accurate evaluation of cardiac status.

Expansion of extracellular fluid volume resulting from sympathoadrenergic and renal mechanisms of compensation is postulated to be the primary cause of clinical cardiac edema. Extracellular fluid may increase approximately 5 to 8 L in adults before peripheral edema becomes evident.[1,3] Generally, an average increase in weight of 1 pound/day indicates fluid retention. Weight gain may be the first evidence of fluid retention in early mild heart failure and is followed by the appearance of transient peripheral edema and organ congestion.

Cardiac edema has several physical characteristics. It is soft, pitting, and symmetrical and initially presents in the dependent parts of the body where venous pressure is highest. In ambulatory patients edema is first noted in the feet and ankles and ascends to include the lower legs. It is most evident at the end of the day and usually resolves after a night's rest. In bedridden patients it is noted first in the presacral area and progresses to include the genital region and medial aspects of the thighs. Facial cardiac edema is rarely seen in adults.

Chronic dependent cardiac edema causes some skin changes. The skin overlying the edematous areas may become reddened, pigmented, and indurated. However, edema by itself rarely interrupts the integrity of the skin or causes ulcers on the lower extremities. When these are present, it may be evidence of underlying peripheral vascular insufficiency.

In advanced heart failure, systemic venous pressure is markedly elevated and arterial pressure is reduced, seriously impairing organ and tissue perfusion. These severe circulatory abnormalities together with acid/base imbalances increase cell membrane permeability. This causes rapid extravasation of fluid throughout the body resulting in the following physical manifestations: anasarca, total body edema, ascites, an accumulation of fluid in the abdominal cavity, and hydrothorax, a pooling of fluid in the pleural space of the thorax. These findings are most frequently observed in patients with chronic, severe, or refractory heart failure. See Chapter 4 for assessment techniques.

Increased tissue oxygen extraction. Oxygen extraction reflects the rate at which tissue cells are able to utilize oxygen delivered by capillary blood. Assuming optimal blood flow, each organ system extracts oxygen at rates depending on organ function and inherent metabolic rate. For example, skeletal muscle requires less oxygen at rest and extracts all oxygen during exercise. Furthermore, it has the capacity to sustain an oxygen debt because of its ability to function by anaerobic metabolism. Other organs such as the heart and central nervous system require a continuous supply of oxygen. The heart extracts 13 ml O_2/dl at rest and adapts to increased myocardial oxygen demand by increasing coronary blood flow by the process of vasodilation rather than by increased oxygen extraction.[12] Cutaneous and renal systems with lower inherent metabolic rates receive relatively high rates of blood flow and extract moderate amounts of oxygen. The extra blood is utilized for nonmetabolic purposes such as glomerular filtration in the kidney and heat loss in the skin. It is postulated that variance in oxygen requirements is an important factor in determining tissue autoregulation of peripheral blood flow.[13] The autonomic nervous system also plays a key role in regulating peripheral circulation.

In heart failure, blood flow to the peripheral tissues is usually diminished secondary to a drop in cardiac output and perfusion pressure. The tissues compensate for slow circulation time by extracting more oxygen per unit of blood flow. This is clin-

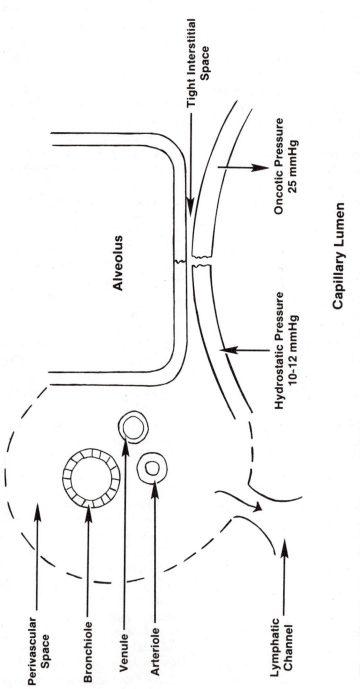

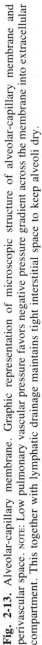

Fig. 2-13. Alveolar-capillary membrane. Graphic representation of microscopic structure of alveolar-capillary membrane and perivascular space. NOTE: Low pulmonary vascular pressure favors negative pressure gradient across the membrane into extracellular compartment. This together with lymphatic drainage maintains tight interstitial space to keep alveoli dry.

ically diagnosed by an increase in the body arteriovenous oxygen difference (A-Vo_2). The normal arteriovenous oxygen difference is 4 ml O_2/dl and represents the average oxygen extraction from body tissue in the basal state.[12]

Increased oxygen extraction is associated with a decline in the affinity of hemoglobin for oxygen, which is caused by an increase in organic phosphate compounds 2,3,diphosphoglycerate (DPG). This decrease in hemoglobin binding of oxygen is reflected by a rightward shift of the oxyhemoglobin dissociation curve and facilitates the release of oxygen to underperfused metabolizing tissues. It represents yet another mechanism whereby the body adjusts to meet tissue metabolic requirements in response to depressed cardiocirculatory function.

ALTERATION IN PULMONARY FUNCTION

Normally, pulmonary capillary hydrostatic pressure is 10 to 12 mm Hg and the oncotic pressure is 25 mm Hg. Consequently, there is an inward pressure gradient of 15 mm Hg that keeps the alveoli dry. Alteration in the ventilatory function of the lung associated with congestive heart failure results primarily from an imbalance of these forces. Within the lung, liquid and colloid move continuously from pulmonary vessels to the interstitial space. This fluid is removed at a constant rate by lymphatic channels that drain into the systemic venous system. This mechanism maintains minimal interstitial fluid volume to facilitate alveolar-capillary gas exchange, and alteration in its function may cause the pulmonary congestion of heart failure (Fig. 2-13).

Elevated pulmonary capillary pressure is the initiating event and is most commonly caused by left ventricular failure and mital stenosis. As the left ventricle fails, end-diastolic pressure rises and is transmitted backward to the left atrium, pulmonary veins, and finally the pulmonary capillary bed. Elevated pulmonary capillary hydrostatic pressure exceeds oncotic pressure at the alveolar-capillary membrane, which favors movement of fluid and protein from the pulmonary capillaries into the

lung tissue. Pulmonary congestion ensues and decreases ventilation by the following pathophysiological processes:

1. Increased tissue fluid coupled with hydrothorax decreases the amount of intrathoracic space available for breathing.
2. Tissue fluid decreases the elasticity or compliance of the lung, thereby increasing oxygen demand and the work of breathing.
3. Tissue congestion interferes with the alveolar-capillary diffusion of oxygen, causing hypoxia and hypercapnia.

During the course of heart failure, pulmonary congestion is thought to progress in stages related to hemodynamic burden, ventricular function, and lymphatic drainage. They are as follows: Stage I, early pulmonary congestion; Stage II, interstitial edema; and Stage III, alveolar edema.[15] During these stages the changes in lung function account for many of the major respiratory symptoms and clinical indicators of the congestive heart failure syndrome (Table 2-7).

Stage I: early pulmonary congestion

During this early phase of pulmonary congestion, an increase in the flow of liquid and colloids from the pulmonary capillaries through the interstitial tissue occurs with a proportional increase in lymphatic drainage. Consequently, there is very little measurable increase in interstitial lung fluid.

According to Ingram and Braunwald, there are few signs and symptoms during this phase.[15] However, it is possible to have the patient report exertional dyspnea, particularly if the congestion is secondary to left ventricular hypofunction. Physical signs are few and may include mild inspiratory rales caused by opening of closed airways. Radiological examination of serial views of the chest may reveal some prominence of the pulmonary veins and arteries secondary to elevated pulmonary vascular volume.

Stage II: interstitial edema (Fig. 2-14)

Generally, interstitial edema occurs when pulmonary capillary hydrostatic pressure exceeds 18 mm Hg. This causes an imbalance of forces at the

Table 2-7. Behaviors symptomatic of respiratory distress in acute congestive heart failure

Behaviors	Clinical indicators	Causes
Nocturnal breathlessness when lying flat Intolerance of a recumbent position at rest Preference for an upright position	Orthopnea	Postural redistribution of pulmonary blood flow Transient pulmonary congestion secondary to increased venous return to the heart
Sudden awakening at night because of extreme shortness of breath and sense of suffocation relieved by sitting upright with the legs dependent	Paroxysmal nocturnal dyspnea	Transient acute alveolar edema secondary to increased pulmonary vascular pressure and increased venous return to the heart Nocturnal depression of the respiratory center Decreased adrenergic stimulation of the left ventricle at rest Bronchospasm caused by congestion of the bronchial mucosa
Reluctance to move about in bed or walk short distances because of extreme fatigue and breathlessness	Severe exertional dyspnea Dyspnea at rest	Severe left ventricular dysfunction with depressed cardiac output and minimal cardiac reserve Pulmonary congestion with interstitial edema and decreased lung compliance
Inability to concentrate Decreased recall of people and recent events	Mental confusion Memory loss	Decreased cerebral perfusion Cerebral hypoxia
Dry nonproductive cough aggravated by exertion and by lying flat Persistent cough at night	Cardiac cough (dyspnea equivalent)	Pulmonary congestion Interstitial edema with stimulation of the interstitial stretch receptors
Verbal pattern of short phrases interrupted by frequent pauses Complaint of shortness of breath Rapid shallow respirations	Dyspnea	Elevated pulmonary capillary pressure resulting from left ventricular failure Pulmonary interstitial edema with decreased lung compliance and increased work of breathing
Expectoration of large amounts of white or pink-tinged frothy mucus	Acute pulmonary edema	Flooding of the alveoli and large airways Marked decrease in lung compliance hypoxia
Inability to sleep Restlessness at night	Insomnia	Mild pulmonary congestion caused by left ventricular failure Mild hypoxia Cheyne-Stokes respiration caused by prolonged circulation time that disturbs the mechanism regulating respirations

capillary membrane leading to an increase in net filtration of fluid from the pulmonary intravascular space into the interstitial space. The rate of fluid filtration from the capillaries into the interstitial space is greater than that removed by lymphatic drainage. Interstitial edema may also occur if systemic venous pressure is sufficiently elevated to inhibit lymphatic drainage.

Interstitial edema first develops in the loose perivascular space around the bronchioles, venules, and arterioles. It decreases the elasticity of the lung tissue and consequently increases oxygen demand and the work of breathing. Perivascular edema also compromises the small airways to increase wasted ventilation and closing volumes, thus contributing to hypoxemia.

Clinical indicators of interstitial edema are quite varied. Increased exertional dyspnea is present because of engorged pulmonary vessels, elevated pulmonary vascular pressure, and reduced lung compliance. Orthopnea may be present if left ventricular function is severely impaired or the patient may complain of a nonproductive cough, frequently referred to as a "dyspnea equivalent."[3]

Attacks of paroxysmal nocturnal dyspnea may also occur. This is caused by postural redistribution of blood flow that increases venous return and pulmonary vascular pressures when the patient is at rest in a recumbent position. It may also occur secondary to congestion of the bronchial mucosa that increases airway resistance and the work of breathing. Pulmonary findings of interstitial edema include tachypnea, rapid shallow respirations secondary to decreased lung compliance, and a dry nonproductive cough resulting from stimulation of the stretch receptors in the interstitium. Moist, fine, crepitant rales are audible over the lung bases.

In cardiogenic pulmonary edema, rales are first noted over the lung base. They spread toward the apices as heart failure worsens. The ascending progression of pulmonary rales is related to the gravity-dependent distribution of pulmonary edema. Because of low pulmonary intravascular pressures, the effects of gravity are greater on the

distribution of blood flow than on tissue forces; consequently, pulmonary vascular pressures are greatest at the base of the lungs and significant elevation first exceeds alveolar pressures in this area. Although compensatory pulmonary arterial vasoconstriction protects the lung from edema, it does so at the expense of pulmonary hypertension and right ventricular overload.

Radiological findings characteristic of interstitial edema include generalized haziness and loss of definition of vascular markings and hilar shadows. Accumulation of fluid in the interlobular septa causes thickening of the septal lines that are described as Kerly B lines.

Stage III: alveolar edema (Fig. 2-14)

As the outward force of pulmonary capillary hydrostatic pressure rises to levels of 25 to 28 mm Hg, it exceeds the inward force of plasma oncotic pressure, resulting in rapid extravasation of fluid out of the intravascular and interstitial space into the alveoli. In early alveolar edema, fluid builds in the corners of the alveoli. The tendency for this to occur has been demonstrated in animal models.[3] These studies suggest that forces resulting from the geometrical configuration of adjacent alveoli serve as a means of collecting liquid.[3,5] The smaller radius of the curvature at the corners of alveoli increases surface tension. This in turn causes more negative interstitial pressures surrounding the corners and leads to a more rapid transfer of fluid into this area. In spite of accumulation of fluid in the corners of alveoli, inflation pressure still maintains the configuration of the gas-exchange unit to preserve some ventilation.

As edema progresses, liquid floods the entire alveolus and it no longer remains open during inspiration. At this stage, the integrity of the alveolar-capillary membrane is disrupted, further adding to the alveolar flooding. Fluid invades the large airways and the patient expectorates frothy pink-tinged sputum. This markedly interferes with oxygen exchange, causing severe hypoxemia, and coupled with severely compromised left ventricular function it constitutes a life-threatening situation.

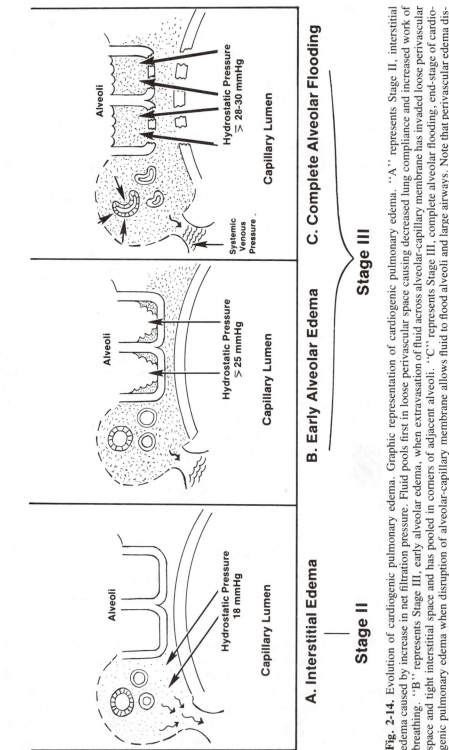

Fig. 2-14. Evolution of cardiogenic pulmonary edema. Graphic representation of cardiogenic pulmonary edema. "A" represents Stage II, interstitial edema caused by increase in net filtration pressure. Fluid pools first in loose perivascular space causing decreased lung compliance and increased work of breathing. "B" represents Stage III, early alveolar edema, when extravasation of fluid across alveolar-capillary membrane has invaded loose perivascular space and tight interstitial space and has pooled in corners of adjacent alveoli. "C" represents Stage III, complete alveolar flooding, end-stage of cardiogenic pulmonary edema when disruption of alveolar-capillary membrane allows fluid to flood alveoli and large airways. Note that perivascular edema distorts bronchioles and pulmonary vessels to further compromise ventilation and perfusion.

Clinical picture

Acute cardiogenic pulmonary edema is the most dramatic and catastrophic indicator of heart failure. It may emerge as the initial symptom of an acute cardiac event such as myocardial infarction or it may indicate exacerbation of chronic heart failure. Regardless of the underlying cause, the clinical picture is generally the same.

The subjective findings include behaviors and verbalizations indicative of extreme restlessness, fear, and anxiety. These patients complain of extreme air hunger and a sense of suffocation; they are unable to tolerate a recumbent position and are often combative.

Respiratory signs include tachypnea, with rates varying from 20 to 40 respirations/minute. The work of breathing is increased, causing high negative intrapleural pressures. This is manifested by dilation of the alae nasi and by inspiratory retraction of the supraclavicular fossae and intercostal spaces. When in a high Fowler's position, these individuals often grasp the side rails in order to mobilize all assessory respiratory muscles.

The chest is dull to percussion and auscultation of the lung reveals wheezing and generalized moist, bubbly rales. It is often difficult to assess heart sounds because of the presence of a loud adventitial noise; however, a third heart sound is frequently present.

The skin is cool, pale, ashen, and markedly diaphoretic. This may reflect hypoxia, diminished cardiac output, and compensatory sympathoadrenergic stimulation.

Vital signs may vary. Generally, the heart rate and blood pressure are elevated because of sympathetic stimulation. As pulmonary edema progresses, accompanied by diminished left ventricular function, the blood pressure falls and cardiogenic shock ensues.

Hemodynamic parameters reveal markedly elevated pulmonary capillary wedge pressure, pulmonary artery pressure, and moderately elevated mean arterial pressure. Systemic vascular resistance is high and right atrial pressure may also be elevated as a reflection of pulmonary hypertension and concomitant right ventricular failure.

Arterial blood gases reflect hypoxemi_ panied by hypocapnia that results from c_ tory hyperventilation. Hypercapnia may __ as heart failure progresses and ventilation fails, or it may reflect the presence of underlying chronic lung disease. Acidemia is a common finding and is related to both diminished ventilation and tissue perfusion.

Radiological examination of the lung fields reveals bilateral confluent densities that start centrally and spread peripherally in a butterfly-wing pattern.[23] Pleural effusions are frequently present and appear on film as a blunting of the costophrenic angles. Cardiac dilation is also a common finding and is diagnosed as an increase in the cardiothoracic ratio greater than 50%. These findings are quite characteristic of acute cardiogenic pulmonary edema; however, because these patients are markedly distressed and difficult to handle, care must be taken to evaluate serial readings of the same view of the chest film to accurately assess the progression or resolution of pulmonary congestion.

Therapeutic interventions   Tx

The therapeutic goals are to (1) increase ventilation and oxygenation, (2) decrease venous return to the heart, and (3) increase peripheral perfusion. Measures taken to increase ventilation and oxygenation include placing the patient in a high Fowler's position with the legs dependent, administration of high concentrations of inspired oxygen usually assisted by mechanical ventilation, and administration of selected drugs. Theophylline is frequently given to combat bronchospasm; however, the side effects of increased heart rate, nausea, and vomiting must be monitored to prevent complications. Morphine sulfate is also used for its narcotic effect and to decrease patient distress and the work of breathing. Morphine also decreases venous and arterial vasoconstriction, thereby reducing preload and afterload.

Measures taken to decrease venous return to the heart include maintaining the patient in a seated position with the legs dependent and administration of rapid-acting diuretics such as furosemide or

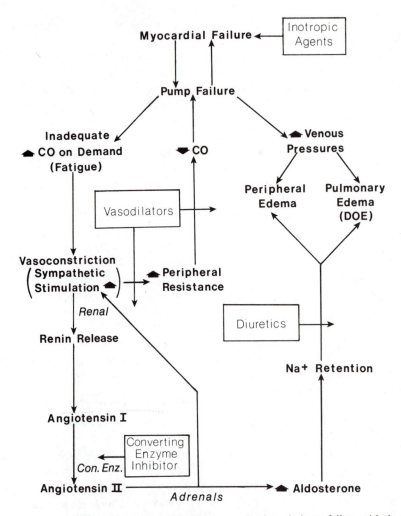

Fig. 2-15. Summary of pathophysiological regulatory mechanisms in heart failure with therapeutic intervention. Schematic diagram of major hemodynamic alterations and compensatory mechanisms that result from myocardial failure. Also shown are sites of action of three major therapeutic interventions: administration of inotropic agents, diuretics, and vasodilators. (From The heart arteries and veins by J.W. Hurst. Copyright © 1982 by J.W. Hurst. Used with the permission of McGraw-Hill Book Company.)

ethacrynic acid. Occasionally application of rotating tourniquets is necessary. The intravenous administration of furosemide also directly produces venodilation before the diuretic effect. Occasionally, oral nitroglycerin may also be used to reduce preload by inducing venodilation. However, oral administration is difficult in these distressed patients, and intravenous use may reduce arterial pressure to dangerously low levels unless controlled by careful arterial pressure monitoring.

Measures taken to increase peripheral perfusion include the use of inotropic, sympathomimetic, and vasodilating agents. The most common agent used to augment contractility is digitalis. Care must be taken before administration to evaluate these patients for possible toxicity. This drug is most helpful to those with rapid heart rates caused by atrial tachycardia or fibrillation. In this situation decreased diastolic filling time often compromises coronary circulation resulting in diminished left ventricular function. Conversion of the rapid rhythm may increase coronary blood flow and improve cardiac function, thereby leading to resolution of pulmonary edema.[15]

Nitroprusside is the vasodilator most frequently used to increase peripheral circulation by reducing systemic vascular resistance and afterload. It is frequently administered in conjunction with a sympathomimetic agent such as dopamine or dobutamine to elevate cardiac contractility and to support mean arterial pressure. The definitive drug therapy for acute cardiogenic pulmonary edema is quite varied and it is essential for clinicians to be conversant with the rationale for administration and side effects to effectively handle these patients. Fig. 2-15 summarizes the physiological mechanisms of heart failure and use of major therapeutic modalities. Chapter 8 gives more detailed information on specific agents.

SUMMARY

The syndrome of congestive heart failure reflects major alteration in cardiovascular function. The degree to which it interferes with homeostatic maintenance is determined by the extent and duration of underlying heart disease, the efficiency of compensatory mechanisms, and the effectiveness of clinical therapeutics.

When cardiac output drops, reflex sympathoadrenergic stimulation increases heart rate and constricts blood vessels to elevate perfusion pressure and to increase venous return. This process acts in concert with the Frank-Starling response to augment myocardial contractility and to support circulation as a short-term compensatory response. As heart failure worsens, sustained hemodynamic burden causes myocardial hypertrophy, and expansion of extracellular fluid volume is evoked by renal compensatory mechanisms. If pump function remains depressed in spite of maximal activation of all compensatory mechanisms, severe pulmonary and systemic congestion results, cardiac reserve becomes markedly depressed, and the heart is no longer able to meet tissue metabolic demands.

Early recognition of key clinical indicators and a comprehensive knowledge of pathophysiology coupled with skilled application of clinical therapeutics will expedite treatment, prevent complications, and maximize health care.

REFERENCES

1. Agus, J.S., and Goldberg, M.: Renal function in congestive heart failure. In Levine, H.J., editor: Clinical cardiovascular physiology, New York, 1976, Grune & Stratton, Inc., pp. 403-444.
2. Braunwald, E., editor: Heart disease: a textbook of cardiovascular medicine, Philadelphia, 1980, W.B. Saunders Co.
3. Braunwald, E.: Clinical manifestation of heart failure. In Braunwald, E., editor: Heart disease: a textbook of cardiovascular medicine, Philadelphia, 1981, W.B. Saunders Co., p. 453.
4. Braunwald, E.: Pathophysiology of heart failure. In Braunwald, E., editor: Heart disease: a textbook of cardiovascular medicine, Philadelphia, 1981, W.B. Saunders Co., p. 453.
5. Broderman, I., and others: Effect of surface tension on circulation in excised lungs of dogs, J. Appl. Physiol. **19:**707, 1964.
6. Burchell, H.B.: Clinical recognition of cardiac hypertrophy, Circ. Res. **34-35**(suppl. 2):116, Aug. 1974.
7. Cannon, P.J.: The kidney in heart failure, N. Engl. J. Med. **296**(1)26, 1977.
8. Cohn, J.N. and others: Neurohumoral control mechanisms in congestive heart failure, Am. Heart J. **102**(3)509, 1981.
9. The Criteria Committee of the New York Heart Association nomenclature and criteria for diagnosis of diseases of the heart and great vessels, ed. 8, New York, 1979, New York Heart Association, Inc.
10. Ganong, W.F.: Review of medical physiology, ed. 8, Los Altos, Calif., 1977, Lange Medical Publications, pp. 522-545.
11. Goldberger, E.: Textbook of clinical cardiology, St. Louis, 1982, The C.V. Mosby Co., p. 282.
12. Grossman, W., and Braunwald, E.: High cardiac output states. In Braunwald, E., editor: Heart disease: a textbook of cardiovascular medicine, Philadelphia, 1980, W.B. Saunders Co., p. 818.
13. Guyton, A.C.: Textbook of medical physiology, ed. 6, Philadelphia, 1981, W.B. Saunders Co., pp. 234, 309.

14. Hurst, J.W., editor: The heart arteries and veins, ed. 5, New York, 1981, McGraw-Hill Book Co.

15. Ingram, R.H., and Braunwald, E.: Pulmonary edema: cardiogenic and noncardiogenic form. In Braunwald, E., editor: Heart disease, a textbook of cardiovascular medicine, Philadelphia, 1981, W.B. Saunders Co., p. 571.

16. Katz, A.M.: Physiology of the heart, New York, 1977, Raven Press, pp. 397-418.

17. Kirschenbarm, M.A., and Stein, J.H.: The effect of inhibition of prostaglandin synthesis on urinary sodium excretion in the conscious dog, J. Clin. Invest. **57:**517, 1976.

18. Ross, G.: Essentials of human physiology, Chicago, 1978, Year Book Medical Publishers, Inc., p. 195.

19. Rutenberg, H.L., and Spann, J.F.: Alteration of cardiac sympathetic neurotransmitter activity in congestive heart failure. In Mason, D.T., editor: Congestive heart failure mechanisms, evaluation and treatment, New York, 1976, Yorke Medical Books, p. 85.

20. Schlant, R.C.: Altered physiology of the cardiovascular system. In Hurst, J.W., editor: Heart failure in the heart arteries and veins, ed. 4, New York, 1978, McGraw-Hill Book Co., p. 537.

21. Sokolow, M., and McIlroy, M.B.: Clinical cardiology, ed. 2, Los Altos, Calif., 1979, Lange Medical Publications, p. 301.

22. Spann, J.F., and Hurst, J.W.: The recognition and management of heart failure. In Hurst, J.W., editor: The heart arteries and veins, ed. 5, New York, 1981, McGraw-Hill Book Co.

23. Spinola, F.H.: Plain film diagnosis of congestive heart failure, J. Med. Soc. N.J. **75:**783, 1978.

24. Spotnitz, H.M., and Sonnenblick, E.H.: Structural conditions in the hypertrophied and failing heart. In Mason, D.T.: Congestive heart failure mechanisms, evaluation and treatment, New York, 1976, Yorke Medical Books, p. 13.

25. Swan, H.J.C., and Parmley, W.: Congestive heart failure. In Sodeman, W.A., and Sodeman, T.M., editors: Pathologic physiology mechanisms of disease, Philadelphia, 1979, W.B. Saunders Co.

26. Tonkon, M.J., Rosen, S.M., and Mason, D.T.: Renal function and edema formation in congestive heart failure. In Mason, D.T., editor: Congestive heart failure, New York, 1976, Yorke Medical Books.

27. Zelis, R. and others: Peripheral circulatory control mechanisms in congestive heart failure. In Mason, D.T., editor: Congestive heart failure mechanisms, evaluation and treatment, New York, 1976, Yorke Medical Books, p. 129.

CHAPTER 3

Underlying causes and precipitating factors in heart failure

LINDA S. PURA
CONCHITA S. SAM

Cardiac performance depends on the interaction of the following mechanisms: (1) diastolic loading or preload, (2) myocardial contractility, (3) systolic loading or afterload, (4) heart rate, rhythm, and conduction, and (5) metabolic state. These factors maintain cardiac output at a level appropriate to meet the body's metabolic demands. Malfunction of these determinants of myocardial performance will ultimately result in heart failure.

In clinical practice, the discriminate classification of the factors causing heart failure will guide the clinician in identifying major patient problems, reaching a definitive diagnosis, and formulating specific interventions. The purpose of this chapter is to present an overview of the major diseases that underlie and precipitate heart failure. The factors that cause heart failure in adults are divided into three subgroups: (1) abnormal loading conditions, (2) abnormal muscle function, and (3) conditions or diseases that precipitate heart failure. Groups 1 and 2 are based on pathophysiological mechanisms. Group 3 is a nonmechanistic category relating possible causes to physiological abnormalities.

ABNORMAL LOADING CONDITIONS
(Table 3-1)

Systolic loading or afterload in the normal heart is intramyocardial wall tension after the onset of muscle shortening and is a key determinant of the quantity of blood ejected by the ventricle. After-load is determined by the tone of systemic arterioles, the elasticity of the aorta and large arteries, the viscosity of the blood, the size and thickness of the ventricle, and the presence of aortic stenosis. Diastolic loading or preload refers to the length of the myocardial fibers before ventricular contraction and is determined by the condition of the mitral valve, the compliance of the ventricle, blood volume, venous tone, and the vigor and timing of atrial contraction. Hemodynamically, preload is reflected by ventricular filling pressure, and, by the Frank-Starling law, the resultant myocardial fiber length is directly related to the force of cardiac contraction. Afterload is reflected by systolic and diastolic arterial blood pressure and by systemic vascular resistance.

Abnormal loading conditions imply a greater than normal burden on the heart because of elevated intramyocardial wall tension and intraventricular volume and pressure. In systolic overload the ventricles generate higher than normal contractile pressures to overcome resistance to the forward flow of blood. Diastolic overload is initially reflected by elevated ventricular end-diastolic volume. Eventually, filling pressures rise beyond those of the normally compliant heart. Over time this causes a decrease in the effective force of ventricular contraction. The definitive cause of diminished contractile performance has yet to be identified. Inflow obstruction, the third condition that contributes to heart failure, is altered blood

Table 3-1. Abnormal loading conditions

Systolic overload	Diastolic overload	Inflow obstruction*
Aortic valvular stenosis	Aortic valvular regurgitation	Mitral stenosis
Pulmonary valvular stenosis	Mitral valvular regurgitation	Tricuspid stenosis
Systemic hypertension	Pulmonic valvular regurgitation	Atrial myxoma
Aortic coarctation	Tricuspid valvular regurgitation	
Pulmonary hypertension	Left-to-right shunts	
	Ventricular septal defect	
	Atrial septal defect	
	Patent ductus arteriosus	
	Aortopulmonary window	
	Coronary arteriovenous fistula	

*Inflow tract lesions exacerbate congestive heart failure by altering loading conditions.

flow from the atria to the ventricles caused by a reduction in the diameter of the valvular opening or interference with the valve leaflets. These abnormal loading conditions trigger the development of chamber dilation and hypertrophy. When this hypertrophic response becomes inadequate, it is likely that the ventricle fails because of marked increase in intramyocardial wall tension.[8] Clinically the patient has manifestations of heart failure.

The right and left ventricles are pumps that work conjointly; therefore pathological events that alter the function of one ventricle will ultimately impair the other. Heart failure is characterized by specific clinical indicators. When left ventricular failure occurs, there is a marked reduction in the forward blood flow manifested by reduced cardiac output and elevated left ventricular end-diastolic pressure. This pressure is transmitted backward from the left ventricle across the mitral valve to the left atrium and the pulmonary circulation (Fig. 2-1). As pulmonary capillary hydrostatic pressure exceeds oncotic pressure, intravascular fluid leaks into the interstitial regions of the lungs, causing pulmonary congestion. Pulmonary congestion reduces lung compliance and gas diffusion and is characterized by insomnia, dyspnea, tachypnea, anxiety, and cyanosis.

In protracted left ventricular failure the right ventricle continues to pump blood against elevated

pulmonary pressures and ultimately fails. Right ventricular failure results in elevated right atrial pressure, which impedes systemic venous return. This increases systemic capillary hydrostatic pressure, which in turn results in peripheral edema and organ congestion. Right ventricular failure is characterized by jugular venous distention, hepatomegaly, hepatojugular reflux, and peripheral edema.

The decreased capacity of the failing ventricles to eject blood diminishes forward flow into the pulmonary or systemic circulation. This is characterized by the clinical indicators of decreased peripheral and pulmonary perfusion. These clinical indicators include weakness, fatigue, decreased cardiac reserve, hypotension, oliguria, and metabolic imbalances. See Chapter 2 for a more detailed discussion.

Conditions producing systolic overload (elevated afterload)

Aortic stenosis (Fig. 3-1, *A*). Constriction of the aortic valve leaflets reduces effective blood flow from the left ventricle. This outflow obstruction may result from rheumatic endocarditis, calcification of a congenital bicuspid or malformed tricuspid aortic valve, atherosclerosis, or degenerative valvular calcification.

Severe aortic stenosis is characterized by reduc-

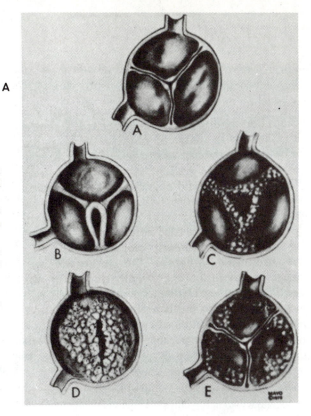

Fig. 3-1. A, Types of aortic valve stenosis. *A,* Normal aortic valve; *B,* congenital aortic stenosis; *C,* rheumatic aortic stenosis; *D,* calcific bicuspid aortic stenosis; *E,* calcific senile aortic stenosis. **B,** In normally functioning aortic valve, systolic pressures of aorta *(Ao)* and left ventricle *(LV)* rise together to same systolic peak *(left diagram).* Aortic stenosis prevents free communication between aorta and left ventricle, resulting in systolic pressure gradient *(right diagram, cross-hatching).* (**A** from Brandenburg, R.O., and others: Valvular heart disease: when should the patient be referred? Pract. Cardio. **5:**50, 1979.)

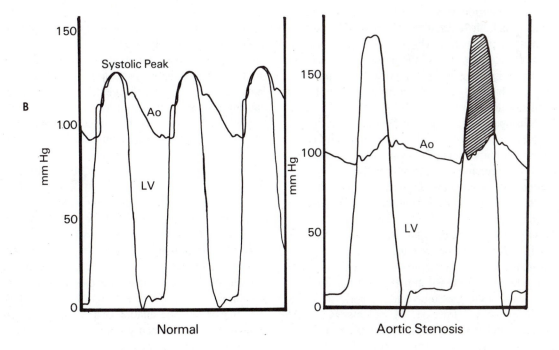

tion of the aortic valve opening to one-fourth the normal size (normal is 2.6 cm² to 3.5 cm²) and a peak systolic ventricular/arterial pressure gradient that exceeds 50 mm Hg.[9,60] The systolic pressure of the left ventricle rises above 150 mm Hg occasionally reaching 350 mm Hg (normal pressure equals 120 mm Hg), while aortic pressure remains normal.[23] (See Fig. 3-1, *B*.) These dynamic changes indicate significant obstruction to left ventricular ejection.

With narrowing of the aortic orifice, pressure overload of the left ventricle stimulates concentric hypertrophy of this chamber. Initially, this compensatory mechanism maintains normal cardiac output despite outflow impedance. However, when the hypertrophic response is no longer effective, cardiac output falls and blood dams up in the left atrium and lungs with pulmonary vascular pressures ultimately exceeding 28 to 30 mm Hg.

Clinical indicators. The major clinical indicators of aortic stenosis in the adult include dyspnea secondary to left ventricular failure, angina, and syncope. Angina is the most common subjective finding in the older individual and is precipitated by exertion and relieved by rest. Angina results from high ventricular wall tension due to concentric hypertrophy, which elevates myocardial oxygen requirements. In the presence of coronary artery insufficiency, this myocardial supply/demand imbalance accounts for myocardial ischemia and severe frequent angina.

Syncope and associated symptoms of dizziness, lightheadedness, or "feeling faint" usually occur during or immediately following physical exertion, and they probably result from inadequate cerebral blood flow. These episodes may also be associated with tachyarrhythmias resulting from myocardial ischemia.

Objective indicators of aortic valvular stenosis include normal blood pressure, unless severe stenosis is present, in which case pulse pressure may be reduced to 30 to 40 mm Hg as a result of decreased systolic pressure rather than elevated diastolic pressure. However, in patients with mild stenosis and associated regurgitation and in older patients with inelastic arterial beds, both systolic and pulse pressures may be normal or widened.[9] The presence of concentric hypertrophy accounts for a forceful, heaving, and prolonged apical impulse, which is displaced downward and to the left. A systolic thrill is usually palpable over the base at the second right intercostal space. The carotid artery pulse is usually not visible, and, when palpated, it coincides with the aortic component of the *second* heart sound (S_2) rather than the first heart sound (S_1) which is the normal finding.

On auscultation, the first heart sound is soft and the fourth heart sound is prominent because of vigorous atrial contraction. Generally, the second heart sound is single as a result of the immobility of the aortic valve. Aortic stenosis is characterized by midsystolic aortic ejection murmur; it has a harsh quality, is loudest over the base, and has a diamond crescendo-decrescendo shape.

Pulmonary stenosis. Stenosis of the pulmonary artery is characterized by fusion and thickening of the valve leaflets with a decrease in the size of the valve orifice. Pulmonary stenosis may be an isolated finding. It is commonly congenital in origin. It is associated with atrial and ventricular septal defects, supravalvular aortic stenosis, patent ductus arteriosus, and tetralogy of Fallot. Although it is rare, it may also be acquired as a result of rheumatic fever or infective endocarditis. The anatomical lesion disturbs right ventricular emptying, causing limited pulmonary blood flow. As a consequence of this outflow resistance, the right ventricle hypertrophies to maintain adequate cardiac output.

With severely stenosed valves, the right ventricle generates excessively high systolic pressures of 75 to 100 mm Hg (normal pressure equals 22 mm Hg) to overcome the outflow resistance; pulmonary artery pressure remains normal, causing a peak systolic pressure gradient between the right ventricle and the pulmonary artery.[5] The major complication in pulmonary stenosis is right ventricular pressure overload and right ventricular failure. If post-stenotic dilation of the pulmonary arteries exists, small aneurysms may form, rupture, and cause significant hemoptysis.

Clinical indicators. Isolated pulmonary valvular stenosis is a relatively common congenital cardiac defect that often permits adult survival.[41a] Mild pulmonary stenosis may cause no symptoms; however, the adaptive response of the right ventricle differs appreciably from patient to patient. In most adolescents and adults with significant valvular stenosis the resting cardiac output is within normal limits, although it does not increase normally with exercise. Individuals with severe pulmonary stenosis may demonstrate diminished right ventricular function because of the degree of ventricular hypertrophy in relation to the amount of coronary circulation, the size of the coronary ostia, and the very high systolic wall pressures that inhibit coronary perfusion. It is possible for asymptomatic individuals to deteriorate very rapidly, with progressive manifestations of systemic vascular congestion—hepatomegaly, fluid retention, ascites, progressive invalidism—and terminating in intractable heart failure. See Fig. 3-2 for cardiovascular findings.

Systemic hypertension. The Framingham study describes hypertension in adults as two repeated, causal, seated systolic pressures above 140 mm Hg and diastolic pressures above 90 mm Hg. This study also shows hypertension to be the major risk factor for 75% of all cases of heart failure reviewed.[31,32] Furthermore, it identifies hypertension as a common cause of cardiovascular morbidity and mortality in the United States.

Essential hypertension. Essential hypertension has an undefined cause and is the prevailing condition in 80% to 95% of affected patients.[32,60] Some of the possible causes include inappropriate renin secretion, increased sympathoadrenergic activity, and excessive sodium retention. It is characterized by elevated peripheral vascular resistance and decreased vascular compliance.

In early hypertension the peripheral resistance may be normal, and the cardiac output may be elevated. As hypertension continues, the peripheral resistance rises and cardiac output falls to normal. As diastolic blood pressure rises and becomes fixed, cardiac output decreases. The plasma volume varies, and plasma renin activity may be normal, suppressed, or elevated. Oparil states that these changes are probably the result of vascular autoregulatory mechanisms.[41]

Later pathological changes include concentric left ventricular hypertrophy with subsequent chamber dilation and generalized atherosclerosis of the aorta and of the coronary, renal, cerebral, and peripheral arteries. Risk factors associated with essential hypertension include hereditary predisposition, salt intake, alcohol intake, smoking, diabetes mellitus, gout, and polycythemia.

Secondary hypertension. Secondary hypertension is the result of disease, organ-related causes, and exogenous agents. (See Table 3-2.)

Clinical indicators. Subjective findings in essential and secondary hypertension may include occipital headaches, tinnitus, dizziness, and epistaxis. These patients may also complain of vague chest discomfort, restlessness, and feelings of nervous tension.

The objective indicators are elevated systolic and diastolic blood pressure (parameters were outlined at the opening of this discussion). It is important to note that care must be taken to check blood pressure in an unstressed, restful environment in order to obtain accurate baseline measurements. It may be necessary to ask the patient to return if hypertension is suspected and if an accurate baseline blood pressure is not obtained at the initial visit. Other physical findings include evidence of left ventricular hypertrophy and organ dysfunction, which may be a primary or secondary result of high blood pressure.

Aortic coarctation (Fig. 3-3). Coarctation of the aorta is a cause of systemic hypertension that can be surgically corrected. The adult form is seen predominantly in males and is described as obstruction to blood flow that results from a stricture of the aortic lumen below the region of the left subclavian artery.[12,58] If untreated, this condition may be associated with aortic valvular abnormalities, hypertension, and degenerative renal disease.

In postductal coarctation blood flow to the lower body is supplied by the left ventricle through the stricture. Because of impedance to blood flow to the lower extremities, the body develops collat-

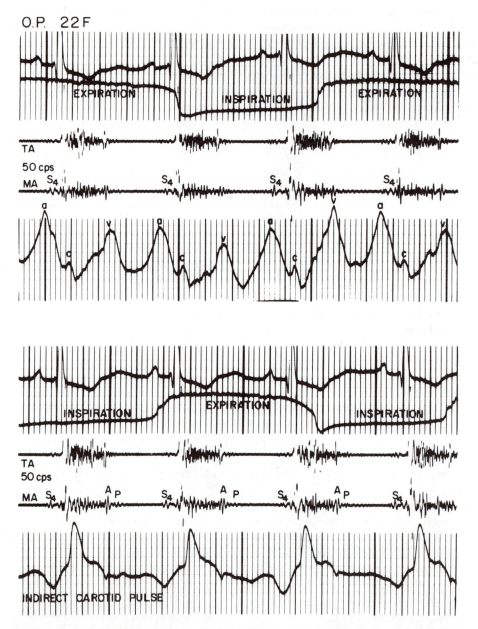

Fig. 3-2. Moderately severe pulmonic valvular stenosis in 22-year-old woman. Long systolic ejection murmur peaks in midsystole. P_2 is delayed and decreased in intensity. A loud, right-sided S_4 gallop that increases in intensity during late inspiration is best recorded at apex and corresponds in time to a prominent jugular venous *a* wave. (From Kaplan, S., and Adolph, R.J.: Pulmonary stenosis in adults. In Roberts, W.C., editor: Congenital heart disease in adults, Cardiovasc. Clin. vol. 10, no. 1, 1979.)

Table 3-2. Pathological mechanisms of secondary systemic hypertension

Causes	Mechanisms	Vascular response
RENAL DYSFUNCTION		
Renovascular disease Renal artery stenosis	Inadequate renal blood flow in post-stenotic vessel triggering renin-angiotensin-aldosterone (RAA) system	↑ blood volume ↑ peripheral vascular resistance ↓ vascular compliance ↑ afterload
Kimmelstiel-Wilson syndrome	Thickened glomerular basement membrane, causing vascular occlusion, and triggering the RAA and salt and water retention	↑ blood volume ↑ peripheral vascular resistance ↓ vascular compliance ↑ afterload
Renal parenchymal disease Glomerulonephritis	Cause unknown; thought to be associated with renal autoregulatory mechanisms	↑ peripheral vascular resistance ↑ afterload
Pyelonephritis	Interstitial scarring and obstruction of intrarenal vessels, possibly triggering RAA and salt and water retention	↑ blood volume ↑ peripheral vascular resistance ↓ vascular compliance ↑ afterload
ADRENAL DYSFUNCTION		
Pheochromocytoma	Increased circulating catecholamines	↑ alpha stimulation of peripheral vessels ↑ peripheral vascular resistance
Cushing's syndrome	Increased secretion of mineralocorticoids; increased secretion of cortisol; salt and water retention	↑ blood volume ↑ vascular compliance ↑ peripheral vascular resistance
Primary and secondary aldosteronism	Inappropriate reabsorption of salt and water from distal tubule and collecting duct in the nephron	↑ blood volume ↓ vascular compliance ↑ blood pressure
NEUROLOGICAL DYSFUNCTION		
Autonomic hyperreflexia	Increased and inappropriate reflex sympathetic stimulation causing severe arteriolar constriction	↑ peripheral vascular resistance ↑ blood pressure

Brain tumors
  Cerebellar
  Posterior hypothalamus
  Brain stem
	Increased catecholamine release	↑ peripheral vascular resistance
		↑ blood pressure

Increased intracranial pressure Cushing response	Stimulation of vasomotor center with intense arteriolar vasoconstriction	↑ peripheral vascular resistance ↑ blood pressure
EXOGENOUS AGENTS		
Oral contraceptives*	Estrogenic portion of agents may alter renal sodium retention mechanism by unknown process	↑ peripheral vascular resistance ↑ blood pressure ↑ blood volume

Sympathomimetic agents
  Dopamine
  Epinephrine
  Caffeine
  Nicotine
  Amphetamines
	Direct stimulation of sympathetic vasoconstriction of peripheral vessels	↑ blood pressure
		↑ peripheral vascular resistance

Steroid therapy	Sodium and water retention	↑ blood volume ↓ vascular compliance ↑ blood pressure

*Oral contraceptives are the most common cause of secondary hypertension.

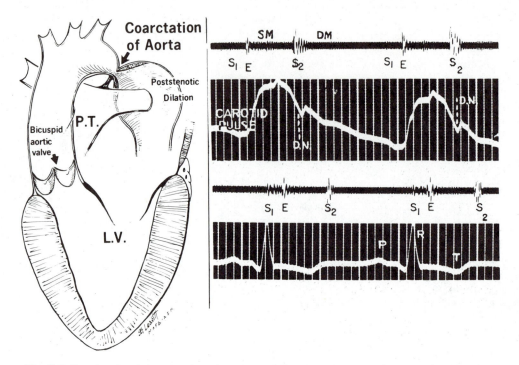

Fig. 3-3. Drawing showing coarctation of aorta and of associated bicuspid aortic valve. Tracings are from 20-year-old man with coarctation of aorta and bicuspid aortic valve. Over aortic area *(upper tracing)*, systolic ejection sound *(E)*, systolic murmur *(SM)*, and early diastolic murmur *(DM)* were present. At apex *(lower tracing)*, prominent ejection sound *(E)* and faint systolic murmur *(SM)* were heard. (From Harvey, W.P.: Auscultatory features of congenital heart disease. In Roberts, W.C., editor: Congenital heart disease in adults, Cardiovasc. Clin. vol. 10, no. 1, 1979.)

CAUSES OF PULMONARY HYPERTENSION

CARDIAC DISORDERS
  Left atrial myxoma
  Mitral stenosis
  Left ventricular failure
  Congenital heart disease
  Left-to-right shunts
  Cor triatriatum

PULMONARY DISORDERS
  Chronic obstructive lung disease
  Interstitial parenchymal lung disease
  Obstruction of pulmonary veins
  Respiratory center depression
  Abnormalities of thoracic cavity

eral circulation by way of the left subclavian artery, internal mammary artery, scapular artery, and intercostal arteries.

The increased resistance to ejection that is produced by the aortic stricture also causes left ventricular hypertrophy and poststenotic dilation of the distal aorta. This is manifested by hypertension in the upper extremities and decreased or imperceptible pressures in the lower extremities.

As the patient ages, hypertension may cause atherosclerosis proximal to the coarctation in both the aorta and the arterial branches. Aortic dilation occurs distal to the narrowing, and the poststenotic vascular intima becomes fibrotic and thickened while the media becomes thinned and distorted. The aorta appears enlarged, tortuous, and often calcified.

Narrowing of the aorta reduces blood flow to organs distal to the stenosis. This affects renal blood flow, which in turn triggers renin-angiotension secretion, causing an increase in systemic vascular resistance. Elevated systolic and diastolic pressures are required to overcome this hemodynamic inequality.

Ultimately aortic coarctation leads to death because of hypertension. Congestive heart failure that is secondary to hypertension increases morbidity and fatalities in patients over the age of 30 with postductal coarctation.[12,60] Hypertensive systolic overload on the left ventricle produces hypertrophy and subsequent dilation with resultant diminished peripheral perfusion and pulmonary congestion. This condition is compounded by hypertensive degenerative changes in the kidney and in the other organ systems.

Clinical indicators. Individuals with this malformation are asymptomatic until hypertension and/or heart failure becomes significant. The characteristic finding is higher systolic pressure in the upper extremities that becomes exaggerated with age. These individuals may also demonstrate marked development of the upper torso in contrast to the hips and legs. They complain of headaches, dizziness, and vague chest discomfort characteristic of hypertension.

Continuous murmurs from collateral vessels may be heard over the back, and pulsations may be felt on the underside of the ribs. Radiographs of the patient's chest may reveal rib notching resulting from enlarged intercostal vessels. When the stricture occurs above the left subclavian artery, the left upper extremity may be cooler and smaller and have a lower blood pressure than the right. Difficulty in swallowing may occur when an anomalous right subclavian artery rises distal to the stricture and passes behind the esophagus to reach the right arm.

Pulmonary hypertension. Systolic pulmonary arterial pressure that exceeds 30 mm Hg (normal pressure equals 18 to 25 mm Hg) constitutes pulmonary hypertension.[3] This condition may be categorized as primary or secondary hypertension. Primary pulmonary hypertension is an uncommon, progressively debilitating disease of unknown cause that acts directly on pulmonary vessels and affects more women than men.[22,60] Secondary pulmonary hypertension is a sequela to cardiac or pulmonary disease. When associated with manifestations of right heart failure it is described as cor pulmonale (see the boxed material on p. 92).

Primary pulmonary hypertension. There have been many theories advanced to explain the origin of primary pulmonary hypertension. They include recurrent episodes of asymptomatic pulmonary embolism, drug hypersensitivity, marked vasospasm, genetic predisposition, and environmental factors such as high-altitude hypoxia.[4] The pathological findings of pulmonary hypertension include fibrous intimal thickening of the smaller pulmonary arteries and arterioles with hypertrophy of the medial muscular layer of the pulmonary artery, resulting in tense noncompliant large vessels and a tense noncompliant vascular bed.[2,9,58] The luminal narrowing of the pulmonary arteries obstructs outflow of blood from the right ventricle, ultimately causing hypertrophy and dilation (cor pulmonale).

Clinical indicators. Primary pulmonary hypertension is fatal in most cases, with death occurring approximately 3 years after the onset of symptoms.[3] Most patients are asymptomatic and are not seen until late in the course of the disease. Individuals complain of exertional dyspnea, syncope, and precordial chest pain, which result from low cardiac output and hypoxemia.

Objective findings reflect pulmonary hypertension and right ventricular hypertrophy. Palpation reveals a left parasternal–right ventricular heave, a prominent jugular venous pulse, and a low-volume carotid pulse. A systolic pulsation in the second left intercostal space is produced by a dilated pulmonary artery. Auscultation over this area reveals an ejection click and a flow murmur, a closely split second heart sound with a prominent pulmonic component, and a right ventricular fourth heart sound.[3] These findings are accompanied by the clinical indicators of marked right ventricular failure—jugular venous distention, hepatomegaly, ascites, and peripheral edema.

Cor pulmonale. Cor pulmonale is pulmonary hypertension with right ventricular failure secondary to intrinsic lung disease, such as emphysema, pulmonary fibrosis, or bronchiectasis, pulmonary vascular disease, such as pulmonary emboli, vasculitis, or tumors, or extrapulmonary causes, such as inadequate chest wall movement or neuromuscular dysfunction.

Clinical indicators—acute cor pulmonale. The term "acute cor pulmonale" describes acute pulmonary obstruction and hypertension that are usually the result of massive embolism. The signs of acute cor pulmonale are characteristic of low-output, left heart failure and severe right ventricular failure. The most common indicators include tachypnea, dyspnea, severe apprehension, and pleuritic chest pain or substernal pressure.

Physical assessment reveals low blood pressure with or without signs of shock. If pulmonary blood flow is markedly reduced, central and peripheral cyanosis may be present. A dilated pulmonary artery may produce a forceful pulsation that may be visualized and palpated at the second left intercostal space. Auscultation may reveal pulmonary rales; a pleural friction rub may be detected if pulmonary infarction occurred; and in massive embolism, accentuated pulmonary component of the

second heart sound and a gallop rhythm may be present.[3] Further indicators of acute right ventricular failure include prominent jugular venous distention and pulsations and a right ventricular heave.

Clinical indicators—chronic cor pulmonale. The cause of pulmonary hypertension in chronic cor pulmonale is related to elevated pulmonary vascular resistance that results from alteration in ventilatory mechanics, gas exchange, and other intrapulmonary events. A discussion of pathophysiology is beyond the scope of this text, however, it is important for the clinician to recognize the clinical indicators of this disease when screening patients with heart failure.

Chronic obstructive pulmonary disease (COPD) is associated with chronic bronchitis with or without pulmonary emphysema. When COPD is associated with right ventricular failure the condition is described as chronic cor pulmonale.[21,39] Individuals with symptoms of chronic bronchitis have a chronic cough with sputum production, recurring chest infections, secondary erythrocytosis, and frequent episodes of right ventricular failure.[39] They have hypoxemia and hypercapnia when at rest and elevated residual volumes, functional residual capacities, and airway resistance. They demonstrate relatively normal total lung capacity and pulmonary compliance. Radiographs of the chest reveal overinflation, increased lung markings, and a large heart.

The emphysematous patient has the dominant symptom of dyspnea and a less frequent cough and sputum production. Erythrocytosis rarely occurs and right ventricular failure tends to develop as a terminal event.[39] Arterial oxygen tensions are normal or slightly depressed, and hypocapnia is common. Lung volumes are large, and pulmonary compliance is high. Chest radiographs show hyperinflation, flattened diaphragms, and a small heart.

The clinical indicators of chronic obstructive pulmonary disease and right ventricular failure are increasing dyspnea and episodes of paroxysmal cough occasionally with syncope. These individuals demonstrate elevated systemic venous pressure with jugular venous distention and pulsation; hepatomegaly; fluid retention with pitting edema and ascites; and signs of right ventricular hypertrophy with a palpable parasternal heave and right ventricular gallop. The lungs reveal diffuse inspiratory and expiratory rhonchi and wheezes.

Conditions producing diastolic overload (elevated preload)

Aortic regurgitation. Aortic regurgitation results from incompetence of the aortic valve during ventricular diastole. This malfunction allows blood from the aorta to flow back across the partially opened valve into the left ventricle, causing volume overload of this chamber. The regurgitant volume may be as much as 60% or more of the forward stroke volume, with most occurring late in diastole.[9]

In acute aortic regurgitation the sudden increase in diastolic volume that results from backflow across an incompetent valve causes a marked increase in left ventricular preload. In the normal-sized heart, the left ventricle is unable to accommodate this volume and end-diastolic pressure rises. As left ventricular end-diastolic pressure rises above left atrial pressure, the mitral valve closes early in diastole. This protects the pulmonary circulation from backward transmission of elevated pressure. Early closure of the mitral valve coupled with tachycardia shortens diastole and is reflected by a much smaller aortic pulse pressure.[9] Furthermore, these individuals exhibit marked tachycardia and a much smaller left ventricle than those with chronic aortic regurgitation.

In chronic aortic regurgitation, the backward flow of blood during diastole increases left ventricular end-diastolic volume and increases the force and fraction of left ventricular ejection by the Starling mechanism. The ventricle dilates in response to increased preload and becomes more compliant. Therefore ventricular end-diastolic pressure does not become significantly elevated until heart failure develops and is accompanied by peripheral vasodilation, which occurs for reasons

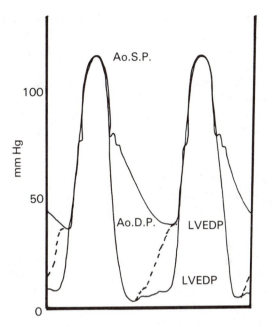

Fig. 3-4. Representation of normal left ventricular end-diastolic pressure *(LVEDP)* and elevated LVEDP *(broken line)* found with acute aortic regurgitation. Aortic pressure tracing demonstrates widened pulse pressure between aortic systolic pressure *(AoSP)* and aortic diastolic pressure *(AoDP)* and its near equalization with elevated left ventricular end-diastole.

unknown. These physiological alterations account for many of the clinical indicators of chronic aortic regurgitation such as low diastolic volume, wide pulse pressure, and prominent peripheral pulses (Fig. 3-4).

The clinical findings of this abnormality depend on the degree of valvular regurgitation and on whether the condition is acute or chronic. A common cause of primary disease of the aortic valve is rheumatic fever.[9] The valve cusps become infiltrated with fibrous tissue. This causes scarring, contracture, and shortening of the valve cusps resulting in aortic regurgitation. Other causes of acquired aortic regurgitation include hypertension, syphilis, and collagen diseases such as seronegative spondyloarthritis and Marfan's syndrome. Patients with chronic aortic regurgitation have the largest end-diastolic volumes of any form of heart disease.[9] This is associated with elevated cardiac output and decreased peripheral vascular resistance.

Clinical indicators—chronic aortic regurgitation. Patients with less significant aortic regurgitation will display more subtle clinical features. Generally there is a latent period of 15 to 20 years between the occurrence of anatomical aortic regurgitation and the development of significant clinical indicators.[21] These individuals may have an excellent capacity for physical exertion because the regurgitant volume decreases when peripheral vascular resistance is reduced. On the other hand, they may develop left ventricular failure or pulmonary edema at rest as the volume of blood returning to the heart increases when recumbent. Early symptoms include an unpleasant awareness of forceful pulsations of the heart, fatigue, dyspnea, and orthopnea. Excessive sweating may also occur as a result of sympathetic stimulation resulting from left ventricular failure. As valvular regurgitation becomes worse, many of the signs associated with severe aortic regurgitation may become apparent. Patients with severe chronic aortic regurgitation display a rhythmic nodding of the head with each heart beat (Musset's sign) and have warm, flushed appearances. Palpation of peripheral pulses reveals a waterhammer-type pulse with abrupt distention and quick collapse. This is visible in the carotid arteries. A bisiferious pulse may also be present and is detected over the femoral and brachial arteries.

The pulse pressure is wide, usually greater than 80 mm Hg (normal pressure equals 30 to 50 mm Hg).[21] The Korotkoff sounds may be heard to zero. The apical impulse is hyperdynamic, diffuse, and displaced laterally and inferiorly.

Auscultation reveals a normal first heart sound and a normal or decreased aortic component of the second heart sound. The murmur is usually a grade three, long, high-pitched, presystolic and/or middiastolic sound. Radiographs of the chest reveal marked increase in heart size, a prominent aortic root, and normal pulmonary venous vascularity.

Clinical indicators—acute aortic regurgitation. Acute severe aortic regurgitation may be caused by infective endocarditis with or without preexisting congenital disease, rheumatic disease of the valve, or trauma to the cusps.[2] In the acute form, the regurgitant volume may be up to 50% or more of volume ejected during systole.[19] The sudden addition of this regurgitant flow to the volume of left atrial contribution severely overloads the normal left ventricle. This causes a rapid rise in diastolic filling pressure to levels as high as 40 to 50 mm Hg.[19]

The clinical manifestations are massive acute pulmonary edema and low cardiac output. These individuals may have a short medium-pitched middiastolic murmur, but it is difficult to detect because of respiratory noise. Early death resulting from severe left ventricular failure is frequent despite intensive medical therapy, with prompt surgical intervention being the treatment of choice.

Mitral regurgitation (Fig. 3-5). Mitral regurgitation refers to lack of coaptation of the valve leaflets, which results in back flow of left ventricular blood volume into the left atrium during diastole. Mitral regurgitation can be either acute or chronic. The most common causes of acute mitral regurgitation are rupture of the papillary muscles or chordae tendineae as the result of myocardial infarction and penetrating or nonpenetrating trauma.[30,47] Rheumatic heart disease or infective endocarditis leads to chronic mitral regurgitation, which is characterized by calcification with shortening and retraction of the mitral valvular leaflets.

During ventricular systole the left ventricle ejects blood back to the left atrium. This causes an increase in left atrial volume and a decrease in the forward stroke volume (Fig. 3-5, *B*). Normal left atrial contribution plus the regurgitant blood volume is redirected to the left ventricle during ventricular filling, increasing the diastolic load. Both the left atrium and the left ventricle are strained by this regurgitation. In chronic mitral regurgitation both chambers dilate and hypertrophy. In time the left ventricle fails, high pressures develop in the left atrium, and pulmonary

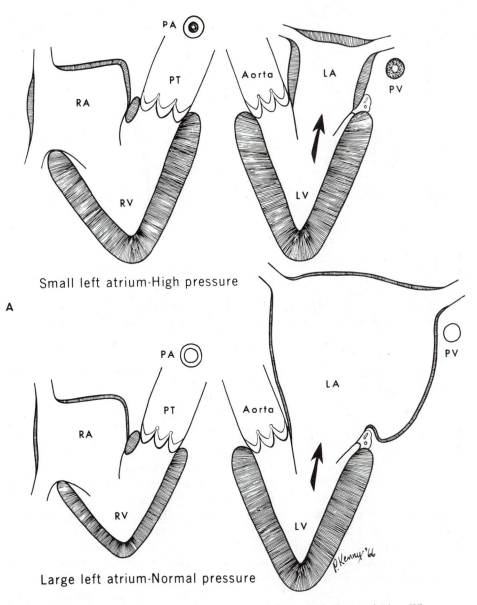

Fig. 3-5. A, Diagram depicting two extremes of spectrum in pure mitral regurgitation. When severe mitral regurgitation appears suddenly in individuals with previously normal or near-normal hearts, left atrium *(LA)* is relatively small and high pressure within it is reflected back into pulmonary vessels and right ventricle *(RV)*. The anatomical indication of this latter physiological event is severe hypertrophy of left atrial and right ventricular walls and marked intimal proliferation and medial hypertrophy of pulmonary arteries *(PA),* arterioles, and veins *(PV)*. At the other extreme, the left atrial cavity is large, and its wall is thin. It is thus able to "absorb" left ventricular *(LV)* pressure without reflecting it back into pulmonary vessels or right ventricle. As a consequence, pulmonary vessels remain normal, and right ventricular wall does not thicken. *PT,* pulmonary trunk; *RA,* right atrium. (**A** from Roberts, W.C., and others: Nonrheumatic valvular cardiac disease: a clinicopathologic survey of 27 different conditions causing valvular dysfunction. In Likoff, W., editor: Valvular heart disease, Cardiovasc. Clin. **5**(2):403, 1973.)

Continued.

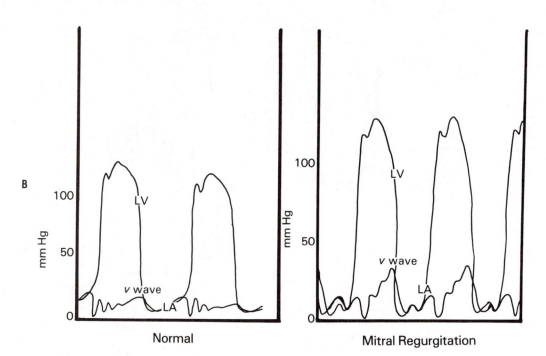

Fig. 3-5, cont'd. B, Mitral regurgitation augments volume of left atrium during left ventricular *(LV)* systolic as evidenced by a tall *v* wave in left atrial *(LA)* pressure.

edema results. By comparison, in acute mitral regurgitation, the left atrium is of normal size and compliance. The regurgitant volume from the left ventricle, propelled backward to the left atrium during systole, causes a rapid increase in left atrial pressures. This leads to acute elevation of pulmonary arterial pressure with subsequent pulmonary congestion. The excessive rise of pulmonary vascular pressure causes the right ventricle to fail, and left ventricular stroke volume is markedly reduced.[9,47]

Clinical indicators. Patients with mild mitral regurgitation may be free of symptoms until an event increases cardiac load and precipitates heart failure. Patients with severe chronic mitral regurgitation and an enlarged left atrium with minimal rise in atrial and pulmonary pressure have symptoms of fatigue and exhaustion related to depressed cardiac output. Those with left atrial and pulmonary hypertension display indicators of right ventricular

failure, including congestive hepatomegaly and ankle edema.[9]

Physical findings are related to left atrial and left and right ventricular enlargement. Hypertrophy of the left ventricle causes the apical impulse to become forceful and displaced to the left and downward. The murmur of mitral regurgitation is pansystolic, and it is best heard at the apex, radiating to the left axilla. It does not vary significantly with respiration and increases in intensity when the individual is squatting and when the blood pressure rises with the use of isometric hand grips; it decreases when the individual is standing. It may be accompanied by a diastolic ventricular gallop that indicates that significant mitral stenosis is *not* present.[21]

When the left atrium dilates, atrial fibrillation frequently develops and may be a source of thrombi and systemic embolization. When chronic mitral regurgitation has caused right ventricular dilation, tricuspid insufficiency may be a sequela and further add to systemic venous hypertension.

Pulmonic regurgitation. Pulmonic regurgitation is incompetency of the primary valvular apparatus. This occurs as the result of the noncoaptation of the pulmonary valvular cusps. Causes of this valvular defect include congenital malformation of the valve or the absence of one or more of the pulmonary valve leaflets. The acquired cause is most commonly the result of valvular ring dilation. This dilation is secondary to pulmonary hypertension or pulmonary artery dilation of any cause. Acquired isolated pulmonary valvular regurgitation may be associated with bacterial endocarditis.

With pulmonary insufficiency, the regurgitant flow from the pulmonary artery plus the normal venous return increases right ventricular diastolic volume. Compensatory mechanisms of dilation and hypertrophy result with decreased ventricular compliance. In time the right ventricular diastolic pressures equal the pulmonary arterial diastolic pressures and right ventricular failure ensues. This is followed by systemic venous congestion and decreased forward flow.

Studies have found that as long as the pulmonary pressures are low in the isolated acquired pulmonary valve regurgitation, the right ventricle is able to tolerate significant volume overload for many years.[19] However, in the face of pulmonary hypertension, the deleterious effects of diastolic overloading and systolic overloading cause right ventricular failure to occur sooner.[21]

Clinical indicators. Isolated pulmonic regurgitation produces an early diastolic decrescendo murmur that is maximal at the same area of aortic regurgitation, to the left of the sternum at the second or third intercostal space and downward along the left sternal border. A chest roentgenogram may show dilation of the pulmonary trunk.

Tricuspid regurgitation. Tricuspid valvular regurgitation is the result of incompetence of the tricuspid valvular leaflets. This is characterized by incomplete valve closure and leads to backward flow of blood from the right ventricle to the right atrium during systole. There are two forms of tri-

cuspid regurgitation, functional and organic. The development of the functional tricuspid regurgitation is a result of right ventricular enlargement, which causes valvular ring dilation and distortion of the chordae tendineae and papillary muscles. The organic form is found in isolated tricuspid regurgitation and is the result of organic disease directly involving the tricuspid valve apparatus, such as rupture or infarction of the papillary muscles or chordae tendineae, infective endocarditis of the leaflets, or fibrosis of the cusps because of carcinoma.[9,60]

With tricuspid regurgitation, the right ventricle is unable to pump all of its volume to the pulmonary circulation. Part of the blood volume is ejected retrograde into the right atrium. During diastole the regurgitant blood plus the usual atrial volume flows into the right ventricle, increasing the diastolic load. The right ventricle adapts by dilation and hypertrophy. Cardiac failure occurs when the hypertrophied ventricle can no longer tolerate the excessive pressures.

Clinical indicators. Tricuspid regurgitation is generally well tolerated; however, when pulmonary hypertension is present, cardiac output drops and the work of the right ventricle increases, causing hypertrophy, dilation, and right ventricular failure. The veins in the neck may show systolic pulsation, which can extend to the earlobes and the eyeballs in severe cases. Venous pulsation may extend to the liver, which will be large and tender. In chronic tricuspid regurgitation the liver is firm and nontender and is associated with ascites, jaundice, and peripheral edema.

The right ventricular impulse is hyperdynamic and has a thrusting quality. On auscultation a pansystolic murmur may be heard at the left sternal border in the fourth or fifth intercostal space; it increases on inspiration. A low-pitched early diastolic murmur may also be present as the result of increased early diastolic filling of the right ventricle.

Severe right-sided heart failure without significant pulmonary congestion occurs not only in tricuspid regurgitation but also in pericardial effusions with tamponade, in constrictive pericarditis, and associated with pulmonary hypertension, secondary to chronic obstructive lung disease.

Left-to-right shunts

A cardiovascular shunt is blood flow through an abnormal communication between the venous and arterial circulation and may be either congenital or acquired.

In left-to-right shunts the arterial blood flow is diverted back to the venous circulation by way of channels between the ventricles, atria, and great vessels and between the coronary arteries and right heart chambers. Left-to-right shunts to the right atrium or right ventricle cause an increase in the right ventricular diastolic volume load. The right ventricle must increase the force of contraction in order to eject an excessively large blood volume into the pulmonary circulation. This may ultimately cause right ventricular failure.

If the left-to-right shunt is found between the aorta and the pulmonary artery, the left ventricle receives a large volume of pulmonary blood flow, and increases its force of contraction, resulting in left sided heart enlargement and eventual myocardial failure.

Ventricular septal defect (Fig. 3-6). In the adult ventricular septal defects are primarily acquired as a result of acute myocardial infarction, bacterial endocarditis initiated by a small congenital ventricular septal lesion, and/or penetrating or nonpenetrating chest trauma.[15,24,44] Few adults are seen with congenital defects because fatalities are highest in early childhood when the lesion is large.

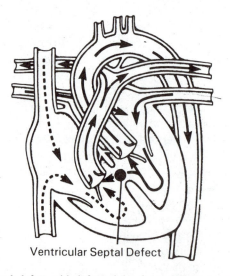

Ventricular Septal Defect

Fig. 3-6. Ventricular septal defect with left-to-right shunt. When a ventricular septal defect is about caliber of aortic orifice, there is free communication between the two ventricles, which allows equalization of pressures between them. Ventricular systolic pressure equals systolic pressure in great arteries. Direction and magnitude of shunt through defect depends on level of pulmonary vascular resistance relative to systemic resistance. When pulmonary resistance is lower than systemic, shunt is in a left-to-right direction and may achieve great magnitude. Right atrium does not participate in shunt. As in any ventricular septal defect with left-to-right shunt, both ventricles and left atrium participate in carrying shunted blood. Right atrium does not participate when defect is small, and left-to-right shunt is of small volume. Pulmonary pressure is normal. Pulmonary arterial vessels may be within a normal range roentgenographically when shunt is small. (From Whaley, L., and Wong, D.: Essentials of pediatric nursing, St. Louis, 1982, The C.V. Mosby Co.)

Those who do survive do so because the communication has spontaneously closed or is clinically unrecognizable.[41a]

The sudden onset of an acquired ventricular septal defect results in an acute left-to-right shunt because the pressure in the left ventricle is higher than in the right. As a result the right ventricle ejects an increased volume of blood into the lungs. This increased volume is returned to the left atrium and ventricle with subsequent volume overload of both ventricles. Increased blood flow through the pulmonary circulation may produce pulmonary hypertension when the pulmonary artery is normal.

The immediate shunting of large volumes of blood from the left to the right ventricle leads to a profound deficit in forward flow, causing hypotension and vascular collapse. The right ventricle is unable to accommodate the sudden volume and filling pressures rise sharply, causing rapid development of right ventricular overload and systemic venous congestion.

Clinical indicators. Acute onset of ventricular septal defect associated with heart failure, although infrequent, may be observed in the adult patient following acute myocardial infarction. The individual may be admitted to the coronary care unit with the classic features of crushing substernal chest pain, diaphoresis, nausea, ECG changes, and elevated cardiac enzymes. The sudden development of neck vein distention, a pansystolic murmur associated with marked elevation in right atrial and pulmonary artery pressure, and a drop in arterial pressure and cardiac output are suspect. With nonoperative management 50% of patients may die within one week and 85% in two months.[13a] The use of vasodilator therapy and intra-aortic counterpulsation may provide hemodynamic stabilization until surgical intervention is feasible.

Atrial septal defect (Fig. 3-7). Atrial septal defect is characterized by an opening in the atrial septum providing a port for blood flow from the left to the right atrium. This lesion is found more frequently in females than in males and may be asymptomatic until the third or fourth decade of life.[19,60] There are several sites where the lesion

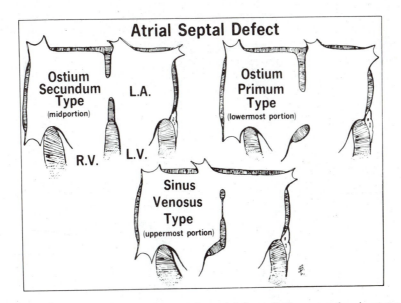

Fig. 3-7. Artist's drawing of three types of atrial septal defects. Ostium secundum is most common type. (From Harvey, W.P.: Auscultatory features of congenital heart disease. In Roberts, W.C., editor: Congenital heart disease in adults, Cardiovasc. Clin. vol. 10, no. 1, 1979.)

may occur. Ostium secundum is located in the center of the septum in the region of the fossa ovalis. It is the most common interatrial opening. Ostium primum is a lesion that is found just above the mitral and tricuspid valve in the lowest portion of the septum; it may be associated with mitral valve prolapse and atrial arrhythmias. Sinus venosus is located at the superior vena cava.[21]

In most atrial septal defects a left-to-right shunt exists as a result of reduced right ventricular pressure that allows preferential flow to the right ventricle when the atrioventricular valves are open and a single-chamber cardiac configuration is present. Over time the right ventricle may hypertrophy in response to pressure overload of pulmonary hypertension and/or incomplete right ventricular emptying. Although life expectancy is shortened in these patients, adult survival is the rule, with many living to advanced ages.[41a]

Clinical indicators. Large atrial septal defects appear early in life and are surgically corrected in childhood. Those individuals with small, simple secundum lesions, which are not detected in childhood, generally demonstrate unremarkable histories and physical examinations as young adults. When complications develop after the third or fourth decade they usually include dyspnea, fatigue, and manifestations of atrial arrhythmias such as fibrillation, flutter, or supraventricular tachycardias.[2a] The diastolic rumbling murmur

heard in children with atrial septal defects is usually not heard in adults. Patients who have developed severe pulmonary hypertension associated with this defect may demonstrate a fourth heart sound originating in the right ventricle and may have murmurs of pulmonary and tricuspid regurgitation. These individuals generally deteriorate, displaying prominent manifestations of right ventricular failure and systemic venous congestion.

Patent ductus arteriosus (Fig. 3-8, *A*). In patent ductus arteriosus, the embryonic ductus arteriosus fails to close shortly after birth and continues as an arterial channel shunting blood between the aorta and the pulmonary artery. The ductus is commonly found near the origin of the left subclavian artery and extends between the aorta and either the bifurcation of the pulmonary artery or the left pulmonary arterial branch (Fig. 3-8, *A*). The incidence of this defect is more prevalent in females than males at a ratio of 3:1.[19,60]

During fetal life the pressure is greater in the pulmonary artery than in the aorta. After birth the aortic pressure exceeds that of the pulmonary artery, causing a left-to-right shunt through the patent ductus. The aortic blood flows into the pulmonary artery, through the pulmonary circulation, and back into the left side of the heart. The amount of blood flow depends on the diameter and length of the ductus and the pressure gradient between the aorta and the pulmonary artery. The excessive

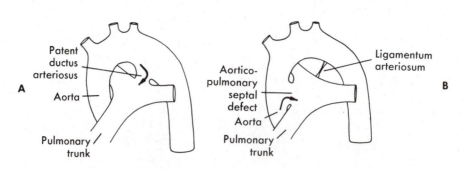

Fig. 3-8. Diagrams of **A,** patent ductus arteriosus, and **B,** aorticopulmonary septal defect. (From Goldberger, E.: Textbook of clinical cardiology, St. Louis, 1982, The C.V. Mosby Co.)

pulmonary venous return to the left side of the heart leads to an increase in the diastolic volume of the left ventricle. This causes dilation and hypertrophy, allowing the left ventricle to eject two or more times the normal cardiac output.[23] Although the heart is able to increase its cardiac output, there is decreased systemic blood supply as a result of the recirculation through the aortopulmonary circuit. In the patient at rest, systemic blood flow is sufficient to meet metabolic demands. However, a moderate increase in activity will precipitate exertional dyspnea and fatigue. As ventricular workload progressively increases, left ventricular dysfunction evolves, and pulmonary congestion develops.

Clinical indicators. A characteristic sign of patent ductus arteriosus is a machinery-like continuous murmur that peaks around the second heart sound and wanes during diastole. This sound denotes the circulation of the aortopulmonary circuit. It is heard best in the first or second intercostal spaces. A thrill may also be felt in this area. Another sign is the wide pulse pressure. This abnormality results from the flow of blood into the pulmonary artery during diastole, causing a drop in the aortic diastolic pressure. The major complications that occur in adults as a result of this malformation are left or right ventricular failure, infective endarteritis, and obliterative pulmonary vascular disease.[9]

Aortopulmonary window (Fig. 3-8, *B*). Aortopulmonary window is an uncommon congenital anomaly that is characterized by a left-to-right shunt that occurs between the aorta and the pulmonary artery. The arterial channel is found just above the aortic and pulmonic valves (Fig. 3-5). Other names for this defect are aortic septal defect, partial truncus arteriosus, or aorticopulmonary septal defect. In this shunt, the pressure gradient causes the blood to flow from the aorta to the pulmonary artery. There is an increase in circulating volume to the lungs and to the left heart. The clinical course reflects that of patent ductus arteriosus, which terminates in left ventricular failure and pulmonary congestion.

Coronary arteriovenous fistulas. Coronary arteriovenous fistulas are usually congenital in origin, but they may be acquired as posttraumatic lesions. In this malformation, either the right or the left coronary artery communicates distally with the right atrium or ventricle, pulmonary artery, coronary sinus, cardiac vein, and, rarely, the left atrium or ventricle. The fistulas bypass the myocardial capillary beds, "stealing" oxygenated blood destined for the heart muscle.

Pathophysiology and flow depend on fistula location, size, and the amount of shunted volume. In the left coronary system optimal coronary blood flow occurs during ventricular diastole, while in the right coronary system lower intramyocardial wall tension and interventricular pressure permit substantial blood flow throughout the cardiac cycle. Therefore flow through the fistula will depend on the lumen size during the receiving chamber's contractile period and the anatomical point of fistula termination. For example, a fistula terminating in an atrial chamber or pulmonary artery will cause a greater left-to-right flow during ventricular systole. The pressure gradient between the aorta and either atria or the pulmonary artery is greater during this time. Clinically a systolic murmur would be heard. Ventricular contraction would cause fistula lumen diminution in the right or left ventricles. Therefore greater shunting into these chambers would occur during diastole, providing a diastolic murmur.

In most patients, the shunt is small with moderate diastolic overloading. Little change is seen in cardiac pressures. Coronary arteriovenous fistulas generally become symptomatic early in life and frequently cause early myocardial infarction; however, an asymptomatic existence may extend into the fifth and sixth decades of life with the prognosis dependent on the magnitude and duration of flow through the fistula.[47]

Inflow obstructions

Mitral stenosis (Fig. 3-9). Mitral stenosis is a pathological lesion with a reduction in the size of the mitral orifice. Normally, in an adult, the mitral

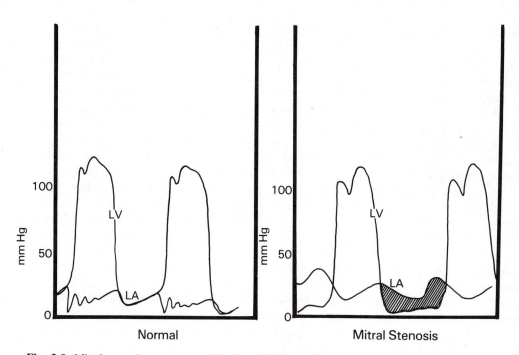

100

mm Hg

50

LV

0

LA

Normal

100

mm Hg

50

LV

0

LA

Mitral Stenosis

Fig. 3-9. Mitral stenosis prevents equilibration of left ventricular and left atrial pressures during diastole, resulting in diastolic pressure gradient *(cross-hatching)*.

orifice measures 4.6 cm.[2,60] Severe mitral stenosis occurs when the opening measures less than 1.0 cm.[2,60] The most common cause of mitral stenosis is rheumatic disease; other causes are congenital defects, left atrial myxoma, and calcified mitral annulus. Mitral stenosis may have the pathological features of valvular leaflet fusion, valvular scarring or thickening and shortening of the chordae tendineae. Mitral stenosis that follows an episode of rheumatic fever takes more than a decade to develop; symptoms are usually manifested after ages 20 to 25.[60] It occurs more commonly in females than in males at a ratio of 2:1.[19,60]

The most significant hemodynamic problem associated with mitral stenosis is the inflow obstruction of left atrial blood volume to the left ventricle and a progressive elevation of atrial diastolic volume. It is possible that incomplete left atrial emptying leads to a reduced, fixed left ventricular filling and resultant decreased, fixed stroke volume

and cardiac output. A compensatory increase in the left atrial pressure occurs to facilitate forward flow through the stenosed value. The left atrium dilates as a response to the increased load. The inflow obstruction, coupled with the continuous propulsion of pulmonary venous blood to the left atrium, causes a rise in the left atrial pressure that results in a diastolic pressure gradient between the left atrium and ventricle (Fig. 3-9). In severe stenosis atrial end-diastolic pressure gradually exceeds that of the ventricle by 5 to 10 mm Hg. This pressure is transmitted backward to the pulmonary capillary bed and causes fluid to accumulate in lung tissue. The pulmonary capillaries undergo intimal thickening, decreasing the capillary lumen size. These intimal changes, characteristic of pulmonary hypertension, create an obstruction to right ventricular ejection. Over a period of years the right ventricular wall thickens, dilates, and fails because of elevated pressure and chronic diastolic overload.

Clinical indicators. The principal symptoms of mitral stenosis is dyspnea resulting from reduced lung compliance. This may be accompanied by cough, hoarseness, and dysphagia as a result of left atrial enlargement. Cough also results from bronchial irritation when the left main stem bronchus is lifted by an enlarged left atrium, dysphagia is caused by posterior displacement of the esophagus, and hoarseness develops from pressure on the left recurrent laryngeal nerve from an enlarged pulmonary artery.[21]

Auscultation of the patient in a left lateral decubitus position reveals a loud first heart sound, an opening snap of the mitral valve, and a soft low-pitched rumbling diastolic murmur accompanied by an apical thrill. There is never a third heart sound in pure mitral stenosis.[9]

Patients with minimal left ventricular involvement and small stroke volumes have normal or reduced arterial pulses; those with marked right ventricular hypertrophy demonstrate the clinical indicators of chronic pulmonary hypertension and severe right heart failure.

Tricuspid stenosis. In tricuspid stenosis, there is an obstruction to right atrial emptying that results from the narrowing of the tricuspid valve orifice. Anatomical features are fusion of the cusps and shortening of chordae tendineae. The most common cause of tricuspid stenosis is rheumatic heart disease. Other causes are right atrial myxoma, carcinoid syndromes, and endocarditis related to drug abuse. Incidence of tricuspid stenosis in women is twice that in men and is usually diagnosed between the ages of 20 and 60 years.

Hemodynamically, there is a diastolic pressure gradient between the right atrium and the right ventricle, although it is small and difficult to elicit since the right side of the heart is a low pressure chamber. This gradient becomes more pronounced during inspiration because of augmentation of venous return. Right-sided heart failure results from the inflow obstruction to right ventricular filling. Right atrial dilation and wall thickening develop to generate the necessary pressure to propel a forward flow into the right ventricle. Over a period of time the right atrium is unable to accommodate venous return. Cardiac output is reduced and fails to increase during exercise. Marked systemic congestion occurs, leading to jugular venous distention, hepatic congestion, ascites, and peripheral edema.

Clinical indicators. Tricuspid stenosis rarely occurs as an isolated lesion; it generally accompanies mitral valve dysfunction. The most common complaints include fatigue, as a result of low cardiac output; discomfort, from hepatomegaly; ascites; and edema. Exertional dyspnea may also be present but is not as dominant as symptoms of systemic venous congestion.

Auscultation of the heart is difficult to interpret because of mitral valve involvement. If the diastolic murmur of tricuspid stenosis is present, it is best heard along the lower left parasternal border in the fourth intercostal space. It is usually shorter, softer, and higher pitched than the murmur of mitral stenosis.

Jugular venous pulses are prominent, and a large *a* wave is present as a result of pressure overload of the atrium. Lung fields are clear in spite of engorged neck veins, and patients are comfortable lying flat.

Atrial myxomas. Atrial myxomas are benign cardiac tumors constituting 30% to 59% of all primary cardiac masses.[11,19] They are usually found in the left or right atrium, arising on narrow pedicles in the fossa ovalis region. Studies have described familial occurrence of these tumors.[48]

Cardiac myxomas frequently act as "ball valve" devices intermittently blocking the AV orifice. They may produce functional mitral or tricuspid stenosis and regurgitation during atrial emptying and postural changes.[54,57] Both right and left atrial tumors may cause right ventricular failure. Left atrial myxomas elevate left atrial and pulmonary capillary pressure. Subsequent pulmonary hypertension overloads the right ventricle, ultimately causing marked right ventricular failure. Fragmentation of right atrial myxomas may cause further pulmonary artery occlusion, thereby increasing pulmonary vascular resistance.

Atrial tumors causing regurgitant defects cause diastolic overload, and the receiving chambers respond to the elevated preload by dilation. If untreated myocardial failure ensues.

Clinical indicators. Cardiovascular indicators associated with atrial myxomas mimic those of tricuspid and mitral valvular disease. Because of "ball valve" movement of the tumors, a differential diagnosis may be established by variation or exaggeration of the findings related to postural changes. Other indicators are nonspecific and include fever, pulmonary and systemic emboli, and evidence of mechanical interference with cardiac function.

ABNORMAL MUSCLE FUNCTION

The heart is primarily a muscle that is organized to function as a pump. It is made up of myocardial fibers that contain actin and myosin filaments. After maximal stretching, these filaments interdigitate and shorten. This overlapping of actin and myosin is the mechanism of myocardial contraction. By the Starling mechanism, when the cardiac muscle is stretched beyond its resting length, the contractile force is increased. However, an excessive ventricular load may alter myocardial function, causing a less forceful contraction. External compression of cardiac muscle, which restricts chamber filling and myocardial fiber stretch, may also interfere with contractile function.

Intrinsic and extrinsic abnormal muscle function are categories of disorders that alter myocardial contractility. Intrinsic causes are conditions that are inherent to the cardiac muscle, while extrinsic factors are external to the myocardium.

Intrinsic causes

Myocardial infarction. Statistical data developed by the American Heart Association indicate that, annually, approximately 1 million people in the United States suffer acute myocardial infarction.[49] Myocardial infarction implies death of cardiac muscle tissue usually associated with refractory substernal chest pain. This is caused by irreversible myocardial damage resulting from obstruction to the oxygen supply by atherosclerosis of one or more coronary arteries. The principal lesion of coronary atherosclerosis is the atherosclerotic plaque or atheroma. The formation of atherosclerosis starts with the accumulation of lipid and fibrous materials within the intima of the blood vessel that later proliferates, leading to wall thickening and lumen narrowing. Thrombin and platelets may aggregate on the plaque, further obstructing blood flow.[60]

Other related causes are coronary thromboembolism, arteritis, venospasm, anomalous vessels, calcium deposits, iatrogenic damage to the myocardium or coronary vessels, and conditions leading to a marked reduction in coronary blood flow, such as hypovolemic shock and pulmonary embolism.[7,27,60]

The presence of ventricular myocardial infarction reduces the size and availability of viable contractile muscle fibers. Heart failure associated with acute myocardial infarction is characterized by ventricular diastolic and pulmonary venous hypertension. This leads to the development of pulmonary congestion. The two mechanisms responsible for pulmonary hypertension are reduced diastolic compliance with augmented resistance to filling and reduced systolic function with subsequent increase in end-diastolic volume and pressure. As the end-diastolic pressure rises, subendocardial blood flow is further compromised, worsening localized ventricular ischemia and extending tissue infarction. This further reduces viable contractile units and increases both systolic and diastolic load.

As ventricular contractile function deteriorates, stroke volume and cardiac output drop. Depressed cardiac output triggers a reflex increase in sympathoadrenergic stimulation and the renin-angiotensin aldosterone mechanism. Accelerated heart rate increases cardiac oxygen requirements, and massive vasoconstriction causes increased resistance to ejection. These events further decrease stroke volume and coronary and systemic tissue perfusion. Metabolic acidosis develops, further depressing myocardial contractility. All these mechanisms intensify the abnormal loading of the damaged myocardium. The inevitable outcome of this cycle is progressive myocardial failure, pulmonary venous congestion, and cardiogenic shock.

When caring for the individual with myocardial infarction, the clinician must observe the patient closely for clinical indicators of heart failure since this condition is a common postinfarction complication. Therapeutic goals are directed toward reduction of myocardial workload. They may be evaluated using the criteria of absent or decreased chest pain, normal heart rate and rhythm, clear lung fields, and normal hemodynamic parameters.

Ventricular aneurysm. Ventricular aneurysm is an outpouching of an area of the myocardium that results in a paradoxical movement during systole. This abnormality results from rheumatic necrosis, penetrating or nonpenetrating trauma, cardiac surgery, or, more commonly, myocardial infarction. Necrotizing injury to the myocardium can lead to the formation of either a true aneurysm or a false aneurysm or "pseudoaneurysm." A true aneurysm is one in which a portion of the ventricular wall is made up of necrosed fibrotic tissue, while a pseudoaneurysm occurs when blood escapes through the ruptured myocardium into the pericardial sac, expanding the sac in that region.[53] The blood stagnates and forms a thrombotic clot and has a greater risk of rupture.[14,50,53] Rupture may occur hours or weeks after myocardial damage. Although rare, peripheral embolism can occur as a result of clots in the aneurysmal dilation, and occasionally, calcifications develop within the dilated wall.

The three complications that develop with true or false aneurysms are heart failure, thromboembolism, and dysrhythmias. Aneurysms resulting from massive myocardial infarctions, especially anteroseptal infarctions, almost always lead to refractory left ventricular failure.[17] The main mechanism of heart failure is related to the loss of viable myocardium and the loss of systolic contractile force. The aneurysmal wall hampers the forward movement of blood, causing a major reduction in the ventricular output. There is retention of blood volume in the aneurysmal pouch, which increases the end-systolic volume in the ventricle. In time the volume load is transmitted to the pulmonary capillary bed, resulting in pulmonary congestion.

Clinical indicators. Clinicians caring for individuals following myocardial infarction or cardiac trauma should watch for indications of ventricular aneurysm. This includes palpation of a second cardiac impulse found medially and superiorly to the point of maximal impulse. The secondary precordial movement is a reflection of the paradoxical systolic expansion of the dilated myocardial wall. This physical assessment plus electrocardiographic evidence of persistent ST segment elevation over the site of the infarcted or traumatized tissue, and the characteristic radiographic finding of bulging of the left ventricular silhouette, should assist the health care team in diagnosing ventricular aneurysm.

Myocarditis. Myocarditis is inflammation of the myocardium. The most common cause in the United States is idiopathic; however, it may also result from an infectious process. Myocarditis may be precipitated by three specific mechanisms: (1) direct myocardial invasion as by coxsackie B virus or, *Trypanosoma cruzi* protozoa (Chagas' disease), (2) production of myocardial toxin as occurs in diphtheria, and (3) stimulation of antibody production as occurs in rheumatic fever.[6] Other causes of myocarditis include toxic chemicals such as lead or arsenic, toxic drugs such as doxorubicin, autoimmune disease such as lupus erythematosus, and metabolic disorders such as uremia.

The inflammation may involve a small portion of the myocardial mass, or it may be distributed over a large area of the heart muscle. The clinical indications of myocarditis depend largely on the number, size, and location of the affected regions. For example, a small focal lesion is usually asymptomatic with no functional impairment, but diffuse myocarditis may lead to profound congestive heart failure. However, focal lesions located in the electrical impulse conduction pathways may lead to dysrhythmias and bundle branch blocks. These disturbances in heart rate, rhythm, and conduction may precipitate congestive heart failure, cardiogenic shock, and sudden death.[6,35,62]

Acute myocarditis occasionally appears as congestive heart failure. Chronic myocarditis usually terminates as congestive cardiomyopathy.[10,19]

Cardiomyopathies. Cardiomyopathies are diseases of the myocardium that are unrelated to other cardiovascular causes. There are three groups in the functional classification: (1) hypertrophic cardiomyopathy, (2) congestive cardiomyopathy, and (3) restrictive cardiomyopathy.

Hypertrophic cardiomyopathy is a disease that is usually genetically transmitted. It is characterized by a marked disorganization of myocardial fibers particularly in the septal tissue. It has been demonstrated that this cellular disorganization may also occur to some extent in normal hearts and in those demonstrating concentric hypertrophy. However, the cellular disorganization is far greater in hypertrophic cardiomyopathy. Examination of these hearts reveals a disproportionate thickening of the ventricular septum with respect to the left ventricular free wall. There is marked increase in myocardial mass with small ventricular cavities and dilated and often hypertrophied atria.[38]

Hypertrophic cardiomyopathy may cause obstruction to the ventricular outflow tract as a result of adynamic septal hypertrophy (ASD). When this occurs it may be accompanied by a form of mitral regurgitation caused by abnormal systolic movement of the anterior mitral valve leaflet (Fig. 3-10). This condition is also called idiopathic hypertrophic subaortic stenosis (IHSS).[38,63]

The degree of obstruction in IHSS is related to clinical manifestations that may range from the asymptomatic individual to the patient in severe congestive heart failure. The most common indicator is dyspnea caused by elevated left ventricular end-diastolic pressure and pulmonary venous hypertension. These pressure abnormalities result from impaired ventricular emptying and increased wall thickness as a result of hypertrophy. Angina pectoris may occur because of an oxygen supply/demand imbalance resulting from increased myo-

cardial muscle mass. Narrowing of the small coronary arteries as a result of elevated intramyocardial wall tension may also contribute to ischemia. Similar to patients with valvular aortic stenosis, these individuals may have a history of exertional syncope because of the inability to increase cardiac output to meet exercise demand.

The auscultatory findings of IHSS with obstruction is a systolic murmur that is harsh and crescendo-decrescendo in configuration. This murmur is caused by both turbulence as blood passes through the narrowed left ventricular outflow tract and mitral regurgitation associated with valvular dysfunction.[63]

Congestive cardiomyopathy is characterized by a massive ventricular dilation. The excessive chamber enlargement leads to a uniform decrease in the ventricular wall motion and gross impairment of the contractile function. There is systolic power failure leading to a diminished ventricular emptying. Ventricular end-diastolic volume overload occurs, and filling pressures increase. Cardiac decompensation results and is accompanied by either pulmonary or systemic congestion. If right ventricular failure is secondary to left ventricular cardiomyopathy, pulmonary arterial hypertension is usually present as well.

Some common examples of congestive cardiomyopathy are the peripartum cardiomyopathy, which is usually seen during the last trimester or the first 6 weeks postpartum, chronic myocarditis, and the alcoholic cardiomyopathy.[3,51,60] Congestive cardiomyopathy is a progressive disease that terminates in fulminating congestive heart failure unless detected early in its course.

Restrictive cardiomyopathy is the third type, characterized mainly by limitation of ventricular filling as a result of diminished ventricular compliance. It is important to note that abnormalities initially occur because of decreased ventricular compliance with contractile dysfunction occurring later. The restrictive process results from infiltrative myocardial disease such as amyloidosis or fibrotic myocardial disease causing tissue thickening by the mechanism of endomyocardial fi-

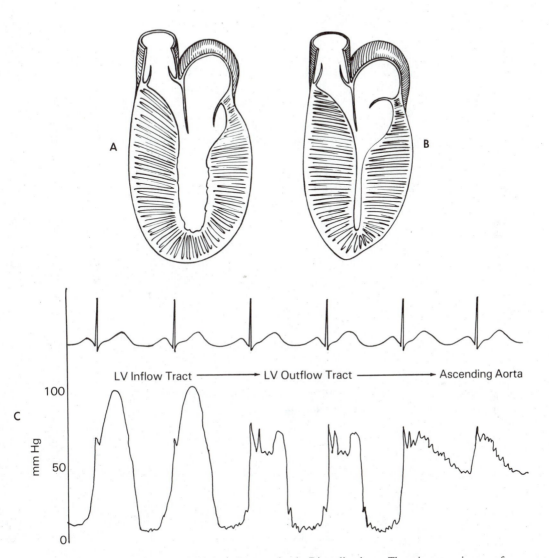

Fig. 3-10. Hypertrophic muscular subaortic stenosis. **A,** Diastolic phase. There is a prominence of ventricular wall, especially in outflow tract. **B,** Systolic phase. Posterior leaflet moves in normal position, but anterior leaflet flutters in relatively open state against hypertrophied ventricular septum, causing subaortic stenosis and mitral insufficiency. **C,** Idiopathic hypertrophic subaortic stenosis (IHSS). Pressure tracings reflecting retrograde withdrawal of catheter from left ventricular inflow tract through left ventricular outflow tract into ascending aorta. (**A** and **B** from Edwards, J.: Classification of congenital heart disease in the adult. In Roberts, W.C., editor: Congenital heart disease in adults, Cardiovasc. Clin. vol. 10, no. 1, 1979.)

brosis or endocardial fibroelastosis. In restrictive cardiomyopathy, the capacity of the ventricles to dilate is greatly limited, and ventricular filling is markedly diminished. Biventricular contractile dysfunction usually develops and is characterized by pulmonary and systemic congestion and diminished peripheral perfusion.

Extrinsic factors

Constrictive pericarditis, pericardial effusion, cardiac tamponade. The heart is covered by a pericardial sac. The fibrous external portion attaches to the diaphragm, sternum, and large blood vessels. The internal portion of the pericardium is composed of two layers: the visceral layer, or the epicardium, is attached to the outer surface of the heart, and the parietal layer lines the external fibrous portion. From 10 to 20 ml of pericardial fluid is found between these two layers.[27] The fluid lubricates these surfaces and prevents friction during cardiac contractions.

Constrictive pericarditis is inflammation of the pericardial sac, which, by a fibrotic process, forms a rigid casing around the heart. When fibrosis restricts cardiac filling, it is called constrictive pericarditis. In this condition cardiac contractility generally is normal, with abnormal filling being the primary defect.

Pericardial effusion is the accumulation of fluid in the pericardial sac. Cardiac tamponade occurs when moderate to large amounts of pericardial fluid compress the heart and restrict chamber filling.

Cardiac tamponade begins when intrapericardial pressure rises to a level equal to right atrial pressure. Since all four cardiac chambers are enclosed in the pericardium, compression will uniformly elevate diastolic pressure and hamper forward flow of blood. Hemodynamically, this is reflected by an equalizing of pressures within the heart chambers.

Clinical indicators—constrictive pericarditis tamponade. The sudden severe chest pain associated with pericarditis simulates that of myocardial infarction. However, pericardial chest pain is aggravated by deep breathing, is associated with

fever, and may be accompanied by a pericardial friction rub. Electrocardiographic findings include ST segment elevation in limb and precordial leads without Q waves. When a patient demonstrates a history of recurrent pericarditis and has clinical manifestations of cardiac compression, constrictive pericarditis may be the underlying cause. If this is the case, it becomes necessary to perform a more extensive differential diagnosis to establish the cause of constrictive pericardial disease.

Indicators of cardiac tamponade may or may not be preceded by pericarditis. Cardiac tamponade is also a complication of surgery and of cardiac trauma. Bedside assessment reveals a deteriorating patient with neck vein distention, distant heart tones, and the presence of pulsus paradoxus, demonstrated by a fall in systolic blood pressure of 10 mm Hg or more during inspiration. If hemodynamic parameters are available, one should observe for equalization of diastolic pressures. Electrical alternans or alternating voltage of the ECG pattern may further reflect accumualtion of fluid in the pericardial sac.

Cardiac trauma. Injury sustained from trauma can cause alterations in the functional or structural integrity of any part of the heart. Cardiac trauma can involve (1) the pericardium, resulting in cardiac tamponade, hemopericardium, and cardiac herniation, (2) the myocardium, causing muscle contusion and rupture, septal perforation, and rupture of either papillary muscle, chordae tendineae, or valves, (3) the coronary vessels, leading to thrombosis, fistula formation, and lacerations, (4) the great vessels, causing acute exsanguination and transection, and (5) the conducting system, leading to dysrhythmias.[8,58,60]

Cardiac insult may result from penetrating injuries caused by knives, bullets, or bone fragments from rib fractures. It may be iatrogenic as a result of perforation from monitoring or diagnostic invasive devices.

Nonpenetrating injuries are blunt cardiac trauma caused by direct or indirect noninvasive external forces, such as blows to the chest, falls, and cardiopulmonary resuscitative procedures. Direct external force is commonly seen in vehicular accidents when the steering wheel directly compresses the heart between the sternum and the spine. Indirect force is associated with any compression of extracardiac structures. An example is the sudden compression of the abdomen that causes an acute upward displacement of abdominal contents. This increases intrathoracic pressure and leads to cardiac injury.

Although unusual, significant cardiomyopathy related to cardiac trauma may develop and terminate in congestive heart failure. The loss of contractile power occurs as a result of the destruction of the integrity of the heart and its accessory parts. This impairment results from compression of the cardiac chambers, loss of myocardial oxygenation, and anatomical damage.

Evidence of cardiac involvement should be diligently sought in any injury of the chest and abdomen or following invasive cardiac procedures. Consequences of cardiac trauma can be catastrophic if not detected early. Characteristic clinical findings include signs of cardiac tamponade, valvular dysfunction, myocardial ischemia, and severe acute right and left ventricular failure.

PRECIPITATING FACTORS

Precipitating factors are conditions that may trigger the occurrence of heart failure in people with preexisting cardiac disease. In these individuals, cardiac function is intrinsically impaired, and cardiac reserve is dependent on functional compensatory mechanisms. When cardiac work load is increased, these mechanisms may no longer be effective; subsequently heart failure develops.

Careful clinical assessment is vital to identifying these precipitating factors. Recognition of them and correlation to underlying heart problems will aid in planning and implementing decisive nursing interventions that may prevent life-threatening cardiac decompensation.[36]

Dysrhythmias

Disorders of the cardiac rate, rhythm, and conduction are among the most important precipitating factors that may initiate congestive heart failure. These dysrhythmias lead to a decrease in cardiac output and an increase in myocardial oxygen consumption.

Tachydysrhythmias. The decrease in diastolic filling time that results from tachydysrhythmias, especially in the presence of mitral stenosis, ventricular hypertrophy, and coronary artery disease, will alter coronary artery perfusion, precipitate myocardial ischemia, decrease cardiac output, and raise atrial pressures. Impairment of cardiac performance ensues as myocardial ischemia is induced because of diminution of coronary perfusion. The clinical syndrome of congestive heart failure results with both pulmonary and systemic congestion.

Bradydysrhythmias. A major determinant of cardiac output is stroke volume or the amount of blood pumped with each heartbeat times the heart rate. Although diastolic filling time is increased with slower rates, individuals with underlying cardiac diseases and marked bradydysrhythmias exhibit a depressed cardiac output. The cardiac output in these individuals may have been previously maintained at maximal levels with normal heart rates because of preexisting dilation and hypertrophy.

Bradydysrhythmias with dissociation between sequential atrial and ventricular contraction, as exemplified by complete or third-degree AV block, result in the loss of the atrial contribution to ventricular filling. This loss further lowers the cardiac output and raises atrial pressures. Atrioventricular synchronization is particularly important when there are abnormalities in ventricular compliance necessitating an enhanced component of atrial filling.

Individuals with concentric hypertrophy, which reduces ventricular cavity size and ventricular filling, will also suffer. The deleterious effect of the bradydysrhythmias, particularly those associated with asynchronicity of atrial and ventricular contraction, is reduction of cardiac output, which further depresses cardiac function and precipitates congestive heart failure.

Intraventricular/atrioventricular conduction defects. Normal ventricular contraction occurs conjointly in a "wringing" effect from apex to base, providing maximum cardiac ejection. The pathological interruption of the pathway of depolarization to either ventricle or a ventricular originated dysrhythmia disrupts the usual ventricular synchronous contractile power. Impairment of myocardial performance results in a decrease of the ejected volume and a rise in atrial pressures. This combination leads to congestive heart failure.

Pulmonary embolism

Pulmonary embolism is occlusion of a pulmonary vessel by agents such as fat globules, air, fibrin, amniotic fluid, foreign bodies, and, most commonly, blood clots originating from distant sources.[18] The most common source of blood clot emboli is the deep veins of the lower extremities. The emboli can be massive, and they can cause obstruction of major pulmonary vessels or a wide section of small arterioles.

Hemodynamic response to embolus is a sudden increase in pulmonary vascular resistance and right ventricular pressures. Mechanical obstruction by the embolus is one of the mechanisms that causes these pressure elevations. A second mechanism is the release of potent vasoactive and bronchoactive agents, such as histamine, serotonin, and prostaglandins, from the platelet aggregation around the embolus. These agents potentiate contraction of the smooth muscle of the pulmonary vascular and bronchial tree.[52]

Pulmonary embolus can result in cardiopulmonary embarrassment in patients with normal heart function, when occlusion of a main pulmonary artery is 50% or greater. However, patients with compromised cardiac contractile function readily decompensate even in the face of small emboli production. Increased impedance to ejection as a result of the pulmonary occlusion and the increased pulmonary resistance places an extraordinary systolic overload on the already burdened heart. Right ventricular failure ensues with sys-

temic congestion and a markedly decreased left ventricular cardiac output.

Anemia

Anemia is defined as a deficiency of red blood cells in the vascular system. Anemia effects a decrease in oxygen transport to the tissues, causing tissue hypoxia. In response to increased plasma volume the cardiac output increases to meet oxygen demand. This is accompanied by low systemic vascular resistance and a high mixed venous oxygen content. Mechanisms that increase cardiac output are (1) decreased left ventricular afterload related to vasodilation and decreased blood viscosity, (2) increased ventricular preload resulting from augmented venous return, and (3) increased myocardial contractility.[19]

A normal heart can adapt to these hemodynamic changes. However, a patient with compromised cardiac status from systolic overload as a result of aortic stenosis or with a diseased myocardium cannot sustain the requirement for increased cardiac output. This additional workload precipitates heart failure. Assessment of hemoglobin in a patient with underlying cardiac problems is critical to prompt intervention since hemoglobin of even 8 to 9 g/100 ml can easily trigger heart failure in patients with underlying heart disease.

Systemic and pulmonic infections

Systemic and pulmonic infections are defined as the invasion and establishment of pathogens in the systemic or pulmonary organs. The initial physiological response to the organisms is a hyperdynamic state. The body releases phagocytes to stop the growth and spread of the pathogens. The clinical presentation of this is fever, which increases the total metabolism. Cardiac output and heart rate increase to meet tissue metabolic demand.

As the infectious organisms die, endotoxins are released. It is likely that local acidosis causes atrioventricular shunting in response to endotoxins with an obligatory increase in plasma volume and a high cardiac output state. Myocardial contractile dysfunction is also a feature that occurs as a metabolic consequence of prolonged or severe sepsis.[10,59] This is a serious complication likely to precipitate profound heart failure.

Endocrine and humoral disorders

Hyperthyroidism-thyrotoxicosis. In hyperthyroidism, the excessive thyroid hormone, thyroxine, directly affects the heart. This may occur either by direct hormone action or may be mediated by catecholamines.[61] The response increases the force of contraction; therefore myocardial metabolic rate and oxygen requirements are increased. It also stimulates the sinoatrial node to increase its rate of discharge. In addition, excess thyroxine appears to make the heart more sensitive to circulating catecholamines, which contribute to the tachycardia and increased force of contraction.[61] Other effects are generalized vasodilation, decreased peripheral resistance, and increased venous return. These factors combine to increase cardiac output to meet the hypermetabolic state.

Paroxysmal or transient atrial fibrillation is a dysrhythmia seen frequently with congestive heart failure. In patients with hyperthyroidism, underlying cardiac disease appears to be the determining factor for this rhythm disturbance. This rhythm disorder alters sequential contraction, further impairing pump function. Therefore masked thyrotoxicosis should be considered in patients with unexplained atrial fibrillation or heart failure that does not respond to the usual medical therapy.[15,29,33]

Hypothyroidism—myxedema. Myxedema, the lack of thyroid hormone, compromises cardiac function in approximately 75% to 80% of patients who remain untreated.[19,61] Cardiac rate, force of contraction, and cardiac output are affected. The decreased heart rate and cardiac output are proportional to the decreased metabolic oxygen requirements. The cardiac walls thicken and enlarge, the chambers dilate, and the myocardial fibers swell. The heart becomes pale, flabby, and dilated. Heart sounds are distant, and electrocardiographic

monitoring reveals diminution of the ECG voltage. These cardiovascular changes are the result of pericardial effusion, myocardial infiltrative disease, and hypothyroid coronary artery disease.

The cardiac enlargement is primarly the result of pericardial effusion not associated with pericarditis and is thought to be related to increased capillary permeability. The effusion content is high in protein and cholesterol.[15,19,34] Hepatic mechanisms responsible for the removal of cholesterol from the circulation are decreased; therefore plasma cholesterol levels are high, resulting in atherosclerosis.[37]

Heart failure results from pericardial effusion and myxedematous infiltration of the myocardium. Lack of myocardial tissue oxygenation further compounds the failure. The myocardium becomes constricted, reducing contractile ability and cardiac chamber size. This, coupled with a slow pulse rate, leads to diminished cardiac output. Pulmonary and systemic congestion occur despite low blood volume.[34] Data collected during assessment demonstrate cardiac enlargement and dilation, significant bradycardia, weak peripheral pulses, distant heart sounds, quiet precordium, displaced apical pulse, and low voltage ECG complexes. These individuals often demonstrate nonpitting facial and peripheral edema and usually do not respond to diuretic or digitalis therapy. Biochemical analysis reveals decreased serum levels of protein-bound iodine, and roentgenograms show an enlarged cardiac silhouette.

Adrenal disorders

Cushing's syndrome. Cushing's syndrome is caused by excessive production of glucocorticoids and androgens as a result of bilateral adrenal hyperplasia. Most patients have truncal obesity, slender extremities, fatigue and weakness, glycosuria, amenorrhea, and purple abdominal striae. Hypertension is present in 80% to 90% of the cases.[60] This syndrome may also be produced by a central mediating lesion such as an ACTH-producing tumor of the pituitary gland. When this occurs the condition is labeled *Cushing's disease*.

The primary significance of this syndrome on the development of heart failure arises from hypertensive sequelae. Before the development of effective treatment, death occurred from accelerated atherosclerosis, myocardial infarction, heart failure, and stroke. Hemodynamic electrocardiographic and radiographic studies reveal no specific abnormalities except those associated with hypertension and hypokalemia.

Hyperaldosteronism. Hyperaldosteronism is a condition associated with hypersecretion of aldosterone. In primary aldosteronism, the stimulus is in the adrenals and occurs from conditions such as benign adrenal adenomas. In secondary aldosteronism, the stimulus is extra-adrenal and may result from renal artery stenosis or from low effective arterial blood volume, which, in turn, stimulates the reinin-angiotensin-aldosterone (RAA) triad, elevating peripheral vascular resistance and expanding blood volume. The outcomes of this syndrome are hypertension and hypokalemia, which may impair cardiac function and result in heart failure.

The major cardiovascular indicators are nonspecific. Hypokalemia may cause electrocardiographic abnormalities such as low-amplitude T waves, U waves, and premature ventricular contractions. There may also be physical and radiographic findings of left ventricular hypertrophy that are suggestive of chronic hypertension.

Pheochromocytoma. Pheochromocytoma is a catecholamine-producing tumor arising in the adrenal medulla. Hypertension is the major cardiovascular indicator of this disorder. The clinical manifestations may include paroxysmal attacks of high blood pressure, headaches, excessive sweating, signs of hypermetabolism, orthostatic hypotension, and unusual blood pressure elevation secondary to trauma or surgery.[60]

Other findings include electrocardiographic changes suggestive of myocardial ischemia resulting from elevated pressure load on the heart. These include transient ST segment elevation or depression, T wave inversion, and alteration as a result of left ventricular hypertrophy. These disappear with resolution of hypertension.

Pheochromocytoma may also be associated with catecholamine-induced inflammatory myocarditis consisting of focal necrosis and fibrosis. This may account for the left ventricular failure and the pulmonary edema that cause almost 50% mortality in patients with this disease.[60]

Hypervolemia

Circulatory hypervolemia can result from heart disease, poor renal function, medications, hormones, and excessive intake of salt. Hormones such as testosterone and diethylstilbestrol (Stilbestrol) cause water retention. Steroids, minoxidil, and indomethacin are also reported to cause fluid retention.[16]

Expanded circulatory volume augments venous return and increases ventricular preload and ventricular filling pressure. In patients with preexisting heart disease, increased filling pressure may exceed cardiac functional capacity, resulting in heart failure.

A thorough assessment will identify the factors that may have precipitated circulatory overload. This should include a detailed medication and diet history, evaluation of fluid intake and output, biochemical analysis, serial body weights, and physical examination for signs of systemic and pulmonary congestion (see Chapter 4).

Obesity

Adult-onset obesity is characterized by normal weight in childhood and adolescence with a gradual increase in weight between 20 and 40 years of age. It is the result of an imbalance in caloric intake and use. The metabolic consequences include decreased sensitivity to insulin with glucose intolerance and elevated blood levels of cholesterol and triglycerides.

A large number of cardiovascular abnormalities are associated with gross obesity. These include increased central blood volume and moderate hypertension. Heart failure is usually chronic and results from increased blood volume and cardiac output, which is proportional to excess body weight. Pulmonary and systemic congestion with dyspnea and edema are related to elevated filling pressure and reduced ventricular compliance. In individuals who sustain a marked reduction in myocardial contractility, the treatment consists of weight reduction, dietary sodium restriction, cardiac glycosides, and diuretics.

Pregnancy

Heart disease still ranks high among causes of death in childbearing.[13,19,40] Pregnancy imposes additional hemodynamic work on the cardiovascular system. It can precipitate heart failure in a woman who has underlying heart disease. Particularly at risk are patients with obstructive valvular disease, which mechanically impedes forward flow.[15]

The pregnant woman with underlying heart disease is at risk at the end of the second trimester. At this time maximum blood volume develops and hemodynamic stress is greatest. The increase in plasma volume reflects changes in the fluid balance. Sodium and water retention are the causes of increased total body water—as much as 8.5 L or 40% above nonpregnant women. This retention results from hormonal changes.[51]

Resting heart rate increases during gestation by approximately 10 to 15 beats per minute.[15,19] This places an added strain on the heart and also elevates oxygen consumption. The heart, already functioning within its limited cardiac capacity, can no longer accommodate the additional load and heart failure ensues, accompanied by pulmonary or systemic congestion. In addition these women are also at risk immediately following delivery when shifts in fluid volume may overload the circulation.

Thiamine deficiency

Inadequate dietary intake of vitamin B_1 or thiamine causes beriberi. Diets low in fat and protein and high in carbohydrates, found most frequently in the Far East, can lead to this disorder. In the United States, the nutritional disorder is commonly related to chronic ingestion of alcohol because thiamine intake is minimal, metabolism of thiamine is impaired, transport of thiamine in the intestines is decreased, and storage of this vitamin in a damaged liver is marginal.[28,35,43]

Beriberi causes depression of the sympathetic nervous system and leads to peripheral vasodilation.[1,19] This is responsible for the hyperkinetic circulating state. Thiamine deficiency causes reabsorption of water by the skeletal muscle and myocardial tissue, thereby decreasing myocardial contractility. It also evokes development of metabolic acidosis, which further depresses contractile function.[4,5,42]

Augmented venous return and deficient contractile power precipitate elevated end-diastolic pressures in the right and left ventricles. In patients with minimal ventricular function, these pressures further limit myocardial contraction. Even in the presence of reduced afterload or reduced systemic vascular resistance, ejection is low.

Heart failure may develop explosively in beriberi as seen with the fulminating form of the disease known as "Shoshin" beriberi. Consumption of highly milled, polished rice and raw seafood potentiate this form of the disease, which is frequently characterized by severe hypotension, tachycardia, and pulmonary edema.[61]

In caring for the individual with congestive heart failure of unknown origin that is unresponsive to digitalis and diuretic therapy, the astute clinician applies transcultural knowledge concerning dietary habits in assisting the health care team in establishing a definitive diagnosis. Congestive heart failure as a result of beriberi will not respond to traditional therapy unless thiamine administration is initiated.

Overexertion/exercise

Physical stress, induced by severe exercise, increases venous return to the heart because of the pumping action of the skeletal muscles. It creates an increase in myocardial workload and increases metabolic heat production; therefore the cardiovascular system has to shut 20% of total cardiac output toward the skin for vasodilation and thermal control.[37] The patient with normal cardiac function compensates by increasing heart rate and contractility to meet these metabolic needs. If there is an underlying depression of cardiac function, the heart cannot achieve maximal contraction to eject the required volume. As a result of reduced ejectile force and diastolic filling time, coronary perfusion is impaired. This may precipitate fatal dysrhythmias and/or acute myocardial ischemia and infarction. Congestive heart failure may follow with marked pulmonary congestion.

Statistics obtained by Waller and others on five men aged 40 to 53 years who ran a distance of 22 to 76 km weekly and who died while running showed that all five men had 76% to 100% narrowing of right coronary, left anterior descending, and left circumflex arteries. Other reports showed one patient who died while jogging had a heart weighing 390 g, a history of myocardial infarction, and 76% to 100% occlusion of left circumflex arteries.[55,56] This evidence reinforces the importance of eliciting historical evidence of exercise tolerance, cardiac risk factors, and compliance to medical therapy in individuals with marginal cardiac function and underlying heart disease.

Paget's disease

Paget's disease is a localized bone disorder characterized by structural abnormality resulting from replacement of the normal bone marrow with highly vascularized connective tissue. This disease is unrelated to Paget's disease in women, which is cancerous dermatosis of the nipple area.[46] Bones extensively affected by Paget's disease are enlarged, easily fractured, and deformed and the overlying skin is warm to palpation. This condition is accompanied by increased blood flow through the affected bone. When the disease is severe the peripheral vascular resistance decreases, and the cardiac output increases above normal levels at rest and after exercise. The mechanism for the local and systemic increase in blood flow is not specific. Presence of arteriovenous communications or an increase in the size and number of arterioles with related venous sinuses are thought to contribute to this phenomenon.[26] Studies have shown that elevated cardiac output was present when serum alkaline phosphatase levels were high or when more than one third of the skeleton was involved.[25,26] Other findings in Paget's disease include the deposition of calcium in arteries, heart valves, and the ventricular septum, producing sclerosis, valvular dysfunction, and atrioventricular or interventricular conduction defects.

In people with preexisting heart disease, the increased blood flow and cardiovascular complications upset the delicate balance of compensation. The burden of increasing workload on an already compromised myocardial function can easily lead to heart failure with either pulmonary or systemic congestion.

Two interesting physical findings that a clinician may observe as a result of increased vascularity are the presence of a bruit and localized warmth over the affected bone.[25]

Other findings of Paget's disease of bone include swelling or deformity of one or more of the long bones, enlargement of the skull, facial pain, headache, backache, and an elevated blood alkaline phosphatase level. The cardiovascular findings are characteristic of high-output states (see p. 53).

Noncompliance to therapeutic regimen

Individuals with existing cardiac disease controlled by medical therapy, be it a drug regimen, dietary sodium restriction, physical activity modification, or a combination of these, are at great risk for cardiac decompensation with the casual reduction or augmentation of therapy. For those people who have previously developed heart failure, lack of compliance to therapy is the most common cause of further cardiac decompensation.[8] Being asymptomatic produces a false sense of well-being and permanent cure. This perception leads to the voluntary modification of treatment. Lack of health education promotes noncompliance, and cultural practices may interfere with adherence to the prescribed therapeutic regimen. Inability to accept changes in role and body image may intensify dissociation from the therapeutic model[33]

The nurse practitioner with a psychosocial and health education knowledge base applies these principles in the nursing process to develop a plan of health care instruction. Implementation of the educational program is initiated to improve patient motivation and foster compliance. Continuous positive reinforcement and patient involvement will assure better adherence to the therapeutic regimen during the course of heart disease.

SUMMARY

It is essential for health care clinicians to be familiar with the major cardiac and noncardiac disorders that underlie and precipitate heart failure. These have been reviewed with emphasis placed on cardiovascular hemodynamic effects and on characteristic clinical indicators. When clinicians are able to identify the factors that may contribute to or precipitate heart failure, the effectiveness of clinical therapeutics will be markedly improved. The information presented in this chapter will provide the knowledge base necessary to accurately assess the individual with heart failure.

REFERENCES

1. Akbarian, M., Yankopoulos, N.A., and Abelman, W.H.: Hemodynamic studies in beriberi heart disease, Am. J. Med. **41**:197, 1966.
2. Alexander, C.S.: Cobalt-beer cardiomyopathy; a clinical and pathological study of twenty-eight cases, Am. J. Med. **53**:395, 1972.
2a. Alpert, J.S., and Braunwald, E.: Congenital heart disease in the adult. In Braunwald, E., editor: Heart disease: a textbook of cardiovascular medicine, Philadelphia, 1981, W.B. Saunders Co.
3. Alpert, J.S., Irwin, R.S., and Dalen, J.E.: Pulmonary hypertension, Curr. Probl. Cardiol. **5**(10):1-39, 1981.
4. Atenski, M.: Thiamine-deficiency-related cardiac failure (letter), Am. J. Dis. Child **134**(11):1098, 1980.
5. Attas, M.: Fulminant beriberi heart disease with lactic acidosis: presentation of a case with evaluation of left ventricular function and review of pathophysiologic mechanisms, Circulation **58**:566, 1978.
6. Barson, W.J., and others: Survival following myocarditis and myocardial calcification associated with infection by coxsackie virus B-4, Pediatrics **68**(1):79, 1981.
7. Boe, I.: Myocardial infarction and ischemic heart disease in infants and children: analysis of twenty cases and review of literature, Arch. Dis. Child **44**:268, 1969.
8. Braunwald, E.: Pathophysiology of heart failure. In Braunwald, E., editor: Heart disease: a textbook of cardiovascular medicine, Philadelphia, 1981, W.B. Saunders Co.
9. Braunwald, E.: Valvular heart disease. In Braunwald, E., editor: Heart disease: a textbook of cardiovascular medicine, Philadelphia, 1981, W.B. Saunders Co.
10. Bruni, F.D.: Endotoxin and myocardial failure: role of the myofibril and venous return, Am. J. Physiol. **235**:H150, 1976.
11. Buckley, H.H., and Hutchins, G.M.: Atrial myxomas; a fifty year review, Am. Heart J. **97**:639, May 1979.
12. Cheitlin, M.D.: Coarctation of the aorta, Med. Clin. North Am. **61**(3):655, 1977.
13. Cole, B.K.: Cardiac disease in pregnancy, Ohio State Med. J. **66**:924, April 1970.
13a. Daggett, W.M., and others: Surgery for postmyocardial infarction ventricular septal defect, Ann. Surg. **186**:260, 1977.
14. Davidson, K.H., and others: Pseudoaneurysm of the left ventricle: an unusual echocardiographic presentation, review of the literature, Ann. Intern. Med. **86**:430, 1977.
15. Davies, H., and Nelson, W.: Understanding cardiology, Woburn, Mass., 1978, Butterworth, Inc.
16. Deglin, J.M., and Murphy, J.: Sodium and water retention associated with indomethacin therapy, Drug. Int. Clin. Pharm. **14**(9):620-21, 1980.
17. Dubnow, M.H., Burchell, H.B., and Titus, J.L.: Post-infarction ventricular aneurysm: clinical morphologic and electrocardiographic study of 80 cases, Am. Heart J. **70**:753, Dec. 1965.
18. Fishman, A.P.: Pulmonary thromboembolism pathophysiology and clinical features. In Fishman, A.P., editor: Pulmonary diseases and disorders, New York, 1980, McGraw-Hill Book Co., p. 809.
19. Fowler, N.O.: Cardiac diagnoses and treatment, ed. 3, New York, 1980, Harper & Row Publishers.
20. Franciosa, J.A.: Hypertensive left heart failure: pathogenesis and therapy, Hosp. Pract. **16**(2):77, 1981.
21. Goldberger, E.: Textbook of clinical cardiology, St. Louis, 1981, The C.V. Mosby Co.
22. Gore, J.M., and Dalen, J.E.: General guidelines for treating pulmonary hypertension, Drug Ther. **6**(10):37, 1981.
23. Guyton, A.: Textbook of medical physiology, ed. 5, Philadelphia, 1976, W.B. Saunders co.
24. Hagan, A.D., and Thorne, J.N.: Ventricular septal perforation following left ventricular angiography, Am. J. Cardiol. **22**:885, 1969.

25. Hamdy, R.: Signs and treatment of Paget's disease, Geriatrics **32**(6):89, 1977.

26. Henley, J.W., Croxson, R.S., and Ibbertson, H.K.: The cardiovascular system in Paget's disease of bone and the resonse to therapy with calcitonin and diphosphate, Aust, N.Z. J. Med. **3**(4):390, 1979.

27. Holloway, N.M.: Nursing the critically ill adult, Menlo, Ca., 1979, Addison-Wesley Publishing Co., Inc.

28. Hoyumpa, A.M., Jr., and others: Intestinal thiamine transport: effect of chronic ethanol administration in rats, Am. J. Clin. Nutr. **31**:938, 1978.

29. Ingbar, S.H.: When to hospitalize the patient with thyrotoxicosis, Hosp. Pract. **10**:45, Jan. 1975.

30. Jackson, D.H., and Murphy, G.N.: Non-penetrating cardiac trauma, Mod. Concepts Cardiovasc. Dis. **45**:123, Sept. 1976.

31. Kannel, W.B., Castelli, W.P. and McNamara, P.M.: Role of blood pressure in the development of congestive heart failure, the framingham study, N. Engl. J. Med., **287**(16): 781, 1972.

32. Kaplan, N.M.: Systemic hypertension mechanism and diagnosis. In Braunwald, E., editor: Heart disease, a textbook of cardiovascular medicine, Philadelphia, 1981, W.B. Saunders Co.

33. Kenner, C.V., Guzzetta, C.E., and Dossey, B.M.: Critical care nursing: mind body spirit, Boston, 1981, Little, Brown & Company.

34. Krueger, J.A., and Ray, J.C.: Endocrine problems in nursing; a physiologic approach, St. Louis, 1977, The C.V. Mosby Co.

35. Lim, C.H., and others: Stokes-Adams attacks due to acute nonspecific myocarditis, Am. Heart J. **90**:172, 1975.

36. Luckmann, J., and Sorensen, K.C.: Medical-surgical nursing; a Psychophysiologic Approach, ed. 2, Philadelphia, 1980, W.B. Saunders Co.

37. Mangs, R.: Runners in the sun, Emergency Med. **13**(15): 135, 1981.

38. Maron, B.J., and Roberts, N.C.: Quantitative analysis of cardiac cell disorganization in the ventricular septum of patients with hypertrophic cardiomyopathy, Circulation **59**:689, April 1979.

39. McFadden, R., Jr., and Braunwald, E.: Cor pulmonale and pulmonary thromboembolism. In Braunwald, E., editor: Heart Disease a textbook of cardiovascular medicine, Philadelphia, 1981, W.B. Saunders Co.

40. Metcalf, J.: The heart in pregnancy: guide to practical considerations, Hosp. Med. **14**:95, Sept. 1978.

41. Oparil, S.: Systemic arterial hypertension. In Willerson, J.T., and Saunders, C.A., editors: Clinical cardiology, New York, 1977, Grune & Stratton, Inc.

41a. Perloff, J.K.: Post pediatric congenital heart disease: natural survival patterns. In Roberts, W.C., editor: Congenital heart disease, Philadelphia, 1977, F.A. Davis Co.

42. Phoraphutkul, C., Gamble, W.J., and Monsol, R.G.: Ventricular performance, coronary flow and myocardial consumption in rats with advanced thiamine deficiency, Am. J. Clin. Nutr. **27**:136, 1974.

43. Regan, T.J., and others: Whiskey and the heart, Cardiovasc. Med. **2**:165, 1977.

44. Rosenthal, A., Parisi, F.F., and Nadas, A.S.: Isolated interventricular septal defect due to nonpenetrating trauma, N. Engl. J. Med. **283**:338, 1970.

45. Sakaibara, S., and others: Arteriovenous fistula: nine operated cases, Am. Heart J. **72**:307, 1966.

46. Shaw, A.B.: Paget's disease, Practitioner **224**(1350): 1323, 1980.

47. Simpson, P.C., and Bristow, J.D.: Recognition and management of emergencies in valvular heart disease, Med. Clin. North Am. **63**(1):155, 1979.

48. Sittanin, P., and others: Atrial myxoma in a family, Am. J. Cardiol. **38**:252, Aug. 1976.

49. Standards and guidelines for cardiopulmonary resuscitation and emergency cardiac care, J.A.M.A. **244**(5):453, Aug. 1980.

50. Sweet, S.E., and others: Left ventricular false aneurysm after coronary bypass surgery: radionuclide diagnosis and surgical resection, Am. J. Cardiol. **43**:154, 1976.

51. Szekely, P.O., and Snaith, L.: Heart disease and pregnancy, Edinburg, 1974, Churchill Livingstone.

52. Vaage, J.: Vagal reflexes in the brochoconstriction occurring after induced intravascular platelet aggregation, Acta Physiol. Sunca. **97**:94, 1976.

53. Vlodavee, Z., Coe, J.L., and Edwards, J.E.: True and false ventricular aneurysms: propensity for the latter to rupture, Circulation **51**:567, 1975.

54. Wallach, J.: Interpretation of diagnostic tests, ed. 3, Boston, 1979, Little, Brown & Company.

55. Waller, B.F., and others: Running to death, Chest **79**:3, March 1981.

56. Waller, B.F., and Roberts, W.C.: Sudden death while running in conditioned runners age 40 years or over, Am. J. Cardiol. **45**:1292, 1980.

57. Waxler, E.B., Kauai, N., and Kasparian, H.: Right atrial myxoma: chocardiographic, phonocardiographic and hemodynamic signs, Am. Heart J. **82**:251, 1972.

58. Wenger, N.K., Hurst, J.W., and McIntyre, M.C.: Cardiology for Nurses, New York, 1980, McGraw-Hill Book Co.

59. Wiles, J.B., and others: The systemic septic response: does the organism matter, Crit. Care Med. **8**(2):55, 1980.

60. Willerson, J.T., and Sanders, C.A., editors: Clinical cardiology, New York, 1977, Grune & Stratton, Inc.

61. Williams, G.H., and Braunwald, E.: Endocrine and nutritional disorders in heart disease. In Braunwald, E. editor: Textbook of cardiovascular medicine, Philadelphia, 1980, W.B. Saunders Co.

62. Wink, K., and Schmitz, H.: Cytomegalovirus myocarditis, Am. Heart J. **100**(5):667, 1980.

63. Wynne, J., and Braunwald, E.: The cardiomyopathies and myocarditis. In Braunwald, E., editor: Heart disease: a textbok of cardiovascular medicine. Philadelphia, 1981, W.B. Saunders Co.

ADDITIONAL READINGS

Adelman, A.G., and others: Current concepts of primary cardiomyopathies, Cardiovasc. Med. **2**:495, May 1977.

Ahmed, S.S., and others: Assessment of left ventricular contractile performance from isovolumetric relaxation phase in man, Cardiology **68**(1):1, 1981.

Anderson, N.E., and others: Clinical significance of right ventricular infarction, N.Z. Med. J. **94**(691):174, 1981.

Baandrup, U., and others: Critical analysis of endomyocardial biopsies from patients suspected of having cardiomyopathy, Br. Heart J. **45**(5):487, 1981.

Barson, W.J., and others: Survival following myocarditis and myocardial calcification associated with infection by coxsackie virus B-4, Pediatrics **68**(1):79, 1981.

Bing, R.J.: Cardiac metabolism: its contributions to alcoholic heart disease and myocardial failure, Circulation **58**(6):965, 1978.

Boucher, C.A., and others: Cardiomyopathic syndrome caused by coronary artery disease, Br. Heart J. **41**(5):613, 1979.

Braunwald, E., editor: Heart disease: a textbook of cardiovascular medicine, Philadelphia, 1980, W.B. Saunders Co.

Bristow, M.R., and others: Dose-effect and structure-function relationships in doxorubicin cardiomyopathy, Am. Heart J. **102**(4):709, 1981.

Brockman, M.D., and others: Myocardial abscess and fatal sepsis caused by group B streptococcus *(S. agalactiae)* in an adult, South Med. J. **72**(12):1629, 1979.

Chesley, L.C.: The control of hypertension in pregnancy, Obstet. Gynecol. Annu. **10**:69, 1981.

Cortis, B.S., Lee, S.S., and Bacalla, M.: Acute myocardial infarction and ventricular fibrillation during pregnancy, I.M.J. **69**:170, Sept. 1981.

Das, U.N.: Possible role of prostaglandins in the pathogenesis of cardiomyopathies, Med. Hypotheses **7**(3):651, 1981.

Dietz, A.J.: Cytomegalovirus infection with carditis, hepatitis, and anemia, Postgrad. Med. **70**(3):203, 1981.

Drake, C.E., and others: ECG changes in hypothermia from sepsis and unrelated to exposure, Chest **77**(5):685, 1980.

Eskridge, R.A.: Septic shock, Crit. Care Q, **2**:55, March 1980.

Ganong, W.F.: Review of medical physiology, ed. 8, Los Altos, 1977, Lange Medical Publications.

Goldberger, A.L.: Congestive heart failure in adults: six considerations in systemic diagnosis, Postgrad. Med. **69**(3):151, 1981.

Gubernan, B.A., and others: Cardiac tamponade in medical patients, Circulation **64**(3):633, 1981.

Haiat, R., and others: Occult pericardial effusion in pregnancy, N. Engl. J. Med. **305**(18):1096, 1981.

Harden, W.R. III: and others: Temporal relation between onset of cell anoxia and ischemic contractile failure, Am. J. Cardiol. **44**(4):741, 1979.

Harmjanz, D., and others: Overcontraction and excess actin filaments: basic elements of hypertrophic cardiomyopathy, Br. Heart J. **45**(5):494, 1981.

Hill, S.L., and others: Changes in lung water and capillary permeability following sepsis and fluid overload, J. Surg. Res. **28**(2):140, 1980.

Horan, M.J., and others: Characteristics and prognoses of apparently healthy patients with frequent and complex ventricular ectopy: evidence for a relatively benign new syndrome with occult myocardial and/or coronary disease, Am. Heart J. **102**(4):809, 1981.

Hubbell, G., Cheitlin, M.D., and Rapaport, E.: Presentation, management and follow-up evaluation of infective endocarditis in drug addicts, Am. Heart J. **102**(1):85, 1981.

Isner, J.M., Del Negro, A.A., and Borer, J.S.: Right ventricular infarction with hemodynamic decompensation due to transient loss of active atrial augmentation: successful treatment with atrial pacing, Am. Heart J. **102**(4):792, 1981.

Legrand, V., and others: Premature opening of pulmonary valve in right ventricular M.I., Acta Cardiol. (Brux.) **36**(4):289, 1981.

Leman, R.B., and others: Heart disease and pregnancy, South Med. J. **74**(8):944, 1981.

Maker, A.B.: A systems approach to nursing the patient with multiple systems failure, Heart Lung **10**(5):866, 1981.

Mandel, W.J.: Cardiac arrhythmias, their mechanisms, diagnosis and management, Philadelphia, 1980, J.B. Lippincott Co.

Marmor, A., and others: Functional response of the right ventricle to myocardial infarction: dependence on the site of left ventricular infarction, Circulation **64**(5):1005, 1981.

Maron, B.J., and Roberts, W.C.: Hypertrophic cardiomyopathy and cardiac muscle cell disorganization revisited: relation between the two and significance, Am. Heart J. **102**(1):95, 1981.

McLarin, C.W., and others: Pseudoanterior myocardial infarction as a manifestation of severe pulmonary embolism, J. Med. Assoc. Ga. **70**:649, Sept. 1981.

McKenna, W.J., and others: Arrhythmia in hypertrophic cardiomyopathy, Br. Heart J. **46**(2):168, 1981.

McManus, B.M., and others: Hemodynamic cardiac constriction without anatomic myocardial restriction or pericardial constriction, Am. Heart J. **102**(1):134, 1981.

Mee, A.S, and others: Congestive (dilated) cardiomyopathy in association with solvent abuse, J.R. Soc. Med. **73**(9):671, 1980.

Pécoud, A., and others: Haemodynamics in phaeochromocytoma, Intensive Care Med. **5:**143, 1979.

Pericarditis with some differences, Emergency Med. **11:**101, Sept. 15, 1979.

Pope, T.L., Jr.: Toxic shock syndrome, Nurse Pract. **6**(5):31, 1981.

Radford, M.J., and others: Ventricular septal rupture: a review of clinical and physiologic features and an analysis of survival, Circulation **64**(3):545, 1981.

Rayburn, W.F., and others: Mitral valve prolapse and pregnancy, Am. J. Obstet. Gynecol. **141**(1):9, 1981.

Rice, C.L., and others: The effect of sepsis and reduced colloid osmotic pressure on pulmonary edema, J. Surg. Res. **27**(5): 347, 1979.

Robinson, J.A.: Septic shock in cardiopulmonary patients, Hosp. Med. **15:**19, Oct. 1979.

Rowley, J.M., and Hampton, J.R.: Diagnostic criteria for myocardial infarction, Br. J. Hosp. Med. **26**(3):253, 1981.

Schulman, P., and others: Left ventricular outflow obstruction induced by tamponade in hypertrophic cardiomyopathy, Chest **80**(1):110, 1981.

Stein, P.D., and others: Performance of the failing and nonfailing right ventricle of patients with pulmonary hypertension, Am. J. Cardiol. **44:**1050, Nov. 1979.

PART II

PATIENT ASSESSMENT

CHAPTER 4

Physical assessment: a tailored approach for patients in heart failure

MAUREEN HARVEY

MAJOR PRINCIPLES OF ASSESSMENT

The physical examination has long been important in establishing a diagnosis. In the fourth and fifth centuries BC, Hippocrates admonished and exemplified the use of concentration and analysis to evaluate information gathered by the five senses. The clinical indicators of heart failure were so obvious and often catastrophic that the syndrome was recognized long before its etiology was elucidated. In ancient times it was known as dropsy. The tendency today to rely heavily on laboratory·measurements and sophisticated diagnostic techniques has left untapped much valuable information the senses can process.

The presence or absence of heart failure can be established by carefully evaluating data collected during the assessment process. In addition, it is possible to differentiate between early, moderate, and late heart failure and between right-sided heart, left-sided heart, and bilateral involvement. These determinations are required to plan and evaluate the patient's care.

An added challenge is the task of uncovering signs of the underlying cause and precipitating event of cardiac decompensation. Often the underlying cause has existed for many months or years, and a precipitating factor has provided the extra burden to unmask the developing disease. A history of having a myocardial infarction despite full return to normal levels of activity may be the underlying cause of failure. The lack of cardiac reserve may become manifested or precipitated when the patient incurs a higher level of cardiac demand. In the patient with known heart failure, the exacerbation may be caused by noncompliance to the treatment regimen, drug side effects, or development of an unrelated illness. These factors must be addressed in order to reverse the trend and bring the demands placed on the compromised heart to a level it can meet.

Another concept that should be appreciated throughout the assessment is that personal interaction can have either a positive or a negative impact on establishing patient rapport. Very few professions are given such license to touch, to probe, to ask intimate questions, and to demand honest self-appraisal. The mere act of sitting next to or on the bed with the patient who is scantily covered may produce high levels of anxiety. Furthermore, the patient who has suspected heart disease may be fearful because of the religious, spiritual, and emotional connotations our society assigns to the heart.[12]

On the positive side, the nature of these interactions tends to bring down barriers and hasten high-quality communication. Both the examiner and the patient are seeking to discover the cause, severity, and implications of the disease. Rarely do two strangers meet with an overt mutual goal of such paramount importance.

Measures may be taken to minimize the negative and maximize the positive aspects of the assessment process. The patient's vulnerability may be reduced and trust enhanced when the examiner:

1. Establishes a relationship before beginning the physical aspects of the examination
2. Is aware of the nonverbal aspects of communication and uses them to advantage
3. Uses a firm and warm but gentle touch
4. Keeps the patient covered
5. Uses frequent eye contact
6. Informs the patient about what is being done
7. Has a calm and reassuring manner
8. Demonstrates confident and organized use of skills

Clues regarding personality as well as mental, social, and emotional status may also be discovered during the examination process. Such observations made about patients are useful in evaluating:

1. Ability to verbalize and express feelings
2. Ability to tolerate pain
3. Impact the illness will have on them, their life-styles, and their families
4. Approaches that will effectively help them cope with the disease and comply with treatment regimens

The purposes of assessment, then, are to identify the type, severity, and cause of heart failure, to establish a therapeutic relationship with the patient, and to collect additional information that will assure that interventions are planned in the manner most acceptable to the patient's personal needs.

This requires a high level of attention and concentration on the part of the clinician. Since it is an integral part of the nursing process, high priority and ample time should be allotted for assessment. Every effort should be made to limit distractions and interruptions. Anything that impairs assessment diminishes care.

The purpose of this chapter is to briefly review the assessment principles, to deliver a detailed presentation of the assessment process as it relates to patients with heart failure, and to describe the major clinical indicators of the syndrome.

GENERAL ASSESSMENT

Focusing on aspects of assessment specifically helpful in evaluating a special population group tends to distort the structure and intent of the process. To reduce this risk, a general description of assessment will precede the detailed description of the process as it relates to heart failure. This overview is meant to be broad and introductory. More in-depth material is abundantly available in the literature.

The goal of the assessment process is to obtain a complete and accurate data base. In order to do so, it is necessary to use a systematic method of evaluation. Developing an organized, comfortable technique and using it repeatedly helps to produce a structured framework within which the information can be collected, communicated, and processed.

The two main vehicles of assessment are the history, or interview, and the physical examination. Although both areas involve collection of objective and subjective data, the history reveals primarily subjective data (those facts or feelings reported by the patient), and the physical examination reveals primarily objective data (manifestations that are observed by the examiner).

History

The goal of the history is to collect subjective data that will be used to diagnose the problem and plan interventions. The key components are:

1. The description of the patient
2. The chief complaint
3. The history of the present illness
4. The past medical history
5. The review of systems
6. The family and social history

The history usually begins with a brief description that sets the stage and allows the reader to visualize the patient. It may include age, sex, level of physical comfort or distress, mental status, occupation, and how the patient entered the health care system. This description is followed by the chief complaint. This is the major reason for seeking medical advice and is recounted in the words of the patient. These statements may be made separately or blended together. Two examples are:

1. Mrs. B is a 60-year-old bank teller brought to the emergency room by ambulance after de-

veloping "trouble catching her breath during a fight with a coworker."

2. Mr. C is a 54-year-old fireman who came to the clinic because of his concern about "feeling weak and tired most of the time for the past few weeks."

The next step in taking a history is to carefully and fully describe the course of the present illness. Initially, it is best to let the patients describe the situation in their own sequence without being led or interrupted. After the patient has finished, necessary data may be obtained with appropriate questions. Such information would include the following:

1. When was the problem first noticed?
2. Had it ever happened before?
3. If so, how frequently?
4. Was anything found to alleviate the problem?
5. What situations seemed to aggravate it?
6. Were there any associated symptoms?
7. What exactly was the character, severity, sequence, and duration of symptoms?

A major portion of the interview will focus on the patient's past history. Areas explored are:

1. Growth and development
2. Childhood disease
3. Adult diseases
4. Previous hospitalizations
5. Immunizations
6. Allergies
7. Medication history

Again it is advantageous to allow patients to verbalize these in their own terms, guiding them with open-ended rather than closed questions. The interviewer may fill in information gaps using prepared lists of questions after the patients have completed their explanations.

The interviewer must assume the lead to obtain information for the review of systems. Most patients will fail to report many pertinent and crucial facts if left to their own recollections and perceptions. To prevent this, the interviewer asks the patient about symptoms related to specific areas. These include:

1. The skin
2. The head and neck
3. The eyes, ears, nose, and throat
4. The cardiopulmonary system
5. The musculoskeletal system
6. The nervous system
7. The gastrointestinal system
8. The genitourinary system
9. Psychological problems

Under each heading there are several standard questions that may be used to guide the interview The box on p. 126 provides a sample format for physical assessment.

The family history may reveal vital information regarding the presence of risk factors, hereditary predisposition, and genetically linked or communicable disease. The social history may reveal further risk factors such as smoking habits, alcohol consumption, diet, drug ingestion, leisure activity, and work responsibility. Determination of marital and family status will provide data regarding stress or support systems.

The nursing history is an integral part of the assessment process and provides more specific information essential to providing comprehensive patient care. It includes the following data:

1. Dietary patterns: likes and dislikes
2. Bowel habits
3. Sleep habits
4. Current level of tolerated activity
5. Hobbies, interests, talents, and skills
6. Languages spoken
7. Religion
8. Economic status
9. Hygiene practices (skin, hair, teeth)
10. Appliances (glasses, dentures, hearing aid)
11. Reactions to previous hospitalizations
12. Attitudes and expectations of health care professionals

The patient is only one source of data available during the assessment process. Others include current and past medical records and input from members of the health care team. When information may be obtained or validated from these sources, it may eliminate the necessity of protracted interviews or repeated questioning of the patient.

FORMAT FOR THE HISTORICAL ASPECTS OF PHYSICAL ASSESSMENT

Informant

Description of patient

Chief complaint

History of present illness

Review of systems; general: State of health, weight, fatigue, fever. *Skin:* Texture, temperature, rashes, growths, sun sensitivity, itching, pigment and color, dryness or sweating, hair, nails. *Head:* Headaches, dizziness, trauma. *Eyes:* Diplopia, acuity, blurring, spots, lacrimation, photophobia, itching, pain, inflammation, infection, discharge, glaucoma, cataract. *Ears:* Hearing, infections, earaches, discharge, tinnitus, vertigo. *Nose:* Discharge, obstruction, colds, allergies, sinus, smell, epistaxis. *Mouth and throat:* Sore throats, hoarseness, dysphagia, bleeding or sore gums, dental, sialorrhea, dryness. *Neck:* Pain, stiffness, injury, thyroid, lumps, lymph nodes. *Cardiopulmonary:* Chest pain, dyspnea, palpitations, cyanosis, cough, hemoptysis, night sweats, edema, murmur, paroxysmal nocturnal dyspnea, orthopnea, wheezing, stridor, syncope, hypertension. *Gastrointestinal:* Appetite, food intolerance, dysphagia, pyrosis, flatulence, nausea, vomiting, pain, bleeding, diarrhea, constipation, melena, stool characteristics, bowel habits, jaundice, rectal conditions. *Genitourinary:* Dysuria, polyuria, oliguria, urgency, frequency, hesitancy, nocturia, hematuria, pyuria, urethral discharge, incontinence, stones, sexual problems, venereal disease. *Male:* Prostate. *Female:* Cata, last menstrual period, duration, amount, menses interval, dysmenorrhea, hypermenorrhea, polymenorrhea, menopause, vaginal bleeding or discharge, dyspareunia, pelvic inflammatory disease, birth control, gravida, para, abortions, complications. *Musculoskeletal:* Muscle pain or cramps; joint pain, swelling or stiffness, weakness; numbness, coldness and discoloration of extremities; back pain; fractures; arthritis; gout. *Nervous:* Seizures, syncope, loss of consciousness, pain, paresthesias, balance, paresis, paralysis, tremor, nervousness, depression, hallucinations, relationships, therapy. *Hematopoietic:* Anemia, bleeding, bruising, dyscrasias. *Endocrine:* Temperature intolerance, thyroid, growth, polyuria, polydipsia, polyphagia and glandular problems

Past history: Immunizations, disease, hospitalization, operations, allergies, injuries, blood transfusions, foreign travel

Family history: Parents, sibs, children, spouse—ages, health, date and cause of death. *Diseases:* Cancer, migraines, tuberculosis, hypertension, coronary artery disease, rheumatic fever, strokes, nephritis or renal arthritis, nervous or mental, epilepsy, hematologic, allergies, diabetes

Social history: Born, sleep, diet, alcohol, tobacco, drugs and vitamins, exercise, religion, Armed Service, education, occupation, marital, environment

From Fowkes, W.C., and Hunn, Y.K.: Clinical assessment for the nurse practitioner, St. Louis, 1973, The C.V. Mosby Co., p. 11.

Family members and significant others may also be excellent resources. It is sometimes helpful to let them remain in the room during the examination. They may add details, discourage denial or misleading responses, and reduce the patient's anxiety. On the other hand, they may also interfere, interrupt, and agitate the patient. Careful observation of these interactional dynamics and early intervention are essential to adjust the situation and maintain a therapeutic patient-examiner relationship.

Physical examination

The physical examination involves the use of all the examiner's senses—sight, hearing, smell, and touch—and may be augmented by use of instruments to increase sensory input. A complete examination includes review of the following areas[5]:

1. General appearance
2. Skin
3. Head
4. Eyes, ears, nose, and throat
5. Neck
6. Cardiovascular system
7. Pulmonary system
8. Nervous system
9. Gastrointestinal system
10. Musculoskeletal system
11. Endocrine system
12. Genitourinary system

The four basic techniques used are inspection, palpation, percussion, and auscultation. These physical assessment skills are developed at the bedside and can become exquisitely sensitive when frequently practiced. The rate at which skill proficiency is achieved is directly related to the effort spent applying them. These are techniques that are learned only by repeated observation and performance. Each physical assessment provides comparative data and increases the experience base of examiners, allowing them to make finer qualitative distinctions of subtle clinical indicators. All that is required to progress is persistence, concentration, and a resource person to verify findings.

Inspection is the first step of physical assessment and should be initiated before other techniques and continued throughout the entire process. If inspection is not performed at the start, before involving the other senses, it is often less effective. While talking to the patient, a conscious effort should be made to note overt visual clues to the underlying condition. Impressions may develop in the following areas[1]:

1. The relationship between chronological and physiological ages
2. Overall level of health, nutrition, and energy
3. The structure and symmetry of the face and musculoskeletal system
4. Ability to move in a coordinated fashion
5. The presence of abnormal postures, movements, or tremors
6. The rhythm and ease of breathing
7. The condition of the skin, hair, and nails
8. The presence of edema, diaphoresis, or abnormal color
9. The presence of venous distention or abnormal pulsations
10. Emotional affect and mental status

Palpation is the second step of assessment and is performed using the most sensitive areas of the hands. Pulsations are most easily assessed with the tips of the fingers, vibrations with the flat of the palm side of the hand, and temperature with the back of the hand. Pressure and gentle probing may be used to identify areas of tenderness. This will elicit responses such as tensing, guarding, or grimacing. Palpation is used extensively to identify organ and vessel size and quality when evaluating the cardiovascular system.

Percussion is the next step of assessment and is especially valuable in assessing the thorax and abdomen. Many variations of the technique are taught, but the most common are the direct and indirect methods. With the direct method, one finger, two fingers, or a percussion hammer is used to tap the skin. With the indirect method, only the flat palmar surface of the distal two phalanges of the nondominant hand is placed on the patient and tapped. The advantage to this technique is that the note may be felt as well as heard. The key to good

Table 4-1. Sounds produced by percussion

Record of finding	Intensity	Pitch	Duration	Quality	Anatomical region where sounds may be encountered
Tympany	Loud	High	Moderate	Drumlike	Air in closed structure vibrates in concert with tissue surrounding it; the gastric air bubble; air in intestine
Hyperresonance	Very loud	Very low	Long	Booming	Air-filled lungs, as in emphysema
Resonance	Moderate to loud	Low	Long	Hollow	Normal lung
Dullness	Soft to moderate	High	Moderate	Thudlike	Liver
Flatness	Soft	High	Short	Flat	Muscle

From Malasanos, L., and others: Health assessment, ed. 2, St. Louis, 1981, The C.V. Mosby Co., p. 17.

percussion is the use of a quick, consistent wrist-snapping motion, not a forearm swing.

The notes elicited vary according to the type of tissue located up to 5 cm below the strike. The five notes heard are tympanic, hyperresonant, resonant, dull or hyporesonant, and flat. They can be distinguished by their pitch, intensity, duration, and quality (Table 4-1).

Auscultation is generally the final step in the classic physical examination and is used to assess the cardiovascular, pulmonary, and gastrointestinal systems. It is performed with a stethoscope to enhance the sound and should be done in a quiet environment so the examiner may concentrate to hear the softer, more subtle sounds.

A systematic approach

These principles and techniques are the foundation upon which a systematic approach to the assessment process is built. The history and physical examination are interrelated procedures conducted in an atmosphere of quiet privacy. The patient needs to feel as comfortable and relaxed as possible and to have trust in the examiner. In an outpatient setting the patient should be allowed to remain clothed during the interview to reduce anxiety.

After achieving this private atmosphere, patients are encouraged to express, in their own words, details of their past and present health history.

During this time the clinician uses skilled listening techniques while making general and detailed observations of the patient's demeanor.

Next the patient disrobes, is draped, and is settled in a comfortable recumbent position. The body should be well aligned to facilitate symmetrical comparison of anatomy. In a calm and organized manner, the examiner proceeds to evaluate the patient from head to toe, using inspection, palpation, percussion, and auscultation. Only that area of the patient being evaluated should be exposed.

Not every patient need be fully assessed on every contact. Judgment as to the severity, elusiveness, or stability of the problem will determine how much depth is necessary. With a patient in stable condition, positive findings in one area may stimulate a more in-depth assessment or a more detailed discussion on related aspects of the history. With a critically ill patient, it is necessary to focus on life-threatening findings. The urgent need for intervention may limit the initial assessment to a cursory interview and a rapid, abbreviated physical examination of the involved organ systems.

When the assessment process is completed, it is important to be sensitive to the impression the patient has regarding his condition. If the findings are serious, examiners frequently communicate this by nonverbal cues. If they fail to explain the results of the examination, the patient will often assume the worst. This increases anxiety, facilitates denial,

Table 4-2. Documenting physical assessment data by category

Category	Data
Neurological	Level of consciousness, ocular signs, motor and sensory function, reflexes
Cardiovascular	Heart rate, rhythm, sounds, pulsations, thrills, vascular pressures, quality of arterial and venous pulses
Pulmonary	Respiratory pattern, breath sounds, cough, sputum, respiratory support devices, pulmonary function parameters
Gastrointestinal	Appetite, diet, bowel sounds, percussion note, palpable masses, size of liver and spleen, abdominal girth, presence of ascites, character of drainage and stools
Genitourinary	Amount, frequency, quality of urine, drainage from the perineal area
Skin	Description of scars, lesions, incisions, wounds, rashes, pigmentation, edema, temperature, color, skin moisture, texture
Paraphernalia	Invasive and support devices such as catheters, intravenous lines, circulatory assist and monitoring equipment
Complaints	Major problems expressed by the patient relating to current and past health problems or hospitalization

fosters noncompliance, and in short is not conducive to a good therapeutic relationship; therefore explanation and reassurance are critical parting gestures.

Upon concluding the assessment, one of the most important tasks is recording and communicating data before it is forgotten or, in the case of a patient with acute heart failure, outdated. Many institutions have preprinted forms to facilitate documentation of the initial assessment, while flow sheets are used for recording continuous physical parameters. When the physical examination is performed head to toe, it is natural to chart findings in that sequence. However, it is much easier to process information and formulate conclusions if findings are grouped by system (Table 4-2). This format also simplifies reference when making comparisons and establishing trends.

It is important that the clinician select an assessment and recording method and use it consistently and repeatedly until it becomes automatic. Although initially this may require referring to a checklist, the steps quickly become internalized. When this technique is used, information is less likely to be overlooked or omitted.

TAILORED ASSESSMENT

When assessment is performed, it should be limited only by the severity of the condition. If a patient has been diagnosed with heart failure, the clinician should not confine the search for manifestations of just that problem because it is probable that unrelated indicators will be missed. In fact, even without a diagnosis to prejudice judgment, the expertise of the observer may bias the evaluation of the patient. Clinicians with cardiovascular expertise may fail to appreciate noncardiac causes of cardiovascular symptoms. Conversely, others may overlook systemic disorders caused by cardiac disease. A full and careful history and physical examination will serve to avoid this pitfall.[6]

It is important that these admonitions be remembered as the remainder of the chapter is examined. The focus of this text is the patient in heart failure; therefore the assessment process is tailored to emphasize clinical indicators that are pertinent to a selected patient population.

Selected history

A major goal of assessing the patient in heart failure is to determine the type and severity of the underlying disease and the extent of the syndrome. In order to achieve this the clinician should be aware of key manifestations and specifically search for them during each phase of the interview.

Major clinical indicators of left-sided heart failure include:

1. Shortness of breath
2. Cough
3. Weakness or fatigue
4. Changes in mental status
5. Diaphoresis and pallor or cyanosis

Right-sided heart failure is more likely to cause:

1. Weight gain
2. Peripheral edema
3. Diuresis at rest
4. Vague gastrointestinal complaints

Although it is useful to separate findings into these groups, patients rarely have unilateral failure.[3,14] Within a short time the syndrome progresses to involve both sides of the circulation. Therefore the interview may be the only way of determining the sequence of symptom development, which will aid in identifying the evolution and cause of cardiac failure.

Clinical indicators of left-sided heart failure. Dyspnea, abnormally uncomfortable breathing, is the most common manifestation of left-sided heart failure. Patients may refer to it as breathlessness, difficulty breathing, or trouble catching their breath. It is important to establish its relationship to position and activity. The classical progression is[3]:

1. Exertional dyspnea
2. Orthopnea
3. Paroxysmal nocturnal dyspnea
4. Dyspnea at rest
5. Acute pulmonary edema

The patient should be carefully questioned regarding the presence of dyspnea and the sequence in which it developed. Reconstructing this progression takes patience and persistence on the part of both the patient and the examiner since it often can be traced back over weeks or years. The patient's earliest recollections may be the inability to continue previously tolerated levels of activity. For example, a patient may have changed from two sets of tennis to one set or from 18 holes of golf to 9 holes because of having developed shortness of breath and/or fatigue.

An effort is then made to quantify the level of dysfunction. Questions asked include:

1. How much activity was required to precipitate the discomfort?
2. How much rest was needed to achieve relief?
3. How many pillows are required to sleep comfortably?
4. Describe the position of comfort at rest.
5. How long is one able to tolerate lying flat?
6. How long after retiring does sudden onset dyspnea occur?

Paroxysmal nocturnal dyspnea is characterized by the following behavior. The patient typically describes awakening suddenly with a feeling of smothering, 2 to 5 hours after falling asleep. This is often accompanied by wheezing, apprehension, and profuse perspiration. It is relieved by sitting bolt upright and walking to a window to deeply inhale "fresh air." The symptoms may resolve in 5 to 60 minutes. Quantifying this period is crucial to determining the extent of nocturnal pulmonary congestion.

Cough is another key finding associated with dyspnea of heart failure. It is usually nonproductive, periodic, nocturnal, and irritating.[3] The patient may expectorate scant amounts of clear mucus; however, in severe pulmonary edema, large amounts of pink, frothy sputum are produced.

Dyspnea and cough are also cardinal features of pulmonary disease. As in heart failure, the patient may have progressive respiratory symptoms strongly related to activity. However, in pulmonary disease a history of heavy smoking and chronic productive cough often precedes the onset of dyspnea. There is a morning cough productive of moderate to large amounts of tenacious yellow sputum and relief is more likely achieved through clearing secretions than by changing position.

When the patient has sudden dyspnea, the differential diagnosis should include heart failure resulting from arrhythmias or coronary insufficiency, acute pulmonary insults, and acute anxiety episodes. Dyspnea localized to the midchest is characteristic of coronary insufficiency, while dyspnea of other origins is more diffuse.[13] When acute pulmonary insults such as pneumothorax or pulmonary emboli are suspected, the examination should reveal related subjective and objective findings. Dyspnea caused by anxiety may be accompanied by a primary complaint of fatigue, frequent heavy sighs, and numbness and tingling around the mouth or hands induced by hyperventilation.

A third manifestation of left-sided heart failure is generalized or exertional weakness and fatigue precipitated by decreased perfusion to the muscles. The feeling may be chronic or intermittent and is often associated with a sense of heaviness in the arms and legs. Exercise may precipitate further compromise in perfusion leading to pain in the legs or intermittent claudication, dizziness, hypotension, and finally syncopal episodes.

Decreased cerebral perfusion, often an early finding of low-output heart failure, may lead to subtle uneasiness or restlessness. Chronically ill patients may complain of insomnia, nightmares, or memory loss. As the syndrome progresses, anxiety, agitation, paranoia, fear of impending doom, or frank psychosis may develop.

When tissue perfusion is compromised in severe heart failure, the signs of tachycardia, diaphoresis, pallor, or cyanosis develop. These indicators are overt and observable by both the patient and the examiner.

Clinical indicators of right-sided heart failure. A key finding in patients with right-sided failure is symmetrical dependent peripheral edema that is more pronounced in the evening. As the disease progresses, it ascends from the ankles to the lower leg, thigh, genitalia, and abdominal wall.[13] Although often unaware of swelling in these areas, the patient may have noticed shoes fit more snugly or leave marks on the feet after removal at night. A ring may be more difficult to remove. Clothes may feel tighter or a larger size may be required. The limbs may feel heavy and weak. These indicators of edema may not be recognized unless the interviewer specifically questions the patient about them.

If the patient has generalized rather than dependent ascending edema, it may indicate hypoproteinemia rather than heart failure. This type of edema is often more pronounced in the eyes and face and is worse in the morning, not the evening. Hypoproteinemia is associated with nephrotic syndrome and liver failure. The relationship between peripheral edema and other clinical findings may help determine the cause of edema. For example:

1. If edema and dyspnea coexist and dyspnea preceded edema, either left-sided failure or lung disease is suspected.
2. If edema and dyspnea coexist and the edema occurred first, either right-sided failure or renal disease is suspected.
3. If ascites and edema coexist and ascites occurred first, liver failure is suspected.
4. If ascites and edema coexist and edema occurred first, either cardiac failure or renal failure is suspected.
5. If jaundice is present, accompanied by edema or ascites, liver dysfunction is suspected.
6. If localized extremity edema occurs in the presence of skin ulceration or abnormal pigmentation, chronic arterial and/or venous insufficiency is suspected.

Each of these findings is observable by the patient. Even ascites may be described as a distended abdomen or "protruding stomach." The task is to establish the historical relationship between them.

Weight gain is a related complaint that most people frequently recognize. An adult may retain 10 to 15 pounds (4 to 7 L of fluid) before pitting edema occurs. However, some patients may gain fluid mass while losing tissue mass and not recognize the change until therapy begins and diuresis results in a markedly lower weight.[13]

A second finding related to fluid retention is diuresis at rest. During the day the patient retains fluid and may experience oliguria because of decreased cardiac output and hormonal compensatory response. When rest decreases the body's metabolic requirements, cardiac function improves. This decreases systemic venous pressure, allowing edema fluid to be mobilized and excreted. Although the oliguric phase may go unrecognized, the client is likely to notice the diuretic phase. Significant nocturia or weight loss during periods of rest at night or during sedentary weekends or vacations may be indications of evolving heart failure.

Gastrointestinal symptoms occur in numerous disorders and are often vague and nonspecific. Right ventricular failure may be accompanied by a feeling of abdominal fullness or discomfort resulting from liver engorgement. On occasion, subcostal pain is so severe that an abdominal catastrophe is suspected. Gastrointestinal manifestations may also be caused by left ventricular involvement. Either group may complain of anorexia or nausea. In severe left ventricular failure a small number of patients may develop hemorrhagic enterocolitis because of depressed splanchnic circulation, and therefore they report abdominal pain, distention, and blood in the stool.

Classifying the severity of heart failure. The preceding descriptions of right- and left-sided failure emphasized the progression of symptoms from early to late forms. This knowledge allows the clinician to evaluate the patient's current level of involvement. By comparing it to past assessments, the disease trajectory may be determined.

A scale to classify and communicate the overall condition of patients with heart disease was devised by the New York Heart Association. It has become a standard tool used across the United States. The functional categories are defined as follows[2]:

Class I   No limitations. Ordinary physical activity does not cause undue fatigue, dyspnea, palpitation, or angina.

Class II   Slight limitation of physical activity. Although the patient is comfortable at rest, ordinary physical activity results in symptoms.

Class III   Marked limitation of physical activity. Although the patient is comfortable at rest, less than ordinary activity will lead to symptoms.

Class IV   Inability to carry on any activity without discomfort. Symptoms are present at rest and increase with activity.

Assigning a patient to one of these categories is only a method of summarizing clinical indicators,

following the trend of illness, and facilitating communication among health care professionals.

Determining causes. The successful management of patients with heart failure depends largely on identifying the underlying cause. Diseases leading to heart failure include:

1. Myocardial infarction or angina
2. Hypertension
3. Valvular dysfunction
4. Pericarditis
5. Rheumatic fever
6. Venereal disease
7. Congenital heart disease
8. Anemia
9. Alcoholism
10. Renal failure
11. Lung disease
12. Pulmonary emboli
13. Endocrine disorders: thyroid disease, diabetes mellitus
14. Chromosomal or congenital disorders: Turner's syndrome, Marfan's syndrome
15. Metabolic disorders: hemochromatosis, glycogen storage disease
16. Collagen diseases: lupus erythematosus, rheumatoid arthritis
17. Sarcoidosis
18. Raynaud's disease
19. Paget's disease
20. Muscular dystrophy
21. Systemic infections

Frequently there is a history of more than one underlying cause of heart failure. At other times, there may be no known specific disease but the patient may report earlier examinations that revealed "a heart problem." If the patient has undergone any recent invasive procedures, complications that might cause failure, such as endocarditis or emboli, should be considered.

On occasion heart failure is the first manifestation of coronary artery disease. In these patients the past medical history may be negative, but the social and family history may reveal the presence of several risk factors. They include cigarette smoking, obesity, high cholesterol ingestion, hypertension, stressed or sedentary life-styles, and a family history of cardiovascular disease.

In addition to the underlying cause, precipitating factors must be ascertained. This is especially important when the onset of failure is sudden or when there has been a dramatic change in clinical status.

Any factor that stresses the cardiovascular system or increases the body's metabolic demand in a patient with underlying heart disease may precipitate cardiac failure. This may result from physical, emotional, or environmental stress or from the development of an unrelated disease. The social his-

Table 4-3. Summary of major historical findings in patients with heart failure

Component of health history	Classification of findings	Types of findings	
		Left ventricular failure	Right ventricular failure
Current and past health history (elicited from client)	Cardinal evidence of heart failure	Dyspnea Decreased exercise tolerance Cough Weakness, fatigue Diaphoresis, pallor Alteration in mental status	Peripheral edema Diuresis at rest Weight gain Vague abdominal complaints Nocturia
	Evidence of underlying disease	Chest pain Congenital heart disease Coronary artery disease Chronic pulmonary disease Rheumatic heart disease Hypertension Diabetes mellitus Recent invasive procedures	
	Evidence of precipitating factors	Chest pain of angina, myocardial infarction, pericarditis, pulmonary embolus Palpitations of tachyarrhythmias Noncompliance with treatment regimen Emotional, physical, environmental, financial stress	
Family and social history (elicited from family)	Evidence of underlying disease	Risk factors for coronary artery disease: Obesity High cholesterol ingestion Stressed/sedentary life-style Familial history of cardiovascular disease, hypertension, diabetes mellitus Cigarette smoking Alcohol ingestion	
	Evidence of precipitating factors	Noncompliance to treatment regimen Major life-style change Sources of emotional, physical, environmental, financial stress	

tory may be helpful in revealing other sources of stress, and the review of systems may reveal symptoms of non-cardiac-related diseases.

A common trigger for cardiac decompensation is tachyarrhythmias and bradyarrhythmias. Although many patients are unaware of moderately slow rhythms, rapid rhythms frequently cause palpitations. Patients should be asked whether throbbing or fluttering sensations in the chest accompany symptoms of chest pain, breathlessness, dizziness, weakness, and fatigue.

In the patient with a history of controlled heart failure, the exacerbation of symptoms may be related to noncompliance with the treatment regimen. This factor frequently goes unrecognized in individuals. In such instances attention to nonverbal clues when discussing the medication history and establishing open lines of communication are helpful.

Coronary artery disease can either cause or precipitate heart failure; therefore patients may have manifestations of angina or myocardial infarction in addition to those of failure. The diagnosis is facilitated when they experience the classic crushing, radiating, substernal chest pain. If the pain is less severe or atypical, the patient may not recognize its importance or report it. When reviewing the present medical history, the examiner is well advised to question the patient about epigastric, arm, neck, or jaw pain that may be related to cardiac ischemia.

Although the range of possible underlying causes and precipitating events is extensive, they are paramount to accurate assessment of the total clinical picture. (Table 4-3 has a summary of pertinent historical findings.) Once identified, treatment can be more specific and more effective.

Selected aspects of the physical examination

Physical examination of the patient with heart failure focuses on the cardiovascular and pulmonary systems. This section emphasizes techniques used to evaluate these two systems and concludes with a description of relevant aspects of gastro-intestinal and skin assessment. In each section findings associated with heart failure are stressed.

CARDIOVASCULAR EVALUATION

Knowledge of the anatomy directs physical assessment. The first step of cardiac assessment is to visualize key landmarks and identify normal heart size and position. The thorax has several bony structures that facilitate very precise descriptions (Fig. 4-1).

About two thirds of the heart lies to the left of the sternum. The right cardiac border runs from the third to the sixth rib along the right sternal border and is mainly comprised of the right atrium and a portion of the right ventricle. The inferior cardiac border sits on the diaphragm, primarily consists of the right ventricle, and extends from the right sternal border at the sixth rib to the fifth intercostal space, midclavicular line. The left cardiac border runs from this point upward and inward to the junction of the second rib at the left sternal border. It is formed by the left ventricle and a superior segment of the left atria (Fig. 4-2).

Inspection of the precordium

To inspect the precordium, the examiner should have the patient lie in the supine position. Standing on the right, the examiner looks across the patient's chest. A bright, mobile light directed tangentially will cast shadows across the chest wall and make subtle findings more visible. Movement may be magnified by placing a pencil, a tongue blade, or the stethoscope over the area and watching it move freely.

In about one half of the adult population, the apical pulse can be seen in or above the left fifth intercostal space just medial to the midclavicular line. It is normally the lowest and most lateral impulse in the chest. Although commonly referred to as the point of maximal impulse (PMI), this term is best avoided since the apical pulsation is not always the largest.

The motion is characterized by a faint lift or heave. This may be associated with retraction of

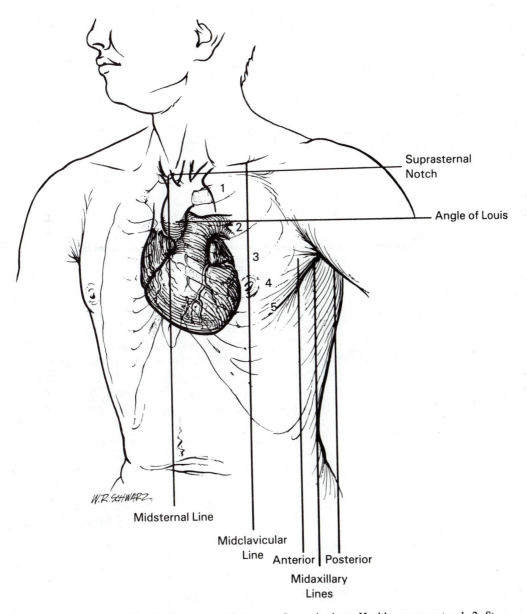

Fig. 4-1. Chest wall landmarks. (From Malasanos, L., and others: Health assessment, ed. 2, St. Louis, 1981, The C.V. Mosby Co.)

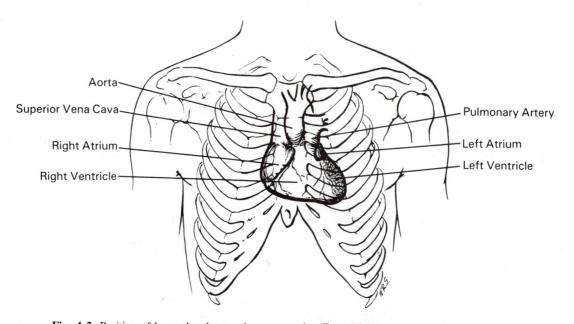

Fig. 4-2. Position of heart chambers and great vessels. (From Malasanos, L., and others: Health assessment, ed. 2, St. Louis, 1981, The C.V. Mosby Co.)

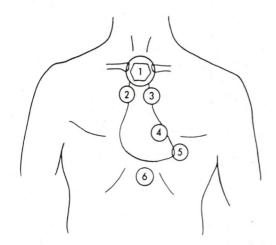

Fig. 4-3. Areas on anterior chest wall that should be routinely palpated. *1,* Sternoclavicular area; *2,* second right intercostal space; *3,* second left intercostal space; *4,* left parasternal area (right ventricular area); *5,* Apical area; *6,* epigastric area. (From Goldberger, E.: Textbook of clinical cardiology, St. Louis, 1982, The C.V. Mosby Co.)

the left lower sternal border. Both movements may be exaggerated in hyperdynamic states and diminished by obesity or increased anteroposterior chest diameter caused by chronic pulmonary disease.[10]

Any motion other than those associated with the apical impulse is abnormal. Increased right ventricular work may result in a diffuse lift seen along the left sternal border, and in severe failure the lower sternum may move outward with each heartbeat. Pulsations seen above the precordium to the left or right of the sternum are abnormal and may indicate pulmonary or systemic hypertension. Epigastric pulsations are normal in some thin individuals and are reflections of the aortic pulse.

Palpation of the precordium

In approximately half of the normal adult population, an apical impulse may be visualized and palpated with a faint, localized tap 2 to 3 cm in diameter at the fifth intercostal space medial to the midclavicular line. It occurs momentarily at the onset of systole. If it is difficult to palpate, the patient may be repositioned from a supine to a high Fowler's or a left lateral position to bring the apex closer to the chest wall. This improves palpation but alters the amplitude and location of impulses (Fig. 4-3).

In heart failure changes in the apical impulse are most frequently associated with left ventricular hypertrophy and dilation.[4] In hyperdynamic states accompanied by elevated diastolic volume, the impulse amplitude increases and is described as a quick thrust followed by retraction. As heart failure progresses and left ventricular enlargement is more pronounced, the impulse duration also increases and is described as a sustained localized, forceful, outward systolic movement. If accompanied by left parasternal retraction, it may be palpated as a rocking motion over the apex. This effect may be perceived if one finger is placed lightly over each of these areas.

In patients with chronic congestive heart failure, the degree of impulse displacement correlates with cardiac size.[7] Cardiac enlargement resulting from elevated pressure load causes an increase in muscle mass and a decrease in compliance. This is reflected by a more forceful, localized impulse that is not markedly displaced. Cardiac enlargement resulting from volume load causes ventricular dilation with little change in compliance. This is reflected by a more diffuse impulse that is displaced downward to the left, and palpation may be performed over the fifth and sixth intercostal spaces.

Right ventricular hypertrophy secondary to left ventricular failure is characterized by a palpable outward impulse along the left sternal border extending from the third to fifth intercostal space. It may be accompanied by an outward movement of the sternum. It is described as a diffuse, brisk, outward early systolic movement located over the left sternal border. Right ventricular failure resulting from tricuspid and/or pulmonary valvular dysfunction or from chronic pulmonary disease causes primary right ventricular hypertrophy. This is characterized by a diffuse lifting pansystolic impulse located along the lower left sternal border; it is frequently associated with pulsation of the pulmonary arteries if there is increased pulmonary blood flow.

The other areas to be palpated are the specific sites where the four valves project their vibrations[10] (Fig. 4-4). They are:

1. The mitral area: fifth left intercostal space medial to the midclavicular line
2. The tricuspid area: fourth left intercostal space at the sternal border
3. The aortic area: second right intercostal space at the sternal border
4. The pulmonary area: first or second left intercostal space at the sternal border

The easiest way to remember these areas is to visualize the heart positioned in the chest and keep in mind that the sound vibrations are like waves that are projected from the valve to the chest in the direction of blood flow. Thus the aortic valve is more to the left but faces the right shoulder. The pulmonic valve is more to the right but faces the left shoulder. The louder the sound, the farther it is projected in that direction.

Many valvular disorders precipitate heart failure and cause abnormal vibrations that are audible as murmurs or palpable as thrills. Palpation is a useful technique to evaluate these vibrations. It also supplements assessment of cardiac status. Thrills are sometimes very subtle, especially when the murmurs are high pitched. To maximize detection, three fingers are placed across one area and left long enough to identify and concentrate on each phase of the cardiac cycle. Mitral and tricuspid thrills may be enhanced with the patient in the left lateral decubitus position. Aortic and pulmonary thrills are more easily evaluated with the patient seated and leaning forward.

The more severe the valvular dysfunction, the more intense the vibration, and the greater the distance it radiates away from the valve. The aortic valve may project its sounds as far as the right neck and shoulder, the pulmonic valve to the left neck and shoulder, the mitral to the left axilla, and the

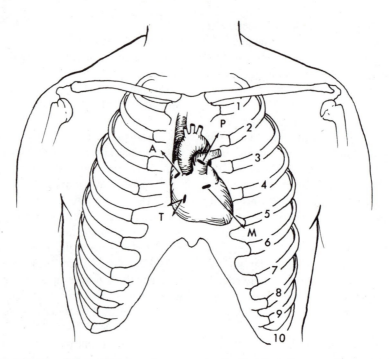

Fig. 4-4. Anatomic and auscultatory valve areas. Anatomic valve areas are represented by solid bars. Arrows show transmission routes of valves to their respective auscultatory sites. *A,* Aortic valve; *P,* pulmonary valve; *M,* mitral valve; *T,* tricuspid valve. (From Papenhausen, J.: Cardiovascular and respiratory assessment for critical care practitioners. In Boarman, C.A., and others: Current practice in critical care, vol. 1, St. Louis, 1979, The C.V. Mosby Co.)

tricuspid to the epigastric areas. When thrills are palpable, the projected distance and the area of maximal intensity should be recorded and related to the phase of the cardiac cycle in which they occur (systole or diastole).

Gallops may be palpated as extra discrete pulsations felt immediately before or after the apical impulse. They may be found over the left sternal border or the apex, depending on the ventricle involved. Both murmurs and gallops are key findings in patients with heart failure.[3,13,14] Because the primary means for evaluating them is auscultation, a description is included in the next section.

Percussion of the precordium

This technique may be used to outline the cardiac silhouette. However, because of the bony structures surrounding the heart, more accurate information regarding heart size and tissue density is available from cardiac roentgenography (Chapter 5).

Auscultation of the precordium

Cardiac auscultation requires a thorough knowledge of the physiological origins of normal heart sounds, a systematic approach to assessment, and an understanding of the significance of abnormal sounds. The examiner is severely limited unless all three skills are developed.

Origins of heart sounds. Normal blood flow through the cardiovascular system is silent except when cardiac contraction causes abrupt acceleration and deceleration of blood flow.[2] The vibrations produced create sound waves transmitted through the chest wall that are detected through a stethoscope. These sounds are described using the following criteria:

1. Pitch or frequency
2. Loudness or intensity
3. Quality or distinguishing characteristics
4. Duration
5. Timing in the cardiac cycle

Heart sounds are created by cardiac contraction; therefore they may be learned, identified, and evaluated by visualizing their relationship to electrical and mechanical cardiac events (Fig. 4-5). Generally, soft sounds are created by acceleration of blood flow through open valves, and louder sounds result from abrupt deceleration when valves close.

Normally no sounds are audible during most of diastole when both the atria and the ventricles are relaxed, the mitral and tricuspid valves are open, and the aortic and pulmonic valves are closed. At the termination of ventricular diastole, the first recorded electrical event, atrial depolarization, causes the first mechanical response, atrial contraction. As a result, blood flow accelerates through open atrioventricular (AV) valves causing a soft, late diastolic vibration called the fourth heart sound (S_4). It may be visualized on the phonocardiogram but is normally too soft to be heard unless amplified (Fig. 4-5).

The second recorded electrical event is ventricular depolarization followed by the mechanical event, ventricular contraction. During this phase all four valves change position. As the AV pressure gradient drops below the ventricular-arterial gradient, the mitral and tricuspid valves close, causing abrupt deceleration of blood flow into the ventricles. This in turn generates vibrations that produce a loud first heart sound (S_1). This marks the beginning of ventricular systole and is the first sound in the cardiac cycle that may be heard without amplification. The phonocardiogram diminishes with opening of the aortic and pulmonary valves because of acceleration of blood across the open valves into the pulmonary arteries and aorta (Fig. 4-5, *Component c*).

The third recorded electrical event is ventricular

depolarization. As the ventricles relax the ventricular-arterial pressure gradient drops below the AV gradient and the aortic and pulmonary valves close. The blood flow into the pulmonary arteries and aorta abruptly decelerates, generating vibrations that produce a loud second heart sound (S_2). This marks the end of ventricular systole and is the second sound in the cardiac cycle that may be heard without amplification.

Following S_2 there is a brief delay when all valves are closed. This is referred to as isovolumetric relaxation. As venous blood fills the atria, the AV pressure gradient falls below the ventricular-arterial gradient, allowing the mitral and tricuspid valves to open. Blood flow accelerates across the open AV valves, producing a soft third heart sound (S_3). This sound is associated with the rapid diastolic filling phase and is normally not audible. As diastolic filling slows, atrial depolarization is initiated and the cardiac cycle is repeated.

To summarize, S_1 is caused primarily by closure of the mitral and tricuspid valves and S_2 by the closure of the aortic and pulmonary valves. They are loud systolic vibrations that are the only sounds normally heard in adults over the age of 30. S_3 and S_4 are soft diastolic vibrations. S_3 occurs in early diastole because of rapid acceleration of blood flow across open AV valves. When this sound is heard in healthy children and young adults, it is considered normal and is termed a physiological S_3. S_4 occurs in late diastole as the atria begin contraction and is rarely audible in normal subjects.

Each sound is created by similar events on each side of the heart. Since mechanical events of the left ventricle are stronger and slightly precede those of the right, the aortic and mitral components are louder and occur just before the pulmonary and tricuspid components. The separation of S_1 usually is too small to perceive; however, a normal separation of S_2 may be audible during inspiration.

A split S_2 results from decreased intrathoracic pressure that augments venous return to the right ventricle, prolonging right ventricular ejection and delaying pulmonary valve closure. The magnified difference in timing becomes audible as a "stud-

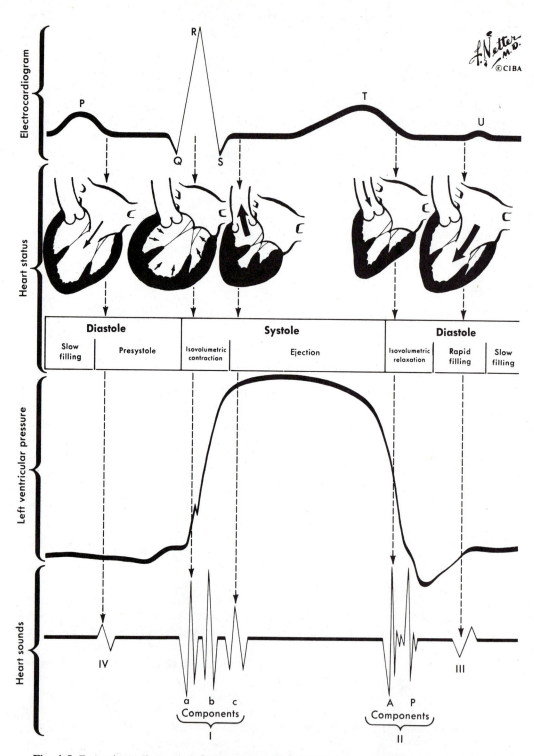

Fig. 4-5. Events in cardiac cycle. (© Copyright 1973 CIBA Pharmaceutical Company Division of CIBA-GEIGY Corporation. Reproduced with permission from the CIBA COLLECTION OF MEDICAL ILLUSTRATIONS by Frank H. Netter, M.D. All rights reserved.)

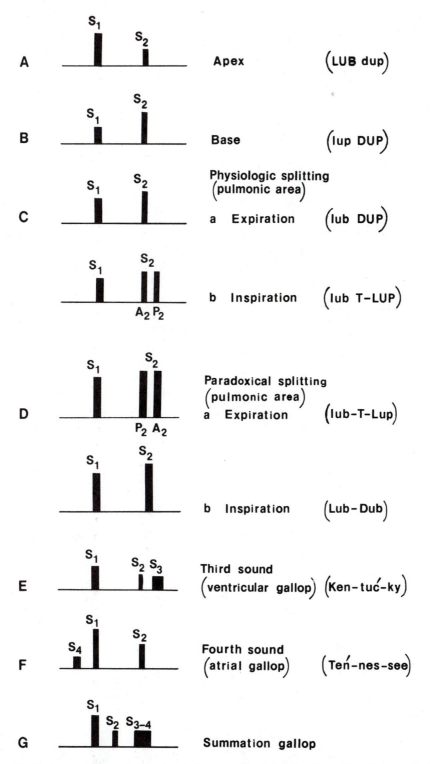

Fig. 4-6. Timing sequence of normal and abnormal heart sounds. (From Papenhausen, J.: Cardiovascular and respiratory assessment for critical care practitioners. In Boarman, C.A., and others: Current practice in critical care, vol. 1, St. Louis, 1979, The C.V. Mosby Co.)

der'' and is described as a split heart sound (Fig. 4-6). There are many causes of asynchronous right and left heart sounds; however, the most common split heard in normal subjects is a split S_2 during inspiration.

Systematic auscultation. Many abnormal heart sounds are soft and transient. In order to hear these subtle sounds, the examination must be conducted in a quiet environment using a carefully selected and properly fitted stethoscope. The patient should be placed in a supine position and draped to allow evaluation of the same four basic areas assessed during palpation; the aortic, the pulmonary, the mitral or left ventricular, and the tricuspid or right ventricular (Figs. 4-3 and 4-4).

Each area is auscultated with the bell and diaphragm. The diaphragm is designed to pick up high-pitched sounds like S_1 and S_2, and the bell detects low-pitched sounds such as S_3 and S_4 murmurs.[10] Care must be taken not to apply pressure to the bell since the taut skin beneath converts it to a diaphragm.

After applying the stethoscope to the chest, the first step is to identify S_1 and S_2. If the heart rate is slow, the distinction is easily made. Since systole is shorter than diastole, there is less time between S_1 and S_2 than between S_2 and the next S_1. When the heart rate is rapid, the difference between the two phases diminishes and other methods must be used to distinguish these sounds.

The following guidelines are useful:
1. S_1 has a slightly longer duration and lower pitch than S_2 (Fig. 4-5).
2. S_1 is caused by mitral and tricuspid closure and therefore is usually the loudest sound heard at the apex and along the left sternal border (Figs. 4-4 and 4-6).
3. S_2 is caused by aortic and pulmonary closure and is louder over the aortic and pulmonic region (Figs. 4-4 and 4-6).
4. Since S_1 marks the onset of systole, it corresponds with the upstroke of the carotid pulse and the QRS complex on the ECG (Fig. 4-5).

After identifying S_1, the examiner focuses atten- tion on each phase of the cardiac cycle, listening to systole (between S_1 and S_2) and to diastole (between S_2 and the next S_1). In order to clearly delineate normal and abnormal sounds, this should be performed at all four valve areas with the bell and the diaphragm.

Abnormal findings. The normal adult findings include a first heart sound (S_1), a second heart sound (S_2), and a split S_2 in the recumbent position that disappears when the individual is upright.[2,10] When other vibrations are heard, they may be evidence of pathological heart function underlying or precipitating heart failure. These sounds may be evaluated by using the following criteria:
1. Sound intensity
2. Area of maximal intensity
3. Position of maximal intensity
4. Relationship to cardiac cycle
5. Relationship to respiratory cycle

S_2 is loudest in the aortic or pulmonary areas; however, right-sided sounds are usually quieter than left-sided heart sounds, which accounts for the softer pulmonary component. To maximize the probability of hearing a split S_2, the examiner listens carefully at the pulmonary area along the high left sternal border at the second to fourth intercostal space and focuses on the relationship of the sound to the respiratory cycle.

Persistent splitting of S_2 (Fig. 4-6). Most patients with a history of heart failure and an audible expiratory split S_2 in both the recumbent and the upright positions are suspect of underlying heart disease.[3] Conditions that lead to persistent splitting of S_2 during both inspiration and expiration are characterized by either a delayed pulmonary component (P_2) or an early aortic component (A_2). When P_2 occurs late it may reflect delayed right ventricular activation secondary to complete right bundle branch block, left ventricular ectopy, or artificial left ventricular pacemaker. A late P_2 may also reflect prolonged right ventricular ejection time resulting from severe right ventricular failure when the ventricle is unable to accommodate elevated venous return, or it may result from pressure overload in pulmonary stenosis or pulmonary embolism. An early aortic component accounts for persistent split S_2 in mitral regurgitation, ventricular septal defects, and massive pulmonary embolism with reduced left ventricular stroke volume.

Paradoxical splitting of S_2 (Fig. 4-6, *D*). Paradoxical splitting of S_2 occurs when a wider split is heard during the expiratory phase of respiration. This occurs when the right ventricle empties before the left and may result from a delayed aortic component or an early pulmonary component. A late A_2 occurs secondary to delayed left ventricular activation and contraction in left bundle branch blocks, right ventricular ectopy, and right ventricular pacemakers. It also accompanies prolonged left ventricular emptying caused by elevated end-diastolic volume of left ventricular failure, coronary artery disease, myocardial ischemia, and myocardial infarction. Other conditions that selectively overload the left ventricle, delaying aortic closure, include valvular aortic stenosis, aortic regurgitation, and severe hypertension.

A rare cause of paradoxical split S_2 is early pulmonary closure resulting from early electrical activation of the right ventricle in type B Wolff-Parkinson-White syndrome.

Gallop rhythms. Third and fourth heart sounds are normally low-pitched, soft diastolic vibrations related to rapid ventricular filling. S_3 occurs early in diastole with the opening of the mitral and tricuspid valves. S_4 occurs late in diastole at the onset of atrial contraction when blood briefly accelerates across the AV valves before they close. Conditions that increase end-diastolic volume and decrease ventricular compliance create resistance to filling that may amplify these vibrations, making them audible as discrete, thudlike sounds called "gallops." The "ventricular diastolic gallop" refers to a pathological third heart sound, and the "atrial presystolic gallop" describes a pathological fourth heart sound. Heart failure secondary to mechanical or functional cardiac disease is the most common condition associated with these gallop rhythms.

Recognition of these sounds requires evaluation using the same criteria previously outlined. The normal heartbeat is described as S_1-lub, S_2-dub.

When a ventricular gallop is present, it is classically described as "lub-dubby," S_1-S_2S_3, and sounds like Ken-tuc-ky[2] (Fig. 4-6, *E*). Musically, it is akin to one half note followed by two quarter notes.

When the S_3 gallop originates in the left ventricle, it is best auscultated using the bell placed over the apex with the patient in the left lateral decubitus position. When S_3 originates in the right ventricle because of right-sided heart disease and failure, it is most audible at the xiphoid or lower left sternal border and may become louder during inspiration because of augmented venous return. Although an S_3 may be differentiated as "right" or "left," the left heart sound predominates and is closely associated with elevated left ventricular filling pressures, left atrial pressures, and pulmonary artery pressures. It may also be detected in high-output failure when diastolic blood velocity and flow across the mitral valve is markedly elevated.

A pathological fourth heart sound or atrial presystolic gallop is a low-pitched sound detected immediately before the onset of systole. It adds an extra vibration just before S_1, is classically described as "delub-dub," S_4-S_1-S_2, and sounds like Ten-nes-see.[2] Musically, it is akin to two quarter notes followed by one half note (Fig. 4-6, *F*).

S_4 is generally difficult to recognize. A right-sided atrial gallop is usually louder on inspiration and may be heard over the left lower sternal border with the patient positioned supine. A left-sided atrial gallop is usually louder on expiration and is heard over the apex with the patient in the left lateral decubitus position. An atrial gallop may be differentiated from a split S_1 because it is heard only with the bell while the high-pitched ejection sounds, S_1 and S_2, are heard with the diaphragm.

The clinical implication of an audible S_4 remains questionable; however, it is generally accepted that atrial gallops are related to decreased ventricular compliance and are not heard in normal subjects. They are often detected in patients with hypertensive cardiac disease, cardiomyopathy, aortic stenosis, and idiopathic hypertrophic subaortic stenosis (IHSS). Furthermore, they are frequently heard in persons with coronary artery disease, acute myocardial infarction, and acute attacks of angina pectoris.

When both S_3 and S_4 diastolic filling sounds are present, a quadruple rhythm may be heard that is described as "delub-dubby," S_4S_1-S_2S_3, and sounds like Ten-ne-tuc-ky.[2] As heart rate increases, S_3 and S_4 merge, producing a single mid-diastolic sound that is louder than S_3 or S_4 alone. This is called a summation gallop and is described as three equally spaced "thuds," lub-dub-dud (Fig. 4-6, *G*).

To auscultate a summation gallop, the clinician places the patient in the left lateral position and holds the bell lightly over the apex at the point of maximal impulse. This rhythm is a characteristic of advanced heart failure.

Murmurs. Murmurs are extraneous abnormal vibrations caused by turbulent blood flow related to narrowed openings restricting forward flow, incomplete valve closure allowing backward flow, or incompetent or irregular vessel walls and high flow rates[2] (Figs. 4-7 and 4-8). The distinguishing characteristics of a murmur include location, timing, duration, pitch, and intensity.

The specific anatomical location should be esti-mated and it should be determined whether the murmur is confined to a fixed area or radiates to other sites on the chest wall. For example, aortic valve dysfunction is generally most easily auscultated at the second left intercostal space with radiation into the neck and down the left sternal border. Mitral dysfunction may be loudest over the apex with radiation into the axilla.

Timing is described by determining the position of the murmur during systole (between S_1 and S_2) and diastole (between S_2 and S_1). The position of the murmur in the cardiac cycle offers further evidence of its origin and may be predicated on the following criteria:

1. A murmur beginning with S_1 is initiated by mitral or tricuspid closure and is usually related to mitral or tricuspid insufficiency.
2. A murmur beginning just after S_1 is initiated by aortic and pulmonary opening and is usually related to aortic or pulmonary disorders.
3. A murmur beginning with S_2 is initiated with aortic and pulmonary closure and is usually related to aortic or pulmonary insufficiency.
4. A murmur beginning just after S_2 is initiated by mitral and tricuspid opening and is usually related to mitral or tricuspid disorders.

The duration describes how long the murmur

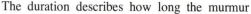
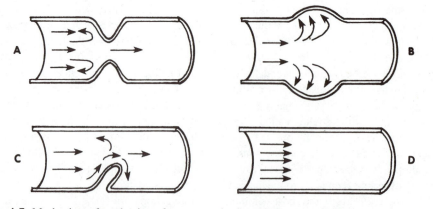

Fig. 4-7. Mechanism of production of murmurs. **A,** Constriction of wall. **B,** Dilation of wall. **C,** Partial impediment of flow, such as that caused by taut membrane. **D,** Increased blood flow (represented by multiple arrows). (From Papenhausen, J.: Cardiovascular and respiratory assessment for critical care practitioners. In Boarman, C.A., and others: Current practice in critical care, vol. 1, St. Louis, 1979, The C.V. Mosby Co.)

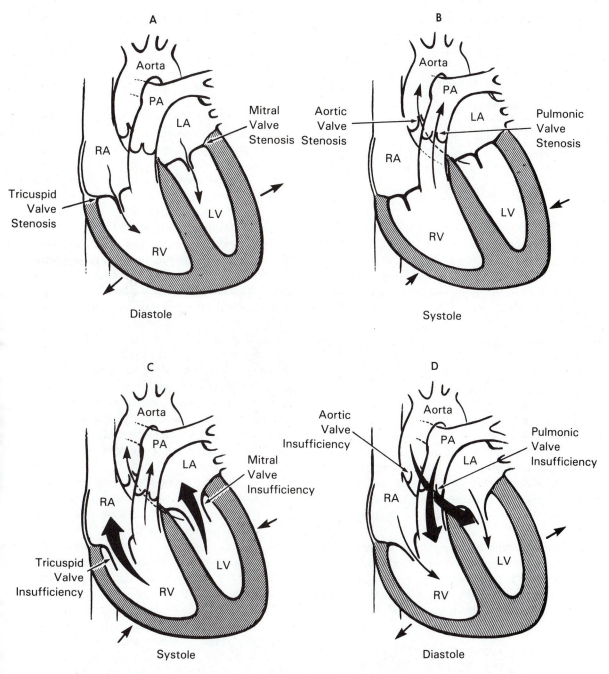

Fig. 4-8. A, Mitral or tricuspid valve stenosis produces diastolic murmur. **B,** Aortic or pulmonary valve stenosis produces systolic murmur. **C,** Mitral or tricuspid valve insufficiency produces systolic murmur. **D,** Aortic or pulmonary valve insufficiency produces diastolic murmur. (From Malasanos, L., and others: Health assessment, ed. 2, St. Louis, 1981, The C.V. Mosby Co.)

lasts during each phase of the cardiac cycle. Murmurs may be continuous throughout the cycle, continuous within a phase of the cycle, or intermittent within a phase of the cycle.[15] They are classically described using the following terms:

Continuous murmur S_1———S_2———S_1

Continuous within a phase
Pansystolic, holosystolic S_1———S_2———S_1

Pandiastolic, holodiastolic S_1———S_2———S_1

Intermittent within a phase
Early systolic S_1———+·—+——S_2

Midsystolic S_1——+——+——S_2

Late systolic S_1——+——+——S_2

Early diastolic S_2——+——+——S_1

Mid-diastolic S_2——+——+——S_1

Late diastolic S_2——+——+——S_1

Each murmur is also evaluated for pitch and quality. Low pitch has a low blowing quality and high pitch has a high whistling quality. Other terms used to describe sound characteristics include "harsh," "rumbling," "grating," and "humming."

Intensity reflects the audibility of the murmur and is closely associated with visual and palpable pulsations. Furthermore, the intensity of a murmur is proportional to the degree of underlying cardiac abnormality and is graded by the following scale:

Grade I	Very faint, heard by experts
Grade II	Faint, but audible with focused concentration
Grade III	Moderately audible, may radiate, not associated with a thrill
Grade IV	Easily audible, may be associated with a thrill
Grade V	Very audible, associated with a thrill, may be heard with the stethoscope lightly touching the chest wall
Grade VI	May be auscultated with the stethoscope off the chest wall, associated with a thrill and marked vascular radiation

The intensity variance of a prolonged murmur may also be described. A crescendo murmur becomes progressively louder in a cycle; a decrescendo murmur becomes progressively softer in a cycle; a crescendo/decrescendo or decrescendo/crescendo murmur is one that varies intensity from loud to soft or soft to loud.

Sound intensity is also related to the extent of radiation and to the respiratory cycle. The louder the murmur, the greater the distance it radiates. When a grade III murmur is auscultated, its area of maximal intensity is localized and the stethoscope is then inched away from that point in the direction of valve projection until the sound can no longer be heard (Fig. 4-4). The relationship of a murmur intensity to the respiratory cycle is used to differentiate left from right-sided murmurs in the same way it is used to differentiate gallops.

When all evaluation criteria are properly used, descriptions of murmurs facilitate diagnosis of disease contributing to heart failure (Table 4-4). The following statements illustrate correct documentation of heart murmurs:

1. A grade III high-pitched, harsh pansystolic murmur heard best at the apex, radiating to the left axilla, enhanced on expiration, and accompanied by a thrill
2. A grade II low-pitched, inspiratory mid-diastolic murmur not associated with a thrill, heard at the left sternal border, fourth intercostal space, with the client supine

Pericardial friction rubs. This finding is classified as extracardiac and is described as a rubbing or scratching sound produced when the pericardial sac becomes inflamed. Generally, these sounds are high pitched and may vary in intensity with the respiratory cycle and position change. They may be localized or general to all auscultatory areas and will change in a matter of hours or days. Pericardial friction rubs detected in persons with heart

failure indicate underlying related cardiac abnormalities. It is a common indicator of pericarditis from postmyocardial infarction and is also
a frequent postsurgical finding in individuals who
have undergone corrective cardiac procedures.

**Clinical significance of auscultatory findings
in heart failure.** Cardiac auscultation is one of the
most sensitive assessment tools for evaluating individuals with heart failure. As noted, this syndrome may alter normal heart sounds, add extra

Table 4-4. Heart murmurs

Murmur	Area (radiation)	Timing	Quality
Innocent systolic ejec- tional murmur	Upper left sternal border	Midsystolic	Increased in supine position Medium pitch Low grade Blowing
Mitral insufficiency	Apex (left axilla)	Pansystolic	Harsh, low
Tricuspid insufficiency	Lower left sternal border (right sternal border)	Pansystolic	Harsh Increase on inspiration
Aortic stenosis	Right sternal border (radiates widely)	Systolic ejection (after S_1 to before S_2)	Crescendo/decrescendo Harsh
Pulmonary stenosis	Left sternal border at second rib (left neck)	Systolic ejection Sound (click)	Crescendo/decrescendo Harsh Increase intensity and increase S_2 split on inspiration
Intraventricular septal defect	Left sternal border	Pansystolic	Heard all over the pre- cordium
Coarctation of aorta	Left midback	Systolic ejection	Increased on inspiration with patient leaning forward
Pericardial friction rub	Mesocardiac area		Scratching sound close to ear
Mitral stenosis	Apex	Mid-diastolic or presystolic (may start with snap)	Faint Increase by lying on left side Not affected by inspiration May have opening snap
Tricuspid stenosis	Left sternal border at fourth rib (apex, xiphoid)	Mid-diastolic	May increase on inspiration Rumbling decrescendo May have opening snap
Aortic insufficiency	Left sternal border at third and fourth ribs and 2 right sternal border	Pandiastolic but ends pre-S_1	Blowing, faint, high pitched Decrescendo Increases on leaning forward
Pulmonary insufficiency	Left sternal border at second rib (toward apex)	Early or pan- diastolic	Decrescendo High pitched, blowing May increase on inspiration
Patent ductus arteriosus	Left sternal border at second rib (neck)	Continuous	Harsh

heart sounds, and be accompanied by abnormal sounds indicating underlying cardiac disease or altered cardiac function. The most common aberration of normal heart sounds secondary to cardiac failure is an altered S_2.[3,13,14] In established left ventricular failure, elevated pulmonary artery pressure may cause more abrupt pulmonary valve closure and enhance that component of S_2. Similarly, elevated pulmonary artery pressure increases impedance to right ventricular ejection, thereby decreasing the effects of inspiration on venous return, causing a persistent, audible expiratory splitting of S_2.

One of the earliest auscultated findings in heart failure is a faint, persistent S_3. As the syndrome evolves, accompanied by elevated end-diastolic volume and decreased compliance, the gallop becomes persistent and palpable. When both the atria and the ventricles are affected, an S_3 and S_4 are audible as a quadruple rhythm, and when accompanied by compensatory tachycardia, they fuse to produce the summation gallop characteristic of advanced heart failure.

Gallop rhythms may also be excellent indicators of the effectiveness of clinical therapeutics.[13] Following the initiation of treatment, the clinician often detects a decrease or disappearance of the extra sounds as early evidence of diminished ventricular load. To realize the full potential of gallops as clinical indicators of the development and resolution of heart failure, it is essential to carefully document all available evaluation criteria.

Heart failure is a frequent symptom of valvular disorders. Murmurs characteristic of pulmonary and tricuspid dysfunction are frequently associated with chronic right ventricular failure, whereas murmurs characteristic of aortic or mitral dysfunction may be associated with acute and chronic left ventricular failure (Table 4-4). Of particular importance is the sudden onset of left ventricular failure secondary to acute anteroseptal infarction associated with a holosystolic murmur. This may indicate severe mitral regurgitation caused by papillary muscle dysfunction or septal rupture caused by severe septal ischemia or infarction.

However, heart failure may also precipitate the onset of regurgitant murmurs. This occurs when cardiac dilation enlarges the valve orifices preventing close approximation of the leaflets. The differential diagnosis is made when the murmur disappears as heart failure resolves.

Examination of blood vessels

Veins

Inspection of venous pulses. Inspection of the neck veins provides valuable data in assessment of heart failure. For proper visualization, the examiner places the patient in a supine position with the neck and upper thorax exposed and the head supported on a small pillow. Both sides are examined; however, the veins on the right are often easier to visualize because of their direct anatomical proximity to the right atrium.

Generally, the most pronounced vessels are the external jugular veins, but their relationship to central venous pressure is dampened because of the semilunar valves. The internal jugular veins are deeper and more difficult to locate but are a more direct reflection of venous pressure. A light directed tangentially across the chest may cause shadows that improve their visibility (Fig. 4-9).

If the venous pressure is elevated, accompanied by engorged vessels, or if the patient is uncomfortable, the head of the bed may be slightly elevated. If the venous pressure is low, the veins may be difficult to locate with the patient supine. To ensure that the vessels are collapsed and not hidden by the anatomy, the examiner may occlude the vein by applying pressure at the point where the vessel disappears under the clavicle. Blood collects in the vein distal to that point, distending the vessel and confirming the existence of low venous pressure.

It is often difficult to distinguish between jugular venous and carotid arterial pulsations because of their close anatomical proximity. This may be facilitated if the examiner is cognizant of the following differentiating features[10]:

1. The normal venous pulsations are diffuse and have three waves, *a, c,* and *y;* the carotid is localized and has one wave.
2. The jugular vein is compressed by minimal pressure; the carotid artery is not.

3. Venous pulsations are obliterated by pressure over the superior aspect of the internal jugular near the jaw; the carotid artery is not.
4. Venous pulsations can be decreased by inspiration and elevating the head of the bed; the carotid pulse is not affected.
5. When one carotid is palpated, the opposite side is observed. If pulsation corresponds with what is being palpated, the pulse is arterial. If not, it is generally venous.

When the neck veins have been identified, they become a valuable source of data in assessing heart failure. Three major goals of this part of the physical examination are:

1. To evaluate the specific types of pulsations as reflections of cardiac function
2. To estimate the central venous pressure by quantifying the degree of distention
3. To observe for a hepatojugular reflux as a key manifestation of right ventricular dysfunction

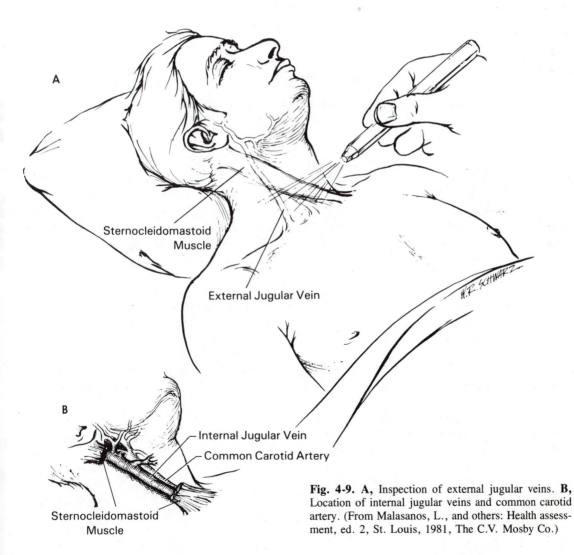

Fig. 4-9. A, Inspection of external jugular veins. **B,** Location of internal jugular veins and common carotid artery. (From Malasanos, L., and others: Health assessment, ed. 2, St. Louis, 1981, The C.V. Mosby Co.)

Sternocleidomastoid Muscle

External Jugular Vein

Internal Jugular Vein

Common Carotid Artery

Sternocleidomastoid Muscle

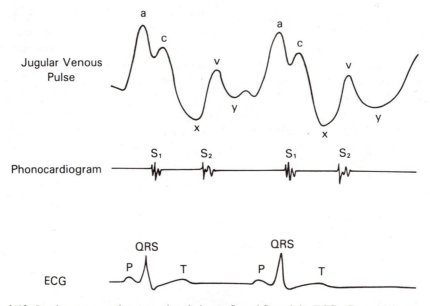

Fig. 4-10. Jugular venous pulse waves in relation to S_1 and S_2 and the ECG. (From Malasanos, L., and others: Health assessment, ed. 2, St. Louis, 1981, The C.V. Mosby Co.)

Evaluation of pulse waves. The normal jugular pulsations are diagrammed in Fig. 4-10. They are reflections of pressure changes in the right atrium and consist of three positive waves *(a, c,* and *v)* and two descents *(x* and *y).*[10]

The *a* wave is normally the largest positive contour and reflects backflow of blood into surrounding veins during atrial systole. It appears as the venous pulsation seen just before the carotid pulse is felt as the first heart sound is heard and may be identified by simultaneously palpating the carotid pulse on the opposite side or by auscultating the heart while observing the neck veins. If the patient is being monitored, the *a* wave may be identified as the impulse occurring immediately after the P wave of the electrocardiogram (Fig. 4-10).

The *c* wave is a reflection of both a carotid percussion wave against the vein and the bulging of the tricuspid leaflets back into the atria during early ventricular systole. It follows the *a* wave but is smaller in amplitude and therefore difficult to visualize (Fig. 4-10).

The tricuspid valve remains closed until well into ventricular diastole, which causes the right atria to fill and its pressure to rise. These events create the *v* wave, which may be visualized as it peaks just after the second heart sound (Fig. 4-9).

The descents are more easily visualized because they are more rapid and abrupt. The *x* descent follows the *c* wave and occurs just before S_2. It results from both the downward movement of the base of the heart during systole and atrial diastole. The *y* descent follows the *v* wave and occurs just after S_2. It coincides with the opening of the tricuspid valve (Fig. 4-10).

Learning the origin of these wave forms helps the clinician to understand alterations that result from pathological conditions causing heart failure. In right-sided failure the high ventricular filling pressures cause more abrupt tricuspid closure with resultant *c* waves.[10] When associated with ventricular dilation and mild tricuspid insufficiency, the backflow of blood across the valve during systole causes large *v* waves. As the right ventricular failure progresses, the *c* and *v* waves become more prominent and the *y* descent more abrupt. Eventually they blend together to one large *cv* wave. In severe tricuspid regurgitation and right ventricular infarction, large *cv* waves may ascend above the neck and appear as pulsating earlobes.

Prominent *a* waves may also appear as prominent neck vein pulsation and are associated with right atrial hypertrophy. Simultaneous atrial and ventricular contraction may also occur continuously during junctional tachycardia or intermittently with atrioventricular dissociations causing the *a* and *c* waves to merge. The resultant *ac* waves are described as cannon waves.

Careful attention to the timing of the pulsations will help to accurately assess etiology. However, one of the common symptoms of heart failure is tachycardia and, unfortunately, the faster the heart rate, the more difficult it is to use this parameter to differentiate waveforms. When this occurs, additional data are necessary. For example, if the abnormal venous pulsation is unilateral, it is more likely to be local in origin than cardiac in origin.

The effect of respirations on pulsation may also help in differential diagnosis of underlying disease. Deep breathing decreases intrathoracic pressure and causes the pressure in the central and jugular veins to drop. The magnitude of venous waveforms, therefore, normally diminishes during inspiration. In the patient with right-sided heart failure, the pulsations paradoxically increase during inspiration. This is because the transient increase in the volume of blood returning to the heart is more than the failing ventricle can handle. The finding is called Kussmaul's sign, and it may also be present in constrictive pericarditis or cardiac tamponade.

Estimating central venous pressure. Central venous pressure (CVP) is used to assess right ventricular competence and circulatory volume status. Since trends in the patient's condition may be reflected by changes in the CVP, it is a parameter for monitoring both the development of the disease and the efficacy of the treatment.

In order to obtain an accurate measurement of vascular pressures with transducers or water manometers, the devices must be level with the zero fulcrum (phlebostatic axis) or the right atrium. The zero position can be approximated by marking the axilla at the junction between the fourth intercostal space and the anteroposterior midpoint. Another technique is to use a site 5 to 6 cm below the sternal angle or angle of Louis.

This zero point is also used to estimate to the CVP by neck vein inspection. Once the level of the right atria has been identified, the patient is placed as flat as tolerated with the head supported but not flexed. While observing the neck veins, the head of the bed should be elevated slowly until the top of the distended internal jugular vein can be seen (Fig. 4-11). The upper portion of the vessel will appear flat and the lower portion will appear full and oscillating.

The central venous pressure is reflected in the horizontal distance between the top of the distended venous column and the estimated level of the right atrium (Fig. 4-12). If the difference between these anatomical reference points is 5 cm and the column is even with the sternal angle, the central venous pressure is recorded as 5. When venous pressure is markedly elevated, external jugular venous distention will extend high into the neck and the veins under the tongue and on the forehead will appear engorged. This finding may also be associated with dilated, visible, superficial thoracic veins in patients with chronically elevated systemic venous pressure.

Hepatojugular reflux. Another application of neck vein assessment is the observation for a hepatojugular reflux. Again, with the patient in a comfortable supine position, head resting on a pillow, the bed is adjusted so that the internal jugulars can be visualized. Sustained firm pressure is then applied over the upper right abdomen for 10 to 60 seconds while the examiner observes for an increase in venous distention or pulsations. Pressure on the abdomen compresses the liver and increases venous return. A competent right ventricle will handle the added load without a visible increase in pressure.

In right-sided heart failure, hepatic compression acts as a temporary fluid challenge by augmenting

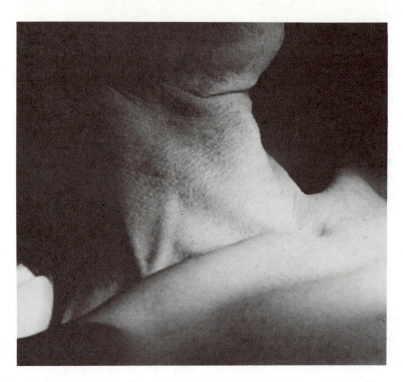

Fig. 4-11. Distended external jugular neck vein of client with right-sided heart failure. (From Papenhausen, J.: Cardiovascular and respiratory assessment for critical care practitioners. In Boarman, C.A., and others: Current practice in critical care, vol. 1, St. Louis, 1979, The C.V. Mosby Co.)

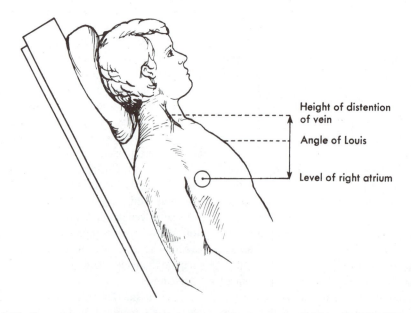

Height of distention
of vein

Angle of Louis

Level of right atrium

Fig. 4-12. Central venous pressure can be estimated by comparing height of angle of Louis and highest point of venous neck vein distention. (From Papenhausen, J.: Cardiovascular and respiratory assessment for critical care practitioners. In Boarman, C.A., and others: Current practice in critical care, vol. 1, St. Louis, 1979, The C.V. Mosby Co.)

venous return. As a result the neck veins distend shortly after the pressure is applied and may collapse again when it is released. This hepatojugular reflux often precedes central venous pressure elevation and is one of the earliest indications of circulatory overload and right ventricular dysfunction.

The test is invalidated if the patient winces, guards, or performs the Valsalva maneuver, because these maneuvers alone can raise the central venous pressure. These variables may be eliminated by instructing the patient to breathe normally during the procedure and by repositioning the hand if compression is painful.

Arteries

Identifying pulse quality. The methodical and thorough evaluation of systemic arterial pulses offers a wealth of information about the cardiovascular system. The arteries most commonly assessed include the temporal, carotid, brachial, radial, ulnar, femoral, popliteal, tibialis, posterior, and dorsalis pedis. To compare features and ascertain localized differences, each is palpated on both the right and the left sides. The brachial or carotid pulses, which are large and close to the skin's surface, are then evaluated to detect more subtle findings. When the carotid pulses are evaluated, the patient's head should be turned toward the side being palpated in order to relax the neck muscles. Taut muscles may mask pulsations.

Using the pads, not the tips, of the fingers, the area of maximal pulsation is located and the following characteristics are evaluated:

1. Rate (beats per minute)
2. Rhythm (regularity)
3. Vessel consistency
4. Volume (strength or amplitude)
5. Contour (shape of the pulsation)
6. Equality

Pulse rate and rhythm are the easiest criteria to evaluate. A classic early sign of heart failure is tachycardia disproportional to exogenous stress. This may be initially detected during arterial pulse assessment and should be related to conditions such as fever, anxiety, and pain. When these variables are removed and tachycardia remains, a more definitive cardiac evaluation should be undertaken.

Abnormal rhythms resulting from anxiety, fever, or cardiac electrical dysfunction also require more definitive assessment, particularly in patients with a history of heart failure.

There is a strong link between the existence of atherosclerosis and the risk of developing heart failure secondary to coronary artery disease. The vessel consistency of a normal artery is smooth, soft, and pliable, whereas sclerotic vessels are described as beaded, tortuous, and ropelike because they feel hard and resist compression. This finding consistent with atherosclerosis is important in individuals with suspected heart failure.

The examiner also identifies the volume and amplitude of the pulse. High-volume pulses are full and difficult to compress, whereas low-volume pulses feel thready and are easily obliterated. Pulse amplitude can be graded on a scale of 0 to 4: 0 indicates the pulse is absent, 1 barely palpable, 2 slightly reduced, 3 normal, 4 abnormally forceful.

Determining the pulse contour is more difficult and requires concentration. The normal pulse starts with a sharp upstroke, makes a smooth, rounded, brief, single peak, and then falls away with a more gradual downstroke. Bounding pulses usually have a sharp upstroke, a short plateau, and an abrupt downstroke. Weak pulses have a gradual upstroke, a prolonged peak, and a gradual downstroke (Fig. 4-13).

Increased pulse amplitude and a bounding quality are associated with the following conditions:

1. High stroke volume in hyperdynamic states
2. High pulse pressure in aortic insufficiency
3. Hypervolemia primary to fluid overload or renal failure
4. High systemic vascular resistance in hypertension

Decreased pulse amplitude and weak quality are associated with these conditions:

1. Low stroke volume in shock and low output states
2. Low pulse pressure in aortic stenosis
3. Hypovolemia in dehydrated or hemorrhagic states
4. Low systemic vascular resistance in anaphylactic or infectious states

POSSIBLE ETIOLOGY

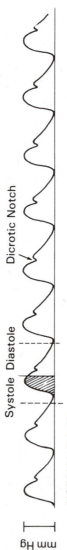

mm Hg

Systole   Diastole   Dicrotic Notch

NORMAL PULSE

Graphic recording of pulse pressure as obtained from electrical transducer. The normal pulse is easily palpable but may be obliterated by pressure. The wave of a single pulsation rises in systole, reaches a summit, and descends more slowly in diastole. The secondary rise in pressure, noted in diastole, is associated with closure of the aortic valve. The point at which the increase in pressure changes the downward slope is known as the dicrotic notch. This may not be palpable. The difference in pressure from the endpoint of diastole to the summit is the amplitude. Normal amplitude (30 to 40 mm Hg) is recorded as 2+. A pulse of greater amplitude is called strong and one of lesser amplitude is weak or faint.

Partial Arterial Occlusion
Myocardial Infarction
Myocarditis
Pericardial Effusion Shock
Stenosis of Valves: Aortic, Mitral, Pulmonic, Tricuspid

SMALL, WEAK PULSE

A weak pulse may be difficult to feel and the vessel may be obliterated easily by the fingers. The pulse may "fade out" (be impalpable). This pulse is recorded as 1+. The pulsation is slower to rise, has a sustained summit, and falls more slowly than the normal. A pulse that is weak and variable in amplitude is called thready.

Hypovolemia
Physical Obstruction to Left Ventricular Output, e.g., Aortic Stenosis

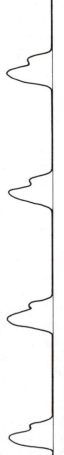

LARGE, BOUNDING PULSE

The large, bounding (also called hyperkinetic or strong) pulse is readily palpable. It does not "fade out" and is not easily obliterated by the examining fingers. This pulse is recorded as 3+

Exercise
Anxiety
Fever
Hyperthyroidism
Aortic Rigidity or Atherosclerosis

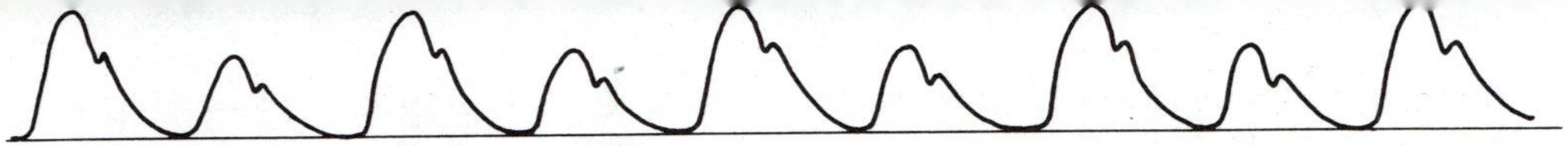

PULSUS ALTERNANS

Pulsus alternans is characterized by alternation of a pulsation of small amplitude with the pulsation of large amplitude while the rhythm is normal.

Left Ventricular Failure
More Significant if Pulse Slow

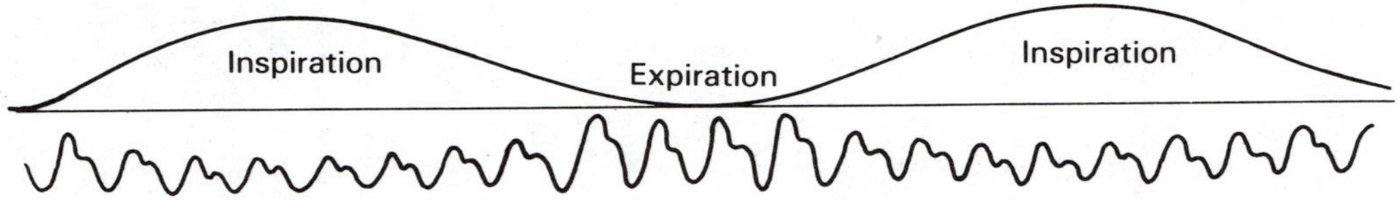

Premature Cardiac Contraction

PULSUS PARADOXUS

Pulsus paradoxus is characterized by an exaggerated decrease (> 10 mm Hg) in the amplitude of pulsation during inspiration and increased amplitude during expiration (see text for measurement with sphygmomanometer).

Inspiration   Expiration   Inspiration

Tracheobronchial Obstruction
Bronchial Asthma
Emphysema
Pericardial Effusion
Constrictive Pericarditis

PULSUS BISFERIENS

Pulsus bisferiens is best detected by palpation of the carotid artery. This pulsation is characterized by two main peaks. The first is termed percussion wave and the second, tidal wave. While the mechanism is not clear, the first peak is believed to be the pulse pressure and the second, reverberation from the periphery.

Aortic Stenosis Combined with Aortic Insufficiency

Fig. 4-13. Comparison of types of arterial pulses. (From Malasanos, L., and others: Health assessment, ed. 2, St. Louis, 1981, The C.V. Mosby Co.)

Many of these conditions may precipitate or cause heart failure. A hyperdynamic circulatory state with moderate vasoconstriction and bounding pulses is characteristic of early heart failure, whereas circulatory collapse with associated weak pulses is characteristic of severe end-stage intractable heart failure.

Comparing pulses to each other for equality of strength can distinguish local from generalized problems. Pulses distal to an obstruction are weak; those proximal may be strong. The quality of a pulse is classified on its distinctive pattern. Those relevant to assessment of patients with heart failure include the following (Fig. 4-13):

1. Pulsus alternans
2. Pulsus bisferiens
3. A dicrotic pulse
4. Pulsus paradoxus

Pulsus alternans is a term used to describe a pulse that has a regular rate and rhythm but alternates in amplitude from beat to beat (Fig. 4-12). It is diagnosed when the frequency of audible heart sounds with the blood pressure cuff inflated to peak systolic range is less than the frequency when the cuff is deflated to midsystolic range. For example, a patient with a heart rate of 80 beats per minute and a systolic blood pressure of 120 mm Hg will have an audible heart rate of 40 beats per minute with the cuff inflated to 118 mm Hg and an audible rate of 80 with the cuff deflated to 100 mm Hg. This is a classic finding in left ventricular failure and is associated with altered functioning of myocardial contractile units and variance in left ventricular preload.[14]

Pulsus bisferiens is a pulse with two sharp peaks separated by a depression (Fig. 4-13). The first is the percussion wave and the second smaller one is the tidal wave. It is not normally palpable but can often be seen when arterial waveforms are recorded from central lines. It generally reflects elevated left ventricular stroke volume and is often detected in patients with both aortic stenosis and aortic insufficiency.

A dicrotic pulse is a similar finding not normally palpable but also visible on arterial waveform recordings. Like pulsus bisferiens, a dicrotic pulse has two peaks; however, the second wave is much weaker and later. It is caused by the closure of the aortic valve just before diastole. The dicrotic pulse is diminished by age and atherosclerosis and becomes exaggerated and palpable in the presence of hyperdynamic states or left ventricular outflow obstruction.

Pulsus paradoxus is an exaggerated drop in systolic pressure during inspiration (Fig. 4-13). Although it can be palpated in severe cases, pulsus paradoxus is best assessed with the sphygmomanometer. The cuff is applied and raised to 20 mm Hg above the systolic pressure. The patient is instructed to breathe out and hold it. The cuff pressure is then slowly lowered until the systolic pressure is located. The deflation is stopped and the patient instructed to breathe in and hold it. If the Korotkoff sounds are no longer heard, the pressure is lowered until they reappear. A difference of 10 mm Hg or less between these two points is normal; more than 10 mm Hg indicates pulsus paradoxus and may reflect cardiac tamponade, constrictive pericarditis, severe lung disease, or advanced heart failure.

Palpation of the arteries offers a complex array of findings associated with cardiovascular disease. Table 4-5 summarizes those manifestations that relate to early and late failure and those that relate to the etiology or precipitating cause of cardiac failure.

Auscultation of blood pressure. Blood flow through vessels is normally linear and inaudible. Turbulent flow through vessels creates sounds called venous hums or arterial bruits.

A venous hum is a continuous low-pitched buzzing noise that may be heard over the jugular veins or in the supraclavicular area. Although it is normal in some young people, it usually reflects turbulent flow. This sound is auscultated with the bell of the stethoscope when the patient is in a sitting position. It is loudest during diastole and can be obliterated or softened by applying pressure over the inferior aspect of the neck vein.

Arterial bruits are associated with obstructing lesions such as atherosclerosis or dissecting aneu-

Table 4-5. Findings in arterial pulse assessment related to heart failure

Clinical indicators	Mechanism
Early	
Tachycardia	Compensatory
Increased pulse volume	Compensatory
Late	
Pulsus alternans	Changes in myocardium
Pulsus paradoxus	Decreased adjustment to respiratory pressure changes
Dicrotic pulse	Hyperdynamic state or decompensation
Decreased pulse volume	Decompensation
CLINICAL INDICATORS RELATED TO ETIOLOGY **OR PRECIPITATING FACTOR**	
Tachycardia	May either be precipitating factor or be related to cause
Ropelike consistency	Atherosclerosis
Increased pulse volume	Hyperdynamic states, aortic valve dysfunction, hypervolemia, renal failure
Decreased pulse volume	Shock
Pulsus bisferiens	Aortic insufficiency and stenosis
Dicrotic pulse	Aortic insufficiency, hypovolemic shock, cardiac tamponade
Pulsus paradoxus	Cardiac tamponade, constrictive pericarditis, severe lung disease

rysms. They are heard best during systole with the bell. Increased cardiac output may increase the sound intensity.

Auscultation of the arteries includes measurement of blood pressure. The systolic pressure reflects the force of left ventricular contraction and should be lower than 104 mm Hg. The diastolic pressure reflects arterial wall tension and vasomotor tone and should be less than 90 mm Hg. The lower limits are more difficult to describe, but generally the blood pressure is not considered abnormally low unless it is accompanied by signs of poor perfusion.

Acute heart failure accompanied by depressed cardiac output lowers blood pressure and narrows pulse pressure. On the other hand, transient diastolic hypertension with pressures in the range of 90 to 120 mm Hg may occur secondary to compensatory sympathetic vasoconstriction. Because systemic vasoconstriction can result from depressed cardiac output, one must look for a change in pressure after the resolution of the episode. If pressure remains elevated, then the underlying or precipitat-ing cause of heart failure is likely to be hypertensive disease.[3,14]

Hypotension in patients with a history of controlled heart failure may be related to clinical therapeutics. Hypovolemia resulting from vigorous diuretic therapy or aggressive vasodilator therapy may cause low blood pressure. Administration of some sympathomimetic agents may markedly elevate pressure. It is therefore important to ascertain a medication history in order to evaluate these variables.

Summary of cardiovascular findings

Cardiovascular assessment is a key component of the physical evaluation of the patient in heart failure. From this assessment conclusions regarding the cause and degree of ventricular involvement may be reached (Table 4-6). It is important that the observations be quantified and carefully documented. The following narrative describes cardiovascular findings in a patient with heart failure.

1. *Precordial inspection and palpation:* There

Table 4-6. Major clinical indicators of heart failure

	Left ventricular failure	Right ventricular failure
CARDIOVASCULAR FINDINGS		
Early signs	Tachycardia	Tachycardia
	Apical impulse deviated to left and downward	Diffuse lift along left sternal border
	Hyperactive apical lift	Paradoxical apical retraction during systole
	Parasternal retractions	Prominent c and v or cv waves
	S_3 loudest over apex on expiration	Abrupt y descent
	Summation gallop over apex (S_4 added to S_3)	Distended neck veins
		Hepatojugular reflux
		S_3 loudest over left sternal border on inspiration
		Summation gallop over left sternal border (S_4 added to S_3)
Late signs	Pulsus alternans	Movement of sternum with systole
	Dicrotic pulse	Kussmaul's sign
	Pulsus paradoxus	Murmurs of pulmonic and tricuspid insufficiency
	Murmurs of aortic and mitral insufficiency	Left ventricular failure
	Hypotension	
	Right ventricular failure	
NONCARDIOVASCULAR FINDINGS		
Early signs	Fine end-inspiratory rales	Spongy tender engorged liver
	Use of accessory respiratory muscles	Palpable spleen
	Speech pattern broken by need to take breaths	Weight gain
	Paroxysmal nocturnal dyspnea	Diuresis during prolonged periods of rest
	Labored breathing on exertion	Hepatomegaly
	Periodic irritating dry nocturnal cough	(When primary right ventricular failure occurs, signs of pulmonary disease are usually overt; see Table 4-4.)
	Cheyne-Stokes breathing during sleep	
	Peripheral pallor and cyanosis	
	Oliguria	
	Decreased memory	
Late signs	Coarse, continuous, diffuse rales	Prominent veins over chest wall
	"Cardiac" wheezes	Symmetrical dependent edema
	Dullness to percussion at bases	Pallor
	Diminished vesicular sounds at bases	Ascites
	Central cyanosis	Central cyanosis
	Clubbing	Jaundice
	Labored breathing at rest	Oliguria
	Cough producing pink, frothy sputum	Decreased level of consciousness
	Decreased level of consciousness	

are no visible pulsations. The apical impulse was palpable 11 cm to the left of the mid-sternal line in the fifth intercostal space and there is an abnormally diffuse prolonged lift. No other pulsations were felt.

2. *Auscultation of the precordium:* The first and second sounds were normal at a regular rhythm of 82 beats per minute. A faint S_3 was heard intermittently during expiration. There was a grade III/VI medium-pitched, mid-systolic murmur heard over the midprecordial area, with no radiation or associated thrill.

3. *Inspection of venous pulsus:* The neck veins were distended 5 cm above the suprasternal notch with the patient at a 45-degree angle. There was a positive hepatojugular reflux and no abnormal venous pulsations.

4. *Palpation of the arteries:* The temporal, carotid, brachial, radial, femoral, popliteal, and pedal pulsus were equal bilaterally at +3 except for the left pedal and popliteal, which were +2. The vessels seemed to have an abnormally hard consistency but were smooth. Although pulsus alternans was not palpable, it was auscultated at a difference of 12 mm Hg (rate 44 at 154 mm Hg, rate 88 at 142 mm Hg systolic). There was no pulsus paradoxus.

5. *Auscultation of the vessels:* The neck vessels were auscultated, revealing no venous hum, but a faint left carotid bruit was heard only during systole. The blood pressure was 166/104 taken early in the examination. Later, supine and sitting pressures on the left arm were read as 154/98 and 142/96 respectively.

PULMONARY EVALUATION

All assessment techniques are used to evaluate the pulmonary system. Inspection, palpation, percussion, and auscultation techniques will be described in general terms and then in terms of significant findings found in persons with heart failure.

The bony thoracic structures that serve as landmarks for cardiac assessment are also used for the pulmonary assessment. The borders of the lung parenchyma and major airways can be traced against them (Figs. 4-14 to 4-16). The trachea descends vertically in the anterior neck and thorax to just below the sternal angle where it divides into the right and left mainstem bronchi. This bifurcation is called the carina.

The apex of each lung extends a few centimeters above the medial aspect of the clavicle. The inferior border rests on the dome-shaped diaphragm. It is located at the sixth rib in the midclavicular line, at the eighth rib in the anterior axillary line, at the tenth rib in the posterior axillary line, and at the tenth posterior intercostal space (Fig. 4-14).

The margins of the lungs move during normal inspiration with the most obvious change noted at the posterior inferior border, which descends from the tenth to the eleventh or twelfth rib (Figs. 4-14 and 4-16).

The anatomy of the thorax guides the selection and sequence of areas for evaluation (Fig. 4-15). Comparisons should be made from side to side before moving up or down. The optimal patient position for this part of the examination is sitting on the edge of the bed with the feet supported.

Inspection of the thorax

Inspection of the thorax reveals two main categories of information: the shape and symmetry of thoracic structures and the characteristics of respiration. Both are clearly visible and may be objectively evaluated.

Thoracic structure. The shape of the normal thorax can be assessed by the following criteria (Fig. 4-15):

1. The chest wall is approximately twice as wide side to side as it is back to front.
2. The chest wall structures are bilaterally symmetrical.
3. The costal angle is normally less than 90-degrees.
4. The ribs join the spinal column at a 45-degree angle.

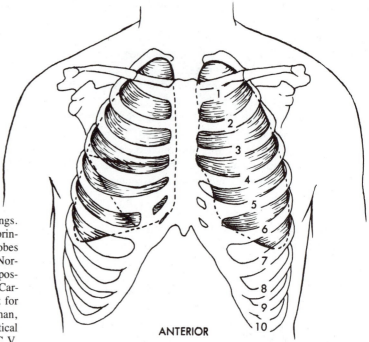

Fig. 4-14. Topographic anatomy of lungs. Notice that behind anterior thorax lie principally upper lobes, whereas lower lobes lie beneath most of posterior thorax. Normal range of motion is indicated in posterior view. (From Papenhausen, J.: Cardiovascular and respiratory assessment for critical care practitioners. In Boarman, C.A. and others: Current practice in critical care, vol. 1, St. Louis, 1979, The C.V. Mosby Co.)

ANTERIOR

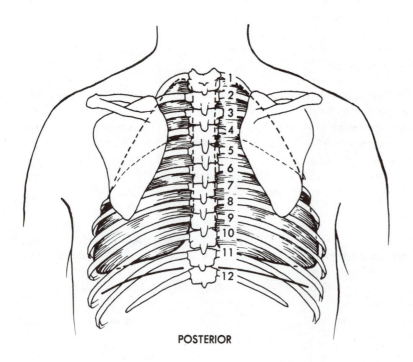

POSTERIOR

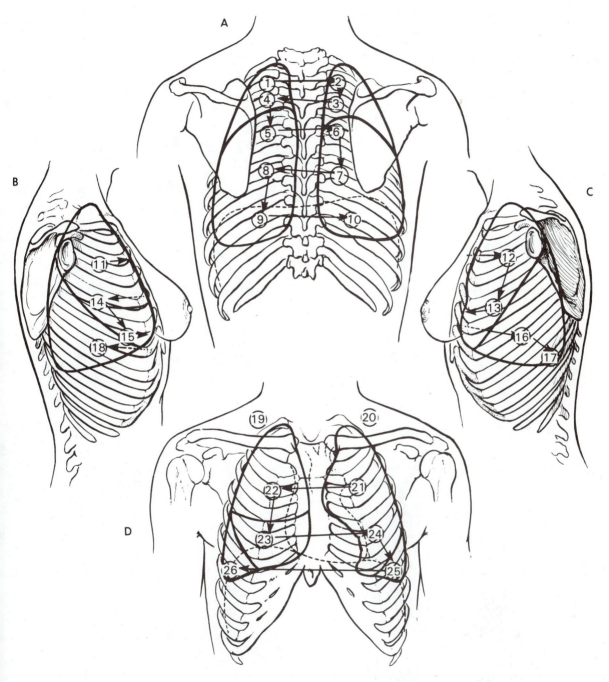

Fig. 4-15. Routine for systematic percussion of thorax. Numbers indicate recommended sequence for percussion and auscultation during a routine screening examination. **A,** Posterior thorax; **B,** right lateral thorax; **C,** left lateral thorax; **D,** anterior thorax. (From Malasanos, L., and others: Health assessment, ed. 2, St. Louis, 1981, The C.V. Mosby Co.)

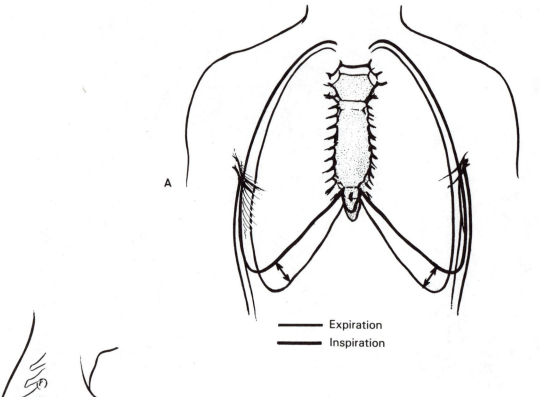

A

_____ Expiration
▬▬▬▬▬ Inspiration

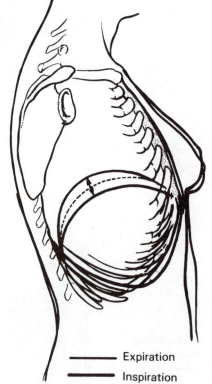

B

_____ Expiration
▬▬▬▬▬ Inspiration

Fig. 4-16. Movement of thorax during breathing cycle. **A,** Anterior thorax; **B,** lateral thorax. (From Malasanos, L., and others: Health assessment, ed. 2, St. Louis, 1981, The C.V. Mosby Co.)

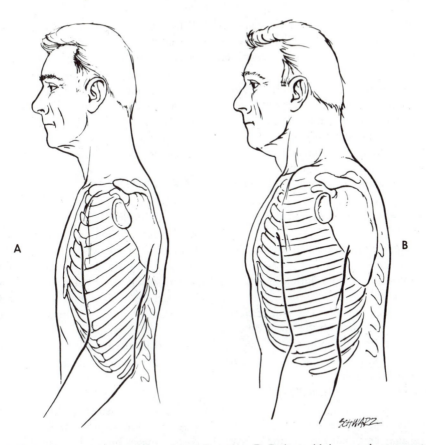

Fig. 4-17. A, Patient with normal thoracic configuration. **B,** Patient with increased anteroposterior diameter. Note contrasts in slope of ribs and development of accessory muscles of respiration in neck. (From Malasanos, L., and others: Health assessment, ed. 2, St. Louis, 1981, The C.V. Mosby Co.)

5. The clavicles join the sternum at about a 90-degree angle.
6. The sternum is approximately even with the ribs in depth (neither depressed nor elevated).
7. The intercostal spaces are fairly equal in size and are slightly depressed (but may not be visible depending on the amount of muscle and adipose tissue outside the chest wall).
8. The spinal column is vertical when viewed from the back and slightly S-shaped when viewed from the side.

Changes in these structures are associated with lung disease. Common findings in chronic airway obstruction include an increase in the costal angle and the rib/spinal angles, an increase in the anteroposterior chest wall diameter, bulging of the intercostal spaces, hypertrophy of the neck muscles, and elevation of the lateral ends of the clavicles, which alters their angle to the sternum (Fig. 4-17).

Acute unilateral changes in the lung may be reflected by loss of chest wall symmetry. For example, an accumulation of air or fluid in the pleural space may cause the intercostal spaces on the affected side to widen and become less concave. This is associated with a tracheal shift away from the affected side. Conversely, a large area of atelectasis may cause the ribs over it to draw together and the tracheal position to shift toward the affected area.

Respiratory pattern. After carefully evaluating the chest wall structure, the examiner focuses on the characteristics of respiration, using the criteria listed below as assessment guidelines[1]:

1. Adult respiratory rate is regular and ranges from 12 to 20 cycles per minute.
2. Sighs or deep breaths average 7 to 10 times per hour.
3. The ratio between inspiration and expiration is 2:3 to 3:5.
4. Muscle contraction associated with respiration is not normally visible.
5. The abdomen moves out during inspiration, especially in men.
6. The ribs move smoothly and symmetrically upward and outward with the lower rib cage moving more than the upper.
7. The arms, neck, and shoulders are normally not involved in respiration.
8. Respiration does not usually interrupt a patient's speech pattern.

In individuals with respiratory distress the expiratory phase may be prolonged and the rib cage may be lifted by the neck muscles during inspiration, causing the whole chest to move up and down as a unit. The use of accessory muscles may be visible first during expiration as abdominal contraction and bulging of the intercostal muscles and later during inspiration as intercostal retractions and neck contractions. The constant demand placed on these muscles causes them to hypertrophy.

In persons who are acutely rather than chronically short of breath, the same muscles may be used to assist breathing, but they will not appear to be hypertrophied. This may be observed in the patient with acute cardiogenic pulmonary edema who characteristically sits upright and supports upper torso weight with the arms to mobilize all accessory muscles. Both groups will break sentences into short phrases because of dyspnea.

When anxiety is the underlying cause of dyspnea, the individual may sigh frequently, whereas dyspnea secondary to organic dysfunction is characterized by impaired ability to breathe deeply.

When pulmonary involvement is localized, the respiratory motion loses symmetry. Pleural effusions, lobar pneumonia, or atelectasis may cause asymmetrical chest movement because of decreased expansion over the involved area.

Palpation of the thorax

The goals of palpation are to confirm findings observed during inspection, to identify areas of tenderness, and to evaluate the transmission of vibrations created when the patient breathes or speaks. They are best accomplished with the individual sitting in a relaxed, upright position.

When the tidal volume is small and breathing is effortless, it may be difficult to evaluate the respiratory pattern by observation. Positioning the hands over the anterior lateral lower chest wall allows the clinician to assess, by palpation, the respiratory rate, rhythm, and inspiratory-expiratory ratio.

Palpation is also valuable in assessing the muscles used for respiration. Less prominent intercostal spaces may be palpated to determine whether they are concave (normal) or convex (from intercostal muscle hypertrophy). The muscles of the neck will feel much larger in patients with chronic dyspnea. When inspiration is seriously labored, inspection of these accessory muscles will easily reveal their use, whereas palpation over the base of these muscles just above the clavicle allows detection of less obvious contractions at earlier stages of dyspnea.

The symmetry of respiration and degree of excursion may also be more accurately assessed by palpation. Standing behind the subject, the examiner places one hand on each hemithorax with the thumbs touching over the center of the lower thoracic vertebrae and the hands extended comfortably, fingers parallel with the ribs. The individual is instructed to take a deep breath while the examiner keeps the fingers stationary on the ex-

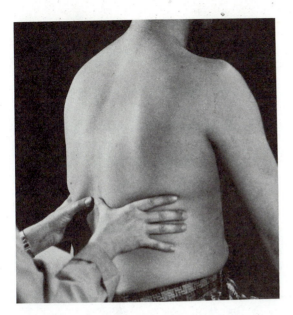

Fig. 4-18. Hand position for palpation of thoracic excursion. (From Malasanos, L., and others: Health assessment, ed. 2, St. Louis, 1981, The C.V. Mosby Co.)

panding chest wall and allows the thumbs to slide passively apart (Fig. 4-18). If motion is uniform, the thumbs will move the same distance.

Identifying areas of tenderness. The thorax is not normally tender to touch. If tenderness is elicited, pericarditis, pleuritis, or rib fractures may be present. This aspect of the physical examination is especially important in determining the origin of chest pain. The other causes of chest pain associated with heart failure, such as myocardial infarction, angina, and pulmonary emboli, do not involve localized tenderness.

Evaluating vibrations. The palmar surface of the hand and fingers are used to palpate inspiratory and expiratory phases for vibrations. When vibrations are detected, there is generally increased turbulence associated with auscultated rales. The sound waves created in the larynx when the patient speaks are normally palpated as faint vibrations in the intercostal spaces. These vibrations are called tactile or vocal fremitus. Sound is transmitted

better through solid tissue than through fluid or air-filled tissue. Conditions that lead to intrapulmonary consolidation, such as interstitial edema, atelectasis, and pneumonia, intensify vibrations, whereas the presence of fluid or air in the extrapulmonary spaces diminishes vibrations. The abnormal findings are described as increased or decreased vocal fremitus.

It is important to realize these vibrations are affected by the quality of the individual's voice. The lower the pitch and higher the intensity, the more prominent the vibrations. To minimize distortion, the person should be instructed to say the same thing over and over in a deep, moderately loud voice as the examiner palpates and compares the various areas of the thorax. Phrases commonly used are "one-two-three" or "ninety-nine."

Percussion of the thorax

Much of the lung tissue is close to the surface of the chest; therefore percussion is a valuable tool for assessing tissue density and determining the level of the diaphragm.

Lung density. Percussion over normal lung tissue elicits different notes, and the examiner must be familiar with these sounds and anatomical tissue density to properly evaluate changes (Fig. 4-19). The note is high pitched when the tissue beneath is less dense and more air filled. This is characteristic in persons with emphysema or pneumothorax. A lower-pitched note indicates increased tissue density, which may be associated with intrapulmonary consolidation of pleural effusions. Percussion may also be helpful in determining the level of pleural fluid. The note will change from resonant over normal lung tissue to dull or flat over the effusion. Pleural effusions are a common finding in persons with moderately severe heart failure and may be initially detected during pulmonary assessment as dull percussion over the lung bases.[1]

Level of diaphragm. The second role of percussion in assessing the pulmonary system is to locate the level of the diaphragm. As the examiner moves down the posterior thorax, resonant notes are heard until the diaphragm is crossed. At this

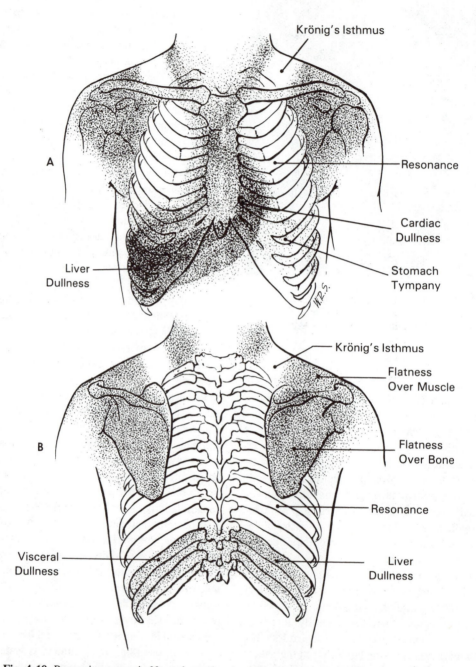

Fig. 4-19. Percussion areas. **A,** Normal anterior chest; **B,** normal posterior chest. (From Malasanos, L., and others: Health assessment, ed. 2, St. Louis, 1981, The C.V. Mosby Co.)

point the note becomes dull or hyporesonant. This technique may be used to determine whether the resting level of the diaphragm is normal (approximately even with the tenth vertebrae). Individuals with late chronic emphysema have flattened depressed diaphragms because of increased lung volume.

After marking the level of the diaphragm on each side, the examiner should ask the person to breathe in and hold it while the new depth is located. Normally the hemidiaphragms move symmetrically downward 1 to 2 cm. If a difference is suspected, it can be magnified by repeating the procedure, having the individual first exhale, then inhale maximally; both sides should descend the distance of two vertebrae.

Auscultation of the thorax

The diaphragm of the stethoscope is designed for auscultation of the normally high-pitched breath sounds. To increase the audibility of the sounds, the patient may be instructed to take a deep breath. To decrease extraneous nasal sounds, the patient should breathe with the mouth open. During evaluation care must be taken to avoid having the patient inadvertently hyperventilate.

The stethoscope is moved through the suggested sequence of positions while the examiner concentrates on inspiration and expiration (Fig. 4-15). Four questions should be answered before moving to a new area:

1. Is the type of sound heard appropriate (vesicular, bronchial, or bronchovesicular)?
2. Is the intensity of the sound normal, decreased, or increased?
3. Are the sounds comparable side to side?
4. Are there adventitious sounds (rales, rhonchi, rubs)?

The clinician then may reassess the same areas by listening to voice sounds instead of breath sounds. The quality and intensity of voice transmission offer information to substantiate impressions gained from previous aspects of the assessment process.

Types of breath sounds. There are three types of breath sounds. They are:

1. Bronchial sounds
2. Vesicular sounds
3. Bronchovesicular sounds

Bronchial sounds are loud, blowing, higher-pitched breath sounds. Inspiration is shorter than expiration and a brief pause separates them. Since they are the result of turbulent flow through the narrow glottis, they are normally heard only over the major airways.

Vesicular sounds are soft, rustling, lower-pitched sounds in which inspiration is longer than expiration and there is no pause between the respiratory phases. They are normally heard diffusely over the lung parenchyma and are created by agitated air flow through the alveoli.

Bronchovesicular sounds are a combination of large airway and alveolar sounds and are found in the midparasternal and interscapular regions. They are louder than vesicular sounds and less harsh than bronchial sounds. The length of the inspiratory and the expiratory phases are equal and there is an almost imperceptible pause between them (Table 4-7).

The first step in assessing breath sounds is to determine if the quality of sound is appropriate for the area being assessed. If bronchial or bronchovesicular sounds are heard over lung periphery, it is abnormal and related to increased tissue density. When there is a consolidating pathological condition with an open major airway leading to it, the bronchial sounds are transmitted further into the lung parenchyma, and the vesicular component is diminished or absent.

Intensity of breath sounds. The intensity of the breath sounds depends on the amount of tissue between the lung tissue and the stethoscope, the density of the lung tissue, and the tidal volume. Sound intensity may be diminished by the following conditions.

1. Obesity
2. Increased anteroposterior chest diameter
3. Depressed tidal volume

Table 4-7. Characteristics of breath sounds

Sound	Duration of inspiration and expiration	Diagram of sound	Pitch	Intensity	Normal location	Abnormal location
Vesicular	Inspiration > expiration 5:2		Low	Soft	Peripheral lung	Not applicable
Broncho-vesicular	Inspiration = expiration 1:1		Moderate	Moderate	First and second intercostal spaces at the sternal border over major bronchi	Peripheral lung
Bronchial tubular)	Inspiration < expiration 1:2		High	Loud	Over trachea	Lung area

From Malasanos, L., and others: Health Assessment, ed. 2, St. Louis, 1981, The C.V. Mosby Co.

4. Pneumothorax
5. Pleural effusion
6. Emphysema

Subtle early changes in the quality and intensity of breath sounds may be difficult to recognize. If the abnormality is localized, bilateral comparison helps to distinguish abnormal findings.

Adventitial sounds. The presence of adventitial sound is abnormal. The major types are rales, rhonchi, and rubs (Table 4-8).

Sounds that are discontinuous and characterized by a series of short sounds similar to popping and crackling noises are called rales. When fine they sound like sandpaper rubbing together and usually result from opening of collapsed, sticky, or congested alveoli. Medium rales sound like a fizzing carbonated drink and are the result of fluid in the bronchioles. Coarse rales are similar to the sound of water boiling and occur when fluid accumulates in the larger airways. Rales develop first during inspiration since air flow is more rapid during this phase.

In general interstitial and alveolar edema is suspected when rales are heard in a person with heart failure. If they are localized and dramatically improve or clear when the individual coughs, they probably reflect atelectasis or an accumulation of secretions.

Rales have important characteristics that should be considered when evaluating pulmonary function of persons in heart failure. First, they evolve rapidly when pulmonary hydrostatic pressure becomes markedly elevated and consequently are an excellent indicator of the progression of heart failure. However, rales resolve more slowly and therefore are a less accurate measure of the resolution of failure.[13] For this reason a patient with left ventricular failure who has been given a diuretic to treat developing rales will generally not demonstrate markedly improved breath sounds until well after the diuresis has occurred.

Second, rales evolve first over the lung bases and ascend up the lung fields as pulmonary vascular pressure rises. Therefore the examiner must examine all areas of the lungs when assessing for the progression and resolution of heart failure and carefully document the extent of lung involvement.

Rhonchi are distinguished from rales by their continuous or sustained quality. They are single long sounds and are caused by air flowing through narrowed openings, much like musical notes produced on wind instruments. They may be high pitched (sibilant) or low pitched (sonorant) and often slowly change pitch to create a musical sound.

Table 4-8. Characteristics of adventitious sounds

Sound	Cause	Description
Rales		
Fine	Produced by air passing through moisture in alveoli	Fine crackling sound occurring at end of inspiration; sound can be simulated by holding lock of hair close to ear and rubbing it between thumb and first finger; fine rales do not clear with coughing
Medium	Produced by air passing through mucus in bronchi or bronchioles	Clicking bubblelike sound occurring midway through inspiration slightly earlier than fine rales; can be simulated by rolling dry cigar between fingers or listening to fizz of newly opened, carbonated drink
Coarse	Produced by passage of air through exudate in trachea and bronchi	Loud bubbling, gurgling sounds occurring during inspiration; coarse rales often clear with vigorous cough
Rhonchi		
Sibilant	Produced by passage of air through bronchi and bronchioles narrowed by secretions, inflammation, or tumors	High-pitched wheezing sound, squeaky or musical in character; sibilant rhonchi are more prominent during expiration although they are audible during inspiration
Sonorous	Produced by passage of air through obstruction in trachea or large bronchi	Low-pitched, snoring sound; sonorous rhonchi may be heard during inspiration or expiration but are most prominent during expiration
Pleural friction rub	Produced by rubbing of visceral and parietal surfaces of the pleura	Grating sound that is usually heard during both inspiration and expiration; may not be audible at all times; often cannot be heard with quiet breathing, becoming apparent only when patient takes deep breath

From Abels, L.F.: Mosby's manual of critical care, St. Louis, 1979, The C.V. Mosby Co., p. 73.

High-pitched rhonchi are commonly described as wheezes because they are caused by narrowing of the lumen. Rhonchi are more likely to be heard during expiration when the airways are smallest. They are associated with early and late alveolar edema, when mucosal edema and free fluid invades the small and large airways.

Transmission of voice sounds. The principle of auscultating voice sounds is based on the relationship of sound transmission to tissue density. Auscultation of normal tissue reveals quiet, somewhat muffled voice sound. Air-filled tissue interferes with sound transmission, causing the voice to be less audible and more muffled, whereas consolidated tissue transmits voice as louder, clearer, and more understandable. To perform this evaluation, the patient is instructed to maintain constant voice intensity and low pitch and to speak the words "ninety-nine" or "one-two-three." If the words are clearly audible over an area of consolidation, the sign is described as bronchophony.[10]

Whispered sounds are barely audible over normal lung tissue, inaudible over air-filled tissue, and clearer over consolidated tissue. Therefore differentiating voice transmission is often easier if the patient is instructed to speak in a whisper. If sound transmission is clear over an area of increased density, the sign is described as whispered pectoriloquy.

A third test of voice transmission is performed by having the patient say "Eēē." This sound assumes a nasal quality, sounds like "Aye" over consolidated tissue, and is described as egophony. Conditions associated with heart failure causing bronchophony, whispered pectoriloquy, and egophony include pulmonary edema, pleural effusion, pneumonia, and atelectasis.

Pulmonary findings in heart failure

There are two categories of pulmonary findings in patients with heart failure. The first category includes findings characteristic of pulmonary congestion secondary to left ventricular failure. The second includes findings related to chronic obstructive pulmonary disease associated with right ventricular failure (cor pulmonale).

Left ventricular failure. The pulmonary manifestations of left ventricular failure begin with pulmonary venous engorgement and interstitial edema, which increases the work of breathing. This is revealed by a more rapid, shallow respiratory rate, slight retraction of the intercostal muscles, and mobilization of the accessory neck muscles. As mucosal edema narrows airway lumina, the expiratory phase increases and is accompanied by high-pitched expiratory rhonchi called "cardiac wheezes."[6] Once alveolar edema evolves, adventitial sounds rapidly develop, unilaterally appearing as fine to medium rales over the right base.[3] Then the left base becomes involved and rales ascend over the lung fields, becoming progressively more diffuse and coarse. In the later stages of left ventricular failure, the rales and wheezes may be audible without a stethoscope and the patient appears severely short of breath. If the patient develops bradypnea rather than tachypnea, it is a grave sign indicating either hypoxic depression of the brain stem or overuse of respiratory depressant drugs such as morphine sulfate.

Pulmonary edema moderately increases the density of lung tissue and leads to signs of consolidation. Because these changes are more subtle than those in more severe forms of consolidation, they must be carefully assessed. Characteristic findings include:

1. Hyporesonant percussion notes
2. Increased palpability of voice sounds (vocal fremitus)
3. Bronchial or bronchovesicular sounds heard over peripheral areas of the lung
4. Increased transmission of the spoken word (bronchophony)
5. Increased transmission of the whispered word (whispered pectoriloquy)
6. "Eēē" to "aye" changes (egophony)

The high pulmonary vascular pressures cause fluid not only to transude into lung tissue but also to pool in the pleural spaces. This condition is called cardiac hydrothorax, and it is observed most commonly in patients with marked elevation in both systemic and pulmonary venous pressures. Hydrothorax usually appears bilaterally. However, pleural effusion confined to the right may be related to underlying disease such as tricuspid stenosis or constrictive pericarditis, which markedly elevate systemic venous pressure. Pleural effusion limited to the left reflects disease such as mitral stenosis, which elevates pulmonary venous pressures.

Pleural effusions produce a demarcated dullness to percussion and egophony at the top of the fluid level. They are also characterized by transmission of both voice and breath sounds over the affected area. As heart failure evolves, pleural effusions intensify shortness of breath and dyspnea because of further reduction in vital capacity. Hydrothorax usually resolves as cardiac function improves and is carefully documented by chest roentgenography.

Right ventricular failure. When right ventricular failure precedes left ventricular failure and is not associated with congenital malformation or valvular abnormalities, the underlying cause is often chronic lung disease, and the condition is

Table 4-9. Physical findings associated with heart failure compared to those of common pulmonary diseases

Disorder	Inspection	Palpation	Percussion	Auscultation
Pulmonary edema	Breathing progressively more labored Cough	Increased	Dull	Bronchovesicular breath sounds Increased transmission of voice sounds
Emphysema	Barrel chest Changes in rib angles Accessory muscle hypertrophy Convex intercostal spaces Prolonged expiratory phase	Decreased vocal fremitus Decreased excursion	Hyperresonant	Diminished vesicular sounds Decreased transmission of voice sounds Rhonchi
Pneumonia	Breathing labored Cough	Increased vocal fremitus	Dull or flat	Bronchial or bronchovesicular sounds Increased transmission of voice sounds Rales
Pleural effusions	Asymmetrical excursion Tracheal deviation away Widening of intercostal spaces	Decreased vocal fremitus Decreased excursion	Dull	Diminished vesicular sounds Decreased transmission of sounds "Eee" to "Aye" changes at top of fluid level
Pheumothorax	Breathing labored Asymmetrical excursion Tracheal deviation away Widening of intercostal spaces	Decreased vocal fremitus Decreased excursion	Tympanic	Diminished vesicular sounds Decreased transmission of voice sounds

diagnosed as cor pulmonale. An in-depth discussion of the clinical indicators of these disorders is beyond the scope of this text; however, the major physical features differentiating common pulmonary diseases from pulmonary edema are summarized in Table 4-9.

INTEGUMENTARY EVALUATION

The skin is one of the largest and most visible organs and may reflect underlying disorders of heart failure. The main techniques used to evaluate the integumentary system are inspection and palpation. Significant findings associated with cardiac failure include:

1. Edema
2. Changes in color and temperature
3. Clubbing
4. Manifestation of conditions underlying or precipitating failure

Edema

Individuals with heart failure often present with dependent symmetrical edema. It is more obvious in the lower extremities after a period of standing or sitting, in the presacral area after reclining, and in the inner aspect of the dependent thigh after lying on one side. To assess these individuals for edema, the medial malleolus, the anterior tibia, the sacrum, and the medial femur are palpated. Evaluating edema is very subjective and several scales have been devised to quantify its severity. One such scale involves pressing the thumb directly down toward the bone for 5 seconds and then observing the area. If an indentation is present after the thumb is removed, it is scored on a scale of 1 to 4[7]:

0	There was no indentation.
+1	There was a slight indentation that quickly disappeared.
+2	There was a moderate indentation that remained 10 to 15 seconds.
+3	There was a deep indentation that lasted 1 to 2 minutes.
+4	There was a deep indentation that lasted several minutes or more.

Common causes of edema other than heart failure include chronic venous insufficiency and renal failure. The differential diagnosis is made by adjunctive diagnostic examination and by establishing the historical relationship between edema and associated findings.

Color and temperature of skin

Color and temperature of the skin are assessed in all areas of the body. The major findings are pallor, decreased temperature, cyanosis, and diaphoresis.

Conditions that cause peripheral vasoconstriction may also lead to generalized pallor and decreased skin temperature. When they are associated with elevated sympathoadrenergic stimulation, diaphoresis develops. When they are associated with peripheral vascular lesions, color and temperature changes are localized and distal to the obstruction.

Cyanosis may or may not be associated with vasoconstriction. Surface capillary beds give the skin a blue appearance when the blood contains more than 5 g desaturated hemoglobin. The total

blood volume is affected when desaturation is secondary to pulmonary dysfunction. Consequently two kinds of cyanosis develop: central cyanosis, observed in warm areas such as the conjunctiva, oral mucous membranes, and circumoral region; peripheral cyanosis, observed in cool areas such as the nose, earlobes, and nailbeds. When vasoconstriction slows capillary blood flow, desaturated blood accumulates in the extremities, causing peripheral cyanosis.

In individuals with acute left-sided heart failure, the skin initially appears cool, moist, and pale, with slight peripheral cyanosis. If pulmonary edema ensues, hypoxemia causes the evolution of central cyanosis and marked diaphoresis may develop.

When individuals develop dependent edema, localized increase in tissue pressure may inhibit perfusion, leading to pallor and decreased skin temperature. Chronic edema may cause changes in pigmentation or redness over the involved areas. It is possible but uncommon for heart failure to be associated with warm, pink, or reddened extremities. This is a characteristic finding in persons with the high-output heart failure and is related to vasodilation, hyperdynamic, and hypermetabolic states[3] (Chapter 2).

Clubbing

Clubbing is a classic finding in persons with chronic central cyanosis and hypoxia; therefore it can occur in chronic heart failure, chronic lung disease, and right-to-left shunts (Fig. 4-20).

Manifestations of underlying causes

The skin may provide information concerning the underlying cause or precipitating factors of heart failure. Xanthomas are skin manifestations of atherosclerosis, a frequent cause of heart failure secondary to coronary artery disease. These lesions are flat, slightly elevated, soft nodules on the eyelids and are often associated with hyperlipidemia. When atherosclerotic lesions of a major peripheral artery decrease perfusion to an extremity, the skin will appear thin, shiny, pale, and hairless.

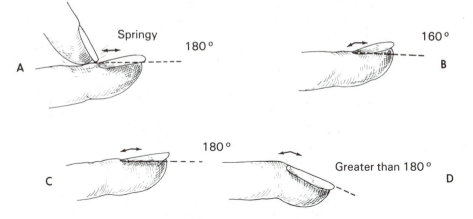

Fig. 4-20. A, Floating nail. **B,** Normal angle of nail; **C,** slight clubbing; **D,** severe clubbing. (From Abels, L.F.: Mosby's manual of critical care, St. Louis, 1979, The C.V. Mosby Co., p. 54.)

The nails are thickened and ulcerations may be present.

When heart failure occurs because of chronic anemia, the skin is pale and cool, and in some cases petechiae are present. When failure is caused by valvular disease, the patient may develop Osler nodes. These are small, discolored, and sometimes painful nodules usually located on the hands. They result from emboli formed on the valves that lodge in the peripheral vessels.

GASTROINTESTINAL EVALUATION

Assessment of the gastrointestinal system involves inspection, auscultation, percussion, and palpation performed in that order. If auscultation is performed after percussion or palpation, manipulation may alter findings by augmenting bowel sounds. If it is possible, the examination is performed with the patient lying flat with the abdominal muscles relaxed. Most abdominal abnormalities associated with heart failure are related to systemic hypertension.

Inspection

Inspection should reveal a symmetrical abdomen without bulges, visible vessels, or distention. Engorged superficial veins and epigastric fullness may reflect portal hypertension and congestive hepatomegaly, whereas bulging masses reflect enlarged organs or tumors. The only visible motion is associated with respiratory movement. In thin individuals, slight epigastric pulsations are observed and reflect movement caused by the aortic pulse wave against the stomach.

Auscultation

Normal bowel sounds are high-pitched gurgling sounds occurring every 5 to 20 seconds. They are most easily recognized with the diaphragm placed over each quadrant for at least 1 to 5 minutes. Charting "no bowel sounds present" without allowing sufficient time for recognition reflects poor assessment technique.

Vascular sounds are low-pitched sounds best heard with the bell. Arterial bruits may occur anywhere in the abdomen and suggest stenotic lesions or aneurysms. A normal venous hum originating from the inferior vena cava and its large tributaries is continuously audible. It is medium pitched and similar to a muscular fibrillary hum. A prominent hum over the periumbilical area may reflect portal hypertension.

Percussion

Percussion should elicit hyporesonant or dull notes over most of the normal abdomen, with hyperresonant notes occurring over the air-filled bowel and tympanic notes occurring over the stomach bubble. Gaseous distention is associated with generalized tympany while peritoneal effusion is associated with dull percussion. This condition is termed ascites and may be associated with chronic severe heart failure. Ascitic fluid seeks the lowest point in the abdomen, producing bulging flanks that are dull to percussion, a protruding, downward-displaced umbilicus, and a shift in the fluid level when the patient is positioned on his side.

Percussion is also used to estimate liver and spleen size. The normal liver has a vertical span of 6 to 12 cm at the midclavicular line and a span of 4 to 8 cm at the midsternal line (Fig. 4-21). Liver size varies slightly with body size, but acute changes usually reflect an underlying pathological condition. The normal spleen extends from the sixth to tenth intercostal space at the midaxillary line. Splenomegaly is usually present when this area is dull to percussion during inspiration.

Congestive hepatomegaly reflects elevated systemic venous pressure secondary to early right ventricular failure and usually precedes edema formation. Splenomegaly may also reflect heart failure; however, it is not a classic sign since heart failure is usually severe and accompanied by endocarditis before the spleen becomes significantly enlarged.[3]

Palpation

Palpation is used to assess the size, position, and consistency of abdominal organs and masses and to identify areas of tenderness. It is of limited value in a patient who is short of breath and unable to lie flat and is even more difficult to perform when ascites or obesity is present.[9]

The organs of most interest in cardiac patients are the liver and spleen. To palpate the liver, the examiner places the left hand under the patient's flank near the eleventh and twelfth ribs and lifts gently. The right hand directed caudally exerts downward pressure just below the rib cage in the upper right outer quadrant. The inferior edge of the

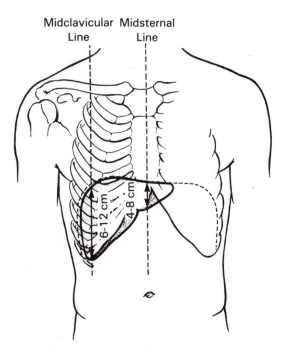

Fig. 4-21. Range of liver span in midclavicular and midsternal lines. Size of liver shows direct correlation to lean body mass. Thus the mean clavicular liver span in men is 10.5 cm and in women is 7.0 cm. (From Malasanos, L., and others: Health assessment, ed. 2, St. Louis, 1981, The C.V. Mosby Co.)

liver is palpated across the costal margin as a sharply defined, smooth, straight surface. During inspiration it descends 1 to 2 cm below the costal margin. If the edge extends below this level, either the diaphragm is abnormally low or the liver may be enlarged. For differential diagnosis the total span of the liver is assessed by percussion.

When the liver is engorged because of right-sided heart failure, its consistency becomes less firm and more "spongy." This reflects venous hypertension and concomitant pooling of blood in the hepatic sinusoids. Hepatomegaly resulting from other causes is generally associated with a firm, nodular, or granular consistency.

If hepatomegaly has developed rapidly and recently, the liver is usually tender to palpation. In chronic heart failure this tenderness disappears, but the liver remains enlarged. In persons with mild right-sided heart failure the jugular venous pressure may be normal at rest but rises to abnormal levels with compression of a congested liver. This sign is *hepatojugular reflux* and is helpful in differentiating hepatic enlargement caused by heart failure from that caused by other conditions.

To palpate the spleen, the left hand is used to lift the patient's left flank while the right hand positioned caudally presses on the upper outer quadrant just below the costal edge. When the patient inspires, the examiner tries to feel the spleen as it descends to the tips of the fingers. The normal spleen is not easily palpated even on inspiration. Splenomegaly makes palpation possible and may be related to advanced heart failure. To confirm its presence, percussion may also be performed.

OTHER RELATED FINDINGS

Assessment of the cardiovascular, pulmonary, integumentary, and gastrointestinal systems reveals most physical changes associated with heart failure. There are some significant findings in heart failure related to altered neurological and renal function.

Neurological alteration

As cerebral perfusion decreases in left ventricular failure, the patient's mental status decreases. The earliest manifestations are insomnia, restlessness, anxiety, decreased attention span, and memory loss. Later the patient becomes obtunded, disoriented, and unresponsive.

Urinary alteration

Renal blood flow is frequently depressed during the course of heart failure, and nocturia occurs relatively early in the evolution of the syndrome. Urine formation is suppressed during the day when the patient is active; this results in part because of redistribution of blood flow away from the kidneys during activity. When the patient is recumbent at night, the deficit in cardiac output is reduced, renal blood flow improves, and diuresis occurs. This pattern of urine production is characteristic of heart failure and is helpful in differentiating urine suppression occurring in renal failure. Oliguria associated with heart failure is a late sign and is related to depressed renal function as a consequence of severely reduced cardiac output. This sign may reflect prerenal azotemia and may be substantiated by biochemical analysis (see Chapters 2 and 5).

REVIEW OF MAJOR CLINICAL INDICATORS

Having examined a myriad of possible physical findings in heart failure, it is important to review the major clinical indicators as they relate to early, late, right, and left ventricular failure (Table 4-6).

Signs of left ventricular failure

In the earliest stages of left ventricular failure, the heart rate and respiratory rate increase to compensate for depressed cardiac output. During this hyperdynamic state, the apical impulse may be displaced outward and downward. As the ventricle dilates, an exaggerated thrust and an S_3 gallop develop. The patient may exhibit restlessness, vague uneasiness, weakness or fatigue, and decreased exercise tolerance and may complain of heaviness in the limbs.

As pulmonary venous congestion occurs, dyspnea on exertion, orthopnea, and paroxysmal nocturnal dyspnea evolve. When fluid invades the pulmonary interstitial space, rales, expiratory wheezes, and a dry, irritating cough develop. Signs of pleural effusion may also be present. As pulmonary congestion interferes with oxygenation, the patient may exhibit insomnia, restlessness, and Cheyne-Stokes respirations during sleep. Peripheral hypoxia is reflected in pale, cool skin and peripheral cyanosis. In patients with chronic illness clubbing may also occur.

As cardiac decompensation progresses, symptoms become more severe. Alveolar edema develops, causing coarse rales and wheezes over both lung fields. This is associated with extreme air hunger, a cough productive of large amounts of pink, frothy sputum, and central cyanosis. As left ventricular output falls, urine production becomes depressed, the skin becomes markedly diaphoretic, the level of consciousness gradually decreases to stupor and coma, and finally blood pressure, heart rate, and respiratory rate fall to life-threatening levels.

Signs of right ventricular failure

When the patient develops right-sided failure, right ventricular dilation and hypertrophy produce a palpable lift and an audible S_3 gallop along the lower left parasternal border. Systemic venous congestion causes distended neck veins, exaggerated jugular pulsations, hepatic tenderness, hepatojugular reflux, and hepatosplenomegaly. Anorexia is also a common complaint.

As the process continues, elevated systemic capillary hydrostatic pressure causes fluid to transude into the tissue interstitial space. This is manifested initially by weight gain and then by the evolution of symmetrical dependent edema. Chronic peripheral edema may cause changes in skin texture and pigmentation.

In later stages of severe chronic heart failure, edema becomes generalized and ascites develops. Poor pulmonary perfusion and stagnant anoxia lead to central cyanosis and alteration in mental status.

Signs of early heart failure

A classic feature of early heart failure is diminished cardiac reserve manifested by decreased exercise tolerance. In these patients it is common for the history to suggest heart failure but for the physical examination to be inconclusive. In such cases if the patient is not in acute distress, a modest amount of physical activity may be used to unmask clinical indicators. Reexamination after the patient has walked around the room or hallway may reveal positive findings that were not present at rest.

Interdependence of the ventricles

Although the pathological condition may be limited to one ventricle, both sides are anatomically and physiologically interdependent and will eventually fail. This occurs in the following manner:

1. Increased backward pressure from one side impedes blood flow from the other.
2. Decreased pumping from one ventricle decreases blood flow to the other because of the waterfall effect.
3. When one chamber hypertrophies, the septum may deviate toward the unaffected side, altering its function.

Because of these factors, a patient who has unilateral failure may show signs of bilateral involvement in a matter of minutes, hours, or weeks. Careful attention to the history and physical examination will help determine the sequence and degree of ventricular involvement.

Occasionally, the waterfall or cascade effect causes a confusing sequence of events.[8] For example, when the patient has acute left ventricular failure, pulmonary symptoms rapidly develop because of pulmonary vascular congestion. When the right side of the heart becomes involved, it is possible that the resultant decrease in right ventricular output may diminish pulmonary vascular congestion enough to temporarily improve the patient's pulmonary symptoms. This phenomenon is rare but may be observed in a critical care setting.

Identifying causes

Identification of the causes of heart failure requires the examiner to keep an open mind and pursue any unusual findings. In addition, specific attention should be given to those conditions commonly associated with heart failure. The more common causes of acute left ventricular failure include coronary artery disease, hypertension, valvular disease, and myocarditis and cardiomyopathies. Right ventricular failure is most commonly caused by left ventricular dysfunction but may also evolve as a result of chronic lung disease, congenital heart disease, tricuspid valvular disorders, constrictive pericarditis, and mitral or pulmonary stenosis. Both ventricles fail when decompensation results from arrhythmias, restrictive pericarditis, tamponade, or chemical insults such as toxins, drug overdoses, electroyte disorders, and acid-base imbalances.

Identifying precipitating events

In many patients the underlying causes have been stabilized or are only slowly progressive. When the condition acutely exacerbates, the precipitating event must be identified to effectively initiate therapy. Examples of these events may include arrhythmias, pulmonary emboli, infections, anemia, and increased emotional and physical stress.

When the patient has been previously diagnosed as having heart failure, the acute episode may be related to the current treatment. If the history reveals the patient is complying with the treatment regimen, it is possible that the therapy is inadequate or that the drug effects are triggering the symptoms. For example, digitalis may cause arrhythmias, diuretics may cause electrolyte imbalances, and antihypertensives may cause hypotension. All of these factors can aggravate heart failure. The drug list should be compiled, reviewed, and assessed for side effects.

USE OF ASSESSMENT DATA IN THE NURSING PROCESS

Too often the experienced clinician becomes very astute in collecting and communicating data but does not synthesize it into an evaluation of the patient's clinical status, a prediction of disease trajectory, and a guideline for care. Performing the history and the physical examination is the first step in this process. From this step potential and existing problems are identified. It takes time and care to arrange problem priorities and to develop a plan of intervention, based on both short- and long-term goals for optimal physical, social, and emotional health care.

Specific interventions to implement each goal are itemized in the care plan. These should include preventive and therapeutic measures.[11] Related teaching activities are also listed to provide progressive organized learning and to ensure continuity of care. Most importantly patients should be

involved in the process. They must have input regarding care. Furthermore, their involvement often stimulates compliance with the treatment regimen. As interventions are implemented, the outcome is continuously evaluated and interventions are adjusted and updated.

There are many standardized forms for recording assessment data, defining problems, and outlining goals and intervention strategies. Many resources are also available with standardized care plans for specific problems. Each institution must select or design a plan best suited to it and then individualize the plan to meet specific patient needs.

SUMMARY

Physical assessment is the primary data source for determining the major clinical indicators of heart failure. It is a complex, continuous process requiring an organized, skilled, methodical approach. It reveals the following data:
1. Major and minor symptoms
2. Major and minor signs
3. Underlying heart disease
4. Underlying related illness
5. Precipitating events
6. Major stress or support systems

The role of skilled nurse clinicians and clinical specialists is pivotal to putting this process into operation. Their contribution to patient care, by incorporating assessment into the comprehensive nursing process, plays a key role in health care maintenance of individuals suffering from congestive heart failure.

REFERENCES

1. Bates, B.: A guide to physical assessment, ed. 3, New York, 1979, J.B. Lippincott Co.
2. Boarman, C.A., and others: Current practice in critical care, vol. 1, St. Louis, 1979, The C.V. Mosby Co.
3. Braunwald, E.: Clinical manifestations of heart failure. In Braunwald, E., editor: Heart disease: a textbook of cardiovascular medicine, Philadelphia, 1981, W.B. Saunders Co.
4. Burchell, H.B.: Clinical recognition of cardiac hypertrophy, Circ. Res. **116**:34-35 (suppl. 2), Aug. 1974.

5. Delp, M., and Manning, R.: Major's physical diagnosis, ed. 8, Philadelphia, 1975, W.B. Saunders Co.

6. Fowler, N.: Cardiac diagnosis and treatment, ed. 3, New York, 1980, Harper & Row Publishers, Inc.

7. Gazes, P.C.: Clinical cardiology: a bedside approach, Chicago, 1975, Year Book Medical Publishers, Inc.

8. Holloway, N.M.: Nursing the critically ill adult, Menlo Park, Calif., 1979, Addison-Wesley Publishing Co., Inc.

9. Kinney, M., and others: AACN's clinical reference for critical care nursing, New York, 1981, McGraw-Hill Book Co.

10. Malasanos, L., and others: Health assessment, ed. 2, St. Louis, 1981, The C.V. Mosby Co.

11. Marriner, A.: The nursing process: a scientific approach to nursing care, ed. 3, St. Louis, 1983, The C.V. Mosby Co.

12. Moss, M.: Coping with physical illness, New York, 1977, Plenum Medical Book Co.

13. Spann, J.F., and Hurst, J.W.: The recognition and management of heart failure. In Hurst, W., editor: The heart arteries and veins, ed. 5, New York, 1981, McGraw-Hill Book Co.

14. Sokolow, M., and McIlroy, M.B.: Clinical cardiology, ed. 2, Los Altos, Calif., 1979, Lange Medical Publications, p. 301.

15. Tilkian, G.G., and Conover, M.B.: Understanding heart sounds and murmurs, Philadelphia, 1979, W.B. Saunders Co.

ADDITIONAL READINGS

Abels, L.F.: Mosby's manual of critical care, St. Louis, 1979, The C.V. Mosby Co.

Anthony, C.P., and Thibodeau, G.A.: Textbook of anatomy and physiology, ed. 10, St. Louis, 1979, The C.V. Mosby Co.

Beeson, P., McDermott, W., and Wyngaarden, I., editors: Cecil textbook of medicine, ed. 15, Philadelphia, 1979, W.B. Saunders Co.

Fowkes, W.C., and Hunn, V.K.: Clinical assessment for the nurse practitioner, St. Louis, 1973, The C.V. Mosby Co.

Hurst, J.W.: The heart, ed. 3, New York, 1974, McGraw-Hill Book Co.

Isselbacher, K.J., Adams, R.D., and Braunwald, E., editors: Harrison's principles of internal medicine, ed. 9, New York, 1980, McGraw-Hill Book Co.

Price, S., and Wilson, L.: Pathophysiology: clinical concepts of disease processes, New York, 1978, McGraw-Hill Book Co.

Selzer, A.: Principles in clinical cardiology: an analytical approach, Philadelphia, 1975, W.B. Saunders Co.

Thompson, J.M., and Bowers, A.C.: Clinical manual of health assessment, St. Louis, 1980, The C.V. Mosby Co.

Willis, F., and Dry, T.: A history of the heart and circulation, Philadelphia, 1948, W.B. Saunders Co.

Zschoche, D.A.: Mosby's comprehensive review of critical care, ed. 2, St. Louis, 1981, The C.V. Mosby Co.

CHAPTER 5

Noninvasive studies and diagnostic adjuncts for heart failure

MARY M. CANNOBIO

The process of assessing patients with congestive heart failure includes the collection of data from diagnostic adjunctive studies. The significance of a comprehensive data base lies in the fact that the information provides the means by which to deliver individualized care to the patient.

Since the various components of the physical assessment process have been addressed in Chapter 4, the focus of this chapter will be to discuss those cardiological investigations that fall under the heading of "noninvasive" studies. This distinction is based on the fact that these procedures do not penetrate the skin surface, and it implies that complications are essentially absent. The exception is the venipuncture, which is necessary to obtain blood specimens for biochemical analysis.

Heretofore, physicians have been responsible for the interpretation and explanation of diagnostic tests. However, as the practice of nursing expands to outpatient as well as inpatient settings, nurses are being required to assume greater responsibility for clinical diagnostics and care. Nursing actions are part of the implementation phase of the nursing process and must be predicated on a firm understanding of the data collected before implementation can occur.

As diagnostic investigations become more sophisticated, nurses are being required to provide detailed explanations to their patients regarding the procedures, and they are required to interpret the results.[25] With this in mind, nurses must be better informed of the studies, in spite of not always being directly involved in the procedure.

The types of information sought through diagnostic studies fall into two main categories: anatomical (structural) and physiological (functional).[23] While both types of information are often obtained in one study, it is important to understand that the principal reason for conducting the study is to obtain the maximal amount of useful information. This chapter will review four commonly used noninvasive studies that assist in the diagnosis and management of heart failure—echocardiography, chest roentgenograms, electrocardiography, and laboratory analysis. In addition, it will address the role of some pulmonary function tests in the evaluation of heart failure and it will provide instructional information for the patient as it relates to the potential health problems that may result from the performance of these procedures.

ECHOCARDIOGRAPHY

Echocardiography is a noninvasive diagnostic technique that visualizes internal cardiac structures and that provides information regarding cardiac function through the use of ultrasound.[18] With this procedure it is now possible to assess and diagnose many types of myocardial, valvular, congenital, and pericardial heart diseases.

Principles of technique

Echocardiography is the transmission of ultrasonic or high-frequency sound waves into the patient's chest by way of a transducer. The trans-

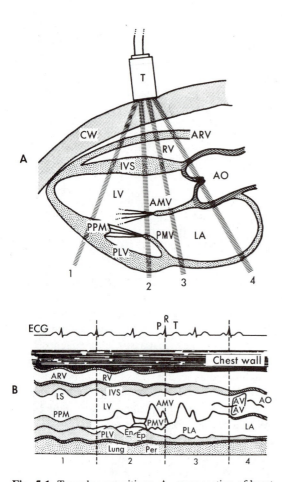

Fig. 5-1. Transducer positions. **A,** cross section of heart and its structures through which the ultrasonic beam passes. **B,** depicts diagrammatically the echocardiogram as the transducer is directed from the apex (position 1) to the base of the heart (position 4). The areas between the dotted lines correspond to the transducer position. *CW,* chest wall, *T,* transducer; *ARV,* anterior right ventricle wall; *RV,* right ventricle; *IVS,* intraventricular septum; *LV,* left ventricle; *Ao,* aorta; *AMV,* anterior mitral valve; *PMV,* posterior mitral valve; *PLV,* posterior left ventricle; *PPM,* posterior papillary muscle; *En,* endocardium; *Ep,* epicardium; *Per,* pericardium. (From Goldberger, E.: Textbook of clinical cardiology, St. Louis, 1981, The C.V. Mosby Co.)

ducer then acts as a receiver of the ultrasonic waves or "echoes." The echoes return after bouncing off the structures and are then electronically displayed through one of the several modes that have been developed.

M mode. The M mode is the basic display pattern for recording ultrasonic echoes. In this mode, the echoes are displayed on an oscilloscope as dots of light that are swept across the oscilloscope screen in a time-motion presentation. Time is represented along the horizontal axis, and distance from the transducer is represented along the vertical axis (Fig. 5-1).

With the patient in a supine or left lateral decubitus position, the M-mode transducer is placed on the surface of the chest at the third or fourth intercostal space along the left sternal border. Direction of the ultrasonic beam is then rotated in an arc from the apex of the heart toward the base in order to best illustrate the cardiac structures[6] (Fig. 5-1). Information about anatomical relationships (such as the right and left ventricles, the aorta, and the left atrium) can be provided. When there is suspicion of valvular disease, the M mode provides a safe and painless means of determining the presence or absence of valve thickening as well as the integrity of the valve leaflets. In addition, cardiac shape, regional wall motion and chamber sizes, including left ventricular size, can be evaluated.

Two-dimensional echo. Cross-sectional echocardiography, also referred to as real time or two-dimensional echocardiography, is a newer technique that allows the ultrasound beam to be moved very quickly, depicting cardiac shape and lateral motion that is not differentiated and often impossible to evaluate with the standard M mode. The recordings are displayed on videotape as a pie-shaped field 60 to 80 degrees wide and 15 cm or more deep[10] (Fig. 5-2).

There are numerous views that are used to obtain the required information. The more commonly used views include the apical four-chamber, the apical two-chamber, the parasternal long-axis, and the short-axis views. In the apical four-chamber

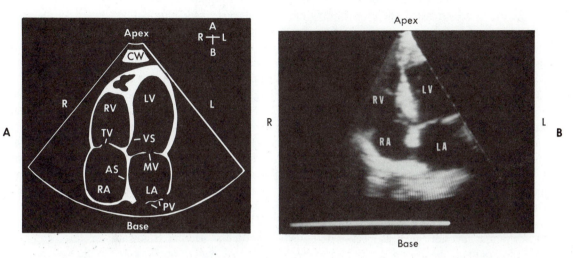

Fig. 5-2. Two-dimensional echocardiography. Apical, four-chamber view of heart. **A,** Diagram illustrates normal echocardiogram. *CW,* chest wall; *RV,* right ventricle; *TV,* triscuspid valve; *AS,* atrial septum; *RV,* right ventricle; *LV,* left ventricle; *VS,* ventricular septum; *MV,* mitral valve; *LA,* left atrium; *PV,* pulmonary valve. **B,** Two-dimensional echocardiogram, apical view from patient with dilated left atrium. (From Goldberger, E.: Textbook of clinical cardiology, St. Louis, 1981, The C.V. Mosby Co.)

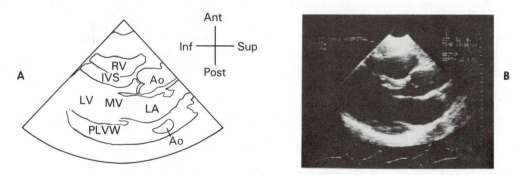

Fig. 5-3. Two-dimensional echocardiography. **A,** Diagram of long-axis view of heart. *RV,* right ventricle; *IVS,* intraventricular septum; *Ao,* aorta; *LV,* left ventricle; *MV,* mitral valve; *LA,* left atrium; *PLVW,* posterior left ventricular wall; **B,** Long axis view of heart. (Courtesy of J. Child, M.D. Non Invasive Labs, Division of Cardiology, University of California, Los Angeles, California.)

view, the transducer is aimed upward toward the base and to the right from the cardiac apex. In this view the four chambers of the heart can be seen with the mitral and tricuspid valves separating the atria from the ventricles (Fig. 5-2). In the parasternal long-axis view, the transducer scans a sagittal section of the heart (apex to base) parallel to the long-axis left ventricle of the heart (Fig. 5-3).

Echocardiography is helpful in the diagnosis of many types of heart disease. For the patient with ventricular failure, the echocardiogram can contribute vital information regarding the myocardium by assessing chamber size, muscle thickness, and motion patterns of the interventricular septum and of the left ventricular posterior wall. In addition, this technique allows quantitative assessment of left ventricular function, such as ejection fraction and cardiac output. Thus, in myocardium damaged by ischemia, areas of hypokinesis, dyskinesis, or akinesis may be detected.

Assessment of ventricular chambers/structures

When reviewing the M-mode echocardiogram, as viewed in Fig. 5-4, one sees five landmarks that are used to identify an echo tracing[1]: the chest wall, the right ventricle, the interventricular septum, the left ventricle, and the left ventricular posterior wall. By using this standard left ventricular echogram, one is able to obtain quantitative infor-

mation regarding the motion patterns of the interventricular septum and left ventricular posterior wall, end-diastolic and end-systolic internal dimensions, and information regarding the wall thickness of the interventricular septum and of the left ventricular posterior wall. This basic information provides the means of defining left ventricular function. In addition, internal dimensions of the right ventricle can also be measured. The boxed material below lists the normal ranges for the left ventricle and left ventricular dimensions.

Interventricular septum. In studying an echocardiogram of the interventricular septum, one looks at the motion or excursion of the septum and at the thickness of the septum during diastole and systole.

Septal motion. Normal excursion of the interventricular septum is toward the left ventricular posterior wall during systole. In the presence of a volume overload, such as seen in mitral or aortic insufficiency where the left ventricular stroke volume exceeds the right ventricular stroke volume, this posterior septal motion appears to be exaggerated.[6] Patients with an anteroseptal myocardial infarction may demonstrate lack of motion of the interventricular septum. Patients with asymmetrical septal hypertrophy resulting from hypertrophic cardiomyopathy may demonstrate either hypokinesis or akinesis of the interventricular septum. In dilated cardiomyopathy both the excursion and thickening of the interventricular septum and

---

LEFT VENTRICLE AND LEFT VENTRICULAR DIMENSIONS

Posterior wall	
Thickness	0.6-1.1 cm
Amplitude of excursion	0.9-1.4 cm
Internal dimensions	
Left ventricular end-diastolic	3.8-5.6 cm
Left ventricular end-systolic	2.6-3.4 cm

the left ventricular posterior wall are decreased, where left ventricular internal dimensions are increased.

Septal thickness. The normal range for diastolic septal thickness is 0.8 to 1.1 cm and is measured at the end of diastole at the inscription of the R wave on the ECG (Fig. 5-4). Disproportionate thickening of the interventricular septum is observed in cardiomyopathic asymmetrical septal hypertrophy and may be present in diseases with right-sided pressure overload, for example, pulmonic stenosis or pulmonary hypertension.[18] Asymmetric hypertrophy of the septum is seen in pressure overload associated with left ventricular disease, which includes aortic valvular disease and hypertensive heart disease.[18]

Paradoxical septal motion. A large number of conditions may produce abnormal or paradoxical interventricular septal motion. These can be brought together in four categories: right ventricular volume overload, intraventricular conduction disturbances, coronary artery disease, and conditions following cardiac surgery.

Left ventricular posterior wall. The left ventricular posterior wall is flat in mid-diastole and moves toward the chest wall (anteriorly) during systole.

Abnormal amplitude of motion. Increases of left ventricular posterior wall excursion are seen in patients with left ventricular overload, and in conditions where the left ventricular posterior wall must compensate for alterations of interventricular septal motion, such as in asymmetrical septal hypertrophy, and coronary artery disease. Decrease in left ventricular posterior wall excursion is seen in patients with coronary artery disease involving the inferolateral wall of the myocardium.

Abnormal posterior wall thickness. The left ventricular posterior wall may be thicker than normal in left ventricular diseases that cause pressure overload, such as aortic valve stenosis, idiopathic hypertrophic subaortic stenosis (IHSS), and hypertensive heart disease. A thinner than normal left ventricular posterior wall may be seen in patients with inferolateral posterior infarction or in patients with dilated cardiomyopathy.

Left ventricular internal dimensions. The measurement of left ventricular internal dimen-

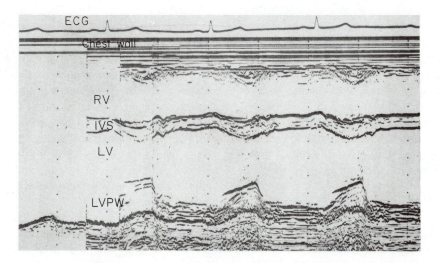

Fig. 5-4. Landmarks used to identify echo tracings: *ECG*, electrocardiography; chest wall; *RV*, right ventricle; *IVS*, intraventricular septum; *LV*, left ventricle; *LVPW*, left ventricular posterior wall. (Courtesy of Non Invasive Labs, Division of Cardiology, University of California, Los Angeles, California.)

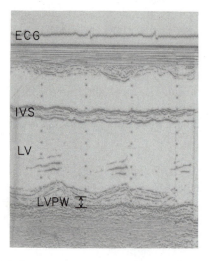

ECG

IVS

LV

LVPW

Fig. 5-5. Patient with dilated left ventricle (6.7 cm) with normal intraventricular septum (1.0 cm). (Courtesy of Non Invasive Labs, Division of Cardiology, University of California, Los Angeles, California.)

sions is important because it affords a quick and reliable assessment of the size of the left ventricle. The left ventricular end-systolic dimensions measure 2.6 to 3.4 cm and the left ventricular end-diastolic dimensions range from 3.8 to 5.6 cm.[10] Measurements greater than 5.6 cm suggest ventricular dilation as may be caused by coronary artery disease, left ventricular volume overload, myopathies, and arrhythmias (Fig. 5-5). Exaggerated septal motion and left ventricular posterior wall motion are characteristic of left ventricular volume overload states, such as aortic insufficiency, and ductus and ventricular septal defects.

CHEST ROENTGENOGRAM

The use of routine roentgen examinations provides important information regarding the size and position of the heart and great vessels as well as alterations in pulmonary circulation and densities of lung tissue.

Radiography of the heart and lungs may often provide the earliest confirmation in the recognition

and diagnosis of cardiac failure.[13,21] It affords the clinician the necessary information regarding anatomical and physiological changes relevant to the diagnosis of heart failure. Interpretation of the chest film should be done systematically in order to avoid overlooking important findings that may contribute to the overall diagnosis of the patient. The boxed material on p. 185 describes one approach to examining the chest roentgenogram.

Common chest film projections include the posteroanterior (PA), lateral, and left and right oblique views. Standard conditions under which the best visualization of the lungs and heart are taken include: (1) placing the patient in an upright position, (2) exposing the film during a deep sustained inspiration, and (3) taking the PA projection with the x-ray tube at least 6 feet from the film (Fig. 5-6). Any alterations in these standard conditions for taking a chest film can readily change the appearance of the heart, lungs, and thorax, thereby giving inaccurate readings.

In clinical situations, such as the intensive care units, it often becomes difficult to obtain good chest films. Because the patient is supine, PA films cannot be obtained and an anteroposterior (AP) projection is used. In this view the x-ray beam enters from the front of the chest, creating a larger cardiac shadow than would normally be seen in the PA views. Often these patients are acutely ill, and they are unable to maintain a sustained inspiration upon command. This results in a distorted cardiac image and unclear visualization of the lung fields and thorax. Therefore, it becomes important that roentgenograms be taken under standard conditions whenever possible and that nurses in the clinical setting be able to compare and contrast chest films to determine progress and/or deterioration of the patient.

The normal cardiac contours that are visualized in the PA view are seen in Fig. 5-7. The radiographic findings for the patient with cardiac failure may vary to some degree, depending on the cause. However, in chronic heart failure certain radiographic changes are commonly observed.

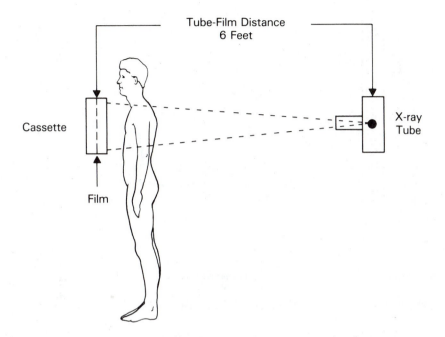

Fig. 5-6. Diagram illustrating the standard 6 foot upright posteroanterior chest roentgenogram.

SYSTEMATIC APPROACH TO INTERPRETATION OF THE CHEST ROENTGENOGRAM

1. **Bony thorax:** ribs—observe for any fractures, rib notching; chest wall—observe for abnormalities such as pectus excavatum, kyphoscoliosis; evidence of prior thoracotomy or sternotomy

2. **Diaphragm:** observe for flattening or elevations of hemidiaphragms; clear visualizations of the costophrenic angles

3. **Tracheobronchial tree:** observe the position of the trachea, the angle of the bifurcation, and the hilum and bronchial tree

4. **Pulmonary vasculature:** observe for normal pulmonary distribution, increased pulmonary vascularity, and decreased pulmonary vascularity

5. **Cardiac silhouette:** observe the size and position of the cardiac borders, any chamber enlargement, and calcifications

6. **Great vessels:** aorta—check for signs of dilation; pulmonary artery—check for signs of dilation and for the presence or absence of the pulmonary trunk

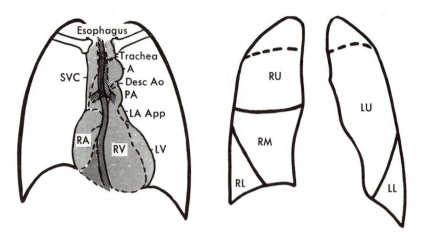

Fig. 5-7. Normal cardiac silhouette. *A,* Aorta, *Desc Ao,* descending aorta; *LA App,* Left Atrial Appendage; *LV,* left ventricle; *PA,* pulmonary artery; *RA,* right atrium; *RV,* right ventricle; *SVC,* superior vena cava. (From Goldberger, E.: Textbook of clinical cardiology, St. Louis, 1981, The C.V. Mosby Co.)

Thorax

Any changes in the size and shape of the thorax, such as scoliosis or pectus excavatum, can alter the position of the heart, making it difficult to determine actual chamber size.

Aorta

A widely dilated ascending aorta may be suggestive of hypertensive disease. However, if the proximal portion of the aorta is dilated, valvular aortic stenosis (poststenotic dilation) is suspected.

Cardiac silhouette

Changes in the cardiac dimensions over a period of time is one of the important radiologic signs used in the evaluation of heart failure. Cardiac enlargement may be generalized to the entire heart or may involve any one of the four chambers.

Ventricular enlargement

Ventricular enlargement on a chest film may be the result of one of two processes: dilation or hypertrophy of cardiac muscle. In dilation the chamber enlargement occurs as a result of increases in volume or because of an intrinsically weakened muscle. Hypertrophy causes enlargement by increasing muscle thickness and ocurs in response to systolic overload or contraction against an abnormally high resistance.[3] On x-ray film one simply sees an increase in the cardiac silhouette but is unable to distinguish which process is occurring.

Left atrial enlargement

Although the left atrium is not part of the normal heart border on the chest film, the left atrial appendage does appear between the pulmonary artery and the apex of the left ventricle. Enlargement of the left atrium appears as a blunting of the left cardiac border in the early stages and as a distinct bulge or convex configuration in the latter stages.[11]

Lung fields

Physiological changes in the pulmonary circulation are the key radiological findings in the progress of heart failure. Pulmonary vascular congestion appears as accentuated vascular shadows produced by blood-filled pulmonary arteries and veins. In a normal upright roentgenogram, blood flow goes to the lower lung fields; however, when pulmonary venous hypertension occurs, blood flow is shifted to the upper lung fields. Progressive prominence of the larger pulmonary veins with upper zone vessel dilation represents important confirmatory signs of early heart failure and is the principal radiographic means of following the progress of the patient.[13]

It cannot be stressed enough that careful attention must be paid to the film technique and that serial tracings must be obtained in order to compare films and to allow for proper evaluation of the vascular changes.

The progressive changes that occur as a result of increased pulmonary congestion are as follows.

Redistribution of pulmonary blood flow. This is one of the earliest signs of pulmonary venous congestion. It manifests itself as distention of the upper pulmonary veins, giving an antler appearance on the plain chest film (Fig. 5-8) with the lower lobe veins remaining normal.

Interstitial edema. This is often mistaken as poor film technique. It appears as a generalized haziness of the lungs that extends to the periphery. Interstitial edema begins to appear when the pulmonary capillary pressure exceeds 25 mm Hg and may appear in one of several varieties.

1. Intraseptal edema. When fluid accumulates in the intralobar septa, Kerly's B lines appear. Kerly's B lines are horizontal linear densities that represent dilated interlobar septa caused by septal edema. They are nonbranching and are usually located at the periphery and in the lower lung fields (Fig. 5-9). They are better exposed on full inspiration and generally disappear once cardiac compensation is restablished. If ventricular failure is recurrent or chronic, the B lines become permanent as a result of fibrosis and are then not a true indicator of pulmonary venous pressure.

2. Perivascular edema represents interstitial fluid of the central and peripheral blood vessels. On the chest film these appear as hazy, ill-defined margins of the hilar and peripheral regions of the lungs (Fig. 5-9).

Table 5-1. Pulmonary capillary wedge presure (Left Atrial) as estimated from the chest film (PA view)

Pulmonary venous markings	Pulmonary capillary wedge pressure (left atrial)
Normal	5-10 mm Hg
1+ Venous redistribution (Equal perfusion of upper and lower fields)	10-15 mm Hg
2+ Venous redistribution (Greater perfusion of upper lung fields: redistribution of pulmonary blood flow)	15-25 mm Hg
3+ Venous redistribution (Interstitial edema)	25-35 mm Hg
4+ Venous redistribution (Pulmonary edema)	Greater than 35 mm Hg

3. Subpleural edema represents interstitial fluid that has extended to the lung periphery. On the film, there appears to be an increase in the thickness and in the density of the interlobar fissures.

Alveolar edema. Pulmonary venous pressures above 25 mm Hg reflect moderate to severe left ventricular failure. Pressures at levels above 25 mm Hg cause transudation of fluid into the alveolar spaces. Radiographically, as fluid fills the alveoli, patch infiltrates begin to appear with hazy mediastinal margins causing the characteristic butterfly appearance (Fig. 5-10, *A*). The alveolar edema accumulates in the perihilar region and is generally bilaterally symmetrical.

Table 5-1 summarizes the estimated pulmonary capillary or left atrial pressures that can be derived from a chest film.

Pleural effusions (hydrothorax). Pleural effusions generally reflect biventricular failure. They may occur unilaterally with right-sided effusions being more common,[17] but more often they will appear bilaterally (Fig. 5-10, *B*). Isolated left-sided pleural effusions are rarely the result of ven-

Text continued on p. 192.

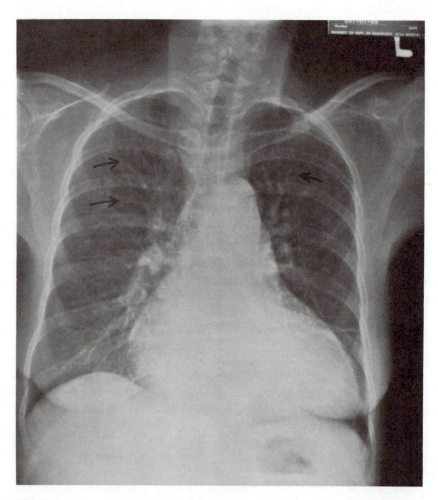

Fig. 5-8. Pulmonary congestion. Upper lobe distention *(arrows)*. Enlarged cardiac silhouette. (Courtesy P. Batra, M.D. Department of Radiology, UCLA School of Medicine, Los Angeles, California.)

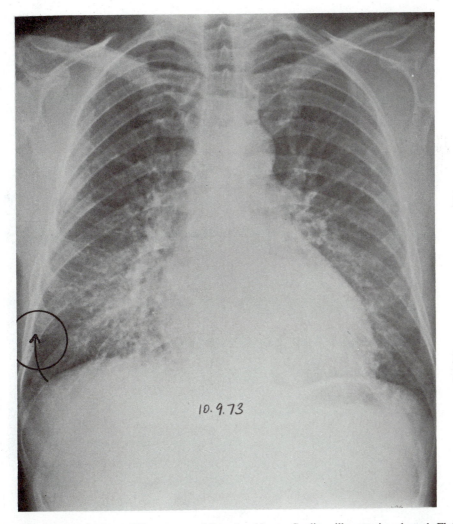

Fig. 5-9. Interstitial edema. Hilar areas are blurred and hazy. Cardiac silhouette is enlarged. Fluid collected within the intralobular septae of the lungs is visible as Kerley's B lines (arrows). (Courtesy P. Batra, M.D. Department of Radiology, UCLA School of Medicine, Los Angeles, California.)

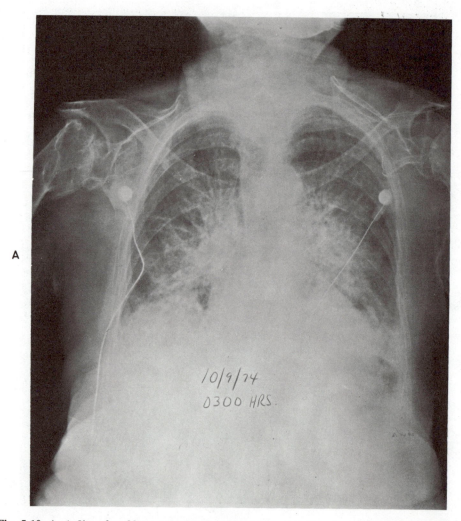

A

10/9/74
0300 HRS.

Fig. 5-10. A, A film of an 83-year-old female with primary alveolar edema with butterfly appearance and hilar haze. (Courtesy P. Batra, M.D. Department of Radiology, UCLA School of Medicine, Los Angeles, California.)

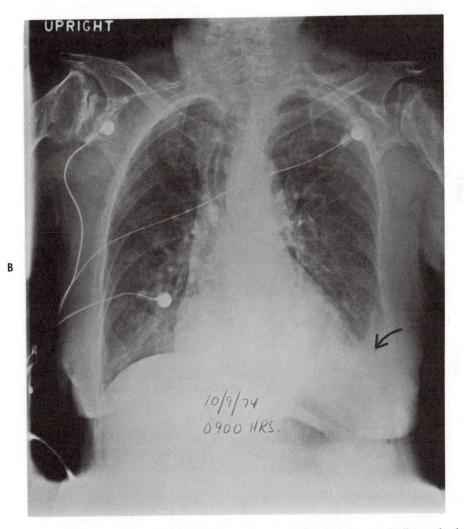

Fig. 5-10, cont'd. B, Following initiation of treatment, perihilar haze has markedly resolved. Enlarged cardiac silhouette and blunting of costophrenic angle *(arrow)*.

tricular failure. If present, or if left-sided effusions exceed the right, the following complications should be suspected: pulmonary infarction, neoplasm, or empyema.[20]

Apart from those radiographic changes that are directly linked with cardiac failure, thought and attention should be given to findings that are associated with the underlying cause. Calcifications associated with mitral or aortic valve disease may be helpful in guiding the diagnosis and treatment of heart failure. Finally, one should not neglect possible secondary complications, such as inflammatory diseases of the lungs or a pneumothorax, that may complicate the picture of congestive heart failure.

ELECTROCARDIOGRAPHY

Because the electrocardiogram (ECG) does not directly reflect intrinsic contractile function, there are no specific ECG changes that contribute to the definitive diagnosis of congestive heart failure. Anatomical dimensional changes and electrical dysfunction associated with the disease process and the treatment modalities are reflected in the ECG. Therefore the ECG can play a critical role in the overall management of the patient with heart failure.

Chamber enlargement

Enlargement of the heart size basically reflects one of two compensatory mechanisms by which the heart responds to the increased workload. Concentric hypertrophy is the result of an increased resistance to ejection (pressure load) that results in the muscle fibers becoming larger and in increased ventricular wall thickness. In contrast, cardiac dilation is the result of increased diastolic volume load. In a dilated chamber, the muscle fibers are stretched, causing the chamber to enlarge.

Conditions such as aortic stenosis, which causes obstruction to left ventricular outflow, can lead to hypertrophy of the left ventricle. Some diseases, however, such as congestive cardiomyopathy, cause stretching of the muscle fiber and can also lead to enlargement of the atria and ventricles. On the ECG tracing, the effect is reflected by increases

in the voltage of the P wave (atria) or QRS complex (ventricle). What is not differentiated is whether the enlargement is the result of dilation or hypertrophy.

Left ventricular hypertrophy. Left ventricular hypertrophy is clinically seen in many cardiac conditions; however, two of the more common causes are valvular heart disease and hypertensive heart disease. Diagnosis of left ventricular hypertrophy is made with reasonable certainty by observing the ECG and is characterized by the following changes (Fig. 5-11):

1. The sum of the S in lead V_1 plus the R in lead V_5 or V_6 is often greater than 3.5 mv (35 mm).
2. A QRS is prolonged as a result of the delayed conduction of the impulse through the ventricles caused by the increase in ventricular muscle tissue.
3. The repolarization process is altered because of delayed conduction through the ventricle. This is illustrated by the accompanying T wave inversions in leads V_4 through V_6.
4. ST-T wave changes are associated with a left ventricular strain pattern and are seen in those leads with tall R waves, *leads I, aV_L,* and leads V_4 through V_6.

Right ventricular hypertrophy. In acquired heart disease, right ventricular hypertrophy is characterized by the following ECG changes (Fig. 5-12):

1. Tall R waves (5 mm or more) in the precordial leads face the right ventricle V_1, V_2 with a concomitant decrease in the depth of the S wave and a small r wave in V_6.
2. Prolongation of the QRS interval does not occur unless an intraventricular conduction defect occurs with the enlarged right ventricle.
3. The T wave is inverted in the right precordial leads, occurring when there is a change in the depolarization forces.
4. The ST segment depression represents a "strain pattern" thought to be the result of long-standing enlargement.

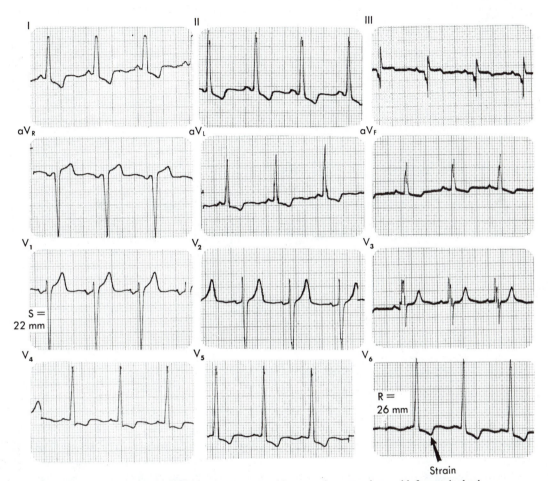

I

II

III

aV~R~

aV~L~

aV~F~

V~1~

S = 22 mm

V~2~

V~3~

V~4~

V~5~

V~6~

R = 26 mm

Strain

Fig. 5-11. Left ventricular hypertrophy. Patient with severe hypertension and left ventricular hypertrophy with strain pattern. Note tall voltage in chest leads, with a strain pattern in leads I, aVl, and V_4 to V_6. Also note tall voltage in lead aVl (R = 16 mm). In addition, note pattern of left atrial enlargement, with biphasic P wave in lead V_1 and broad, notched P wave in lead II (P mitrale). (From Goldberger, A.L., and Goldberger, E.: Clinical electrocardiography: a simplified approach, ed. 2, St. Louis, 1981, The C.V. Mosby Co.)

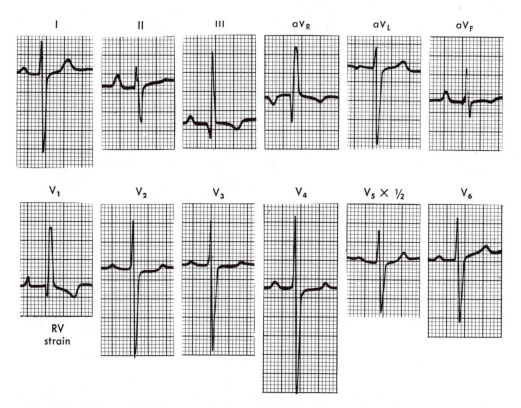

Fig. 5-12. Right ventricular hypertrophy. Sometimes with right ventricular hypertrophy lead V_1 shows tall R waves as part of the qR complex. Note peaked P waves (leads II, III, and VI) as a result of right atrial enlargement. Also note prolonged P-R interval (0.24 sec), which indicates first degree block. (From Goldberger, A.L., and Goldberger, E.: Clinical electrocardiography: a simplified approach, ed. 2, St. Louis, 1981, The C.V. Mosby Co.)

Atrial hypertrophy. Atrial contraction and function are observed in height and shape of the P waves on the ECG. Left atrial hypertrophy produces distinct changes in the P wave. Broad notched P waves lasting 0.12 second or more in duration reflect left atrial hypertrophy and are suggestive of mitral and/or aortic disease. The amplitude of the P wave may be normal or peaked. It may be biphasic with a broad terminal negative deflection in lead V_1. It is sometimes referred to as P mitrale, a term first used to describe this pattern when seen in patients with mitral stenosis (Figs. 5-13 to 5-15). In contrast, the presence of a prominent tall P wave of greater than 2.5 mm in lead II

and III with a peaked upright P wave in V_1 is indicative of right atrial hypertrophy (Figs. 5-16 and 5-17). Right atrial hypertrophy occurs most commonly in the presence of chronic pulmonary disease and may be a finding associated with concomitant right ventricular failure.

Additional ECG changes

Voltage. While a common finding in chronic heart failure, low limb lead voltage may also reflect pericardial disease, emphysema, or diffuse myocardial injury. It may also occur as a normal finding.[9]

Q waves. Although these usually suggest

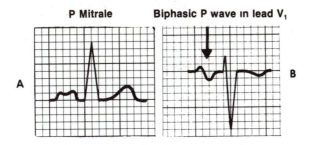

Fig. 5-13. Left atrial enlargement. Left atrial enlargement may produce **A,** wide, humped P waves in one or more of extremity leads (P mitrale pattern) and/or, **B,** wide, biphasic P waves in lead V_1. (From Goldberger, A.L., and Goldberger, E.,: Clinical electrocardiography: a simplified approach, ed. 2, St. Louis, 1981, The C.V. Mosby Co.)

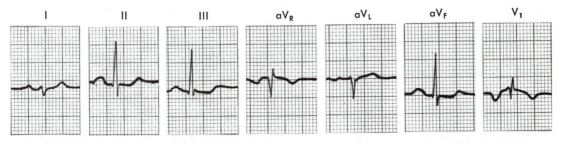

Fig. 5-14. Left atrial enlargement. Example of broad, humped P waves in patient with left atrial enlargement (P mitrale) pattern. (From Goldberger, A.L., and Goldberger, E.: Clinical electrocardiography: a simplified approach, ed. 2, St. Louis, 1981, The C.V. Mosby Co.)

ischemic heart disease, noninfarctional Q waves may occur in diseases that cause myocardial fibrosis, such as alcoholic cardiomyopathy or hypertrophic subaortic stenosis. Q waves with persistent ST elevations and the clinical signs of heart failure should arouse the suspicion of a ventricular aneurysm.[8]

Tachycardia. Reflective of a compensatory attempt to improve output of blood in the failing heart, rapid heart rates may also reflect the toxic effects of drugs, such as digitalis and aminophylline, as well as progression of the disease process.

Arrhythmias. A myriad of arrhythmias may be observed in the patient with cardiac failure. A major source of ineffective mechanical pumping, arrhythmias are representative of precipitating events, underlying disease as well as toxic effects of many pharmacological agents.[16]

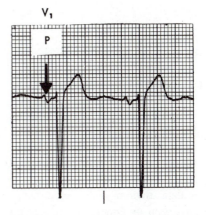

Fig. 5-15. Left atrial enlargement. Example of wide, biphasic (initially positive, then negative) P wave in case of left atrial enlargement. (From Goldberger, A.L., and Goldberger, E.: Clinical electrocardiography: a simplified approach, ed. 2, St. Louis, 1981, The C.V. Mosby Co.)

P pulmonale

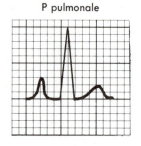

Fig. 5-16. Right atrial enlargement. Tall narrow P waves indicate right atrial enlargement (P pulmonale pattern). (From Goldberger, A.L., and Goldberger, E.: Clinical electrocardiography: a simplified approach, ed. 2, St. Louis, 1981, The C.V. Mosby Co.)

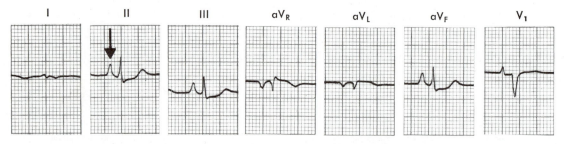

Fig. 5-17. P pulmonale. Note tall P waves, best seen here in leads II, III, aVf, and V_1 in client with right atrial enlargement (P pulmonale). (From Goldberger, A.L., and Goldberger, E.: Clinical electrocardiography: a simplified approach, ed. 2, St. Louis, 1981, The C.V. Mosby Co.)

Additionally, an all too frequent cause of arrhythmias is noncompliance with drug therapy. Failure to comply with drug therapy may be the result of the patient's lack of understanding regarding the purpose of the therapy or of a misunderstanding in the methods of administration. In either case it becomes important to assess the underlying reason for noncompliance and correct the situation with detailed instruction.[15]

Intermittent rhythm disturbance may include atrial fibrillation or flutter, ventricular premature beats, ventricular tachycardia, and complete AV block. Because of the constant introduction of new pharmacological agents used in the treatment of cardiac failure, it becomes essential that clinicians remain well informed of the current drug therapies

and their potential deleterious effect on the intraventricular conduction system of the heart.

Table 5-2 gives a summary of the most common arrhythmias seen in congestive failure with a possible clinical cause.

LABORATORY ANALYSIS

Diminished cardiac output in cardiac failure affects all body systems, particularly the kidney, liver, and lungs. The result of these effects on laboratory analysis can be numerous, but they are generally dictated by the underlying cause, treatment, and progress of the patient in congestive heart failure.

Although it is not always possible to remember all normal laboratory values, it is important to be-

Table 5-2. ECG changes seen in congestive heart failure with varying causes

Disorder	ECG changes	Arrhythmias
CORONARY ARTERY DISEASE		
Myocardial infarction	Q, QS waves	Premature ventricular contractions; ventricular fibrillation; AV disturbances
Myocardial ischemia	Inverted T waves	Accelerated rhythms
VALVULAR HEART DISEASE		
Mitral stenosis	Broad, notched P waves; right ventricular hypertrophy with pulmonary hypertension	Atrial fibrillation
Mitral regurgitation	Broad, notched P waves; left ventricular hypertrophy; nonspecific ST-T wave abnormalities	Atrial fibrillation; premature atrial contractions
Aortic stenosis	Inverted T waves Left ventricular hypertrophy	Atrial fibrillation; left bundle branch block; complete AV block
Aortic regurgitation	Left ventricular hypertrophy	AV conduction disturbances
CARDIOMYOPATHIES		
Idiopathic hypertrophic subaortic stenosis	Nonspecific ST-T wave abnormalities Left ventricular hypertrophy	Bundle branch block; ventricular and atrial arrhythmias

come familiar with the basic ones that reflect the status of the patient. It is also important to understand the purpose of the test, the cost to the patient, the risks involved, and any complications that may result from the procedure.

For the patient with congestive heart failure, the most frequently used biochemical tests to determine clinical status include blood chemistries, hematological screen, and urinalysis. Although they are not classified as a biochemical test, pulmonary function tests will be discussed in this section. Table 5-3 lists the common laboratory studies that are used in the evaluation and management of congestive heart failure.

Blood chemistries

Serum electrolytes. Electrolyte imbalances do occur in congestive heart failure and may reflect complications of failure as well as the use of diuretics and other drug therapy. While all electrolytes are clinically relevant, disturbances in so-dium and potassium are particularly significant with respect to changes in blood volume and cardiac status.

One of the outstanding features of heart failure is depressed cardiac output and inability to meet tissue metabolic requirements. A drop in the cardiac output will decrease renal perfusion, initiating a series of compensatory responses. A decrease in renal blood flow stimulates the release of aldosterone from the adrenal cortex. In the distal renal tubules, aldosterone acts to conserve sodium by increasing the reabsorption of water and sodium, thereby augmenting fluid retention.[2]

In patients with severe congestive heart failure, an increase in total body water dilutes body fluids and is reflected by a decrease in the serum sodium. This hyponatremic state occurs in spite of a high total body sodium and is the result of an expanded extracellular fluid volume. Persistent low serum sodium stimulates the secretion of the antidiuretic hormone (ADH), leading to further water reten-

Table 5-3. Laboratory tests used in the management of congestive heart failure (CHF)

Laboratory test	Clinical causes in CHF	Normal values
SERUM ELECTROLYTES		

Sodium (Na^+)	↓ Dilutional hyponatremia:
	    Diuretics—ethacrynic acid; thia-
	      zides, furosemide
	    Na^+ restriction
	    Overhydration
	    Hepatitis with ascites
	    Vomiting
	  Dehydration
		136-142 mEq/L

Potassium (K^+) (plasma)	↓ Hypokalemia:
	    Diuretics—ethacrynic acid; thia-
	      zides, furosemide
	    Dehydration
	    Diabetic acidosis
	    Stress
	    Gastric suctioning, vomiting
	↑ Hyperkalemia
	    Oliguria, anuria
	    Parenteral administration of IV K^+
	    K^+ sparing diuretic—spironolac-
	      tone, triamterene
		3.8-5.0 mEq/L

Chloride (Cl^-)	↓ Hypochloremia
	    Loss of Na^+, K^+
	    Metabolic acidosis
	    Diarrhea
	    Diuretics—ethacrynic acid thiazides,
	      furosemide
	    Gastric suction, vomiting
		96-103 mEq/L

Serum CO_2	Metabolic acidosis Metabolic alkalosis	22-32 mEq/L
URINALYSIS		

Urine output	Decreased urine output:
	    Hypovolemia
	    Dehydration
	    Cardiogenic shock
		25 ml/hr
		600 ml/24 hr

pH	↑ (Alkalinity): metabolic alkalosis K depletion ↓ (Aciduria): metabolic acidosis	4.6-8.0
Specific gravity	↑ 1.010: Excessive fluid intake ↑ 1.035: Decreased fluid intake	1.016-1.035

Glucose	↑ Glycosuria
	    Diabetes mellitus
	    Thiazide diuretics
		Negative

Protein (qualitative)	Mild proteinuria (1-2 g/day): Hypertension	Negative

Table 5-3. Laboratory tests used in the management of congestive heart failure (CHF)—cont'd

Laboratory test	Clinical causes in CHF	Normal values

Red blood cells	Hematuria:
	    Infective endocarditis
	    Congestive heart failure
		Negative

PULMONARY FUNCTION TESTS		
Vital capacity	Decreased Left ventricular failure Mitral stenosis Pulmonary hypertension	4000-5000 ml
Total lung capacity	Decreased Left ventricular failure	6 L
Residual volume	Normal or slightly increased Left ventricular failure	1.2 L
Maximum breathing capacity	Decreased left ventricular failure Decreased lung compliance	Males: 125-150 L/min Females: 100 L/min
BLOOD CHEMISTRIES		
Blood urea nitrogen (BUN)	↑ Decreased blood flow Diuretics—thiazides	8-18 mg/dl
Uric acid	↑ Diuretics—ethacrynic acid, thiazides, fuosemide	Male: 2.1-7.8 mg/dl Female: 2.0-6.4 mg/dl
Creatinine	↑ Prerenal failure—inadequate renal blood flow	0.6-1.2 mg/dl

Serum glucose	↑ Hyperglycemia:
	    Myocardial infarction
	    Diabetes mellitus
	    Stress
	    Diuretics—thiazides
		70-110 mg/dl

ENZYMES, ISOENZYMES		
Creatine phosphokinase (CPK)	↑ Moderate to high—myocardial infarction	Male: 35-135 IU/L Female: 55-170 IU/L
Isoenzyme CPK-MB	↑ Mild—myocardial ischemia ↑ Marked—myocardial infarction	
Lactate dehydrogenase (LDH)	↑ Myocardial infarction Liver disease	80-120 Wacher units 150-450 Wroblewski units 71-207 IU/L
Serum glutamic-oxaloacetic transaminase (SGOT)	↑ High levels—myocardial infarction, liver necrosis Mild to moderate levels—CHF, dissecting aneurysm, liver congestion	10-40 Karmen units

Continued.

Table 5-3. Laboratory tests used in the management of congestive heart failure (CHF)—cont'd

Laboratory test	Clinical causes in CHF	Normal values
HEMATOLOGIC SCREEN		
Red blood cell count (RBC)	↑ Polycythemia (secondary)—congenital heart disease	Male: $4.6\text{-}6.2 \times 10^6/\mu l$ Female: $4.2\text{-}5.4 \times 10^6/\mu l$
White blood cell count (WBC)	↑ Mild to moderate—infections (mainly bacterial)	$4500\text{-}11,000/\mu l$
Neutrophils	↑ Mild to moderate—inflammatory process, catecholamine release (drugs, stress), tissue destruction (myocardial infarction)	
Hemoglobin (Hb)	↓ Anemia (high output failure) Hemorrhage ↑ Hemoconcentration Dehydration	Male: 13.5-18.0 g/100 ml Female: 12.0-16.0 g/100 ml
Hematocrit (Hct)	↓ Overhydration Loss of RBC ↑ Hemoconcentration	Male: 40%-50% Female: 35%-45%
Erythrocyte sedimentation rate	↑ Infections Myocardial infarction Disease states causing cell destruction	Male: 0-15 mm/hr Female: 0-20 mm/hr
Prothrombin time	Prolonged prothrombin time Drugs—Anticoagulants, Salicylates, Quinidine Right ventricular failure Drugs—Barbiturates, Vitamin K	12-14 sec
ARTERIAL BLOOD GASES		
pH	↑ 7.45 (alkalosis) ↓ 7.35 (acidosis)	7.35-7.45
P_{CO_2}	↑ Respiratory acidosis Pulmonary edema Excessive dosage of narcotics Hypoventilation ↓ Respiratory alkalosis Pain anxiety Fever Hyperventilation	33-45 mm Hg
HCO_3	↓ Metabolic acidosis Myocardial infarction Diabetic ketoacidosis Diabetic ketoacidosis Pulmonary edema Cardiogenic shock ↑ Metabolic alkalosis Diuretics—ethacrynic acid; furosemide; thiazides Antacids	24-28 mEq/L
P_{O_2}	↓ Hypoxemia Pulmonary edema Cardiogenic shock	80-100 mm Hg

tion. Diuretics are used to enhance the renal excretion of total body sodium and water, and they may also contribute to hyponatremia if fluid intake is not restricted.[19] Patients who are on long-term diuretic therapy and low-sodium diets may also develop a dilutional hyponatremia. Care should be taken, however, in replacing sodium orally or parenterally because of the risk of pulmonary edema, which can occur rapidly in the patient with marginal ventricular function. Other situations that can contribute to a low serum sodium include hyperglycemia, hepatic failure with ascites, and acute renal insufficiency.[23] It becomes clear that clinicians must frequently monitor serum sodium levels in both the acute setting as well as with patients who are receiving long-term diuretic therapy. Apart from the laboratory results, one must be alert to symptoms such as headaches, apathy, tachycardia, and generalized weakness, which may accompany significant hyponatremia.[22]

Certain diuretics exert their major action on the ascending limb of Henle's loop and result in a loss of potassium and hydrogen and an increase in bicarbonate absorption. (See Chapter 8.)

Hyperkalemia, elevated serum potassium level, is not a primary disturbance in low-output heart failure; however, it may occur secondary to depressed effective arterial blood volume, which decreases renal blood flow and lowers glomerular filtration rate (see Chapter 2). However, hypokalemia, low serum potassium level, may complicate heart failure as a result of the use of diuretics, such as thiazides and furosemide.[19] These agents may lead to excessive excretion of potassium. It is important to note that hypokalemia may predispose digitalis toxicity, and because most patients with congestive heart failure are taking this drug, this may present a major clinical problem.

BUN, creatinine, uric acid. Any impairment of kidney function may be reflected by elevated levels of blood urea nitrogen (BUN), uric acid, and creatinine. The BUN may rise in conditions such as congestive heart failure and dehydration. This generally results from excessive diuretic therapy. In replacing fluids, clinicians must be alert to

early clinical changes that indicate overhydration. Such changes may include distended neck veins, increases in right atrial and pulmonary wedge pressure, and pulmonary congestion. Once hydration is established, the BUN should return to normal, if kidneys are functioning normally.

Uric acid is an end product of metabolism and is cleared by glomerular filtration. Therefore patients with congestive heart failure with decreased creatinine clearances may develop hyperuricemia. Diuretics, particularly the thiazides, are also known to cause elevated uric acid values by impairing uric clearance from the kidney. Elevations of serum creatinine may also reflect impaired renal function associated with low-output heart failure.

Glucose. Serum glucose levels may be mildly increased as a result of the suppression of insulin caused by the hypokalemia that is brought on by the loop diuretics. Patients with congestive heart failure may also have elevated serum glucose levels as a result of the release of stress-related catecholamine. As part of sympathoadrenergic compensation, catecholamines are released, causing the breakdown of stored glycogen and promoting the synthesis of glucose. While this may be a significant finding in all cases of congestive heart failure, patients who are diabetic or borderline diabetic may manifest elevated blood glucose levels and require supplmental insulin administration and close monitoring of blood sugars.

Enzymes

Structural damage to the liver may occur as a result of hepatic congestion from chronic severe heart failure. Slight elevations in the serum bilirubin and serum glutamic-oxaloacetic transaminase (SGOT) levels reflect liver dysfunction. Hepatic necrosis may also be associated in cases where there is marked increase in SGOT and lactate dehydrogenase (LDH) levels; however, myocardial damage may also contribute to elevated enzymes. Therefore one must be careful to differentiate the cause of the increase.

Cardiac isoenzymes. Cardiac isoenzymes are tissue-specific forms of substances found in the myocardial muscle. Cardiac isoenzymes used in the diagnosis of acute myocardial infarction are lactic dehydrogenase (LDH) isoenzymes and creatinine phosphokinase (CPK) isoenzymes. LDH has five isoenzymes that are numbered 1 to 5. When acute myocardial infarction occurs, 80% of affected individuals exhibit a marked elevation in LDH_1 within 48 hours following the episode.[24]

CPK has three isoenzymes, CPK-MM, CPK-MB, and CPK-BB. The fraction that is specific for myocardial damage is CPK-MB. This substance becomes elevated 4 to 8 hours after onset of chest pain of acute myocardial infarction and reaches peak activity at 24 hours.[26] It is suggested that blood samples be drawn at the onset of symptoms and every 3 to 6 hours thereafter for the first 24 hours. This will help to establish a trend analysis of the isoenzyme patterns, and it may be particularly useful in diagnosing myocardial infarction as a precipitating factor of heart failure.

Arterial blood gases

Arterial blood gases determine the acid-base balance of body fluids resulting from respiratory and metabolic components. The respiratory component may be monitored by observing for changes in the partial pressure of carbon dioxide (Pco_2). Changes in Pco_2) may occur as a result of changes in the rate and depth of ventilation. The metabolic component may be monitored by looking at the bicarbonate concentrations (Hco_3). The basic mechanism for controlling the metabolic acid-base balance is in the kidney. The Pao_2 measures the arterial oxygen tension in the blood and gives a reliable estimate of pulmonary oxygen transport.

Left ventricular failure is commonly characterized by hypoxemia with a decreased oxygen saturation resulting from alterations in ventilation-perfusion ratios.

In the clinical situation of congestive heart failure, the alveoli become filled with fluid, causing a drop in the Pao_2 (hypoxemia). In a compensatory attempt to increase the Po_2, the patient will increase the respiratory rate and depth, causing hyperventilation. This will result in a drop in the Pco_2 with a mild respiratory alkalosis. With deterioration or pulmonary edema, hypoventilation may occur, elevating the Pco_2. In the presence of advanced alveolar edema in which all lung fields are involved, arterial gases will show a severe oxygen deficit.

Hematological screen

Complete blood count. The components of the complete blood count (CBC) that assist in the evaluation and subsequent management of the patient with congestive heart failure include hematocrit (Hct), hemoglobin (Hb), sedimentation rate, and white blood count (WBC).

The Hct is the volume of packed red cells in 100 ml of blood. The Hb is the oxygen-carrying component of the red blood cell (RBC). The normal values for the Hct and Hb are listed in Table 5-3.

While not specific to the diagnosis of congestive heart failure, the Hb and the Hct may reflect a precipitating cause, aggravation of a disease process and/or effects of treatment. As an example of cause, patients with high-output failure resulting from anemia may have low Hb or low Hct. The cause of the anemia may be blood loss, or hemolysis, which results in decreased oxygen-carrying capacity.

Secondary polycythemia is a condition in which the red cell mass increases in response to pathological stimulus.[23] It commonly occurs in patients with chronic lung disease or cyanotic congenital heart disease with hypoxemia. In the setting of congestive heart failure, it occurs as a result of increased blood viscosity precipitated by an increase in red cell mass, causing sluggish flow and poor oxygen delivery.[22]

The sedimentation rate, which reflects the speed with which the red cells settle in uncoagulated blood, is characteristically low in congestive heart failure. It is postulated that this results from a decrease in fibrinogen levels, reflecting impaired liver function. While the sedimentation rate is not a specific test for heart disease, its main value is as a reflection of the inflammation process. It may be elevated in acute myocardial infarction, bacterial endocarditis, and Dressler's syndrome, conditions that may precipitate or underlie heart failure.[12]

The normal WBC is usually 4500 to 11,000 μ/L. Included in the WBC report is the percent of each of the different types of white cells (leukocytes) in the blood sample. This is commonly referred to as the differential. Elevated WBCs and extreme shifts to the left are indicative of infection. However, a high-normal or slightly elevated leukocytosis may be the result of stress-related catecholamine release. This may occur in the setting where tissue destruction has occurred secondary to myocardial ischemia.

Clotting profile. Part of the normal clotting profile includes the prothrombin time. Of the 12 clotting factors found in the blood, the prothrombin time measures four factors (Factors XII, IX, XI, and VIII). Decreases in any of these factors result in a prolonged prothrombin time. Because all factors except Factor XII are synthesized in the liver, any damage to the liver secondary to congestion or necrosis can disrupt the normal clotting factors and prolong the prothrombin time. Mild or moderate elevations generally do not cause bleeding; however, if other coagulation or platelet problems exist, spontaneous bleeding can occur into the skin, stool, or urine. Care must be taken to protect these patients from traumatic arterial punctures, and venipunctures as well as intramuscular injections.

Apart from intrinsic disruption of clotting factors, many patients with congestive heart failure are placed on long-term prophylactic anticoagulant therapy, especially in the presence of atrial fibrillation secondary to underlying mitral valve disease. These patients must be carefully instructed in anticoagulation therapy to avoid the risk of hemorrhage. Instructions should clearly outline the purpose, dosage, side effects, complications, and treatment. In addition, the need to keep laboratory appointments to regularly check prothrombin time levels must be stressed. This often presents a problem for the patient who is without transportation, lives a long distance from the hospital, or is without funds. In order to assist with compliance,

attempts to solve these problems should be made before the patient leaves the clinical area.

Urinalysis

Certain clinical indicators elicited from both the patient's history and the urinalysis stem from variations in renal clearance. Oliguria, which tends to occur during the day in the ambulating patient, is related in part to decreased renal blood flow, aldosterone secretion, and renal congestion. Nocturia, which may be an early sign of congestive heart failure, occurs during the night as a result of redistribution of blood volume. During the night with recumbency, the volume of urine may be 30% to 50% greater than during the day, and there is a tendency for diuresis.

Upon chemical examination of the urine, mild albuminuria of 1 to 2 g/L is common with a specific gravity being higher during phases of sodium and water retention and during periods of diuresis.[14] It is not uncommon to find white blood cells in the urine sediment, but the presence of red blood cells is less common in uncomplicated congestive heart failure.[23] Decreased creatine clearance in urine collected over a 24-hour period reflects decreased glomerular filtration. Low urine sodium levels may indicate retention of body sodium even in the presence of a low or normal serum sodium level.

Pulmonary function tests

The most significant role of pulmonary function tests is to differentiate dyspnea secondary to primary pulmonary insufficiency from pulmonary congestion caused by left ventricular failure. Vital capacity and maximum expiratory flow rates are indicators of maximum ventilation that the patient can voluntarily achieve. Patients with pulmonary congestion resulting from left ventricular failure will have decreased vital capacities but will maintain normal maximum expiratory flow rates. Total vital capacity tends to be less than 70% of normal in a patient who is dyspneic.

In isolated right ventricular failure, the pulmonary function tests are usually normal, unless there is associated lung disease caused by pulmonary hypertension.

HEALTH CARE IMPLICATIONS

The diagnosis of heart failure must be made quickly and early in the course of the disease if the patient is to survive. The role of the clinician in detecting indicators of cardiac decompensation has generally been limited to identifying the prominent physical findings. However, with the evolution of a more sophisticated, technological practice, investigative studies are essential in prognosticating impending crisis. For this reason, patient assessment skills must also include a working knowedge of diagnostic studies. This is also necessary to explain the purpose and technique to the patient and family, identify errors in technique, and report changes that may alter the treatment regime of the patient.

The major health care problems related to noninvasive studies fall into the categories of poor patient cooperation and faulty procedural technique. These contribute to inaccurate diagnostic results, often necessitating repeated studies. Most patient problems occur because individuals do not understand the important of the examination or are operating from misinformation or myths. For example, many patients object to numerous venipunctures because they fear loss of blood, leading to sustained fatigue and weakness. A simple explanation of the origin of these symptoms of heart failure coupled with the importance of information gained from blood analysis will help discredit this myth. In this way, the clinician may evoke patient cooperation by explaining the purpose of the procedure. The exception is the semilucid or unconscious patient. In this situation, the family may be of assistance.

Echocardiograms, while generally a painless procedure, can be fatiguing. Patients are instructed to maintain one to two positions for a period lasting from 40 minutes to 1 hour, depending on the tracings to be obtained and the skill of the technician.

Preparation of the patient before the procedure can ensure cooperation and often helps in procuring a better tracing.

Faulty techniques can be costly in terms of both patient care and money. Therefore clinicians must be familiar with what constitutes good technique and work with the technicians to obtain the best examination.

SUMMARY

The following guidelines summarize the basic responsibilities of the nurse clinician when dealing with noninvasive studies.

1. Prepare the patient by delivering a clear explanation of the procedure as well as carrying out required preparations, such as keeping the patient from eating or drinking or withholding medications.
2. Possess a firm understanding of the prescribed study, which includes rationale for use, general knowledge of procedure, expected results, complications, and associated side effects.
3. Assist or perform the prescried study as delineated by the nursing role. For example, echocardiograms and chest roentgenograms are done by technicians; nurse clinicians assist with handling the patients, particularly when the procedures are done at the bedside, and they intervene when the procedure poses a threat to patient integrity.
4. Interpret the studies as delineated by the nursing role. For example, skilled nurse clinicians, practitioners, and specialists are often required to recognize significant electrocardiographic, chest roentgenogram, and laboratory findings.
5. Perform nursing actions and interventions based on interpretation of the findings. This may include communication and documentation of the results as well as administration of medication or other therapeutic modalities as delineated by the clinical nursing role.

REFERENCES

1. Benchimol, A.: Noninvasive techniques in cardiology for the nurse and technician, New York, 1978, John Wiley & Sons, Inc.
2. Braunwald, E.: Clinical manifestations of heart failure. In Braunwald, E., editor: Heart disease: a textbook of cardiovascular medicine, Philadelphia, 1981, W.B. Saunders Co., p. 493.
3. Braunwald, E.: Pathophysiology of heart failure. In Braunwald, E., editor: Heart disease: a textbook of cardiovascular medicine, Philadelphia, 1981, W.B. Saunders Co., p. 453.
4. Burke, S.R.: The composition and function of body fluids, ed. 3, St. Louis, 1980, The C.V. Mosby Co.
5. Clark, N.T.: Pump failure, Nurs. Clin. North Am. 7(3):529, 1972.
6. Feigenbaum, H.: Clinical application of echocardiography, Prog. Cardiovasc. Dis. **14**:531, 1972.
7. Fowler, N.: Cardiac diagnosis and treatment, ed. 3, New York, 1980, Harper & Row Publishers Inc.
8. Goldberger, A.L.: Congestive heart failure in adults: six considerations in systematic diagnosis, Postgrad. Med. **69**(3):151, 1981.
9. Goldberger, A.L., and Goldberger, E.: Clinical electrocardiography, ed. 2, St. Louis, 1981, The C.V. Mosby Co.
10. Goldberger, E.: Textbook of clinical cardiology, St. Louis, 1981, The C.V. Mosby Co.
11. Harris, E.A., and others: Intensive care of the heart and lungs, ed. 2, London, 1972, Blackwell Scientific Publications Inc.
12. Hurst, J.W.: The physician's approach to the patient with heart disease. In Hurst J.W., and others, editors: The heart arteries and veins, ed. 5, New York, 1982, McGraw-Hill Book Co.
13. Jefferson, M.A., and Rees, S.: Clinical cardiology radiology, London, 1973, Butterworth Publishers Inc.
14. Kee LeFever, J.: Clinical implications of laboratory studies in critical care, Crit. Care Q. **2**(3):1, 1979.
15. Kenner, C.V., Guzetta, C.E., and Dossey, B.M.: Critical care nursing: body-mind-spirit, Boston, 1981, Little, Brown & Co.
16. Mayer, G.G., and Kaelin, P.B.: Arrhythmias and cardiac output, Am. J. Nurs. **72**:1597, 1972.
17. Meszaros, W.T.: Lung changes in left heart failure, Circulation **57**:859, 1973.
18. Morganroth, J., and Josephson, M.E.: Echocardiography: methodology and basic measurement characteristics, Pract. Card., pp. 126-140, April 1978.
19. Perez-Stable, E.C., and Materson, B.J.: Diuretic therapy of edema, Med. Clin. North Am. **55**:359, 1971.
20. Perloff, J.K.: The clinical manifestations of cardiac failure in adults, Hosp. Pract. **70**:43, 1970.
21. Sokolow, M., and McIlroy, M.D.: Clinical cardiology, ed. 2, Los Altos, CA, 1979, Lange Medical Publications.
22. Spooner, B., Gross, B.W., and Hasko, B.A.: Diverse implications of laboratory values in congestive heart failure, Crit. Care Q. **2**(3):37, 1979.
23. Tilkian, S.M., and Conover, M.H.: Clinical implications of laboratory tests, ed. 3, St. Louis, 1981, The C.V. Mosby Co.
24. Van Dijk, J.M., and others: Differential diagnosis of chest pain: use of 150 enzyme LDH level as a criterion, Postgrad. Med. **65**(1):189, 1979.
25. Waxler, R.: The patient with congestive heart failure: teaching implications Nurs. Clin. North Am. **11**(2):297, 1976.
26. Yiongson, J.G., and Woods, G.L.: Cardiac isoenzymes: clinical implications and limitations, Crit. Care Q. **2**(3):47, 1979.

CHAPTER 6

Clinical applications of radionuclide angiography in congestive heart failure

NANCY PANTALEO STÜDER
PREDIMAN K. SHAH
DANIEL S. BERMAN

Until recently, accurate and objective assessment of cardiac function required invasive procedures like cardiac catheterization and contrast angiography. However, recent advances in noninvasive techniques like echocardiography and radionuclide angiography have made it possible not only to assess cardiac anatomy but also to accurately determine important variables of cardiovascular function. In this chapter, we will briefly review the technical aspects of radionuclide angiography and its clinical application in the assessment of patients with known or suspected congestive cardiac failure. The main objective of this chapter is to familiarize the clinician with the nuclear noninvasive diagnostic tests available in the assessment and treatment of individuals with congestive heart failure.

TECHNICAL CONSIDERATIONS

Over the last few years, the availability of safe and suitable radiotracers, as well as technological developments in the field of gamma cameras and minicomputers, has made it feasible to perform radionuclide angiography not only in special nuclear medicine laboratories but also at the bedside of critically ill patients during supine or sitting exercise. Extensive details regarding the equipment and the techniques used are beyond the scope of this chapter and are described elsewhere.[1,5]

There are two principal methods of performing radionuclide angiography: these are the first-pass and the equilibrium techniques (Table 6-1).

First pass method

In this method, a suitable radiotracer (usually a nonparticulate technetium-99m agent such as technetium-99m pertechnetate, technetium-99m pyrophosphate, or technetium-99m sulfur colloid) is injected as a bolus into either a peripheral or a central vein. The sequential passage of the radiotracer through the right side of the heart, the lungs, and the left side of the heart is imaged by a gamma scintillation camera, which is appropriately positioned over the chest in any desired position, for example, right anterior oblique, left anterior oblique, or anterior. The data are generally stored on magnetic tape for subsequent processing. The whole imaging process is completed within a few seconds and repeat imaging requires additional bolus injections of radiotracer. The data can be processed to determine left as well as right ventricular ejection fractions and can be used to provide a cinematic display of images that allow assessment of regional ventricular wall motion.*

We gratefully acknowledge the valuable secretarial assistance of Connie Coffman and Joyce Nunn and the valuable computer assistance of Sharon Hulse and David Brown.

*References 6, 10, 12, 18, 30.

Table 6-1. Comparison of methods for radionuclide angiography

	First-pass method	Equilibrium method
Radiotracer	99mTc pertechnetate 99mTc pyrophosphate 99mTc diphosphonate	99mTc labeled albumin or 99mTc labeled autologous RBC
Administration	Requires rapid bolus injection of tracer	Nonbolus IV injection of tracer is sufficient
Advantages	1. Acquisition time is very brief (a few seconds) requiring little patient cooperation 2. Optimal separation of various cardiac chambers achieved without overlap 3. Intracardiac shunt can be detected 4. Pulmonary transit time can be determined	1. Repeated imaging can be performed up to 4-6 hours after tracer injection and hence imaging can be performed in multiple views as well as systematically 2. High spatial resolution for regional wall motion analysis
Disadvantages	1. Repeat imaging requires repeat radiotracer injection 2. Spatial resolution for regional wall motion is not optimal	1. Acquisition time is long but can be reduced with modification of technique and use of high-sensitivity collimators 2. Overlap of cardiac structures is a problem requiring careful positioning of the cardiac chambers

Equilibrium method

The equilibrium method has been variously named as equilibrium radionuclide ventriculography, angiography, and multiple-gated blood pool scintigraphy. This method employs the intravenous injection of a radiotracer that stays within the intraventricular compartment, such as technetium-99m labeled albumin or autologous erythrocytes labeled in vivo or in vitro with technetium-99m.[11,16] Unlike first-pass scintigraphy, the equilibrium method does not require bolus injection. From 3 to 5 minutes after injection, the radioactivity equilibrates within the cardiovascular blood pool, and imaging is begun by using a gamma scintillation camera attached to a minicomputer. Imaging is always performed in at least the 45 degree left anterior oblique view, with the exact degree of obliquity adjusted to allow maximal separation of the left and right ventricles. To minimize the overlap by the left atrium, slight caudal tilt is also added to the imaging distributor. Additional views routinely used to evaluate regional wall motion of all portions of the left ventricle include the anterior view and the 70-degree left anterior oblique view (Fig. 6-1). With the

multiple gated technique, the electrocardiographic R-R interval is divided into 14 to 64 equally spaced intervals spanning onset of systole to end-diastole. Through the use of the minicomputer, the gamma camera images each cardiac cycle during these evenly spaced intervals (frames) and stores them in computer memory. Data from the corresponding parts of multiple cardiac cycles are added together until radionuclide count density per frame has been achieved for adequate spatial and temporal resolution. Traditionally each imaging view spans several hundred beats over 4 to 6 minutes of acquisition time. However, recent studies indicate that the acquisition time can be reduced to 1 to 2 minutes per view without significant loss of information content.[15,19]

The variables of cardiac function that can be determined from either form of radionuclide angiography include:

1. Left ventricular volumes, ejection fraction, ejection and filling rates, and regional wall motion
2. Right ventricular ejection fraction and regional wall motion
3. Pulmonary blood volume and intracardiac shunt

4. Relative stroke volume of the two ventricles, providing an index of valvular regurgitation
5. Cardiac output

Left ventricular ejection fraction is the single most important description of global ventricular function, and, of all the parameters measured by radionuclide angiography, it receives the most attention. Determination of ejection fraction is usually performed with a count-based approach as determined by the following equation:

$$EF = \frac{EDC - ESC}{EDC - bkg}$$

That is, the ejection fraction equals the radioactive counts at end-diastole (EDC) minus the radioactive counts at end-systole (ESC) divided by the background corrected radioactive counts (bkg) at end-diastole (see also Fig. 6-2). In general, after data acquisition from either the first-pass or the equilibrium method, the regions of interest, for example, the left or right ventricular blood pools, are identified, and the edges are determined using various semiautomatic algorithms or light pen assignment. Following appropriate background subtraction, the end-diastolic and the end-systolic frames with corresponding counts are determined, and ejection fraction is automatically computed. The various frames can be displayed in a rapid sequence, closed-loop, flicker-free movie format for visual display of regional wall motion.

The normal ranges for left and right ventricular ejection fractions vary slightly from laboratory to laboratory.[16] In our laboratory, which uses the multiple gated equilibrium imaging technique, the normal left ventricular ejection fraction ranges from 0.54 to 0.78 with a mean of 0.64 ± 0.08 SD,

WALL MOTION EVALUATION

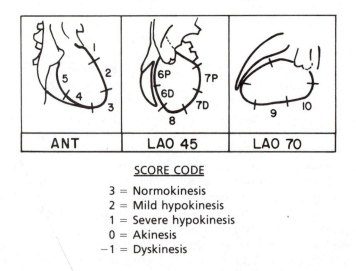

SCORE CODE

3 = Normokinesis
2 = Mild hypokinesis
1 = Severe hypokinesis
0 = Akinesis
−1 = Dyskinesis

Fig. 6-1. Three radionuclide views and the scoring system used in our laboratory. In the anterior view *(Ant)*, segment *1* = anterobasal segment; *2* = anterior wall, *3* = apex; *4* = inferior wall; *5* = inferobasal segment. In the LAO 45 degree, *6P* represents proximal septum, *6D* the distal septum, *(4)* the inferoapical segment, *7D* the distal posterolateral segment, *7P* the proximal posterolateral segment. In the LAO 70 degree, segments *1* and *2* represent the anteroseptal wall, segment *3* the apex; segment *4* represents the inferior wall, and segment *5* represents the posterobasal segment. A score ranging from 3 to −1 is assigned by concensus to each of the segments.

whereas the right ventricular ejection fraction ranges from 0.39 to 0.58 with a mean of 0.48 ± 0.05 SD.

The validity of radionuclide determined ejection fraction has been established by multiple comparisons with that determined by contrast angiography. In addition, the nuclear techniques have demonstrated a high degree of temporal intra- and interobserver reproducibility.[4] Unlike contrast ventriculography, the nuclear count–based method does not rely on assumptions regarding the geometric shape of the ventricle in the calculation of ejection fraction. For this reason, and because of their highly objective value, these techniques have now replaced the contrast ventriculogram as the standard for ejection fraction measurements.

Left ventricular regional wall motion, as assessed from radionuclide angiograms, also compares favorably to that determined from contrast angiography. Currently under development are quantitative methods for assessment of regional wall motion.[17] These methods offer the promise of providing an objective and reproducible measurement of regional ventricular function.

Left ventricular volumes from radionuclide angiograms may be determined using standard area-length geometric techniques[2,23] or alternatively using count changes irrespective of geometric formulae.[25,29] Both methods have shown good correlation with angiographically determined left ventricular volumes.

CLINICAL APPLICATIONS

Noninvasive radionuclide angiography can be applied in conjunction with routine clinical, electrocardiographic, and radiographic assessment of

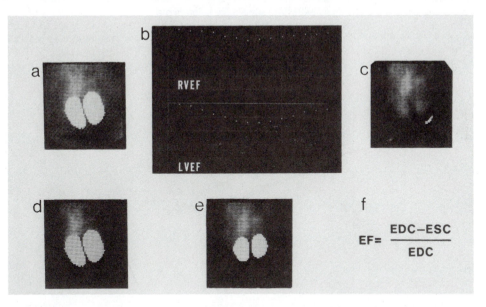

Fig. 6-2. Steps involved in one method of computer analysis of ejection fraction. **A,** Operator draws regions of interest over left ventricle and right ventricle. **B,** Activity versus time curves are generated for the left ventricle and the right ventricle, and end-diastolic and end-systolic frames are selected. **C,** Operator selects a paraventricular background ROI, and subtracts background counts from the end-diastolic and end-systolic frames. **D,** Regions of interest drawn over the left ventricle and right ventricle in end-diastolic frame. **E,** Regions of interest drawn over the left ventricle and the right ventricle in end-systolic frame. **F,** Ejection fractions calculated using this formula.

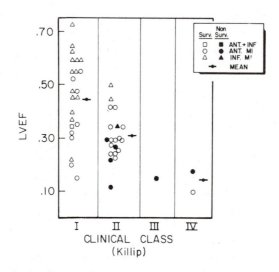

Fig. 6-3. The distribution of left ventricular ejection fraction (LVEF) among a group of patients with acute myocardial infarction. Patients in Killip Class I have no clinical signs of left ventricular failure, whereas patients in Killip Class II have signs of mild left ventricular failure. Pulmonary edema is present in Killip Class III and shock in Killip Class IV. Note that there is a wide range of LVEF among patients in Killip Class I and II, with many patients in Killip Class I demonstrating reduced LVEF (<0.54).

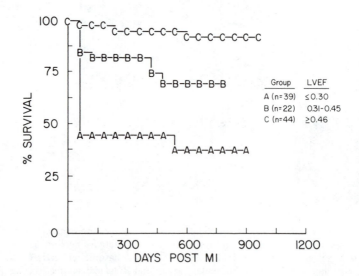

Fig. 6-4. The prognostic influence of left ventricular ejection fraction (LVEF) infarction is illustrated in the relationship of LVEF to postinfarction survival. Note that patients in Group A with severely reduced LVEF of ≤0.30, have a 30% survival compared to patients in Group C with LVEF ≥0.46 who have a 95% survival.

patients who are known or suspected to have congestive heart failure, and it can address these clinical problems:

1. Detecting the presence and severity of cardiac dysfunction
2. Predicting a prognosis based on
   a. Determining the etiological structural basis for heart failure
   b. Determining the response to therapeutic interventions (surgery, drugs, balloon counterpulsation, etc.)
3. Aiding in decision making for timing and appropriateness of surgical intervention
4. Excluding cardiac causes of clinical indicators that simulate those of congestive heart failure

Assessment of severity and prognosis of heart failure in myocardial infarction

Radionuclide angiography has been extensively used in the evaluation of acute left ventricular dysfunction following myocardial infarction.[22,24,26,28] In general it has been observed that left ventricular ejection fraction is depressed in over 90% of patients with anterior myocardial infarction and in about 50% of patients with inferior myocardial infarction. In general, the greater the clinical severity of left ventricular failure as assessed from Killip classification,[14] the lower is the left ventricular ejection fraction. However, it is important to note that a sizable proportion of patients not exhibiting clinical signs of left ventricular failure actually are shown to have variable degrees of depression in left ventricular ejection fraction (Fig. 6-3). In some cases, profound reduction of left ventricular ejection fraction occurs despite the total absence of clinical indicators of congestive heart failure. Of particular importance has been the observation that a severely depressed left ventricular ejection fraction (≤ 0.30) is of adverse prognostic value as indicated by a high mortality, for example, 54% in comparison to the 4% mortality observed in patients with a left ventricular ejection fraction exceeding 0.30[28] (Fig. 6-4). Thus assess-

ment of left ventricular ejection fraction provides important information regarding the severity of infarction as well as its implications for short-term survival.

Detection of right ventricular infarction as a cause of systemic venous hypertension and low-output state

A very useful application of radionuclide angiography has been the detection of predominant right ventricular dysfunction that complicates 40% to 50% of patients with inferior myocardial infarction[28] (Fig. 6-5). This syndrome can produce signs of right ventricular failure, manifested by systemic venous hypertension as well as a low cardiac output, and hypotensive state.[27] The recognition of this syndrome is important in view of its favorable prognosis when appropriately treated by volume infusion and/or inotropic-vasodilator therapy. Chronic persistent right ventricular failure may be the outcome of predominant right ventricular infarction. The diagnosis can be suspected from the results of a radionuclide angiogram.

However, it should be recognized that scintigraphic evidence of predominant right ventricular

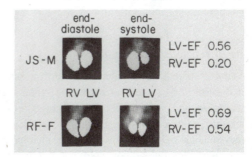

Fig. 6-5. The top panel demonstrates 45 degree LAO gated blood pool image of a patient with inferior myocardial infarction complicated by predominant right ventricular dysfunction as indicated by normal left ventricular ejection fraction with a depressed right ventricular ejection fraction. The panel at the bottom represents a patient with an uncomplicated inferior infarction with normal LVEF and RVEF.

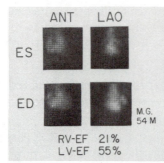

ANT   LAO

ES

ED

M.G.
54 M

RV-EF   21%
LV-EF   55%

Fig. 6-6. Gated blood pool images demonstrating evidence of predominant right ventricular dysfunction in a patient with chest pain and shock. Pulmonary angiography confirmed extensive emboli.

dysfunction may also be observed in other causes of right ventricular failure, such as precapillary pulmonary hypertension as in chronic obstructive pulmonary disease (COPD), pulmonary embolism, primary pulmonary hypertension, and right-sided valvular heart disease (Fig. 6-6). Therefore the correct cause of predominant right ventricular failure can only be deduced from consideration of additional clinical, radiological, ECG, echocardiographic, and other scintigraphic details (e.g., pyrophosphate scintigraphy).

Detection of ventricular aneurysm as a cause of refractory heart failure

About 10% to 15% of patients develop a localized diastolic and systolic deformity of their left ventricle secondary to a transmural myocardial infarction. This deformity, called a ventricular aneurysm (Fig. 6-7), not only fails to contribute to systolic ejection of blood but, by expanding in systole, in fact wastefully expends some of the contractile effort of the normally contracting myocardium, thereby contributing to or worsening congestive heart failure. When congestive heart failure from a localized ventricular aneurysm becomes severe and refractory to medical treatment, surgical resection offers the possibility of clinical improvement and amelioration of heart failure.

Although diagnosis of a ventricular aneurysm may be suspected clinically or from an ECG and a chest roentgenogram, invasive contrast ventriculography is frequently necessary for definitive diagnosis. It has been clearly shown, however, that the definitive diagnosis can now be made accurately by noninvasive radionuclide angiography.[7-9,13]

Differentiation of cardiomyopathies

Cardiomyopathy is a generic term that is used to describe a variety of diseases that produce predominant dysfunction of myocardium without any etiological relationship to valvular heart disease, congenital heart disease, systemic hypertension, or coronary artery disease. In general, three basic pathophysiological types have been described, each generally caused by relatively specific disease states (Table 6-2). The three pathophysiological types of cardiomyopathy can often be easily differentiated from radionuclide angiography (Table 6-2 and Fig. 6-8).[20] For example, a patient may come into the hospital with clinical indicators suggestive of congestive heart failure that might be considered to be secondary to poor left ventricular function or valvular heart disease until a high ejection fraction and a thickened septum characteristic of idiopathic hypertrophic subaortic stenosis is found on radionuclide angiography. This differentiation is of critical value since the prognosis and management of this type of cardiac muscle disease is quite different from other forms of cardiomyopathy.

Acute volume overload as a cause of severe heart failure

In acute mechanical volume overload resulting from acute severe valvular regurgitation, such as acute mitral regurgitation caused by myocardial infarction or bacterial endocarditis, acute aortic regurgitation caused by endocarditis, or aortic dissection, or intracardiac shunt as a result of postmyocardial ventricular septal rupture, the patient may exhibit clinical indicators of severe left ventricular failure. In these instances, the diagnosis can often be suspected clinically and confirmed by cardiac catheterization. Radionuclide

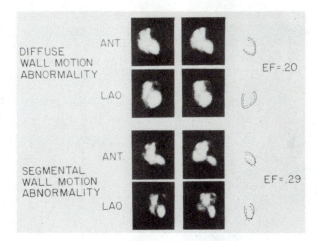

Fig. 6-7. Two different patterns of wall motion abnormality are illustrated; both are associated with depressed global left ventricular ejection fraction. The top panel demonstrated diffuse generated hypokinesis consistent with a cardiomyopathy whereas the bottom shows localized apical dyskinesis consistent with an apical aneurysm.

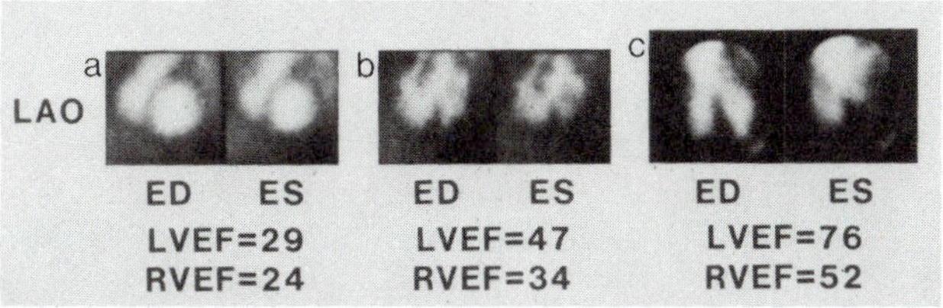

Fig. 6-8. Representative examples of gated blood pool images of three patients with different forms of cardiomyopathy. **A,** Congestive cardiomyopathy. **B,** Restrictive cardiomyopathy; **C,** hypertrophic cardiomyopathy. (See text for details.)

Table 6-2. Cardiomyopathies

	Congestive (dilated)	Hypertrophic	Restrictive
Cause	Idiopathic; alcoholic; postviral ischemic; peripartum; late stages of hypertrophic types; sarcoidosis; collagen diseases; infiltrative diseases	Idiopathic, in association with pheochromocytoma; lentigines, neurofibromatosis; Friedreich's ataxia	Idiopathic; ischemic; amyloidosis; hemochromatosis; endomyocardial fibrosis; eosinophilic heart disease (Loeffler)
Findings on RNA	Dilated chambers; diffuse hypokinesis; markedly depressed left and right ventricular ejection fraction*	Small chambers; thickened septum; hypercontractile ventricles, high ejection fraction	Normal to small chambers; normal to slightly depressed ejection fraction

*Right ventricular size and ejection fraction may be disproportionately less abnormal compared to that of the left ventricle in ischemic cardiomyopathy.

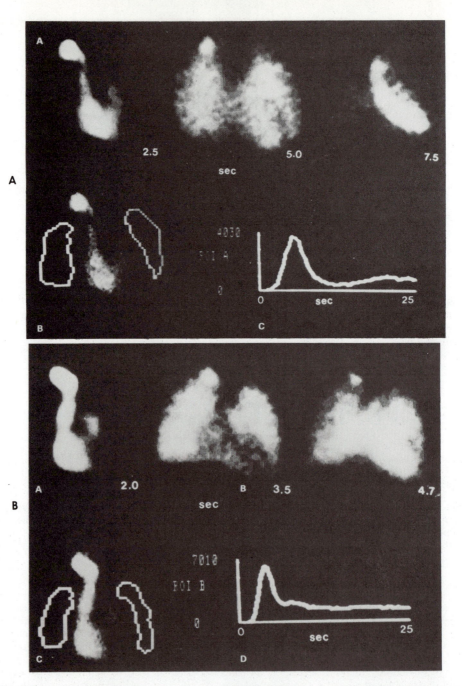

Fig. 6-9. A, Normal radionuclide angiogram. *A,* Selected frames of anterior projection that show clear visualization of radioactivity within the superior vena cava, right atrium, right ventricle, pulmonary artery, lungs, left side of the heart, and aorta. Regions of interest are marked over both lung fields far from central circulation, *B.* Pulmonary time-activity curve is displayed in *C.* **B,** Left-to-right shunt. Clear visualization of the superior vena cava, right atrium, right ventricle, and pulmonary artery (2.0 seconds). The lung fields are seen in *B* (3.5 seconds). The left side of the heart and the aorta are not clearly seen, and there are persistent levels of activity in the lung fields (4.7 seconds, *A*). Regions of interest over both lung fields are seen in *C.* An abnormal pulmonary time-activity curve showing rapid transpulmonary transit time and early recirculation as a result of left-to-right shunting is shown in *D.* (From Treves, S.: Sem. Nucl. Med., **10**[1]:16, Jan. 1980.)

angiography can provide a clue to this diagnosis by demonstrating normal or hypercontractile left ventricle with normal to high ejection fraction in the face of clinical indicators of severe heart failure (Fig. 6-9). When only one ventricle is involved with the volume overload, as seen in valvular insufficiency, a marked difference in the stroke counts of the two ventricles also points to the correct diagnosis (see below). In ventricular septal rupture, the diagnosis and assessment of the severity of the left-to-right shunt can be made using first-pass radionuclide angiography.[3] Accurate diagnosis of these mechanical lesions is critical since early aggressive surgery can be life-saving in this group of patients.

Atrial myxoma versus mitral stenosis as a cause of pulmonary congestion

While echocardiography is a highly accurate technique for differentiation of mitral stenosis from atrial myxoma as a cause of pulmonary congestion and other symptoms, radionuclide angiography can also be used successfully to diagnose the presence of a myxoma[21] (Fig. 6-10).

Detection of left ventricular thrombus in cardiomyopathy and postinfarction left ventricular dysfunction

Individuals with chronic heart failure and poorly contracting dilated chambers or ventricular aneurysms have a high frequency of systemic embolization from clots forming in either the left atrium or the left ventricle, the detection of which may rationalize the institution of prophylactic anticoagulant therapy. Demonstration of filling defects in the apex of the left ventricle, indicative of a mural thrombus, is possible with radionuclide angiography (Fig. 6-11), although two-dimensional echocardiography is more established value in this regard.

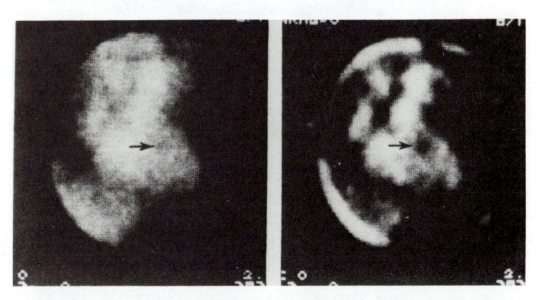

Fig. 6-10. Unprocessed and computer-processed diastolic right antierior oblique gated radionuclide cardiac images in a patient with a large left atrial myxoma. A blood pool defect *(arrow)* is clearly defined in the region of the left ventricle in the computer-processed image on the right. This defect is poorly defined in the unprocessed image on the left. (From Pohost, G.; Circulation **55:**88, 1977.)

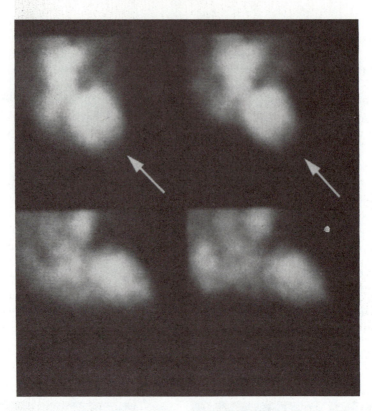

Fig. 6-11. Gated blood pool images of a patient with dilated left ventricle with diffuse generalized hypothesis secondary to multiple infarcts demonstrated an apical filling defect *(arrow)* consistent with mural thrombus.

Determination and quantification of valvular regurgitation

Since severe valvular regurgitation frequently results in or contributes to the development of heart failure and is amenable to surgical treatment, it is important to evaluate its role in the clinical presentation of a patient with heart failure. Although invasive catheterization and angiography can make this distinction, noninvasive nuclear angiography may also prove to be of value in the detection and estimation of the severity of valvular regurgitation. Using the ratio of left and right ventricular stroke counts, an abnormally high ratio has been correlated with the presence of valvular regurgitation.[8] However, further work in this area is

necessary to more clearly define the accuracy and the ultimate role of radionuclide angiography in this regard.

Decision regarding surgical intervention for heart failure

The main surgically correctable causes of congestive heart failure include valvular disease, ventricular aneurysm, congenital heart disease, intracardiac shunts, AV fistulas and hypertrophic cardiomyopathy. Surgical outcome for these lesions is generally unfavorable if diffuse severe left ventricular dysfunction is present, identified by an ejection fraction of ≤ 0.20 to 0.25. Therefore noninvasive determination of left ventricular contrac-

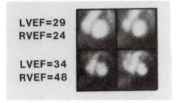

LVEF=29
RVEF=24

LVEF=34
RVEF=48

Fig. 6-12. Gated blood pool images in 45 degree LAO view before and after hydralazine therapy for chronic heart failure demonstrated. Hydralazine-induced reduction in ventricular size associated with improved ventricular function.

tile pattern and ejection fraction may help the decision-making process in regard to whether the patient should actively be considered for invasive evaluation for possible surgery or whether further invasive workup for consideration of surgery should be avoided.

Evaluation of the effects of therapeutic interventions on ventricular function in congestive heart failure

The noninvasive and repeatable nature of radionuclide angiography makes it very attractive for the objective assessment of ventricular function in response to pharmacological, mechanical, and surgical treatment (Fig. 6-12). In general, ejection fractions, chamber size, and contractile patterns can be easily evaluated but in the future, it may be possible to actually determine stroke volume and cardiac output on a routine basis.

HEALTH CARE IMPLICATIONS

The goal of health care is to assist the patient in achieving and maintaining optimum physical and mental health. The nuclear cardiology studies may be a major instrument toward attaining that goal; however, they may also pose a threat to the patient's well-being by causing unnecessary anxiety or misconceptions.

Fluid-filled catheters in critical care units (CCU) provide a system whereby leaky electrical current may increase the potential for ventricular fibrilla-

tion induced by electricity. The critical care clinician should not only be responsible for the patient's comfort during bedside scans but also for the patient's safety. Therefore after the patient is comfortably positioned under the camera and the procedure fully explained, the clinician should check to see that all electrical equipment is grounded. In addition, all electrical equipment should be checked weekly for current leakage.

One of the most important requisites for all clinicians working in the intensive care unit CCU, (ICU), or outpatient setting is their responsibility for patient education. In preparation for the exercise test, patients should be asked not to eat or drink for 3 to 4 hours before the test. This is to ensure that blood is not diverted to the gastrointestinal tract for digestion but will remain within the skeletal muscle and heart muscle during the exercise stress test. Many patients are taking cardiac medications and are asked to temporarily discontinue them before the test. A drug such as propranolol is usually stopped 48 hours before the test. Nurse clinicians should contact the patient's physician before the discontinuation of any cardiac medications. It is normal procedure for patients to sign a consent form before the test is performed. Nurse clinicians can assist the patient in completing this form by answering questions and explaining the procedure. These simple explanations accomplished before the test can help alleviate anxiety and confusion that may arise during the test.

Patients should be told that skin preparation (shaving off hair, alcohol cleansing, etc.) is common practice before the test is begun, to facilitate placement of small electrodes on the chest. These electrodes are then connected to an ECG monitor so cardiac rhythm may be continuously observed during the course of the test, which consists of exercise on a bicycle.

Patients should be reassured that a physician will supervise the test and communicate with them regarding development of symptoms. If the patients experience chest pain, arm pain, shortness of breath, or light-headedness, they are instructed to notify the physician immediately. The physician will decide when the test should be stopped depending on the symptoms, blood pressure, electrocardiogram and degree of fatigue that develops.

Following the exercise, patients are allowed to rest until their heart rate, electrocardiogram, and blood pressure have returned to baseline. It is common for them to inquire as to the results of the test immediately. Nurse clinicians may provide support at this time by explaining that the attending physician will be notified of the results within a 24-hour period and a final written report will be sent within a few days. This type of communication may help allay immediate anxiety. However, if not, interventions should be directed toward reassurance and facilitating immediate physician-patient communication. Those nurses who are in collaborative practice with physicians and are in attendance during the procedure generally have the authority to provide this explanation.

SUMMARY

The widespread availability of noninvasive radionuclide angiography with its technical refinements has been a welcome addition to the armamentarium of the clinician as well as the investigator in evaluating patients with a variety of cardiovascular disorders that can adversely affect the efficiency of the heart and result in heart failure. It would be incorrect to assume that radionuclide angiography will totally replace invasive contrast angiography; nevertheless, this technique has considerably enhanced our understanding of cardiovascular function and with the continued interest and improvement in instrumentation, its applicability is bound to expand in a more meaningful fashion. Further refinements in technology are likely to overcome the major shortcomings of the currently available imaging systems, that is, high cost and bulk. In this context, the recently introduced nuclear stethoscope, which uses a scintillation probe that is less bulky and less expensive, appears to be particularly promising.

REFERENCES

1. Ashburn, W.L., Schelbert, H.R., and Verba, J.W.: Left ventricular ejection fraction: a review of several radionuclide angiographic approaches using the scintillation camera, Prog. Cardiovasc. Dis. **20**:267, 1978.
2. Ashburn, W., Kostuk, W., Karliner, J., and others: Left ventricular ejection fraction and volume determinations by radionuclide angiography, Semin. Nucl. Med. **3**:166, 1973.
3. Askenazi, J., Ahnberg, D., Koingold, E., and others: Quantitative radionuclide angiography: detection and quantitation of left to right shunts, Am. J. Cardiol. **37**:382, 1976.
4. Berman, D., and Mason, D.T.: Gated cardiac blood pool scintigraphy in the assessment of ventricular function. In Mason, D.T.: Advances in heart disease, New York, 1978, Grune & Stratton, Inc., p. 153.
5. Berman, D.S., Maddahi, J., Garcia, E.V., and others: Assessment of left and right ventricular function with multiple gated equilibrium cardiac blood pool scintigraphy. In Berman, D.S., and Mason, D.T., editors: Clinical nuclear cardiology, New York, 1981, Grune & Stratton, Inc., p. 224.
6. Bodenheimer, M.M., Bonka, V.S., Fooshea, C.M., and others: Quantitative radionuclide angiography in the right anterior oblique view: comparison with contrast ventriculography, Am. J. Cardiol. **41**:718, 1978.
7. Botvinick, E., Shames, D., and Hutchinson, J.C.: Noninvasive diagnosis of a false left ventricular aneurysm with radioisotope gated cardiac blood imaging, Am. J. Cardiol. **37**:1089, 1976.
8. Dymond, D.S., Jarriett, P.H., Britton, K.E., and Spurrell, R.A.J.: Detection of postinfarction left ventricular aneurysm by first pass radionuclide ventriculography using a multi-crystal gamma camera, Br. Heart J. **41**:68, 1979.
9. Friedman, M.L., and Cantor, R.E.: Reliability of gated heart scintigrams for detection of left ventricular aneurysm: concise communication, J. Nucl. Med. **20**:720, 1977.
10. Hecht, H.S., Mirell, S.G., Rolett, E.L., and Blahd, W.H.: Left ventricular ejection fraction and segmental wall motion by peripheral first-pass radionuclide angiography, J. Nucl. Med. **19**:17, 1978.
11. Hegge, F.N., Hamilton, G.W., Laison, S.M., and others: Cardiac chamber imaging: a comparison of red blood cells labeled with Tc-99m in vitro and in vivo, J. Nucl. Med. **19**:129, 1978.
12. Jengo, J.A., Mena, I., Blaufuss, A., and Criley, J.M.: Evaluation of left ventricular function (ejection fraction and segmental wall motion) by single pass radioisotope angiography, Circulation **57**:326, 1978.
13. Katz, R.J., Simpson, A., DiBianco, R., and others: Noninvasive diagnosis of left ventricular pseudoaneurysm, Am. J. Cardiol. **44**:372, 1979.

14. Killip, T. III, and Kimball, J.T.: Treatment of myocardial infarction in a coronary care unit, Am. J. Cardiol. **20**:457, 1967.

15. Maddahi, J., Berman, D., Silverberg, R., and others: Validation of a two minute technique for multiple gated scintigraphic assessment of left ventricular ejection fraction and regional wall motion (abstract), J. Nucl. Med. **19**:669, 1978.

16. Maddahi, J., Berman, D.S., Diamond, G., and others: Evaluation of left ventricular ejection fraction and segmental wall motion by multiple gated equilibrium cardiac blood pool scintigraphy. In Cady, L., editor: Computer techniques in cardiology, New York, 1978, Marcel Dekker, Inc., pp. 389-416.

17. Maddox, D.E., Wynne, J., Uren, R., and others: Regional ejection fraction: a quantitative radionuclide index of regional left ventricular performance, Circulation **59**:1001, 1979.

18. Marshall, R.C., Berger, H.J., Costim, J.C., and others: Assessment of cardiac performance with quantitative radionuclide angiography, Circulation **56**:820, 1977.

19. Pfisterer, M.E., Matthias, E., Ricci, D.R., and others: Validity of left ventricular ejection fractions measured at rest and peak exercise by equilibrium radionuclide angiography using short acquisition times, J. Nucl. Med. **20**:484, 1979.

20. Pohost, G.M., Fallon, J.T., and Strauss, W.H.: The role of radionuclide techniques in patients with myocardial disease in nuclear cardiology. In Willerson, J.T., editor: Cardiovascular clinics, Philadelphia, 1979. F.A. Davis Co., p. 149.

21. Pohost, G.M., Pastore, J.O., McKusick, K.A., and others: Detection of left atrial myxoma by gated radionuclide cardiac imaging, Circulation **55**:88, 1977.

22. Reduto, L.A., Berger, H.J., Cohen, L.S., and others: Sequential radionuclide assessment of left and right ventricular performance after acute transmural myocardial infarction, Ann. Intern. Med. **89**:441, 1978.

23. Resych, S.K., Scholtz, P.M., Newman, G.E., and others: Cardiac function at rest and during exercise in normals and in patients with coronary heart disease: evaluation by radionuclide angiocardiography, Ann. Surg. **187**:449, 1978.

24. Rigo, P., Murray, M., Strauss, H.W., and others: Left ventricular function in acute myocardial infarction evaluated by gated scintiphotography, Circulation **50**:678, 1974.

25. Ritchie, J.L., Sorensen, S., Kennedy, W.J., and Hamilton, G.W.: Radionuclide angiography: noninvasive assessment of hemodynamic changes after administration of nitroglycerin, Am. J. Cardiol. **43**:278, 1979.

26. Schelbert, H.R., Hennina, H., Ashburn, W.L., and others: Serial measurements of left ventricular ejection fraction by radionuclide angiography early and late after myocardial infarction, Am. J. Cardiol. **38**:407, 1976.

27. Shah, P.K., Shellock, F., Berman, D., and others: Predominant right ventricular dysfunction in acute myocardial infarction: frequency, clinical, hemodynamic and scintigraphic findings, Circulation **62**(suppl. III):313, 1980.

28. Shah, P.K., Pichler, M., Berman, D.S., and others: Left ventricular ejection fraction determined by radionuclide ventriculography in early stages of first transmural myocardial infarction, Am. J. Cardiol. **45**:542, 1980.

29. Slutsky, R., Karliner, J., Ricci, D., and others: Left ventricular volumes by gated equilibrium radionuclide angiography: a new method, Circulation **60**:556, 1979.

30. Steele, P., Kirch, D., Mathews, M., and Davies, H.: Measurement of left heart ejection fraction and end-diastolic volume by a computerized, scintigraphic technique using a wedged pulmonary arterial catheter, Am. J. Cardiol. **34**:179, 1974.

CHAPTER 7

Physiological basis and clinical application of bedside hemodynamic monitoring

MAGDA BUNOY
PREDIMAN K. SHAH

This chapter discusses an important aspect of the management of a patient with congestive heart failure. The fundamental value of hemodynamic monitoring is to provide direct measurement of important descriptors of the heart as a pump and of the factors that regulate the performance of the heart as a pump. The clinical and practical utility of these measurements depends upon an understanding of the normal cardiac physiology and its alterations in the patient with congestive heart failure. The quantitative and qualitative analysis of hemodynamic data yields clinically useful information that not only aids in making the proper diagnosis but also allows selection of appropriate therapy, the effects of which can be quickly and accurately monitored. The hemodynamic measurements can also provide useful prognostic information, particularly in patients with congestive heart failure resulting from acute myocardial infarction.

The contents of this chapter are particularly directed toward the critical care clinicians who will be taking care of patients undergoing bedside hemodynamic monitoring. It is the intent of this chapter to provide relevant information that will allow the critical care clinician to:

We gratefully acknowledge the editorial assistance of Patricia Allen, the secretarial assistance of Joyce Nunn and Beverly Yoshioka, and the artwork of Lance Laforteza.

1. Describe the basic physiological principles of hemodynamic monitoring including: cardiac output and determinants thereof and intracardiac and peripheral arterial pressures.
2. Describe the techniques of hemodynamic monitoring, that is, procedures for insertion of balloon-tipped flotation catheter (Swan-Ganz catheter) and arterial cannula; describe the techniques for the determination of cardiac output.
3. Correctly identify and describe pressure tracings.
4. Identify normal and abnormal values of hemodynamic variables.
5. Recognize the complications of hemodynamic monitoring.
6. Describe the clinical application of hemodynamic monitoring in the patient with congestive heart failure by: (a) recognizing the specific hemodynamic alterations of the various clinical syndromes associated with congestive heart failure, (b) selecting the appropriate therapy, and (c) assessing the response to therapy as reflected by changes in the hemodynamic variables.
7. Present the health care management of the patient with heart failure undergoing hemodynamic monitoring with emphasis on identifying health care problems and nursing interventions.

PHYSIOLOGICAL PRINCIPLES OF HEMODYNAMIC MONITORING

Since an understanding of the factors that affect tissue perfusion and the mechanical performance of the heart as a pump is essential to the rational application of techniques of hemodynamic monitoring for the patient with congestive heart failure, these factors will be briefly reviewed.

Cardiac output

The cardiac output (CO) is the volume (liters) of blood ejected by the heart during each minute, and this in turn is the product of the stroke volume (SV) and the heart rate per minute. The SV is the volume (milliliters) of blood ejected by the ventricle during each beat and is equivalent to the difference between the end-diastolic volume (EDV) and the end-systolic volume (ESV) of the ventricle. For comparison of measurements between individuals of different sizes both CO and SV are divided by the body surface area and expressed as cardiac index (CI) and stroke volume index (SVI) respectively.[24,49]

Determinants of cardiac output. The pump performance of the heart as reflected by the SV is principally determined by three factors: (1) preload, (2) afterload, and (3) contractility.[5,7,38]

Preload. Preload may be defined as the end-diastolic stretch of the muscle fiber, which in the intact ventricle is related to the EDV. The physiological studies of Frank and Starling showed that the force of contraction of the muscle is related to the initial length of the muscle fiber. Ventricular volume and pressure are related to each other in a curvilinear fashion and their relationship is determined chiefly by the compliance or its inverse descriptor, the stiffness, of the muscle. The determination of ventricular volume until recently required angiographic or thermodilution techniques, but recent advances in echocardiography, digital angiography, and radionuclide angiography hold promise for easier and noninvasive determination of ventricular volumes. Meanwhile, it is common in clinical situations to measure directly or indirectly the left ventricular end-diastolic pressure (LVEDP) and accept it as a reasonable surrogate measure of fiber length or EDV. However, changes in left ventricular pressure volume relationship resulting from altered states of compliance can pose serious constraints on the validity

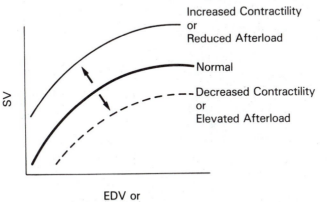

Fig. 7-1. Diagram represents curvilinear relationship between preload as depicted by ventricular end-diastolic volume *(EDV)* and overall pump function as depicted by stroke volume *(SV)* (Frank-Starling ventricular function curve). Curve is shifted upward and to left by increasing contractility or reduced afterload, whereas reduced contractility and elevated afterload produce downward and leftward displacement. *EDP,* Ventricular end-diastolic pressure. *PCW,* Mean pulmonary capillary wedge pressure. *PA_{EDP},* Pulmonary arterial end-diastolic pressure.

of EDP as a reflector of true EDV. The curvilinear relationship of preload and SV is commonly referred to as the ventricular function curve or the Frank-Starling curve (Fig. 7-1). In the intact heart a measurement of ventricular output (SV) and of ventricular filling (fiber stretch) is required to plot the Frank-Starling curve. The LVEDP is equivalent to the mean left atrial pressure (LAP) and to the mean pulmonary capillary wedge pressure (PCWP) in the absence of an obstruction at the level of the mitral valve as, for example, in mitral stenosis. In turn the pulmonary artery end-diastolic pressure (PA_{EDP}) is equivalent to the mean PCWP in absence of elevated pulmonary vascular resistance. Both the PA_{EDP} and the PCWP are conveniently determined at the bedside and commonly used as indirect measurements of LVEDP or preload.[24,38,41]

As seen in Fig. 7-1, for a given EDV a subsequent contraction generates a corresponding SV, and an increase in EDV (more diastolic fiber stretch) causes an increase in SV. By plotting the generated SV at increasing levels of EDV, one creates a ventricular function curve (Fig. 7-1). The curve reaches a plateau, indicating that the relationship is nonlinear, and eventually the SV does not continue to increase despite an increasing EDV. In the clinical setting the SV is plotted against the PCWP or the PA_{EDP}, because it is more convenient to use these variables instead of LVEDP or LVEDV to approximate end-diastolic fiber length.[5,24,38]

The ventricular diastolic volume is related to the ventricular diastolic pressure, as is shown in Fig. 7-2. The normal curve *A* shows that this relationship allows relatively large changes in the diastolic volume to be accompanied by relatively small changes in the ventricular diastolic pressure. This diastolic pressure volume relationship refers to the compliance of the relaxed ventricle. Certain disease states, such as ischemia, myocardial infarction, hypertrophy, or infiltrative diseases, may give rise to a decrease in ventricular compliance as is seen in curve *B*. As compared with curve *A*, curve *B* demonstrates a much greater increase in diastolic pressure for a given increase in diastolic

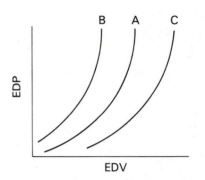

Fig. 7-2. Pressure and volume relationship (compliance curve) of left ventricle under normal circumstances *(A)*, with curves *B* and *C* representing situations where compliance is reduced or increased respectively. See text for details. *EDV,* Ventricular end-diastolic volume. *EDP,* Ventricular end-diastolic pressure.

volume. Conversely, the compliance may be increased as, for example, in chronic volume overload resulting from valvular regurgitation. In this situation, as depicted in curve *C*, for a given change in diastolic volume the corresponding changes in diastolic pressure are small. Careful review of these figures shows that a change in EDP may be indicative of a corresponding change in EDV or compliance or both.

The preload is influenced by the total circulating blood volume, the distribution of the blood volume, and the atrial contraction. When the circulating blood volume is depleted as in instances of hemorrhage, the venous return to the heart decreases and the ventricular EDV falls; consequently there is a decrease in SV and CO. For a given total blood volume, the ventricular EDV is influenced by the distribution of blood between the intrathoracic and extrathoracic compartments, and this is influenced by body position. When the individual is supine the venous return is greater. An elevation of intrathoracic pressure tends to impede venous return to the heart, thus diminishing the intrathoracic blood volume and reducing CO. The resting venous tone also affects the EDV. The smooth muscle in the venous walls responds to a variety of neural and humoral stimuli. Venoconstriction increases the venous return to the heart, as does the pumping action of skeletal muscle during exercise, which squeezes blood out of the veins. A vigorous and appropriately timed atrial contraction augments ventricular filling and the EDV and EDP. The atrial kick is of particular importance in patients with ventricular hypertrophy or diminished left ventricular compliance, whose resistance to ventricular filling tends to be increased.[12,24,38,49]

Afterload. Ventricular afterload is the tension developed during systole. It is directly related to the product of the intraventricular pressure and the ventricular cavitary radius and inversely related to the ventricular wall thickness. Thus changes in afterload may result from alterations in systolic pressure, cavity dimensions, or wall thickness.

In addition to these factors, the afterload is also governed by the outflow impedance against which the ventricles eject. Peripheral arteriolar resistance is the major component of the outflow impedance. By measuring the mean driving pressure and the mean flow, one can calculate the resistance to ejection. The effect of variations in outflow impedance on the SV is critically dependent upon the underlying state of myocardial function. A rise in outflow resistance produces little change in the SV in the presence of normal myocardial function. But with increasing severity of myocardial dysfunction, a rise in outflow resistance results in a greater fall in the SV. Changes in aortic outflow impedance may also influence SV in another way. In the presence of mitral or aortic regurgitation or left-to-right intracardiac shunt the forward fraction of the total left ventricular SV is determined by the aortic outflow impedance. Increase of outflow impedance may reduce the forward fraction of the total SV without necessarily affecting fiber shortening or the total SV. The rationale for the use of vasodilators in congestive heart failure is partly related to the convese of this impedance-SV relationship. For example, reduction in outflow impedance results in a greater SV in the presence of significant myocardial dysfunction and a greater proportionate forward SV in the presence of regurgitant lesions.[12,24,38,41]

Contractility. This term is somewhat more difficult to define in precise terms. However, a change in cardiac function that cannot be attributed to alteration in preload or afterload is attributed to a change in contractility, an inherent force of contraction. Several variables have been proposed as valid measurements of contractility but most of these variables have subsequently been shown to be modified by altered loading conditions as well. Maximum velocity of fiber shortening extrapolated to zero load (V_{max}) has been proposed as a measure of contractility; more recently it has been demonstrated that the ratio of end-systolic pressure and end-systolic volume (Sagawa index) is a more accurate descriptor of the contractile state of the myocardium. A detailed description of these variables is beyond the scope of this chapter and the reader is referred elsewhere.[5,12,24,38]

Examination of Fig. 7-1 shows that an upward and leftward shift of the Frank-Starling curve implies a higher SV for a given EDP or EDV. This shift may occur not only because of an increased contractility but also because of a reduced afterload. Similarly a downward and rightward shift of this curve may result from depressed contractility or increased afterload.

Myocardial contractility is related to a number of factors, including the quantity of norepinephrine released by sympathetic nerve endings, the concentration of other circulating catecholamines, the presence of exogenously administered inotropic agents, pharmacological depressants, or physiological depressants, and a loss of ventricular substance as occurs in myocardial infarction.*

Systemic arterial pressure

Systemic arterial pressure determines the perfusion pressure of various organ systems and is predominantly a product of the CO and the systemic vascular resistance (SVR). In general a drop in CO is compensated by an increased SVR in an attempt to maintain the arterial blood pressure within a normal range. The SVR in turn is determined by the caliber of the peripheral arterioles, which is modulated by the smooth muscle tone, the

---

*References 6, 12, 14, 24, 38.

electrolyte and water content within the walls of the arterioles, and the viscosity of blood. The smooth muscle tone is regulated by local and systemic metabolic, humoral, and neural factors, Increased peripheral arteriolar tone may result from sympathetic stimulation, alpha-adrenergic catecholamines, and angiotensin, whereas decreased smooth muscle tone may result from parasympathetic stimulation, local hypoxia, hypercapnia, acidosis, and accumulation of potassium ions and adenosine. Determination of systemic arterial blood pressure is important, therefore, not only as an indicator of organ perfusion pressure but also for indirect determination of SVR.[23,24] While sphygmomanometry is the standard technique for determination of systemic arterial pressure, accurate measurements are difficult or impossible to obtain in the presence of severely reduced blood pressure or during a state of intense peripheral vasoconstriction. In these circumstances direct determination of intra-arterial pressure is necessary; in addition, this allows continuous monitoring of pressure in seriously ill patients. Furthermore, rapidly fluctuating blood pressure and use of intravenous vasopressor or vasodilator therapy requires accurate and continuous monitoring of arterial pressure, which can best be performed by intra-arterial pressure monitoring.*

TECHNIQUES OF HEMODYNAMIC MONITORING
Insertion of Swan-Ganz balloon-tipped pulmonary artery flotation catheter
(Fig. 7-3)

Right-sided heart catheterization with the Swan-Ganz catheter can be performed under fluoroscopic guidance or more commonly at the bedside by pressure monitoring. The catheter can be inserted into the central venous system via the basilic, brachial, subclavian, internal jugular, or femoral veins.† Table 7-1 summarizes the variables measured by hemodynamic monitoring.

---

*References 11, 12, 19, 24, 38.
†References 8, 12, 23, 40, 43, 45.

Table 7-1. Variables measured by hemodynamic monitoring

Right-sided catheterization with Swan-Ganz catheter	Intra-arterial catheterization
1. Right atrial pressure (approximates right ventricular end-diastolic or filling pressure)	Systolic arterial pressure (approximates left ventricular systolic pressure in the absence of obstruction at the level of the aortic valve)
2. Pulmonary artery systolic pressure (reflects right ventricular pressure)	Diastolic arterial pressure
3. Pulmonary artery diastolic pressure (approximates the pulmonary capillary wedge pressure)	Mean arterial pressure
4. Pulmonary capillary wedge pressure (approximates left atrial pressure, which reflects left ventricular end-diastolic pressure unless there is obstruction at the level of the mitral valve)	
5. Cardiac output by thermodilution	

Procedure
1. Identify an appropriate indication for insertion of Swan-Ganz catheter.
2. Obtain informed consent for the procedure from the patient.
3. Clean and prepare the insertion site with antiseptic scrub.
4. Isolate the insertion site with widely covering sterile drapes.
5. Ensure that the operator scrubs and wears a sterile gown and a mask. (For procedures performed under fluoroscopy, everyone in the room should wear a lead apron.)
6. Have a sterile, fluid-filled, accurately zeroed and calibrated transducer connected to a waveform-displaying oscilloscope on

which the patient's ECG is continuously monitored.

7. The operator should connect the right atrial and pulmonary arterial ports of the Swan-Ganz catheter to the pressure transducer by means of fluid-filled, air-free, stiff pressure tubing with intervening three-way stopcocks.

8. Flush both lumina of the catheter, eliminating all air bubles from the system and keeping the lumina fluid-filled before insertion.

9. Test the inflation of the balloon under sterile water, making sure that there is no air leak and that the balloon inflates concentrically. For the 7F Swan-Ganz catheter, the inflation volume is generally 1 to 1.5 ml.

10. Following proper local anesthesia, a suitable vein is punctured percutaneously or exposed by cutdown. Using an introducer assembly for percutaneous technique or cutdown venostomy, the tip of the catheter with the balloon deflated is inserted into the vein. The catheter is advanced gently and steadily while the pressures from the PA port and the ECG are monitored on the oscilloscope until the tip is the superior or inferior vena cava, near or in the right atrium.

11. Entry of the catheter tip into the thorax is associated with increased respiratory fluctuation in pressure. This usually occurs after advancement of the catheter tip for approximately 15 to 20 cm from the jugular or subclavian vein, 50 cm from the left antecubital fossa, 40 cm from the right antecubital fossa, and 30 cm from a femoral vein. At this point the balloon is inflated to the recommended volume printed on the catheter shaft (usually 1 to 1.5 ml on a 7F Swan-Ganz catheter).

12. Under continuous pressure and ECG monitoring, carefully advance the catheter from the right atrium into the right ventricle, then into pulmonary artery, and finally into a "wedge" position. This usually takes 10 to 20 seconds.

13. If after advancing the catheter with the balloon inflated the pulmonary artery pressure is not obtained, deflate the balloon and withdraw the catheter into the right atrium (confirm by pressure monitoring or fluoroscopy) and repeat the procedure.

14. Failure of a balloon flotation catheter to enter the right ventricle or pulmonary artery is rare but may occur in patients with an enlarged right atrium or right ventricle, particularly if the CO is low or tricuspid incompetence is present. Deep inspiration by the patient during advancement may facilitate passage of the catheter. Use of fluoroscopy, while not routinely necessary, may be quite helpful in such cases.

15. Pulmonary artery pressure will usually be observed as soon as the balloon traverses the pulmonic valve.

16. Once the balloon becomes lodged in the "wedge" position, deflate the balloon.

17. After deflation of the balloon, the catheter tip tends to recoil toward the pulmonic valve and may sometimes slip back into the right ventricle. In such a case reinflate the balloon and advance the catheter by 2 to 3 cm.

18. Should the catheter become too soft to advance it may be stiffened by slowly injecting 5 to 10 ml of sterile cold solution (saline or 5% dextrose) into the PA port as the catheter is advanced through the peripheral vessel.

19. If the pulmonary capillary wedge pressure is obtained at a volume substantively less than the recommended inflation volume or if the pulmonary artery pressure does not reappear after deflation of the balloon while in "wedge" position, the catheter should be gradually withdrawn with the balloon deflated until the volume required for wedging is equal or nearly equal to the full inflation volume. The final position of the catheter

may be checked by fluoroscopy or from an overpenetrated chest radiogram..

20. Secure catheter in place and apply sterile dressing.

Insertion of intra arterial cannula

Systemic intra-arterial catheterization and monitoring of pressure are readily accomplished at the bedside. Appropriate and accurately calibrated equipment for hemodynamic monitoring and recording must be available. The usual sites for intra-arterial catheter insertion are the radial, brachial, axillary, and femoral arteries. Before any artery is catheterized, the circulation must be checked to ensure adequate blood supply to the extremity involved.*

Procedure

1. Locate selected artery by palpation and make markings of its depth and position.
2. Prepare skin surface and drape.
3. Anesthetize puncture site.
4. Perform percutaneous or cutdown arteriotomy under strict sterile conditions.
5. Introduce appropriate cannula into the artery. For the radial artery, a 1½-inch long 20-gauge cannula is more frequently used, whereas the femoral artery requires a longer, 3- to 6-inch, and larger (18-gauge) cannula.
6. When there is a free retrograde flow of blood through the needle lumen, advance the plastic cannula into the artery and remove the metal cannula.
7. Blood should be spurting freely from plastic cannula.
8. Connect cannula to fluid-filled, air-free appropriately zeroed and calibrated pressure trandsucer.
9. Secure the catheter in place and apply sterile dressing.

Determination of cardiac output

The three common methods of determining CO are the (1) Fick method, (2) the dye dilution

*References 3, 8, 12, 15, 19, 38, 43.

method, and (3) the thermodilution method. However, the Fick and dye dilution methods are not practical for rapid and serial measurement of cardiac output at the bedside. Hence these two methods will be discussed very briefly.

Fick method. According to the Fick equation:

$$CO = \frac{O_2 \text{ consumption (ml/min)}}{\text{arterial } O_2 \text{ content (vol \%)} - \text{venous } O_2 \text{ content (vol \%)}}$$

where CO is the cardiac output in liters per minute and O_2 consumption is the amount of oxygen consumed by the body per minute in the basal state.

$$\frac{\text{Blood } O_2 \text{ content}}{(\text{ml}/100 \text{ ml})} = \frac{Hb \times 1.38 \times O_2 \text{ saturation}}{100}$$

where Hb is the amount of hemoglobin/100 ml of blood (g/100 ml) and 1.38 equals the milliliters of O_2 carried by fully saturated 1 g of Hb.

Arterial O_2 content is measured from peripheral arterial blood, whereas the mixed venous O_2 content is measured from the pulmonary arterial blood since that represents a uniform mixture of venous return from all parts of the body.[12,23,24]

Dye-dilution technique. The dye-dilution technique utilizes the principles introduced and developed by Stewart and Hamilton.[12,23,24] If an unknown volume (V) exists in a compartment to which a known amount (A) of a uniformly mixing indicator is added, then V can be determined as follows:

$$V = \frac{A}{\text{Concentration of the indicator}}$$

The same principle when applied to a circulating volume of fluid is modified so that when a known amount of an indicator is added and allowed to mix, its concentration is sampled downstream and the volume flow per minute can then be calculated as:

$$\frac{\text{Volume flow/unit time}}{(CO)} = \frac{\text{Amount of indicator}}{\text{Average concentration of the indicator integrated over the first passage time of the indicator}}$$

NORMAL VALUES AND FORMULAS FOR HEMODYNAMIC VARIABLES

Mean right atrial pressure (RAP)	4-6 mm Hg
Right ventricular pressure (RVP)	Systolic 20-25 mm Hg Diastolic 4-6 mm Hg
Pulmonary artery pressure (PAP)	Systolic 20-25 mm Hg Diastolic 8-12 mm Hg
Mean pulmonary capillary wedge pressure (PCWP)	8-12 mm Hg
Mean left atrial pressure (LAP)	8-12 mm Hg
Left ventricular pressure (LVP)	Systolic 110-120 mm Hg Diastolic 8-12 mm Hg
Systemic arterial pressure	Systolic 110-120 mm Hg Diastolic 70-80 mm Hg
Mean arterial pressure	70-105 mm Hg

$$MAP = \frac{\text{systolic} + 2\ \text{diastolic}}{3}$$

Cardiac output   4-8 L/minute
$CO = \text{Heart rate} \times SV$

Cardiac index   2.5-3.5 L/minute/M²

$$CI = \frac{CO}{BSA}$$

Systemic vascular resistance   800-1200 dynes/second/cm^{-5}

$$SVR = \frac{(MAP - RAP)}{CO} \times 80$$

Pulmonary vascular resistance   60-100 dynes/second/cm^{-5}

$$PVR = \frac{\text{Mean PA} - \text{Mean PCW}}{CO} \times 80$$

Total pulmonary resistance   200-300 dynes/second/cm^{-5}

$$TPR = \frac{\text{Mean PA}}{CO} \times 80$$

Stroke volume   55-100 ml/beat

$$SV = \frac{CO}{HR}$$

Stroke volume index   35-45 ml/M²/beat

$$SVI = \frac{\text{Stroke volume}}{BSA}$$

Stroke work index   45-75 Gm M/M²/beat
$SWI = (MAP - PCW) \times SVI \times .0136$

Thermodilution method. Thermodilution was introduced by Fegler in 1954 as a method for measurement of blood flow. It represents an application of the indicator dilution principle in which a known change in the heat content of the blood is induced at one point of the circulation and the resulting change in temperature detected at a point downstream. Cardiac output is calculated from the thermodilution curve by the following equation:

$$CO = \frac{(1.08)\ (60)\ V_I\ (T_B) - T_I)}{\Delta T_B\ (t)\ dt}$$

where:

1.08 = factor derived from specific heat and specific gravity of 5% dextrose divided by specific heat and specific gravity of blood

60 = seconds/minute

V_I = 10 ml (volume of injectate)

T_B = initial blood temperature (°C)

T_I = initial injectate temperature change

$\Delta T_B\ (t)\ dt$ = integral of blood temperature change (°C × second)

In contrast to the dye dilution, the thermodilution technique uses cold (negative heat) solution as an indicator. The addition of the thermistor to the balloon-tipped flotation catheter by Swan and Ganz made it considerably easier and practical to measure CO at the bedside. The thermodilution method makes it possible to perform repeated, rapid, and serial CO measurements at short intervals.*

In clinical practice the procedure for measuring CO by thermodilution includes the following:

1. A Swan-Ganz thermodilution catheter with a thermistor must be in place in the pulmonary artery.
2. An accurately calibrated CO computer must be available.
3. The catheter cable of the computer should be connected to the thermistor port of the balloon-tipped flotation catheter and the injectate cable to the thermometer should be immersed in the beaker containing the injectate solution.

---

*References 8, 16, 18, 23, 30, 40, 42, 45.

4. Sterile beaker with 10-ml syringes filled with sterile 5% dextrose in water and placed in a basin of crushed ice and water should be available.
5. Temperature of the injectate should be between 0° and 4° C.
6. The cold solution should be injected into the right atrial port (proximal lumen) as rapidly as possible. The CO will be calculated by the computer and the measurement shown on the digital display in liters per minute.
7. Three successive measurements are usually made with the average used as the CO measurement.
8. Triplicate CO determinations have a reproducibility (coefficient of variation) of 4% using 10 ml of cold injectate and a bedside computer. Although slightly greater variability (5.5%) has been observed when room temperature injectate has been used, recent studies suggest that accuracy or reproducibility of cardiac output determination is not significantly affected when room temperature injectate is used.
9. Monitor injectate volume as part of intake and output.

The boxed material on p. 227 shows normal values and formulas for hemodynamic variables.

NORMAL PRESSURE TRACING

It is essential from the standpoint of accuracy of hemodynamic monitoring to carefully analyze the pressure tracings before measuring pressure values. Pressures from the cardiac chambers and great vessels are usually transmitted through a fluid-filled catheter to a transducer. This translates the hydrostatic pressure into an electrical signal that can be recorded or displayed as a deflection.

Nurses and physicians must be familiar with the characteristics of the various pressure tracings. They should also be aware of the sources of errors that may distort the pressure tracing such as catheter whips and systolic amplification in the peripheral artery. Figs 7-3 through 7-9 show the normal pressure tracings recorded from the right-sided

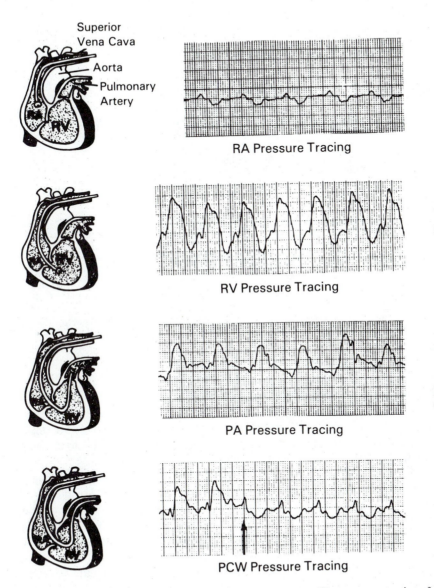

Fig. 7-3. Sequential passage of the Swan-Ganz catheter and corresponding pressure tracings from RA, RV, PA, and pulmonary wedge position as catheter enters each area during insertion.

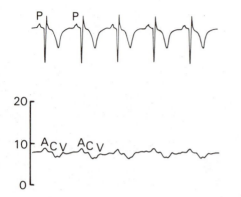

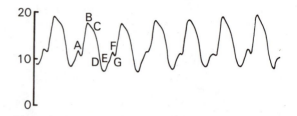

Fig. 7-5. Right ventricular pressure tracing, divided into seven phases: *A*, isovolumetric contraction; *B*, rapid ejection; *C*, slow ejection; *D*, isovolumetric relaxation; *E*, rapid filling; *F*, diastasis; *G*, end-diastole (point at which end-diastolic pressure is measured).

Fig. 7-4. Right atrial pressure tracing showin *a, c,* and *v* waves. *A* wave is produced by atrial systole and corresponds to PR interval of ECG. *C* wave is caused by closure and bulging of tricuspid valve into right atrium during isovolumetric phase of right ventricular contraction and immediately follows R wave of ECG. *X* descent results from ''pulling down'' of atrioventricular valve ring during ventricular ejection. *V* wave is caused by right atrial filling during ventricular systole; *y* descent results from right atrial emptying following opening of tricuspid valve.

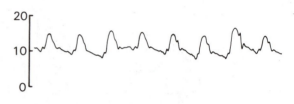

Fig. 7-6. Pulmonary arterial pressure tracing. Normal pulmonary artery tracing begins with steep upstroke to summit resulting from right ventricular ejection. Then it is followed by gradual fall in pressure until pulmonic valve closes (represented by dicrotic notch), after which pressure continues to gradually decline to lowest point (diastolic level).

cardiac chambers, pulmonary artery, pulmonary capillary wedge, peripheral artery, and thermodilution cardiac ouput curve. For simplicity, only general descriptions will be made of the normal pressure tracings.

Atrial pressure tracings (RA, LA, and PCW) (Fig. 7-4). The *a* wave is produced by atrial systole. It occurs in sinus rhythm and coincides with the PR interval of the electrocardiogram. The *c* wave is a sharp inflection caused by atrioventricular valve closure. The *x* descent results from atrial relaxation.

The *v* wave results from passive atrial filling, whereas atrioventricular valves are closed during ventricular systole; the *y* descent results from atrial emptying following opening of the atrioventricular valves.

The left atrial *a, c,* and *v* waves are similar in contour and magnitude to the PCW, *a,* and *c* waves. However, the left atrial pressure waves

precede those of the PCW waves because of the time delay for retrograde transmission of the pressure waves from the LA to the pulmonary capillary bed.[12,49]

Ventricular pressure tracings (right and left ventricle) (Figs. 7-5 and 7-6). The ventricular pressure tracing begins with a rapid upstroke to the summit, followed by a rapid downstroke. The phases of the ventricular pressure tracing are isovolumetric contraction, maximal ejection, reduced ejection, isometric relaxation, rapid filling, diastasis, and end-diastole.[12,49]

Arterial pressure tracings (pulmonary artery, aorta, or peripheral artery) (Figs. 7-7 and 7-8). The normal arterial pressure tracing starts with a steep rise to the summit because of ven-

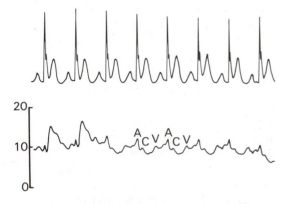

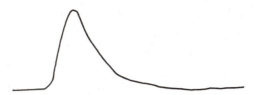

Fig. 7-9. Thermodilution cardiac output curve.

Fig. 7-7. Pulmonary capillary pressure tracing. The *a, c,* and *v* waves of the pulmonary capillary wedge tracing are similar in contour to the left atrial tracing. However, because of time delay for retrograde transmission of pressure waves from left atrium to pulmonary capillary bed, the PCW is delayed in timing compared to left atrial pressure. The *a, c,* and *v* waves represent physiological events analogous to those of right atrium.

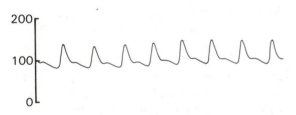

Fig. 7-8. Peripheral arterial pressure tracing showing steep upstroke and descent of pressure characterized by dicrotic notch (closure of aortic valve).

tricular ejection. This rise in turn is followed by a gradual fall in pressure until the valve (pulmonic or aortic) closes, shown on the pressure tracing as the dicrotic notch. Beyond the dicrotic notch, the pressure tracing is characterized by a continued decrease in pressure as blood pours into the pulmonary or peripheral arterial system without further resupply.[12,49]

Thermodilution cardiac output curve. The thermodilution cardiac output curve starts with a positive upward deflection to the summit, followed by a gradual downward deflection that falls to the baseline (Fig. 7-9).*

CLINICAL APPLICATION

Bedside hemodynamic monitoring is clinically useful as an aid in the diagnosis and assessment of the severity of congestive heart failure, diagnosis of certain pathophysiological mechanisms of heart failure, selection of appropriate modality of therapy, and rapid and sequential assessment of response to therapy. In addition, beside hemodynamic monitoring aids in the prediction of prognosis in acute myocardial infarction and in the diagnosis of hypovolemia, pulmonary embolism, septic shock, and pericardial disease, all of which may produce clinical indicators simulating congestive heart failure. Hemodynamic monitoring is of particular value in acute myocardial infarction, circulatory collapse, and respiratory failure. It is also useful during surgery, because it provides continuous monitoring of a rapidly fluctuating state of cardiovascular performance, which can be thoughtfully optimized with the help of therapeutic interventions. The clinical situations in which hemodynamic monitoring can be of considerable value in the management of the patient are as follows:

1. Complications of acute myocardial infarction
   a. Severe heart failure—low-output syndrome
   b. Shock (cardiogenic vs hypovolemic)
   c. Acute mitral regurgitation
   d. Ventricular septal rupture
   e. Right ventricular infarction

---

*References 8, 16, 18, 24, 45.

f. Recurrent or continuing myocardial ischemia

g. Patient requiring parenteral vasodilator, inotropic therapy, or intra-aortic balloon pumping

2. Perioperative state
   a. Before and during surgery in "high-risk" patients
   b. Postoperative low-output state
   c. Patients undergoing hypotensive anesthesia

3. Other states
   a. Patients with extensive trauma and burns
   b. Patients suspected of massive pulmonary embolism
   c. Patients suspected of acute cardiac tamponade
   d. Evaluation of intensive therapeutic strategies in patients with chronic refractory heart failure
   e. Patients with acute respiratory failure requiring positive end-expiratory pressure
   f. Research tool for clinical investigation

The value of bedside hemodynamic monitoring is that it:

1. Allows precise measurement of (a) cardiac function and dysfunction, (b) degree of dysfunction, and (c) mechanism of dysfunction

2. Aids in diagnosis of specific clinical syndromes, such as hypovolemia, acute mitral regurgitation, ventricular septal rupture, cardiac tamponade, right ventricular infarction, septic shock, acute pulmonary embolism, (Table 7-2)

3. Allows selection of appropriate therapeutic intervention based on the hemodynamic profile (Table 7-2)

4. Allows rapid assessment of response to therapy

5. Aids in predicting a prognosis in patients with acute myocardial infarction (Table 7-3)

Diagnostic value

The salient hemodynamic findings in selected clinical disorders are summarized in Table 7-2. While in the majority of these disorders diagnosis is generally suspected or obvious based on clinical and radiological assessment, often the clinical features may overlap or be ambiguous. In this case hemodynamic data serve to confirm or refute the clinical diagnosis.

Left ventricular failure (Table 7-2). Typical hemodynamic indicators of left ventricular failure include an elevated PCW and a depressed SV and CO. However, it should be realized that compensatory adjustments over time or effective therapy may keep these hemodynamic variables only marginally abnormal or within the normal range. Under these circumstances, however, stress-induced abnormalities of hemodynamic variables can frequently be demonstrated. In severe cases arterial pulsus alternans may be an additional useful sign.*

Acute right ventricular infarction (Table 7-2). This syndrome occurs in approximately 40% of cases with inferior infarction and a characteristic hemodynamic profile may be seen in about 50% of these cases, although volume loading may unmask these abnormalities in the remaining patients. The hemodynamic findings include elevated RA pressure, which equals or exceeds a normal or mildly elevated PCW. The RA pressure may show inspiratory increase (Kussmaul's sign) and tracing may show a steep y' descent, whereas the RV pressure tracing may show a square root sign of diastolic dip and plateau, simulating constrictive pericarditis. In some cases pulsus paradoxus may be present, simulating cardiac tamponade. Low SV and CO occur frequently in this syndrome, sometimes producing frank syndrome of shock.[23,27,41]

Hypovolemia (Table 7-2). Inadequate left ventricular filling and EDV may result from low total blood volume or inappropriate peripheral distribution of a normal blood volume. By virtue of inadequate preload, left ventricular SV and CO decrease. Profound drop in CO may produce shock. Hemodynamic findings indicate reduced left ventricular filling pressure as indicated by low PCW. Although the optimum level of preload varies from individual to individual as well as with the status of left ventricular function and compliance, patients with reduced left ventricular function and compliance generally produce the highest SV at relatively higher than normal levels of preload as

---

*References 6, 8, 10, 20, 23, 26.

Table 7-2. Salient hemodynamic profile in specific clinical disorders

	RA	PCW	PA	CO	BP	Comments
Hypovolemia	↓	↓	↓	↓	↓	Orthostatic ↑ HR and/or ↓ BP
LV failure	—	↑		↓	—	Severe cases may show pulsus alternans
RV infarction	↑	—	Normal	↓		RA ≥ PCW, steep *y* descent in RA, low PA and RV pulse pressure, diastolic dip and plateau pressure in RV
Acute MR	—	↑ Large *v* waves	↑	↓	—	Disproportionately large *v* waves on PCW tracings
Acute VSD	—↑	—↑	—↑	RV output high LV forward output low	—	O_2 step-up from RA to RV or PA, early recirculation on thermodilution curve
Acute tamponade	↑	↑	↑	↓		Pulsus paradoxus and diastolic pressure equilibration RA = PCW = PA_{EDP}
Massive PE	↑	—	↑	↓	↓	$PA_{EDP} \gg$ PCW
Septic shock	—	—	—	↑	↓	High cardiac output, low vascular resistance in early stages
Noncardiac Pulmonary edema	—	—	—	—	—	Normal or near normal PCW

↓	= Reduced		↑	= Elevated
LV	= Left ventricular		RA	= Right atrial pressure
RV	= Right ventricular		PCW	= Pulmonary capillary wedge pressure
VSD	= Ventricular septal defect		PA	= Pulmonary arterial pressure
PE	= Pulmonary embolism		CO	= Cardiac output
MR	= Mitral regurgitation		PA_{EDP}	= Pulmonary arterial end-diastolic pressure
—	= Within normal limits or no characteristic change		PE	= Pulmonary embolism

judged from PCW. Although there are considerable individual variations, the optimum SV in acute myocardial infarction may be obtained at PCW of 14 to 18 mm Hg. Higher levels of PCW generally produce symptomatic pulmonary congestion without further increases in SV.[8,10,17]

Acute mitral regurgitation (Table 7-2). Acute mitral regurgitation may result from a variety of causes, including endocarditis and acute myocardial infarction. Generally, severe acute mitral regurgitation produces marked elevation of left atrial and PCW pressures with marked accentuation of *v* waves in PCW tracings, which are often reflected even onto the PA tracing.*

Acute ventricular septal rupture (Table 7-2). This complication may also occur following acute myocardial infarction and produce clinical indicators simulating acute mitral regurgitation. However, the diagnosis is easily confirmed by simultaneous withdrawal of blood from RA and PA for detection of an oxygen step up.†

Acute cardiac tamponade (Table 7-2). This syndrome results from pericardial fluid under ten-

*References 10, 20, 23, 38, 39.
†References 8, 10, 23, 39, 43.

Table 7-3. Prognostic implications of hemodynamic subsets in acute myocardial infarction

	PCW (mm Hg)	CI (L/minute/M²)	% mortality	Suggested hemodynamic treatment
Subset I	≤18	>2.2	3	Observation
Subset II	>18	>2.2	9	Diuretics and/or vasodilators
Subset III	<18	<2.2	23	Volume, ↑ HR if slow
Subset IV	>18	<2.2	51	Diuretics, vasodilators with or without inotropes and/or IABP

HR = heart rate; IABP = intra-aortic balloon pumping.

sion and produces a characteristic hemodynamic profile. There is elevation and equalization of filling pressures of RV and LV as reflected in elevation and equalization of RA and PCW pressures. In addition, an exaggerated respiratory decline in systolic blood pressure of >10 to 15 mm Hg (pulsus paradoxus) is frequently detected. Diastolic compression of cardiac chambers impedes ventricular filling resulting in low SV and CO that, when severe, produces shock.[8,10,23,27]

Acute massive pulmonary embolism (Table 7-2). Severe pulmonary embolism may produce a syndrome simulating congestive failure and cardiogenic shock. However, unlike shock from severe left or biventricular failure, pulmonary embolism produces an elevation of PA systolic and diastolic pressures without primary alteration of PCW. Thus PA$_{EDP}$ exceeds the PCW by more than 5 mm Hg. However, pulmonary embolism may exist without such hemodynamic alterations.[8,23]

Septic shock (Table 7-2). Although the diagnosis of septic shock is generally not difficult on clinical grounds, hemodynamic data often provide the first or a confirmatory clue. The early phase of septic shock (warm phase) is generally characterized by elevated CO and markedly reduced SVR. However, in advanced cases low CO and high SVR are more frequently observed.

Noncardiac pulmonary edema (Table 7-2). Pulmonary edema from increase in capillary permeability occurs in a variety of clinical disorders including septic shock and narcotic overdose and is associated with normal or near-normal cardiac function as assessed from PCW. In contrast, pulmonary edema from heart failure is characterized by a markedly elevated PCW (>25 to 30 mm Hg). Noncardiac pulmonary edema often produces the clinical picture called adult respiratory distress syndrome (ARDS).

Prognostic value (Table 7-3)

Several studies have emphasized the prognostic value of objectively determined parameters of ventricular function in acute myocardial infarction. It is generally known that the greater the clinical severity of left ventricular failure, the higher is the mortality in acute myocardial infarction. However, it has also been pointed out that clinical assessment of the severity of left ventricular failure may not only be relatively insensitive but may also demonstrate a temporal lag with respect to hemodynamic signs of heart failure, particularly in the early hours of acute myocardial infarction. These considerations and others have persuaded some physicians to recommend routine hemodynamic monitoring in all patients with acute myocardial infarction. Besides offering diagnostic information (as discussed earlier), hemodynamic variables show strong prognostic value for short-term survival as shown in Table 7-3.[2] Using PCW and CI, Forrester, Chatterjee, and their colleagues were able to classify patients with acute myocardial infarction into four subsets with differing mortality rates.[9,10,17,36]

Table 7-4. Hemodynamic basis for clinical features in acute congestive heart failure

Clinical presentation	Hemodynamic basis
PULMONARY CONGESTION ⟶	ELEVATED PCW
Minimal to mild	14-18 mm Hg
Moderate	18-25 mm Hg
Severe	>25 mm Hg
ORGAN HYPOPERFUSION ⟶	LOW CARDIAC INDEX
Mild	2.2-2.5 L/minute/M²
Moderate	2-2.2 L/minute/M²
Severe	<2 L/minute/M²

Therapeutic value

Knowledge of precise hemodynamic perturbations in various clinical disorders allows for a more rational approach toward the optimization of clinically relevant hemodynamic variables. As discussed earlier, pulmonary congestion is related to elevated PCW, whereas manifestations of clinical organ hypoperfusion and shock are related to a depressed CO with or without a low blood pressure (Table 7-4). The object of treatment of congestive heart failure is to reduce the elevated PCW, optimize the depressed SV and CO, and maintain an adequate perfusion pressure. The agents that can accomplish these objectives are shown in Table 7-5. As is apparent in critically ill patients, rapidly acting and potent medications are generally necessary to favorably optimize the abnormal hemodynamic and, eventually, the clinical state, and this requires precise knowledge and repeated assessment of hemodynamic variables. This bedside hemodynamic monitoring provides not only diagnostic information for selection of proper therapy but also a rapid access to repeated assessment and follow-up in response to selected therapy. Based on hemodynamic subsets in acute myocardial infarction, appropriate general therapeutic recommendations can be made (Table 7-5).*

*References 9, 17, 20, 39, 46.

Table 7-5. Objects of treatment of congestive heart failure

Object	Result	Medical therapy
To reduce high PCW	To relieve pulmonary congestion	Diuretics, vasodilators
To increase depressed CI	To improve tissue perfusion	Vasodilators, inotropic drugs
To maintain adequate blood pressure	To maintain tissue perfusion	Inotropic-vasopressor drugs

COMPLICATIONS OF INVASIVE BEDSIDE MONITORING

Although invasive hemodynamic monitoring is of considerable value in the management of critically ill patients, there is a finite, albeit low, risk of complications associated with it, the true incidence of which is difficult to ascertain.

Table 7-6 lists the reported complications. The complications may be related to the technique and site of insertion of monitoring catheters, the passage of the catheter through the heart, inappropriate monitoring and maintenance of indwelling catheters, and erroneous measurements and interpretation of hemodynamic variables.[37]

Table 7-6. Complications of hemodynamic monitoring

Swan-Ganz catheterization	Pressure monitoring intra-arterial
Sepsis: local, systemic, endocarditis	Arterial spasm, thrombosis, embolism
Thrombosis or phlebitis of the vein	Bleeding and hematoma
Hematoma formation	Arterial dissection
Pneumothorax if subclavian route is used, less common when internal jugular route is used	Trauma to neighboring structures
Arrhythmias: atrial or ventricular during passage through atrium or ventricle	Local and systemic sepsis
Transient right bundle branch block or complete heart block with preexisting left bundle branch block	
Pulmonary embolism and infarction	
Pulmonary artery rupture, bronchopulmonary fistula	
Embolism of clot, air, fragments of balloon	
Coiling and knotting of catheter	
Balloon rupture	

Complications associated with Swan-Ganz catheterization

The Swan-Ganz catheter can be inserted into the central circulation via the antecubital vein, the jugular and subclavian veins, or the femoral vein. Insertion through the antecubital vein may be performed percutaneously or by surgical cutdown. Complications associated with antecubital insertion are few and include local and systemic sepsis and phlebitis, inability to advance the catheter because of venospasm or angulation of veins at the level of the shoulder, and displacement of catheter during arm movement.

In recent years the percutaneous insertion of these catheters via the internal jugular vein has become popular; however, complications associated with this route include air embolism, thrombophlebitis, injury to the carotid artery, and less commonly pneumothorax.[13,21] Similarly, insertion via the subclavian vein, although providing a short, direct route into the central circulation, is also associated with risks of pneumothorax, hemothorax, injury to the subclavian artery and brachial plexus, air embolism, and subcutaneous and mediastinal emphysema. Insertion through the femoral vein is relatively safer, since injury to vital organs is rare. However, risks include thrombophlebitis, local and systemic sepsis, and movement of the catheter with movement of the lower extremity.

Complications resulting from the passage of the Swan-Ganz catheter through the right side of the heart include atrial and ventricular arrhythmias and transient right bundle branch block, which in a patient with prior left bundle branch block may result in complete heart block.[26] These complications underscore the need for careful ECG monitoring during catheter insertion.

Intracardiac knotting of the catheter can occur but fortunately does not result in serious complications to the patient.[31] The risk of knotting is greatest when bedside insertion is performed in patients who have enlargement of the right side of the heart with low cardiac output, high right-sided heart pressures, and tricuspid regurgitation. In all these instances continued and persistent manipulation of the catheter without fluoroscopic guidance may lead to looping and knotting of the catheter within the right side of the heart. The examiner can reduce the risk of knotting by insertion of the catheter under fluoroscopic guidance in such patients and by resisting the temptation of persistent advancement of the catheter beyond an estimated length required to reach the pulmonary artery. Experienced operators may open intracardiac knots by using a flexible guide wire or they may need to perform venostomy to remove the tightened knot.[31]

Pulmonary embolism and infarction from long-term Swan-Ganz catheterization may result from permanent wedging of the catheter with the balloon inflated or deflated.[44] This complication can be avoided by limiting the time during which the catheter is allowed to stay in wedge position to 20 to 30 seconds. Constant attention to pulmonary artery pressure monitoring must be maintained so that catheter tip migration into wedge position and consequent damping of the pulmonary artery pressure tracing can be quickly recognized. Then the wedging can be remedied by gently withdrawing the catheter 1 to 2 cm at a time till a high-fidelity undamped pulmonary artery pressure tracing is restored.

When catheter wedging is achieved with inflation of the balloon by less than 1 ml of air, the catheter tip is likely to be too far into the pulmonary arterial bed. Spontaneous migration and wedging of the catheter are then possible.

Rupture of a pulmonary artery branch with serious exsanguinating hemorrhage may result from inappropriate inflation of the balloon, especially in patients with elevated pulmonary artery pressures or in those taking anticoagulant medication.[34] Rarely, massive in situ thrombosis of the pulmonary artery may result from Swan-Ganz catheterization.[25,50]

Rupture of the latex balloon occurs not infrequently and this may predispose to air embolization. Mechanical trauma to tricuspid and pulmonic valves may predispose to formation of aseptic and infected vegetations in addition to disruption of the valvular tissue.[21,32,33]

Multiple avenues for bacterial contamination with invasive hemodynamic monitoring remain a constant hazard. This underscores the importance of adopting strict, aseptic, and sterile technique, both during initial insertion and during continued care of indwelling catheters. Among the various sources of bacterial contamination are the patient's skin, the operator and the assistant, and monitoring equipment including tubings, stopcocks, and pressure transducers.[22,35,47,48]

To improve the safety of use of Swan-Ganz catheters, the following guidelines are suggested:

1. Keep "wedge" time to a minimum, especially in patients with pulmonary hypertension (preferably 10 to 15 seconds).
2. When the balloon is reinflated for recording wedge pressure, the inflation medium (carbon dioxide or air) must be added slowly under continuous monitoring of the pulmonary artery pressure waveform. Inflation *must* be stopped immediately when the pulmonary artery pressure tracing is seen to change to pulmonary wedge pressure.
3. If fluoroscopy is available (as in the cardiac catheterization laboratory), refloat the catheter tip from the central pulmonary artery for each wedge pressure measurement.
4. Make a careful note of the balloon inflation volume. If "wedge" is recorded with a balloon volume significantly below that indicated on the catheter shaft, pull the catheter gradually into a position in which full or near full inflation volume produces a wedge tracing.
5. Anticipate spontaneous catheter tip migration toward the periphery of the pulmonary bed. To avoid possible damage to the pulmonary artery, monitor the pressure tracing during every balloon inflation.
6. Spontaneous catheter tip migration into wedge position may also induce pulmonary infarction. Continuous or frequent monitoring of the catheter tip pressure is therefore necessary.
7. Do not use liquids for balloon inflation; they may be irretrievable and may prevent balloon deflation.
8. Keep a syringe on the balloon lumen of the catheter to prevent accidental injection of liquids into the balloon.

Health care responsibilities

Health care action	Health care rationale
1. Assess patient's level of orientation and understanding and present a brief and simple explanation of the environment, equipment, and personnel. If family members are present, give them the same explanation, including visiting privileges.	Allay fear and anxiety
2. Explain procedure and role of the patient during the procedure of insertion and monitoring of hemodynamic variables.	Supplements physician's explanation to further allay fears and anxiety
3. Check chart for signed consents for insertion of intra-arterial and balloon-tipped (Swan-Ganz) catheters.	
4. Assemble equipment for hemodynamic monitoring under strict aseptic conditions and bring to the bedside.	
5. Calibrate transducers and check function and safety of other equipment necessary for hemodynamic monitoring.	
6. Take vital signs and assess clinical status of the patients before insertion procedure. Document findings in nursing record.	Baseline information
7. Instruct and/or assist the patient to assume the most comfortable position for the procedure.	
8. Assist with pulmonary artery catheterization and monitoring:	
a. Assist physician into sterile gown and gloves.	
b. Assist physician in sterile preparation of insertion site.	
c. Prepare solution for flushing and wiping the catheter.	
d. Assist physician with instrumentation as necessary.	
e. Display and monitor pressure waveforms during insertion of catheter.	
f. Monitor ECG continuously during insertion and inform physician of any arrhythmias.	
g. Assess clinical status and vital signs every 15 minutes during insertion and as needed.	
h. Support physical and emotional needs of the patient.	
i. Obtain initial hemodynamic variables (RA, PA, PCW).	Baseline information
j. Apply sterile dressings and secure catheter.	
k. Obtain written medical guidelines.	
l. Display clear and stable PA pressure waveform on the oscilloscope continuously.	Pressure waveform showing location of catheter
m. Measure cardiac output.	Baseline information
n. Aspirate gently when withdrawing blood specimen from pulmonary artery catheter.	Forceful aspiration may withdraw arterialized blood from the arterial side of the capillary system instead of mixed venous sample.
o. Inflate balloon very slowly when measuring PCW. (Read instructions with catheter as to recommended medium of inflation, amount, and technique.)	Inflating balloon too fast may rupture balloon and damage the blood vessel.

Health care responsibilities—cont'd

Health care action	Health care rationale
9. Intra-arterial catheterization and monitoring.	Indicates arterial occlusion and interrupted or decreased blood supply.
a. Assess circulation, color, sensation, and movement of extremity distal to intended site of insertion and compare to the other extremity. Document findings. Report any variances to physician.	
b. Prepare equipment and supplies.	
c. Immobilize extremity.	
d. Assist physician with preparation of site of insertion and the required instruments.	
e. Support physical and emotional needs of patient.	
f. Obtain initial intra-arterial pressure measurement.	
g. Apply sterile dressing and secure catheter.	
h. Obtain written medical orders for management of variances in blood pressure.	
i. Display a clear and stable arterial pressure waveform.	
j. Check pulses, color, movement, and sensation of extremity with the insertion site every hour and as needed during monitoring. Report variances to physician. Document findings in nursing record.	
10. Initiate written nursing care, taking into consideration individual needs of patient.	Gives evidence that planning has been done to make sure that patient receives appropriate nursing care
	Serves as method of communication for all nursing staff concerned with patient.
11. Take pressure readings at end of expiration.	Avoids transmission of fluctuating levels of intrathoracic pressure to intravascular pressures
12. Flush lines with heparinized solution every hour and as needed	Maintains patency of lines and prevents clot formation
13. Measure hemodynamic variables including cardiac output and systemic vascular resistance every hour and as needed.	
14. Check calibration of transducers in reference to the mid-axillary line before each reading.	Ensures accurate measurements
15. Display clear and stable ECG signal and pressure waveforms on the oscilloscope at all times.	Shows location and proper function of lines
16. Inspect insertion sites for any bleeding, redness, and swelling.	Ensures detection of infection and complications
17. Change dressings at insertion sites every 24 hours and as needed.	Ensures infection control
18. Observe strict aseptic technique during flushing of lines, drawing of blood specimens, and measuring of cardiac output.	
19. Keep physician informed of variances in hemodynamic variables, changes in pressure waveforms, and clinical status of the patient.	Ensures total assessment of patient

Continued.

Health care responsibilities—cont'd

Health care action   *Health care rationale*

20. Integrate hemodynamic measurements with the clinical assessment of patient. *Do not depend on hemodynamic variables to evaluate patient.*

21. Assess and support physical and emotional needs of patient and family during hemodynamic monitoring.
    a. Anxiety
    b. Fear
    c. Sensory and sleep deprivation
    d. Fatigue
    e. Restricted mobility

Ensures better cooperation and participation of patient and family in the care process.

Complications of the intra-arterial pressure monitoring

Cannulation of a radial artery is generally free of any major complications. The reported complications include bleeding and hematoma formation, dissection, local and systemic sepsis, vascular insufficiency to the hand resulting from spasm or thrombosis, and a possible, though unproven, risk of cerebral or coronary embolism from vigorous retrograde flushing of arterial cannula.[12,15,19,28]

HEALTH CARE IMPLICATIONS

Before attempting to discuss the nursing management of a patient with congestive heart failure undergoing hemodynamic monitoring, it is essential to emphasize that monitoring and care of any patient with hemodynamic monitoring should only be done by a trained critical care clinician with a working knowledge of the principles, techniques, clinical application, complications, and nursing implications of hemodynamic monitoring.

The nursing management of a patient with acute congestive heart failure varies little from the care of any critically ill patient; therefore this discussion only details the health team responsibilities rele-

vant to hemodynamic monitoring. (See boxed material, pp. 238-40, and health care plan, pp. 241-244.)

SUMMARY

A careful understanding of the determinants of cardiac performance leads to a more rational and optimal clinical application of bedside hemodynamic monitoring. Hemodynamic monitoring aids in the diagnosis, assessment of severity, selection of therapy, and prompt assessment of response to therapy in critically ill patients. Although its advantages are substantive, hemodynamic monitoring should only be considered to have a complementary role in the overall clinical and noninvasive assessment of critically ill patients. The temptation of heavy reliance on hemodynamic variables as the sole guides to clinical management of the patient with serious disregard for clinical assessment should be avoided.

Although the relative safety of hemodynamic monitoring justifies its widespread use, indiscriminate performance of hemodynamic monitoring by personnel without adequate background skills and training should be discouraged.

HEMODYNAMIC MONITORING STANDARD HEALTH CARE PLAN

Potential problems	Nursing diagnosis	Expected outcome	Nursing activities
1. Anxiety caused by diagnosis, procedures, and highly technical environment	Coping, ineffective individual Fear	Verbalizes fears and concerns regarding diagnosis and asks questions pertinent to procedures and technical environment Verbalizes acceptance of hemodynamic monitoring as an aid to diagnosis and therapy The client will receive emotional support from staff	Assess patient's level of orientation and understanding. Present a clear and simple explanation of procedures, diagnosis, and environment. Emphasize that pain medication as needed and local anesthetic will be given. Perform nursing duties with calm and organized demeanor. Respond quickly to call lights and alarm signals.
2. Feelings of loss of control resulting from necessary medications and temporary dependence on others	Disturbance in; self-concept, self-care deficit: bathing/hygiene; powerlessness	Verbalizes acceptance of temporary dependence on others for care Verbalizes ability to cope with restricted activity Expresses dislike for dependent role	Allow patient to express feelings. Encourage independence within physician's orders and patient's tolerance. Allow patient to participate in care and make decisions if possible.
3. Discomfort caused by pain at insertion site and restricted movement in extremities with catheters	Comfort alteration: pain; impaired physical mobility	Verbalizes comfort and relief of pain Accepts restriction of movement on the extremities with the catheters	Administer pain medication as needed per physician's order. Explain need for restricted movement. Immobilize affected arm with padded armboard.
4. Potential disorientation and abnormal behavior resulting from sensory and sleep deprivation	Sensory perceptual alterations; sleep pattern disturbance	Oriented to time, place, and person Early detection of and prevention of abnormal behavior	Orient patient to time, place, and personnel. Observe for any signs of confusion, agitation, and withdrawal.

Continued.

HEMODYNAMIC MONITORING STANDARD HEALTH CARE PLAN—cont'd

Potential problems	Nursing diagnosis	Expected outcome	Nursing activities
5. Fatigue caused by frequent measurements of hemodynamic variables		Verbalizes feeling and need for rest	Schedule activities to allow for rest periods. Provide a quiet and restful environment.
6. Family anxiety	Coping, ineffective family: compromised	Verbalizes feelings and concerns. Calmly visits with patient at intervals. Appears relaxed	Allow family to visit as frequently as possible. Delegate one nurse to listen to family. Enlist help of clergyman of choice if desired.
7. Potential complications (Table 7-6)	Injury, potential for (Table 7-6)	Strong palpable pulses, warm extremities, adequate capillary filling, and good mobility	Check extremities for pulses, color, temperature, sensation (such as numbness and pain), movement, and capillary fillings before insertion, during monitoring, and after discontinuance of catheters.
a. Circulatory impairment in extremities with catheters	Alteration in peripheral tissue perfusion	No signs of infection at insertion sites; no inappropriate rise in temperature	Observe strict aseptic technique in the assembling of equipment, flushing of lines, drawing of blood specimen, and measuring of CO. Change dressings at insertion sites every 24 hours and as needed.
b. Infection (local and systemic)	Impairment of skin integrity: actual		Inspect insertion sites for redness, swelling, and drainage during dressing change.

HEMODYNAMIC MONITORING STANDARD HEALTH CARE PLAN—cont'd

Potential problems	Nursing diagnosis	Expected outcome	Nursing activities
c. Bleeding from insertion sites and catheter connectors	Potential for fluid volume deficit	No bleeding from insertion sites and catheter connectors	Apply pressure dressings to insertion sites.
			Tighten all catheters and tubing connectors.
d. Pulmonary infarction resulting from spontaneous wedging of the PA catheter in a small branch of the pulmonary artery		No clinical or radiographic evidence of pulmonary infarction	Display pulmonary artery catheter tip pressure waveform at all times.
			Keep balloon deflated when not measuring PCW.
			Deep breathing and coughing may dislodge overwedged catheter.
			Advise physician to reposition catheter.
e. Pulmonary embolism	Potential for impaired gas exchange	No clinical signs of pulmonary embolism	Check hemodynamic monitoring system for any clots or air bubbles.
			Aspirate for clots and air bubbles before flushing catheters.
			If there is no resistance to PA balloon inflation, do not introduce any more air; balloon may be ruptured.
f. Arterial embolization	Potential for altered tissue perfusion	No clinical signs of compromised circulation in all systems	Inspect system for clots and air bubbles frequently.
			Flush arterial catheter with heparinized solution free of air bubbles.

Continued.

Potential problems	Nursing diagnosis	Expected outcome	Nursing activities
g. Arrhythmias caused by manipulation of pulmonary artery catheter tip during insertion and slippage of catheter tip to the RV during monitoring	Potential for alterations in cardiac output	Prevention of arrhythmias during insertion and monitoring	Monitor PA pressure and ECG at all times. Keep balloon inflated during insertion and any time catheter tip slips from PA to RV.
h. Balloon rupture		Balloon not ruptured by overinflation or too rapid inflation	Inflate balloon slowly when measuring PCW. Use recommended amount of air.
8. "Damping" of pressure tracings because of air bubbles, clots, and kinks in the tubing or catheter		Clear pressure tracings on oscilloscope; no air bubbles, clots, and kinks in the catheter or tubing	Inspect catheter and tubing for clots, kinks, and air bubbles frequently. Aspirate for clots and air bubbles. Flush system with heparinized solution free of air bubbles every hour and as needed.
9. Dislodgement of PA catheter from the pulmonary artery to the right ventricle		Oscilloscope shows PA pressure waveform and appropriate action taken if catheter slips from PA to RV	Inflate balloon if intact. Monitor ECG rhythm closely. Advise physician to reposition catheter.
10. Inappropriate measurements and waveforms		Clear and well-defined pressure waveforms and accurate measurements	Analyze pressure waveforms carefully. Record if necessary. Check position of patient and transducers. Recalibrate transducers and check oscilloscope. Integrate hemodynamic measurements with the clinical assessment of the patient.

REFERENCES

1. Abernathy, W.S.: Complete heart block caused by the Swan-Ganz catheter, Chest **65:**349, 1974.
2. Afifi, A., Chang, P.C., Liu, V.Y., and others: Prognostic indexes in acute myocardial infarction complicated by shock, Am. J. Cardiol. **33:**826, 1974.
3. Bedford, R.F.: Percutaneous radial artery cannulation: increased safety using teflon catheters, Anesthesiology **42:**219, 1975.
4. Bouchard, R.J., Gault, J.H., and Ross, J., Jr.: Evaluation of pulmonary arterial end-diastolic pressure as an estimate of left ventricular end-diastolic pressure in patients with normal and abnormal left ventricular performance, Circulation **44:**1072, 1971.
5. Braunwald, E., and Frahm, C.J.: Studies on Starling's law of the heart. IV. Observations on the hemodynamic functions of the left atrium in man, Circulation **24:**633, 1961.
6. Braunwald, E., Ross, J., Jr.: The ventricular end-diastolic pressure: appraisal of its value in the recognition of ventricular failure in man, Am. J. Med. **34:**147, 1963.
7. Brobeck, J.R., Jr., editor: Best and Taylor's physiological basis of medical practice, ed. 10, Baltimore, 1979, The Williams & Wilkins Co.
8. Buchbinder, N., and Ganz, W.: Hemodynamic monitoring: invasive techniques, Anesthesiology **45:**146, 1976.
9. Chatterjee, K.: Effects of vasodilator therapy in severe pump failure in acute myocardial infarction on short term and late prognosis, Circulation **53:**797, 1976.
10. Chatterjee, K., and Swan, H.J.C.: Hemodynamic profile of acute myocardial infarction, In Corday, E., and Swan, H.J.C., editors: Myocardial infarction, Baltimore, 1973, The Williams & Wilkins Co.
11. Cohn, J.N.: Blood pressure monitoring in shock: mechanism of inaccuracy in auscultatory and palpatory methods, J.A.M.A. **199:**972, 1967.
12. Daily, E.K., and Schroeder, J.S.: Techniques in bedside hemodynamic monitoring, ed. 2, St. Louis, 1981, The C.V. Mosby Co.
13. Daily, P.O., Greipp, R.B., and Shumway, N.E.: Percutaneous internal jugular vein cannulation, Arch. Surg. **101:**534, 1970.
14. Diamond, G.A., and Forrester, J.S.: Effect of coronary artery disease and acute myocardial infarction on left ventricular compliance in man, Circulation **45:**11, 1972.
15. Downs, J.B., Rackstein, A.D., Klein, E.F., and others: Hazards of radial artery catheterization, Anesthesiology **38:**283, 1973.
16. Fegler, G.: Measurement of cardiac output in anesthetized animals by a thermodilution method, Am. J. Exp. Physiol. **39:**153, 1954.
17. Forrester, J.S., Diamond, G.A., Chatterjee, K., and others: Medical therapy of acute myocardial infarction by the application of hemodynamic subsets, N. Engl. J. Med. **295:**1356, 1404, 1976.
18. Ganz, W., and Swan, H.J.C.: Measurement of blood flow by thermodilution, Am. J. Cardiol. **29:**241, 1972.
19. Gardner, R.M., Schwartz, R.N., Wong, H.C., and others: Percutaneous indwelling radial artery catheters for monitoring cardiovascular function, N. Engl. J. Med. **290:**1227, 1974.
20. Gazes, P.C., and Gaddy, J.E.: Bedside management of acute myocardial infarction, Am. Heart J. **97:**782, 1979.
21. Green, J.R., Jr., and Cummings, K.C.: Aseptic thrombotic endocardial vegetations: a complication of indwelling pulmonary artery catheters, J.A.M.A. **225:**1525, 1973.
22. Greene, J.R., Jr., Fitzwater, J.E., and Clemmer, T.P.: Septic endocarditis and indwelling pulmonary artery catheters, J.A.M.A. **233:**891, 1975.
23. Grossman, W., editor: Cardiac catheterization and angiography, Philadelphia, 1974, Lea & Febiger.
24. Guyton, A.C.: Circulatory physiology: cardiac output and its regulation, Philadelphia, 1963, W.B. Saunders Co.
25. Laprin, E.S., and Murray, J.A.: Hemoptysis with flow directed cardiac catheterization, J.A.M.A. **220:**1246, 1972.
26. Lassers, B.W., George, M., Anderton, J.L., and others: Left ventricular failure in acute myocardial infarction, Am. J. Cardiol. **25:**511, 1970.
27. Lorell, B., Leinbach, R.C., Pohost, G.M., and others: Right ventricular infarction: clinical diagnosis and differentiation from cardiac tamponade and pericardial constriction, Am. J. Cardiol. **43:**465, 1979.
28. Lowenstein, E., Little, J.W., III, and Lo, H.H.: Prevention of cerebral embolization from flushing radial artery cannulas, N. Engl. J. Med. **285:**1414, 1971.
29. Luck, J.C., and Engel, T.F.: Transient right bundle branch block with "Swan-Ganz" catheterization, Am. Heart. J. **92:**263, 1976.
30. Maruschak, G.F., Meathe, E.A., Schauble, J.F., and others: A simplified equation for thermal dilution cardiac output, J. Appl. Physiol. **37:**414, 1974.
31. Mond, H.G., Clark, D.W., Nesbitt, S.J., and others: A technique for unknotting an intracardiac flow-directed balloon catheter, Chest **67:**731, 1975.
32. O'Toole, J.D., Wurtzbacher, J.J., Wearner, N.E., and others: Pulmonary valve injury and insufficiency during pulmonary artery catheterization, N. Engl. J. Med. **301:**116, 1979.
33. Pace, N.L., and Horton, W.: Indwelling pulmonary artery catheters: their relationship to aseptic thrombotic endocardial vegetations, J.A.M.A. **233:**8983, 1975.
34. Pape, L.A., Haffajee, C.I., Markis, J.E., and others: Fatal pulmonary hemorrhage after use of the flow-directed balloon-tipped catheter, Ann. Intern. Med. **90:**344, 1979.
35. Prachar, H., Dittel, M., Jobst, C., and others: Bacterial contamination of pulmonary artery catheters, Intensive Care Med. **4:**79, 1978.

36. Rahimtoola, S.H., Loeb, H.S., Ehsani, A., and others: Relationship of pulmonary artery to left ventricular diastolic pressures in acute myocardial infarction, Circulation **46:**283, 1972.

37. Ronan, J.A., Steelman, R.B., DeLeon, S.C., and others: The clinical diagnosis of acute severe mitral insufficiency, Am. J. Cardiol. **27:**284, 1971.

38. Rushner, R.F.: Cardiovascular dynamics, Philadelphia, 1970, W.B. Saunders Co.

39. Swan, H.J.C.: What is the role of invasive monitoring procedures in the management of the critically ill? Cardiovasc. Clin. **8:**103, 1977.

40. Swan, H.J.C., Ganz, W., Forrester, J.S., and others: Catheterization of the heart in man with the use of a flow-directed balloon-tipped catheter, N. Engl. J. Med. **283:**447-451, 1970.

41. Swan, H.J.C., Forrester, J.S., Diamond, G., and others: Hemodynamic spectrum of myocardial infarction and cardiogenic shock: a conceptual model, Circulation **45:**1097, 1972.

42. Swan, H.J.C., and Ganz, W.: Guidelines for use of balloon-tipped catheters, Am. J. Cardiol. **34:**119, 1974.

43. Swan, H.J.C., and Ganz, W.: Use of balloon flotation catheters in critically ill patients, Surg. Clin. North Am. **55:**501, 1975.

44. Swan, H.J.C., and Ganz, W.: Complications with flow-directed balloon-tipped catheters, Ann. Intern. Med. **91:**494, 1979.

45. Swan-Ganz flow directed monitoring catheter specifications: Santa Ana, Calif., 1977, Edwards Laboratories.

46. Vandermoten, P., Bernard, R., de Hemptinne, J., and others: Cardiac output monitoring during the acute phase of myocardial infarction: accuracy and precision of the thermodilution method, Cardiology **62:**291, 1977.

47. Walrath, J.M., Abbott, N.K., Caplan, E., and others: Stopcock bacterial contamination in invasive monitoring systems, Heart Lung **8:**100, 1979.

48. Weinstein, R.A., Stamm, W.E., Kramer, L., and others: Pressure monitoring devices: overlooked source of nosocomial infection, J.A.M.A. **236:**936, 1976.

49. Yang, S.S., Bentivolio, L.G., Maranhas, V., and others: From cardiac catheterization data to hemodynamic parameters, ed. 2, Philadelphia, 1978, F.A. Davis Co.

50. Yorra, F.H.M., Oblath, R., Jaffe, H., and others: Massive thrombosis associated with use of the Swan-Ganz catheter, Chest **65:**682, 1974.

ADDITIONAL READINGS

Bernstein, W.H., Fierer, E.M., Laszlo, M.H., and others: The interpretation of pulmonary artery wedge pressures, Br. Heart J. **22:**37, 1960.

Chambers, D.A., Kaplan, J.A.: Tracings of left heart failure— not mitral regurgitation, Anesthesiology **47:**395, 1977.

Critical care nursing policy and procedure manual, Los Angeles, 1981, Cedars-Sinai Medical Center, Department of Nursing.

Folse, R., and Braunwald, E.: A method for the determination of the fraction of left ventricular volume ejected per beat and of the ventricular end-diastolic and residual volumes, Circulation **25:**674, 1962.

Gebbie, K.M., and Lavin, M.A., editors: Classification of nursing diagnoses, St. Louis, 1975, The C.V. Mosby Co.

Gordon, M.: Nursing diagnoses and the diagnostic process, Am. J. Nurs. **76:**1298, 1976.

Kaplan, J.A., and Miller, E.D.: Internal jugular vein catheterization, Anesthesiol. Rev. **3:**21, 1976.

Katz, J.A., Cronan, L.H., Barash, P.G., and others: Pulmonary artery flow-guided catheters in the perioperative period: indications and complications, J.A.M.A. **237:**2832, 1977.

Luchinger, P.C., Seipp, H.W., Jr., and Patel, D.J., Relationship of pulmonary artery wedge pressure to left atrial pressure in man, Circ. Res. **21:**315, 1962.

Manjuran, R.S., Agarwag, J.B., and Roy, S.B.: Relationship of pulmonary artery diastolic and pulmonary artery wedge pressures in mitral stenosis, Am. Heart. J. **89:**207, 1975.

Mayers, M.: Standard care plan, Palos Verdes, Calif., 1975, El Camino Hospital.

Millar, S., editor: Methods in critical care, Philadelphia, 1980, W.B. Saunders Co.

Popkess, S.A.: Diagnosing your patient's strength, Nursing '81 **11:**34-37, July, 1981.

Smith, R.N.: Invasive pressure monitoring, Am. J. Nurs. **78:**1514, 1978.

PART III

PATIENT INTERVENTION

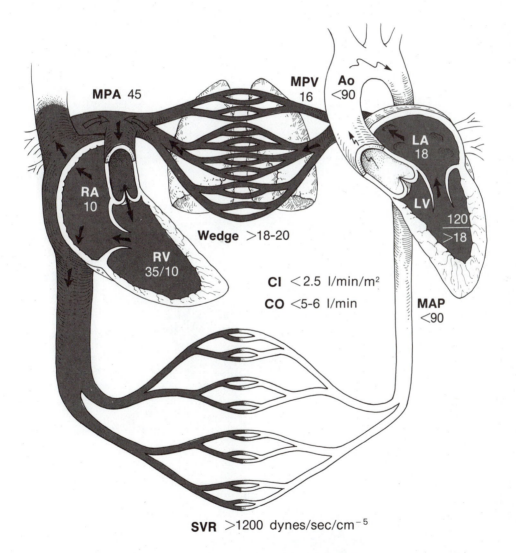

Clinical congestive heart failure

CHAPTER 8

Drug therapy for congestive heart failure

LISA M. TAORMINA-PAPLANUS
CHARLEEN A. STREBEL
CYDNEY R. MICHAELSON

The pharmacological management of congestive heart failure has been the cornerstone of therapy for close to 200 years. It began as a folk remedy with the administration of a mixture of herbs identified by William Withering as an effective treatment for the condition of "dropsy." Withering isolated the herb foxglove, digitalis leaf, and observed and documented its ability to effect pronounced diuresis in individuals with congestive heart failure.[63] Foxglove, administered as the cardiac glycoside digoxin, remains an important agent used in management of this syndrome.

Treatment of congestive heart failure begins with the identification and elimination of underlying causes and precipitating factors of heart disease. The rationale for drug therapy is based on manipulation of the major components of myocardial function; these are preload, afterload, contractility, heart rate, rhythm, conduction, and metabolic state. The primary goal of drug therapy is reduction of cardiac work and an increase in cardiac output and cardiac reserve.

Preload and contractility are intrinsic properties of the myocardium; afterload and heart rate are generally regulated by extrinsic mechanisms. Classic management of heart failure includes the use of digitalis to improve contractility, the manipulation of preload by administration of diuretics and dietary salt, and water restriction. Over the past 10 years, the use of vasodilators to reduce afterload has been added as an important adjunct in the management of both acute and chronic heart failure (Fig. 8-1).

The purpose of this chapter is to present the prescriptives for use and the actions of inotropic agents, vasodilators, and diuretics in the setting of acute and chronic heart failure. The implications for health care and patient education are included along with an overview of the major agents in each drug category. Information regarding specific agents and modes of administration are included in the tables, while more comprehensive material on pharmacodynamics is available in pharmacology textbooks.

INOTROPIC AGENTS

The rationale for use of inotropic agents in the therapy of heart failure is to improve depressed cardiac contractility, boost stroke volume, and generate increased cardiac output. Heart rate and stroke volume are two major determinants of cardiac output; an increase in either will promote an increase in ventricular output. In the setting of heart failure, sympathoadrenergic stimulation is a primary mechanism of compensation, causing elevated heart rate and peripheral vascular resistance. This increased heart rate serves to elevate myocardial oxygen demand and to decrease diastolic filling time, thereby depressing coronary artery perfusion and further contributing to myocardial dysfunction. Therefore augmentation of stroke volume through enhancement of contractil-

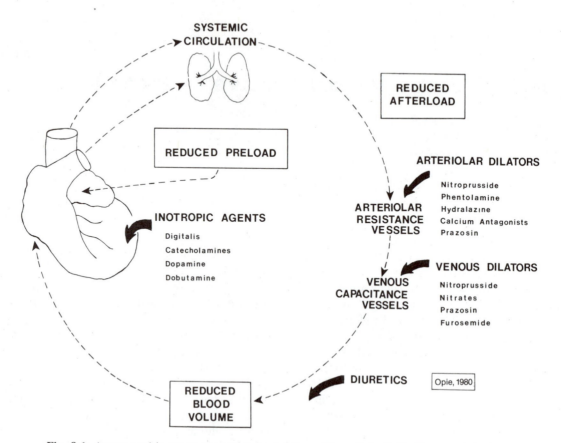

Fig. 8-1. Agents used in severe congestive heart failure. (From Opie, L.H.: Drugs and the heart vasodilating agents, Lancet **3:**966, 1980.)

ity may be accomplished by administering selected inotropic agents. These include digitalis glycosides and sympathomimetic agents.

Digitalis glycosides

Digitalis is the most important and the most widely used positive inotropic drug. It increases contractility of heart muscle and affects the electrophysiological properties of conductivity, refractoriness, and automaticity. Therefore it functions both as a positive inotropic agent and as an antiarrhythmic agent.

Digoxin

Action. Digoxin is the digitalis glycoside used most widely to treat heart failure. Its direct effect on the myocardium occurs in the following man-

ner. Digitalis inhibits the membrane-bound Na^+,K^+-ATPase enzyme. This enzyme normally provides the energy for the Na^+,K^+ pump across the myocardial cell membrane. When the pump is inhibited, intracellular Na^+ accumulates, displaces protein-bound calcium, and promotes movement of extracellular calcium from the sarcolemma and T tubules into the cell. As the concentration of free intracellular Ca^{++} ions increases it promotes more efficient excitation-contraction coupling, resulting in a more rapid and forceful myocardial contraction. Thus the degree of inhibition of membrane-bound Na^+,K^+ ATPase enzyme by digitalis determines the magnitude of its inotropic effect.[1]

Digoxin also exerts an effect on the electrical properties of myocardial tissue. It increases conduction velocity through the atria and ventricles while decreasing the speed of conduction through the atrioventricular (AV) node and the Purkinje fibers. Furthermore, it decreases refractoriness in the atria and in the ventricles and increases refractoriness in the AV node. (See Table 8-1.)

These effects are best appreciated clinically in the setting of atrial fibrillation with a rapid ventricular response. With adequate digitalization, the AV node becomes increasingly refractory to bombardment of impulses from the atria. In addition, the speed of conduction through the node is slowed, resulting in a less frequent ventricular response. This allows more efficient filling of the ventricles and should result in a net increase in cardiac output.

Cardiac slowing is not a significant feature of digoxin action in the *normal* heart, but commonly tachycardia decreases when digoxin improves contractility and relieves heart failure. However, clinically it would be an error to administer digoxin to a patient in heart failure accompanied by a reflex sinus tachycardia resulting from constrictive pericarditis, cardiac tamponade, or thyrotoxicosis. In these settings, myocardial contractility is not severely impaired and toxic doses of digoxin would be required to slow the heart rate. The approach in this setting should be directed toward alleviating the underlying causes and treating the rapid heart rate with other agents.

Absorption, half-life, excretion. Approximately 55% to 75% of oral digoxin is absorbed from the gastrointestinal tract. (However, the absorption of some modern suspensions reaches almost 100%.) It has a half-life of about 36 to 48 hours, and it is excreted essentially unchanged in individuals with normal kidney function. This causes daily loss of about one third of the body stores. For patients with normal kidney function who have not previously received digoxin, the administration of daily maintenance therapy without a loading dose results in the development of steady-state plateau concentrations after 4 to 5 days. With daily maintenance therapy, a steady-state is reached when daily loss is matched with daily intake.[10] Because of the high degree of tissue binding, digoxin is very

Table 8-1. Electrophysiological effects of digitalis

Property	Response
PACEMAKER AUTOMATICITY	
SA node	→ ↑*(↑ after atropine or toxic doses)
Purkinje fibers	↑
EXCITABILITY	
Atrium	→†
Ventricle	Variable†
Purkinje fibers	↑†
CONDUCTION VELOCITY	
Atrium, ventricle	↑ (slight)†
AV node	↓
Purkinje fibers	↓
EFFECTIVE REFRACTORY PERIOD	
Atrium	↓ (↑ after atropine)
Ventricle	↓
AV node	↑
Purkinje fibers	↓

From Moe, G.K., and Farah, A.E.: Digitalis and allied cardiac glycosides. In Goodman, L.S., and Gilman, A. editors: The pharmacological basis of therapeutics, ed. 5, New York (Copyright © 1975 by The MacMillan Publishing Co., Inc.)
*The arrows indicate the direction, not the magnitude, of the changes indicated: ↑, increased; →, no significant change; ↓, decreased.
†Decreased with high toxic doses of digitalis

difficult to remove from the body; extreme caution is essential when administering the drug.

Dosage. When digoxin is used in the treatment of heart failure, the desired inotropic effects are generally reflected by subjective changes in circulatory status, improvement of congestive symptoms, and increased cardiac reserve. Therefore it is quite difficult to establish a dosage schedule to elicit a specific response. This situation is compounded by the following factors: (1) there has been no positive evidence to establish a relationship between inotropic effectiveness and serum digoxin levels; (2) the arrhythmogenic toxic effects of elevated serum digoxin levels in subjects with normal serum potassium levels varies substantially from patient to patient; and (3) because of the high degree of tissue binding, toxic levels of digoxin are quite difficult to remove from the body. For this reason, the drug dose is arbitrarily set for all patients.[32,52,53]

The current trend of administering digitalis glycosides reflects conservatism and caution. When instituting digitalis therapy for chronic heart failure, particularly in elderly patients, the favored approach is daily maintenance therapy without a loading dose. This approach to therapy is then followed by the monitoring of clinical effects, arrhythmogenic effects, blood levels, and evidence of systemic and cardiac toxicity. Great care is taken to use the agent only when necessary, to avoid concurrent drug effects, and to be alert to all factors that may alter drug sensitivity.

Benefits in heart failure. Digitalis benefits patients in heart failure by slowing conduction of impulses through the AV node and the Purkinje fibers as well as by increasing the AV nodal refractory period. This, in concert with the inotropic mechanisms, increases both the force and the velocity of myocardial contraction and shortens the duration of systole. It promotes more complete emptying of the ventricles, reducing heart size.

The hemodynamic effects include an increase in stroke volume, a decrease in ventricular end-diastolic volume and filling pressures, and a drop in central venous and pulmonary capillary wedge pressures. Cardiac output increases in relation to filling pressures and are reflected by a shift upward and to the left when plotted on the left ventricular function curve (Fig. 8-2). These alterations should diminish systemic and pulmonary venous congestion, improving circulatory function.

An increase in contractility resulting from the inotropic effect of digitalis is associated with an increase in myocardial oxygen consumption. However, in the setting of heart failure, this may be offset by hemodynamic effects that reduce filling pressure and ventricular distention, resulting in decreased heart size and intramyocardial wall tension. By Laplace's law, a drop in wall tension reduces myocardial oxygen requirements.

The inotropic effect of digitalis is a mechanism

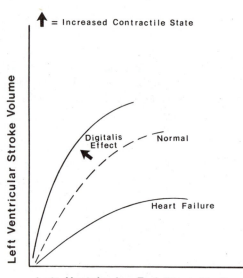

Fig. 8-2. Effect of digitalis on left ventricular function.

that is only partially understood. This drug does not reverse the underlying cause of heart failure and cannot cure heart disease. It acts primarily as an agent to augment the contractile component of cardiac function. In order for the effect to be clinically relevant, improvement of myocardial contractility has to result in improvement of circulation as a whole. The patient should demonstrate by improved renal perfusion and moderate diuresis, decreased congestive symptoms, and increased cardiac reserve. Digitalis is frequently used with diuretics and/or vasodilators to optimize hemodynamic effect.

Prescriptives for use. The effectiveness of digitalis on the failing heart depends on the setting in which it is used. It is most effective in heart failure associated with low cardiac output caused by ischemic, hypertensive, rheumatic, or congenital heart disease. Excellent responses are often seen in patients with rheumatic mitral stenosis accompanied by atrial fibrillation with a rapid ventricular response. Lesser degrees of benefit may be observed with aortic valvular disease or mitral insufficiency.[56]

Generally, it is less effective and not recommended for patients in sinus rhythm with heart failure that results from valvular stenotic lesions, subvalvular stenosis, and high-output states, such as anemias and thyrotoxicosis. The inotropic effect of digitalis may be useful in heart failure associated with acute myocardial infarction; however, because of its effects on myocardial oxygen consumption, administration requires great caution and vigilance. It is contraindicated in heart failure resulting from cardiac tamponade and constrictive pericarditis.

Acute heart failure. The development of better diuretics and vasodilators has lessened the need for digitalis in acute heart failure with sinus rhythm. The major indication for digitalis is the combination of acute congestive heart failure precipitated by rapid atrial fibrillation. Immediate electrical cardioversion is indicated if these arrhythmias are accompanied by hypotension.

A classic situation in which digitalis exerts a major hemodynamic effect is valvular disease with sudden onset of atrial fibrillation and a concomitant reduction in cardiac output. For example, with mitral stenosis, high left atrial pressures are required to squeeze adequate volume across a stenotic orifice. This causes left atrial dilation and hypertrophy, predisposing to the development of atrial arrhythmias. Preservation of optimum ventricular diastolic filling time becomes imperative to the maintenance of adequate cardiac output. The genesis of rapid atrial fibrillation abolishes the critical contribution of "atrial kick," in addition to abruptly curtailing left ventricular filling time. This may reduce cardiac output by as much as 35% to 50%. Digitalis slows impulse conduction through the AV node and increases the nodal refractory period. By slowing the ventricular response to rapid atrial bombardment, it improves diastolic filling and may precipitate conversion to normal sinus rhythm with restoration of optimal atrial contribution to cardiac output.

Digitalis is also useful in the setting of congestive heart failure with atrial fibrillation without valvular heart disease.[46] With digitalis therapy and with slowing of the ventricular response or subsequent conversion to normal sinus rhythm, the improvement in cardiac output may be quite dramatic.

Some authorities believe that digitalis has not demonstrated benefit in isolated mitral stenosis with normal sinus rhythm unless ventricular failure has supervened.[10] Yet others think that prophylactic digitalis used in mitral stenosis with normal sinus rhythm is helpful simply by avoiding the harmful effects of sudden atrial fibrillation.

Of clinical importance with regard to use of digitalis in the treatment of acute heart failure are (1) its ventricular arrhythmogenic potential in unstable ischemic heart disease and (2) the inability to titrate to the end point of ventricular function. Therefore it is understandable how the relatively new parenteral sympathomimetic agents with selective inotropic effects are replacing digitalis in the acute management phase of ischemic heart disease, where low output is a major presenting symptom.

In most acute care facilities, the current treatment trend, seems to be a shift away from the use of digitalis in the management of the patient in acute heart failure, except in those situations discussed earlier with the drug being used cautiously in the management of the patient in chronic heart failure.

Chronic heart failure. Although there are some promising oral inotropic agents under investigation, digitalis remains the only oral inotrope available for treatment of the patient with chronic heart failure. The classic protocol for these individuals has been rest, dietary sodium restriction, digitalis, and diuretics. The greatest benefit of digitalis has been seen in the patient with chronic heart failure and chronic atrial fibrillation.[46] This situation is particularly common in mitral valve disease but is not infrequent in other types of valvular disorders, cardiomyopathies, and ischemic heart disease.[13] In moderate to severe chronic heart failure, most patients derive therapeutic improvement from the use of digitalis in combination with diuretics and oral vasodilators.

The controversy regarding the use of digitalis in chronic heart failure centers on its long-term administration to patients with normal sinus rhythms.

Findings in a study by Lee and others have demonstrated that patients with chronic heart failure and with normal sinus rhythm who derived benefit from digoxin therapy had more severe heart failure, with greater left ventricular dilation and a prominent third heart sound.[38] The data suggest that long-term digoxin therapy is clinically beneficial in patients with normal sinus rhythms and a third heart sound. It is also beneficial for those with heart failure that persists despite diuretic treatment. It is less beneficial in those individuals who have improved with diuretics alone. The study concludes that chronic heart failure with sinus rhythm and a third heart sound failing to improve with diuretics is an indication for use of digitalis. There has been no comparison of digitalis with afterload reduction in these studies.

Factors altering digitalis sensitivity
(Table 8-2)

Cardiac disease. Digitalis effects are modified by the type and severity of underlying heart disease. Severe heart disease with focal ischemia, myocardial fibrosis, and ventricular dilation enhances automaticity of the Purkinje cells predisposing to ventricular arrhythmias. Caution must be exercised when digitalis is administered to these individuals because the electrophysiological aberrations in impulse formation and conduction may interact with the drug to promote increased ventricular automaticity.

Controversy exists regarding the role of digitalis in the setting of acute myocardial infarction. Much of the debate focuses on research done on the healthy heart. Digitalis, by its inotropic action, increases myocardial oxygen consumption, thereby increasing oxygen requirements. In the failing heart, digitalis reduces ventricular dilation and wall tension, thereby decreasing myocardial oxygen requirements. In acute myocardial infarction accompanied by heart failure, the diminution of the heart size and the wall tension should result in a net reduction of myocardial oxygen demand.[28] However, the data have yet to be collected to support universal use of the drug in this setting.

In acute rheumatic carditis where congestive heart failure coexists with delayed AV conduction, the administration of digitalis presents a therapeutic dilemma. Administration may be indicated to augment contractility but carries with it a risk of impaired conduction. Careful monitoring of the electrocardiogram and documentation of rhythm trends are required to avoid the side effects of second- and possibly third-degree heart block.

Systemic disease

Thyroid disease. Thyroid disease alters digitalis sensitivity. In hypothyroidism, the pharmacokinetics are altered, resulting in prolonged half-life of serum digoxin, and in hyperthyroidism the half-life is decreased.[20] The resistance to digitalis in hyperthyroid disease has not been clearly defined, but it is thought to be related to increased autonomic neural tone, which generally influences the effect of digitalis on the heart. For this reason, the drug is not recommended as a first-line treatment for atrial fibrillation or for rapid atrial rhythms associated with thyrotoxicosis. The recommended therapy is beta blockade with correction of the underlying cause of high output failure.

Renal failure. Renal failure seriously affects digitalis sensitivity by influencing absorption and elimination and predisposing to rapid shifts in electrolytes. Since water-soluble digoxin is removed from the body in the unaltered state by the kidneys, individuals with reduced renal function receiving this agent are highly susceptible to a toxic response. Pronounced reduction in glomerular filtration rate prolongs the half-life of digoxin, increasing serum concentration. In the presence of azotemia toxicity may be avoided by careful monitoring of renal function, by limited use of a loading dose, and by reduction of the maintenance dose.

Patients undergoing hemodialysis are prone to rapid shifts in potassium levels and to altered magnesium levels. This may also seriously affect digitalis sensitivity. To avoid these problems it is essential to closely monitor serum electrolytes and to control intake of magnesium-containing antacids in patients taking digitalis.

Pulmonary disease. Patients with pulmonary disease and heart failure are generally more sensitive to digitalis than those without lung disease. Research is highly suggestive that pulmonary dis-

Table 8-2. Factors and mechanisms altering digitalis sensitivity

Disorders	Mechanisms
SYSTEMIC DYSFUNCTION	
Renal failure	Reduced excretion
Low/lean body mass	Reduced binding to skeletal muscle
Chronic cardiac disease	Impaired intracellular calcium ion transport
Chronic pulmonary disease	Hypoxia, acid-base disturbances
Myxedema	Prolonged half-life
Hyperthyroidism	Decreased half-life
Acute hypoxemia	Sensitized to digitalis arrhythmias
Age	Increased sensitivity
ELECTROLYTE DISTURBANCE	
Hyperkalemia/hyponatremia	Reduced digitalis binding
Hypokalemia	Increased digitalis binding
Hypomagnesemia	Increased sensitivity to toxic effects
Hypercalcemia	Increased sensitivity to digitalis effect
Hypocalcemia	Decreased sensitivity to digitalis effect
CARDIAC DYSFUNCTION	
Myocardial fibrosis	Possible increased ventricular automaticity
Acute myocardial infarction	Possible increased sensitivity to inotropic effect resulting in elevated MVO_2 (myocardial oxygen consumption)
Acute rheumatic carditis	Danger of conduction block
Chronic ischemic cardiomyopathy	Decreased sensitivity
DRUG THERAPY	
Potassium-losing diuretics	Increased sensitivity
Quinidine	Decreased renal clearance; reduce digitalis dose 30% to 50% with concomitant administration
Beta blockade	Potentiates effect on AV conduction
Verapamil	Potentiates effect on AV conduction
Barbiturates, phenylbutazone, phenytoin	Increased hepatic metabolism possibly decreases blood levels
Beta-sympathomimetic amines	Increased ventricular automaticity and ectopy
Anesthesia	Promotion of ventricular ectopy
Analgesics: morphine; meperidine	

ease predisposes to manifestations of digitalis toxicity at relatively low serum concentrations.[10]

There is a high incidence of arrhythmias especially during episodes of acute respiratory failure. It is proposed that hypoxemia lowers the threshold for digitalis-induced arrhythmias by sympathetic discharge and catecholamine release and by altering acid-base and electrolyte balance.[46] However, lung disease is not a contraindication for the use of digitalis. It is indicated as an agent of choice when pulmonary disease is associated with atrial fibrillation and left ventricular failure. When right ventricular failure coexists, diuretic therapy is also employed.[46] It is important for these patients and their health care clinicians to be aware of the effect of the lung disease on digitalis to maximize therapeutic drug action and effect proper compliance.

Advanced age. Advanced age has been linked to digitalis sensitivity. Several factors contribute to this condition. These include decreased skeletal muscle mass, which diminishes the apparent volume of drug distribution; the presence of more severe heart disease; lung disorders; and impaired renal and hepatic function.[46] For these reasons, the aged should be treated with smaller doses of digitalis accompanied by careful monitoring for clinical indicators of toxicity.

These individuals are also at risk for drug interaction with medications taken concurrently. A careful assessment of drug history and counseling regarding the importance of compliance is absolutely essential to ensure optimal therapeutic benefit.

Electrolyte abnormalities. Disturbance of electrolyte and acid-base balance significantly alters digitalis sensitivity. The electrolytes that most clearly influence digitalis sensitivity include potassium (K^+), magnesium (Mg^{++}), and calcium (Ca^{++}).

Digitalis and potassium compete for the digitalis binding sites on cell membranes. Increased extracellular potassium ions inhibit digitalis binding to Na^+, K^+ ATPase, decreasing the inotropic effect and suppressing digitalis-induced ectopic rhythms. Therefore animals and humans with elevated

serum potassium levels can tolerate large doses of digitalis without developing toxic ectopic activity; however, the positive inotropic effect is minimized.[42,61]

Low serum potassium levels increase digitalis binding to the cell membrane sites and enhance the toxic arrhythmogenic effects. When this occurs, ectopic complexes and rapid rhythms may appear after administering very small doses of the drug. Furthermore, hypokalemia has a primary arrhythmogenic effect by both decreasing the effective refractory period of Purkinje cells and shortening the coupling interval of ventricular extrasystoles.[10] Therefore individuals receiving digitalis who become potassium depleted are at high risk for developing ectopic ventricular rhythms accompanied by supraventricular tachycardia with block and/or AV junctional tachycardias.[57]

In the setting of compensated heart failure, these rhythms may precipitate acute pulmonary congestion and seriously compromise myocardial perfusion. To reduce the risk of digitalis intoxication, clinicians must carefully monitor blood chemistries and electrolytes and be alert to situations that predispose to hyperkalemia and hypokalemia. These include diuretic therapy, particularly with agents promoting rapid and sustained potassium loss; low cardiac output states and episodes of hypoxemia, which alter acid-base balance; rapid administration of carbohydrates; the use of insulin; and dialysis therapy.

Hypomagnesemia increases digitalis sensitivity, as does hypokalemia, while administration of magnesium-containing salts suppresses digitalis-induced arrhythmias. The physiological function of the ion is poorly understood. It is known that Mg^{++} is instrumental in the transport of Na^+ and K^+ across the cell membrane; therefore it is possible that the mechanism of digitalis toxicity may be similar to that which occurs with hypokalemia.[48]

Some of the causes of hypomagnesemia that predispose to digitalis toxicity are long-term administration of diuretic agents; gastrointestinal disorders such as malabsorption syndromes, diarrhea, and bowel resection; diabetes mellitus; inadequate diet; excessive alcohol intake; prolonged nasogastric suction; and protracted secondary aldosteronism characteristic of chronic heart failure.

Hypercalcemia increases digitalis sensitivity. The interaction of the calcium ion and the digitalis is related to the effect of digitalis on the Na^+, K^+ ATPase enzyme. Digitalis inhibits the membrane-bound enzyme, allowing accumulation of intracellular sodium to displace bound calcium ions. This promotes an exchange of intracellular sodium ion for extracellular calcium ion. Calcium ion facilitates the excitation contraction coupling mechanism, resulting in a more forceful and rapid contraction. Furthermore, it alters the membrane potential of the myocardial cells, promoting increased ventricular automaticity.

Because of the additive effect of calcium and digitalis, caution should be exercised when administering calcium to digitalized patients. This is particularly important during cardiopulmonary resuscitation when large amounts of parenteral calcium may be administered.

Hypocalcemia causes insensitivity to digitalis, so when treating hypocalcemia it is advisable to carefully monitor electrolytes and to correct low serum calcium levels before increasing the dose of digitalis. If the dose is increased first and the calcium levels are corrected later, the possibility of developing digitalis toxicity is increased.

The effect of acid-base status on digitalis sensitivity is complex. Alterations in serum potassium concentrations that accompany shifts in hydrogen ion concentration affect binding of digitalis and development of toxic-induced arrhythmias. Acid-base status also affects serum levels of calcium ion, which also alters digitalis sensitivity. However, it has not been clarified whether acidosis and alkalosis, independent of electrolyte and hydrogen ion imbalance, directly alter digitalis sensitivity.[10]

Concurrent drug effects. Concurrent drug administration may prevent absorption or may interact with digitalis to alter sensitivity. Oral absorption of digoxin may be decreased by certain agents such as cholestyramine, neomycin, propantheline, and nonabsorbable antacids and Kaolin (Kaopectate). Drugs that affect metabolism or excretion of digitalis may also affect the incidence of toxicity. For example, diuretic agents increase the incidence of digitalis toxicity by promoting electrolyte disturbance. Potassium-wasting diuretics include furosemide, ethacrynic acid, and thiazides.

Catecholamines and sympathomimetic agents such as epinephrine, isoproterenol, and high-dose dopamine may interact with digitalis to promote a high incidence of toxic arrhythmias. These agents have the inherent property of precipitating ectopic activity; therefore the risk is additive when administered with digitalis preparations. On the other hand, administration of antiarrhythmic agents may mask electrophysiological indicators of toxicity creating the impression of cardiotoxic resistance.[9]

Arrhythmogenic anesthetic agents may interact with digitalis to promote ventricular ectopy. They may also alter the absorption and excretion of the drug by their pronounced systemic effect. Two such agents are succinylcholine and cyclopropane.[22,45] Adverse digoxin reaction has also been linked to the use of analgesic agents such as meperidine and morphine. These agents are often used concurrently with anesthetic agents; therefore the incidence of arrhythmias in digitalized patients may be significant during induction and postoperative recovery.

In a recent study by Cogan, administration of nitroprusside and hydralazine to patients with chronic congestive heart failure who were receiving digoxin therapy was associated with an increase in the renal clearance of digoxin. The operative mechanisms were improved circulation and improved renal hemodynamics, which increased drug metabolism and excretion with a resultant decrease in serum digoxin levels.[17] The issue of raising the digoxin maintenance dose to increase or to maintain therapeutic blood concentrations in this setting requires further investigation. Currently, concomitant administration of vasodilators in the acute setting requires close observation of serum digoxin levels and clinical indicators of reduced digoxin effect.

Perhaps the most striking drug interaction altering digitalis sensitivity is between digoxin and quinidine sulfate. Quinidine administration induces a twofold rise in serum digoxin level in patients receiving maintenance digoxin therapy. The alterations induced by quinidine are the results of (1) a reduction in the volume of distribution of digoxin as quinidine displaces it from the tissue binding sites; (2) a reduction in the total body clearance of digoxin; and (3) a reduction in the renal clearance of digoxin.

To avoid digoxin toxicity, it is crucial to halve the dose if quinidine therapy is instituted. Likewise, a patient with therapeutic digoxin blood levels who is receiving both digoxin and quinidine may need more digoxin if quinidine is to be discontinued. Quinidine is also thought to prolong the half-life and raise the blood levels of digitoxin. The digitalis-quinidine interaction has been responsible for many clinical cases of digoxin toxicity; therefore patients should be closely observed and interviewed to elicit clinical indicators of toxicity (anorexia, vomiting, diarrhea, palpitations), changes in cardiac rhythms, and changes in serum concentrations of potassium, calcium, and digoxin. Monitoring may also be necessary each time the quinidine dose is changed. Most importantly, to ensure continuity of treatment, clinicians must accurately communicate all aspects of drug therapy to colleagues and to patients who are administering and receiving these agents.

Digitalis toxicity. Digitalis toxicity occurs with unacceptably high frequency. Approximately one out of every five individuals may exhibit clinical indicators associated with drug-induced toxicity. It occurs most frequently in the elderly with advanced heart disease, atrial fibrillation, and associated pulmonary and renal dysfunction—factors that increase digitalis sensitivity. Conversely, other factors may predispose to decreased drug sensitivity (see the boxed material on p. 259). When this occurs, clinicians may increase maintenance doses before identifying the complicating variables. Consequently, in both situations individuals are at risk to develop toxic reactions to therapy.

Table 8-3. Cardiac arrhythmias characteristic of digitalis toxicity

Common arrhythmias	Uncommon arrhythmias
Ventricular bigeminy, trigeminy	Sinus arrest
Multiform ventricular extrasystoles	Bidirectional tachycardia
Ventricular tachycardia	

AV conduction disturbances
  Mobitz type I Wenckebach
    phenomenon
  Complete heart block
	Atrial flutter
	Atrial fibrillation

Junctional rhythms
  Escape
  Tachycardias	

Atrial tachycardia with block	

The clinical indicators of digitalis toxicity include systemic and cardiac manifestations. Both may occur as initial symptoms; however, because of the production of a chemically purer substance, the noncardiac side effects are becoming relatively less common. The most common cardiac features of toxicity are arrhythmias. (See Table 8-3.) Generally, increased ventricular automaticity with bigeminy and trigeminy is first noted; however, multiformed ventricular extrasystoles and paroxysmal atrial tachycardia with AV block may portend toxicity. There may also be AV conduction disturbances as well as Wenckebach phenomenon, complete heart block, and junctional escape rhythms. Sinus arrest is uncommon, and a slow pulse without accompanying clinical indicators is generally a poor sign of digitalis toxicity.[12]

The systemic indicators of toxicity include gastrointestinal symptoms of anorexia, nausea, vomiting, and diarrhea; however, abdominal pain or a tight, bloated feeling are also important, but rarely emphasized, findings. Special attention should be given to fatigue and other central nervous system symptoms, especially in the elderly, since these may easily be attributed to the individual's poor health. Varying degrees of mental confusion, hallucinations, restlessness, insomnia, apathy, drowsi-

---

FACTORS GENERATING LOW SERUM DIGOXIN/DIGITOXIN LEVELS

1. Dosages
   a. Inadequate or missed
   b. Noncompliance
2. Poor gastrointestinal absorption
   a. Malabsorption
   b. Bowel resection
   c. Drug interference: kaolin, cholestyramine, neomycin, *p*-aminosalicylic acid
3. Disruption of enterohepatic flow (especially for digitoxin)
   a. Cholestyramine therapy
   b. Biliary drainage
4. Increased hepatic metabolism
   a. Barbiturates
   b. Phenylbutazone
   c. Phenytoin

Table 8-4. Systemic indicators of digitalis toxicity

Body locus	Clinical indicators
Gastrointestinal system	Anorexia, nausea, vomiting, diarrhea, abdominal pain, bloating
Central nervous system	*Fatigue,* confusion, lethargy, insomnia, apathy, drowsiness, psychotic episodes, headaches, neurological facial pain, paresthesias
Eyes	Blurred vision, altered or indistinct color perception, amblyopia, diplopia, scotomas, halos, flickering, retrobulbar neuritis
Endocrine system	Gynecomastia in men (rarely)
Skin	Allergic reactions, urticarial or scarlatiniform (rarely)

---

ness, and extreme weakness have been noted secondary to digitalis toxicity. In the setting of heart failure, it is quite difficult to distinguish these from symptoms of low cardiac output.

Visual complaints may be the initial symptom in some individuals. These include altered or indistinct color perception, blurred vision, scotomas, flickering, amblyopia, diplopia, and halos. Allergic skin lesions are rare, and gynecomastia is occasionally seen in men. (See Table 8-4.)

Management of digitalis toxicity. Successful management of digitalis toxicity is predicated on early recognition of associated arrhythmias. These may include occasional ventricular ectopy, marked first-degree heart block, or atrial fibrillation with a slow or sudden regularization of a more rapid ventricular response. If the arrhythmia is not life-threatening, the required intervention may be limited to temporary withdrawal of digitalis and electrocardiographic monitoring until the arrhythmia resolves. Rhythm disturbances that impair cardiac output because they are too fast or too slow require immediate vigorous intervention. The most dangerous of these is ventricular tachycardia. Subjects who develop this rhythm associated with digitalis toxicity usually do not survive.[10,12]

Ventricular ectopy resulting from digitalis toxicity may be treated with lidocaine and phenytoin. These agents have little effect on the sinoatrial rate, and atrial and AV or His-Purkinje system conduction. Phenytoin may in fact improve sinoatrial and AV conduction.

Other antiarrhythmic agents have been employed to manage these toxic arrhythmias; however, each carries a higher risk than lidocaine or phenytoin. Propranolol, because of its antiadrenergic effects, decreases automaticity; however, its use is particularly undesirable with congestive heart failure, because of depression of myocardial contractility with subsequent hemodynamic deterioration. Quinidine and procainamide are useful in reducing enhanced ventricular automaticity, but they carry high risk for depressing the entire conduction system as well as reducing myocardial contractility.

Potassium administration is recommended to treat ventricular ectopy secondary to digitalis toxicity when hypokalemia is present. Preferably, potassium should be given orally; however, if necessary it may be slowly administered intravenously when appropriately diluted. It is important to emphasize that potassium may be contraindicated when digitalis has impaired AV conduction since elevated serum potassium concentrations may potentiate the problem. Furthermore, its use must be limited in patients with impaired renal function.

Experimental supplies of incomplete antibodies have recently become available. These bind both tissue and serum drug and immediately reverse the toxicity. If their substance proves to be nontoxic and if it is made widely available, it will probably become the treatment of choice.

Digoxin levels. When electrocardiographic changes suggest digitalis toxicity, serum blood concentrations are obtained by radioimmunoassay to determine whether or not the drug level is inappropriately elevated. The blood samples should be drawn before the regular daily dose or, at the earliest, 2 hours after an intravenous dose and 6 hours after an oral dose. It is at this time that optimal equilibrium has been achieved and serum concentrations reflect tissue drug levels. In patients with depressed myocardial function more time should be allowed for equilibrium to occur.[38] Because of the many factors altering the effect on any digoxin level (see Table 8-2) absolute serum concentrations may not correlate directly with drug effects. Therefore an unexpected low level may require evaluation of compliance and a review of other causes of altered digitalis sensitivity. Furthermore, these factors may limit the role of digoxin levels as being absolutely diagnostic for digitalis toxicity.

Relative contraindications. Generally, acute myocardial infarction and chronic lung disease with hypoxemia are settings not conducive to administration of digitalis. Hypoxemia may increase the arrhythmogenic properties, and myocardial infarction and ischemia may be extended by the inotropic properties of the agent. In acute myocarditis with failure, digitalis may be more likely to contribute to arrhythmias and not help the failure. Renal failure requires a lower dose, judicious monitoring of serum potassium levels, and vigilant observation for clinical indicators of toxicity.

In hypertensive heart disease, the primary problem is elevated afterload, so the preferred therapy is use of vasodilators. Digitalis is generally not indicated unless atrial fibrillation is present; then verapamil may be the agent of choice since it will reduce both ventricular rate and afterload. Particular caution is necessary when a patient is taking

Table 8-5. Pharmacological properties of selected cardiac glycosides

Agent	Absorption	Excretion	Onset of action	Peak effect	Half-life	Therapeutic plasma level	Toxic plasma levels
Digoxin	55%-75% GI	Principally renal; some GI	5-30 min	1-5 hr	36-48 hr	0.8-1.6 ng/ml	2.4 ng/ml
Digitoxin	90%-100% GI	Principally hepatic; some renal excretion of metabolites	30 min-2 hr	4-12 hr	4-6 days	14-26 ng/ml	34 ng/ml
Ouabain	Unreliable	Renal; some GI	5-10 min	½-2 hr	21 hr	—	—

Table 8-6. Dosage of selected digitalis glycosides

Agent	Administration	Digitalizing quantity (given in divided doses)	Maintenance quantity (daily dose)
Digoxin (Lanoxin)	Oral	1.5 mg (0.5-2 mg)	0.5 mg (0.125-0.75 mg)
	Intravenous	1 mg (0.5-1.5 mg)	0.5 mg (0.125-0.75 mg)
Digitoxin	Oral	1.0-1.5 mg over 24-48 hr	0.1-0.2 mg
	Intravenous	1 mg (0.5-1.5 mg)	0.1 mg (0.1-0.1 mg)
Ouabain	Intravenous only (slowly)	0.5 mg (0.12-0.25 mg)	—

Adapted from Hahn, A.B., Barkin, R.L., and Oestreich, S.J.K., Pharmacology in nursing, ed. 15, St. Louis, 1982, The C.V. Mosby Co., p. 574.

other drugs that inhibit AV conduction, and digitalis should be avoided in patients who require direct current countershock because life-threatening arrhythmias may develop.

Review of agents (see Tables 8-5 and 8-6)

Digitoxin. Digitoxin is the chief active glycoside of *Digitalis purpurea,* purple foxglove, and it is the active ingredient in digitalis leaf. It is a longer-acting compound than digoxin and is virtually completely absorbed in the gut. Because it is chiefly metabolized and excreted in the liver and gut, blood levels are not significantly altered by poor renal function. Furthermore, omission of a dose has little effect on blood levels.

The major disadvantage of this compound is the long half-life when compared to digoxin (4 to 6 days digitoxin, 36 to 48 hours digoxin). It is contraindicated in patients with reduced liver function.

This may occur in those individuals with chronic heart failure accompanied by venous hypertension and hepatic congestion. Side effects, contraindications, and implications for health care are similar to digoxin.

Ouabain. Ouabain is the most rapidly acting of the cardiac glycosides in clinical use. The plasma half-life is 21 hours in subjects without renal impairment, and its onset of action after intravenous injection is 5 to 10 minutes, with the peak effect occurring in 90 minutes.[34] It is primarily excreted unchanged by the kidneys and is also metabolized in the gastrointestinal tract.

According to Goodman and Gilman, use of this agent is infrequent and probably more hazardous than digoxin.[20] Because it is so irregularly and poorly absorbed from the gastrointestinal tract, it must be administered parenterally and is confined to use in critical-care settings. Its side effects, contraindications, and health care considerations are the same as digitalis.

Amrinone. Amrinone, a new drug under investigation, is a nonglycosidic, nonadrenergic, positive inotropic agent that is being tested in the management of patients with refractory heart failure who are receiving digitalis. In a recent study, amrinone induced hemodynamic improvement in patients with congestive heart failure and coronary artery disease and was associated with no evidence of myocardial ischemia or increased myocardial oxygen consumption.[7] It is postulated that amrinone's effect on cardiac contractility accounted for increased cardiac output significantly more than a fall in preload or afterload.[7,60]

The mechanism of amrinone's positive inotropic effect remains uncertain. It is believed that the myocardial contractile state is improved in a manner not related to Na^+, K^+-ATPase activity (as with digitalis) or alterations in adenosine 3,5-cyclic monophosphate and phosphodiesterase (as with catecholamines).[60] Catecholamines seem not to be required for amrinone to exert a positive inotropic effect. These properties also appear to be additive to those of digitalis. In this study, amrinone served to increase or maintain cardiac output at a reduced filling pressure in patients at rest, generating a sense of well-being that enabled the subjects to engage in their own exercise training program. After 4 weeks, an increase in exercise capacity was quite apparent. The patients treated with amrinone no longer experienced orthopnea or paroxysmal nocturnal dyspnea, and some were able to return to a gainful existence.[60]

Further studies examined the clinical and hemodynamic effects of long-term amrinone therapy in patients with refractory heart failure.[43,55] The results demonstrated amrinone-dependent hemodynamic benefits during long-term therapy without tachyphylaxis. Amrinone was given intravenously followed by oral maintenance therapy. The average unit oral dose was 1 to 3 mg/kg. Some nausea and anorexia were experienced after the initial intravenous bolus injection, but they subsided within a few hours. Ventricular arrhythmias associated with too rapid intravenous injection (1 mg/minute) were eliminated as well as the gastrointestinal effects by slower (0.2 mg/minute) administration.[60] Finally, thrombocytopenia (platelet count less than $150,000/mm^3$) had been reported as a significant side effect of amrinone. Lowering the dose to 2 mg/kg and combining low-dose amrinone with hydralazine proved beneficial in averting this side effect.[43,55]

It is advised that clinicians closely monitor future clinical investigation of this agent. It has caused significant thrombocytopenia and alteration in gastrointestinal and liver function. Currently, research is directed toward developing a second generation of agents similar to amrinone that will provide more effective hemodynamic response with fewer side effects.

Health care implications. To obtain the desired effect of digitalis in the setting of heart failure is a difficult goal to accomplish. From the information presented, the reader may conclude that a multitude of variables may supervene to alter the effect of therapy. It is essential for health care professionals to internalize this material and to operationalize the concepts when delivering care to individuals undergoing therapy. The following points have been included to facilitate this process.

Assessment

1. Assess for underlying cause and precipitating factors in heart failure.
2. Observe and elicit data from patients regarding the clinical indicators of resolving or progressing heart failure (peripheral edema, weight gain, shortness of breath, fatigue, exertional dyspnea).
3. Monitor serum electrolytes, blood chemistries, and blood gases when indicated. Special attention should be given to creatinine levels as evidence of renal function, especially in the elderly.
4. Obtain a careful drug history before and during maintenance digitalis therapy.
5. Monitor electrocardiograms for evidence of cardiotoxicity.

6. Assess for central nervous system effects such as confusion, apathy, drowsiness, and lethargy.
7. Observe and assess for visual abnormalities characteristic of digitalis toxicity (impaired color perception, blurred vision, scotomas, halos).
8. Assess for gastrointestinal abnormalities characteristic of digitalis toxicity that occur after initiating therapy (nausea, vomiting, diarrhea, abdominal bloating, feeling of fullness, anorexia).
9. Assess for patient's attitude and environmental factors that may contribute to or interfere with drug compliance. See Chapter 12 for detailed information on patient education.

Intervention
1. Carefully calculate drug dosage before administration.
2. Meticulously document the amount, frequency, route of administration, and therapeutic response.
3. Judiciously communicate clinical status to all health care professionals caring for the patient. This is absolutely essential to preserve digitalis sensitivity and to avoid drug interaction.
4. Plan a patient-family teaching program regarding the desired inotropic and arrhythmogenic drug effects, monitoring for these effects, and toxic manifestations. Emphasize the importance of regular professional health care supervision. Discuss the goal of therapy

Table 8-7. Location of sympathetic receptor sites and vasoactive response

Site	Receptor	Elicited response when receptor stimulated*
HEART		
SA node	beta$_1$	↑ automaticity
Atria	beta$_1$	↑ contractility ↑ conductivity
AV node	beta$_1$	↑ conductivity ↑ automaticity ↓ refractory period
His-Purkinje network	beta$_1$	↑ automaticity
Ventricles	beta$_1$	↑ contractility
VASCULATURE		
Vein/peripheral arterioles	alpha	Constrict
Skin and mucosal arterioles	alpha	Constrict
Renal arterioles	alpha	Constrict
Pulmonary arterioles	alpha and beta$_2$	Constrict and dilate
Skeletal muscle arterioles	alpha and beta$_2$	Constrict and dilate
Abdominal viscera arterioles	alpha and beta$_2$	Constrict and dilate
Coronary arterioles	alpha and beta$_2$	Constrict and dilate
LUNG		
Bronchial smooth muscle	beta$_2$	Relax

*↑, increase; ↓, decrease.

in terms of return to an optimal health state. Include the importance of compliance to all aspects of the treatment regime: weight control, dietary restrictions, exercise tolerance, and stress-related activities.

Sympathomimetic agents

Sympathomimetic amines are inotropic agents used to treat severe heart failure accompanied by low cardiac output states. These drugs simulate sympathetic nerve stimulation and the response of specific adrenergic receptor sites (Table 8-7). There are three major types of receptors: alpha-adrenergic, beta-adrenergic, and dopaminergic. Alpha effects are exerted largely on peripheral arterioles, causing vasoconstriction of the skin and of the mesenteric and renal circulations, elevated blood pressure, reflex bradycardia, and increased afterload. Beta-sympathomimetic effects reflect the response to two types of beta-adrenergic receptors, beta$_1$ (β_1) and beta$_2$ (β_2). Beta$_1$ receptors are located predominately in the heart and cause increased myocardial contractility, elevated heart rate, and accelerated AV conduction. Beta$_2$ receptors are located in the bronchi, blood vessels, and uterus. Beta$_2$ effects result in bronchial relaxation and vasodilation of peripheral arterioles. Beta$_2$ receptors also activate renin, which promotes renal-mediated peripheral vascular constriction. Dopaminergic receptors promote vasodilation of the mesenteric and renal circulation.

Benefits in heart failure. A major compensatory mechanism in heart failure is activation of the sympathoadrenergic system. Initially, this supports circulation by augmenting heart rate and contractility and by mediating selective vasoconstriction. However, as heart failure persists, this mechanism loses its cardiac effectiveness. Two important factors may elicit this response. First, the myocardium requires higher levels of exogenous norepinephrine (catecholamines) to maintain rate and contractility. Second, depletion of endogenous or cardiac stores of norepinephrine interferes with sympathetic augmentation of contractility. These factors contribute, in part, to pump failure and support the rationale for administering supplemental catecholamine and digitalis preparations; however, it must be emphasized that while sympathomimetic amines augment cardiac function by increasing heart rate and contractility, they may do so at the expense of increasing myocardial oxygen consumption.

A major therapeutic objective of treating low-output heart failure associated with acute myocardial infarction is to enhance cardiac output and peripheral perfusion without significantly increasing myocardial oxygen demand. This may be accomplished by administering selected agents, such as dopamine and dobutamine, to augment contractile function, by using vasodilators to decrease afterload, and by avoiding selected alpha and beta agonists, which significantly elevate heart rate and peripheral vasoconstriction. It is requisite for clinicians to be familiar with the various sympathomimetic amines, their primary adrenergic effect, and the indications for their use in heart failure. Table 8-8 summarizes the properties of these agents.

Prescriptives for use
Acute heart failure
Beta agonists

DOPAMINE. (See the box on p. 266.) Dopamine is the immediate precursor of norepinephrine. It indirectly exerts an inotropic effect by stimulating release of norepinephrine. It is characterized by its dose-dependent effects on alpha, beta, and dopaminergic receptors. At lower doses, between 2 to 10 μg/kg/minute, it may be very effective in treating low-output acute heart failure. Beta$_1$ stimulation increases contractility while dopaminergic receptors will preserve renal perfusion despite mildly elevated peripheral vascular resistance. This is particularly useful in conditions associated with increased vascular tone. The major clinical limitations arise at higher doses, 10 to 20 μg/kg/min when beta$_1$ and primary alpha effects result in tachyarrhythmias and marked peripheral vascular constriction. For this reason, in severe congestive heart failure the dose should be closely monitored and kept within strict bounds. Dopamine is also indicated when an inotropic effect is needed together with an increase in renal blood flow, as manifested in patients with low cardiac output that

Table 8-8. Selected sympathomimetic agents: organ response

Agent	Alpha	Organ response	Beta$_1$	Organ response	Beta$_2$	Organ response
Dopamine*						
≤2-5 µg/ kg/minute	0	↔ PVR ↓ or ↔ BP	+++	↑ Contractility ↑ CO ↔ HR	++	↔ or ↑ vasodilation (renal blood flow ↑ through stimulation of dopaminergic receptors causing ↑ UO)
5-10 µg/ kg/minute	+++	↑ PVR ↑ BP	++++	↑↑ Contractility ↑ CO ↑↑ HR	+	Less ↑ vasodilation (renal blood flow may ↓ causing ↓ UO)
≥10-20 µg/ kg/minute	++++	↑↑ PVR ↑↑ BP	++++	↑↑ Contractility ↑ CO (may ↓) ↑↑ HR	0	No ↑ vasodilation (no dopaminergic effect resulting in oliguria)
Dobutamine						
2-10 µg/kg/ minute	+	↔ PVR (↑ with high doses) ↔ BP	++++	↑ Contractility ↑ CO ↔ HR	++	↑ vasodilation
≥20 µg/kg/ minute	+	↑ PVR	++++	↑ Contractility ↑ CO ↑↑ HR	0	↓ vasodilation
Isoproterenol (Isuprel)	0	↔ PVR ↓ BP (with high dose)	++++	↑ Contractility ↑ CO ↑↑↑ HR	++++	↑↑ vasodilation
Prenalterol (under investigation)	0	↔ PVR ↔ BP mean	+++	↑ Contractility ↔ HR	0	↔ vasodilation
Phenylephrine (Neo-Synephrine)	++++	↑↑ PVR ↑↑ BP	0/+	↔ Contractility (↑ with high doses) ↓ CO ↓ HR	0	↓ vasodilation
Epinephrine	+++	↑ PVR ↑ BP	++++	↑ Contractility ↑↑ CO ↑↑ HR	++	↑ vasodilation
Norepinephrine (Levophed)	++++	↑↑ PVR ↑↑ BP	++	↑ Contractility ↔ or ↓ CO ↑ HR (↓ with high doses)	0	↔ vasodilation
Ephedrine	++++	↑↑ PVR ↑↑ BP	+++	↑ Contractility (↓ with high doses) ↑ CO ↔ HR (↑ with blocked vagal reflexes)	+	↑ vasodilation

*Dopamine is the only sympathomimetic agent that stimulates dopaminergic receptors located in coronary, intracerebral, mesenteric, and renal vascular beds.

↑, increase; ↓, decrease; ↔, unchanged; 0, no effect; +, least effect; ++++, greatest effect; *PVR*, peripheral vascular resistance; *BP*, blood pressure; *CO*, cardiac output; *HR*, heart rate, *UO*, urinary output.

Drug: **Dopamine (Intropin)** (alpha and beta agonist—norepinephrine precursor)

Mixture: 200 mg/250 ml D$_5$W—800 μg/ml
400 mg/250 ml D$_5$W—1600 μg/ml double-strength solution

Dose: Therapeutic dose = 2-10 μg/kg/minute
Low dose = 1-5 μg/kg/minute = predominantly beta effect
Moderate dose = 5-10 μg/kg/minute = dopaminergic effect
High dose = 10 μg/kg/minute = predominantly alpha effect

Protocol: Used to decrease LVEDP and to raise cardiac output in a setting of low arterial pressure; continuously monitor hemodynamic parameters and urine output; deliver with infusion pump; discard solution after 24 hours; incompatible with alkaline solutions.

Precautions: Beta-receptor effects are blocked by propranolol; it will cause bradycardia and hypotension with phenytoin; do not use in setting of pheochromocytoma; uncorrected tachyarrhythmias; or ventricular fibrillation

Dopamine diluent chart: 200 mg/250 ml D$_5$W = 800 μg/ml = 800 μg/60 μgtt

Weight		Dosage: μg/kg/minute																				
lb	kg	2	2.5	3	3.5	4	4.5	5	5.5	6	6.5	7	7.5	8	8.5	9	9.5	10	11	12	13	14
88	40	6	8	9	11	12	14	15	17	18	20	21	23	24	26	27	29	30	33	36	39	42
99	45	7	8	10	12	14	15	17	19	20	22	24	25	27	29	30	32	34	37	41	44	47
110	50	8	9	11	13	15	17	19	21	23	24	26	28	30	32	34	36	38	41	45	49	53
121	55	8	10	12	14	17	19	21	23	25	27	29	31	33	35	37	39	41	45	50	54	58
132	60	9	11	14	16	18	20	23	25	27	29	32	34	36	38	41	43	45	50	54	59	63
143	65	10	12	15	17	20	22	24	27	29	32	34	37	39	41	44	46	49	54	58	63	68
154	70	11	13	16	18	21	24	26	29	32	34	37	39	42	45	47	50	53	58	63	68	74
165	75	11	14	17	20	23	25	28	31	34	37	39	42	45	48	51	53	56	62	68	73	79
176	80	12	15	18	21	24	27	30	33	36	39	42	45	48	51	54	57	60	66	72	78	84
187	85	13	16	19	22	26	29	32	35	38	41	45	49	51	54	57	61	64	70	77	83	89
198	90	14	17	20	24	27	30	34	37	41	44	47	51	54	57	61	64	68	74	81	88	95
209	95	14	20	21	25	29	32	36	39	43	46	50	53	57	61	64	68	71	78	86	93	100
220	100	15	19	23	26	30	34	38	41	45	49	53	56	60	64	68	71	75	83	90	98	105
242	110	17	21	25	29	33	37	41	45	50	54	58	62	66	70	74	78	83	91	99	107	116

μgtt/minute

Drug:	**Dobutamine (Dobutrex)** (beta agonist)
Mixture:	250 mg/250 ml D_5W = 1 mg/ml (may be diluted in only 50 ml if necessary)
Dose:	2.5-10 μg/kg/minute
Protocol:	Short-term inotropic support in heart failure secondary to depressed contractility; does not have potent pressor effects so may be ineffective in hypotensive states not related to cardiac function; deliver with infusion pump; continuously monitor hemodynamic parameters
Precautions:	Stenotic valvular and subvalvular lesions; incompatible with alkaline solutions

Dobutamine diluent chart: 250 mg/250 ml D_5W = 1 mg/ml = 1 mg/60 μgtt = 1000 μg/60 μgtt

Weight lb	Weight kg	Dosage: μg/kg/minute 2	2.5	3	3.5	4	4.5	5	5.5	6	6.5	7	7.5	8	8.5	9	9.5	10	12	14	16	18	20
88	40	5	6	7	8	10	11	12	13	14	16	17	18	19	20	22	23	24	29	34	38	43	48
99	45	5	7	8	9	11	12	14	15	16	18	19	20	22	23	24	26	27	32	38	43	49	54
110	50	6	8	9	11	12	14	15	17	18	20	21	23	24	26	27	29	30	36	42	48	54	60
121	55	7	8	10	12	13	15	17	18	20	21	23	25	26	28	30	31	33	40	46	53	60	66
132	60	7	9	11	13	14	16	18	20	22	23	25	27	29	31	32	34	36	43	50	58	65	72
143	65	8	10	12	14	16	18	20	21	23	25	27	29	31	33	35	37	39	47	55	62	70	78
154	70	8	11	13	15	17	19	21	23	25	27	29	32	34	36	38	40	42	50	59	67	76	84
165	75	9	11	14	16	18	20	23	25	27	29	32	34	36	38	41	43	45	54	63	72	81	90
176	80	10	12	14	17	19	22	24	26	29	31	34	36	38	42	43	46	48	58	67	77	86	96
187	85	10	13	15	18	20	23	26	28	31	33	36	38	41	44	46	48	51	61	71	82	92	102
198	90	11	14	16	19	22	24	27	29	32	35	38	41	43	46	49	51	54	65	76	86	97	108
209	95	11	14	17	20	23	26	29	31	34	37	40	43	46	48	51	54	57	68	80	91	103	114
220	100	12	15	18	21	24	27	30	33	36	39	42	45	48	51	54	57	60	72	84	96	108	120
242	110	13	17	20	23	26	30	33	36	40	43	46	50	53	56	59	63	66	79	92	106	119	132

μgtt/minute

is accompanied by oliguria and adequate mean arterial pressure.

DOBUTAMINE. (See the box on p. 267.) Dobutamine is a synthetic cardioactive derivative of dopamine that stimulates beta$_1$, beta$_2$, and alpha-adrenergic receptors. It acts directly on the heart and does not depend on the release of endogenous norepinephrine. It is considered the most effective sympathomimetic agent for short-term management of acute low-output pump failure that is *not accompanied by hypotension.* Cardiac output is improved by its strong beta$_1$ effect and further facilitated by its mild beta$_2$ vasodilating effects. This agent demonstrates a low incidence of drug-induced tachycardia and peripheral vasoconstriction; thus it is less likely to elevate myocardial oxygen requirements. Because dobutamine has minimal alpha effects, it may not achieve adequate pressor effects in severe hypotensive states. Furthermore, dobutamine does not act on dopaminergic receptors to promote renal vasodilation; however, it increases renal perfusion indirectly by elevating cardiac output. It also causes a redistribution of blood flow in favor of coronary and skeletal muscle beds, over mesenteric and renal vascular beds.

COMBINATION THERAPY. Combination therapy of vasodilators with sympathomimetic amines is frequently used to treat acute left ventricular failure. In acute anteroseptal infarction, when pump failure results from diastolic overload as a result of sudden mitral regurgitation secondary to papillary muscle rupture, the therapeutic regime may require parenteral administration of nitroglycerin to reduce preload and dobutamine to increase contractility. The therapeutic goal is to augment cardiac output, increase peripheral perfusion, reduce regurgitant volume, relieve acute pulmonary congestion, and preserve the myocardium. Nitroglycerin not only reduces preload but improves myocardial oxygen supply by elevating subendocardial blood flow.

In acute left ventricular failure characterized by depressed myocardial function secondary to cardiac surgery, the agents dobutamine or low-dose dopamine may be necessary to wean the patient from cardiopulmonary bypass. These agents are also used in conjunction with an arteriolar dilator, such as nitroprusside, to diminish peripheral vascular resistance, which may be significantly elevated during the perioperative state. The primary therapeutic objective is to decrease aortic impedance and augment contractility until the heart muscle recovers from the depressive effects of surgery. See Chapter 14 for more information on care of the surgical patient.

Administration of dobutamine and nitroprusside is frequently used to augment myocardial contractility and to reduce afterload in the setting of low-output left ventricular failure secondary to myocardial ischemia and infarction. The goal of therapy is to elevate contractility, decrease afterload, increase peripheral perfusion, and preserve the myocardium. Parenteral administration of sodium nitroprusside decreases afterload and, in combination with the inotropic property of dobutamine, or low-dose dopamine, effects a net increase in cardiac output without hypotension. (See Fig. 8-2.)

Sympathomimetic support may also be indicated in the setting of acute inferior wall infarction complicated by right ventricular infarction and failure. In a recent study, acute right ventricular infarction accompanied by shock was treated with aggressive volume expansion and dopamine.[37] However, the patient continued to demonstrate low cardiac output and developed tachycardia secondary to high-dose dopamine. Counterpulsation was added to maintain adequate arterial pressure, with no substantial increase in cardiac output. Finally, the use of dobutamine and counterpulsation effected an increase in cardiac output and peripheral perfusion. Thus the combination of sympathomimetic therapy and mechanical support yielded favorable results in this patient.

ISOPROTERENOL. *Isoproterenol* has predominant beta$_1$ and beta$_2$ action. It is a synthetic catecholamine with a chemical structure related to norepinephrine. It directly stimulates the heart to augment contractility, increase heart rate, and increase myocardial oxygen consumption. Furthermore, it promotes vasodilation in renal and mesenteric beds, reducing peripheral vascular resistance. Because of its potent cardiac tachycardia and increased myocardial oxygen consumption effects, it is not an agent of choice in low-output pump failure secondary to myocardial infarction. Rather, this agent is used to treat hemodynamically unstable bradycardias not responsive to atropine, and it is indicated to raise heart rate in the setting of complete heart block with a slow ventricular response until pacemaker therapy may be established. An isoproterenol infusion may also be used to support a very sick patient with low cardiac output immediately following open-heart surgery.[56] However, the rhythm must be closely monitored for onset of sinus tachycardia and ventricular ectopy, which heralds termination of therapy. Because of its arrhythmogenic effects, this agent is contraindicated in the setting of digitalis-induced cardiotoxicity. (See box below.)

Alpha agonists. These sympathomimetic agents, which have predominate alpha effects, include norepinephrine, epinephrine, phenylephrine, ephedrine, and methoxamine. Generally, their marked peripheral vasoconstrictive properties and mild inotropic effects limit their use in heart failure. (See Table 8-8.) This is indeed the case when acute

Drug:	**Isoproterenol (Isuprel)** (beta agonist)
Mixture:	1 mg/250 ml $D_5W = 4/\mu g/ml = 4 \mu g/60 \mu gtt$
Dose:	2-20 μg/minute of a 1:250,000 solution
Protocol:	Short-term chronotropic and inotropic support in AV heart block with symptomatic bradycardia; bronchospasm resolution during anesthesia; cardiac catheterization to simulate exercise; to effect peripheral vasodilation when central venous pressure and blood volume are elevated or normal; continuously monitor hemodynamic parameters and electrocardiographic patterns; deliver with an infusion pump
Precautions:	Markedly elevates myocardial consumption; use cautiously in coronary insufficiency, hyperthyroidism, and known sensitivity to sympathomimetics and pre-existing cardiac arrhythmias with tachycardias; should not be used concurrently with epinephrine since both are potent cardiac stimulants and are likely to precipitate fatal arrhythmias

Isoproterenol diluent chart: 4 μg/60 μgtt
Titrate to increase heart rate

8 $\mu gtt = $ .5 μg/min	135 $\mu gtt = $ 9 μg/min
15 $\mu gtt = $ 1 μg/min	150 $\mu gtt = $ 10 μg/min
23 $\mu gtt = $ 1.5 μg/min	165 $\mu gtt = $ 11 μg/min
30 $\mu gtt = $ 2 μg/min	180 $\mu gtt = $ 12 μg/min
38 $\mu gtt = $ 2.5 μg/min	195 $\mu gtt = $ 13 μg/min
45 $\mu gtt = $ 3 μg/min	210 $\mu gtt = $ 14 μg/min
60 $\mu gtt = $ 4 μg/min	225 $\mu gtt = $ 15 μg/min
75 $\mu gtt = $ 5 μg/min	240 $\mu gtt = $ 16 μg/min
90 $\mu gtt = $ 6 μg/min	255 $\mu gtt = $ 17 μg/min
105 $\mu gtt = $ 7 μg/min	270 $\mu gtt = $ 18 μg/min
120 $\mu gtt = $ 8 μg/min	285 $\mu gtt = $ 19 μg/min
	300 $\mu gtt = $ 20 μg/min

left ventricular failure is precipitated by hypertensive disease or myocardial infarction. The alpha effects increase afterload and cardiac work, ultimately worsening heart failure.

PHENYLEPHRINE AND METHOXAMINE. Phenylephrine and methoxamine are powerful alpha agonists and have little inotropic and chronotropic effect. Because of their potent vasoconstrictive properties, they elevate blood pressure, which stimulates baroreceptor vagal response, producing a pronounced reflex bradycardia. For this reason, they may be effective in converting paroxysmal tachy-cardia to normal rhythms. If these rhythms are precipitating factors in acute heart failure, then these agents may be indicated; however, long-term use is contraindicated, especially in the setting of ischemic heart disease, hyperthyroidism, and hypertension. (See the box below.)

NOREPINEPHRINE. Norepinephrine (Levophed) may be required in selected settings for its pressor effects. In severe low-output failure characterized by marked hypotension and cardiogenic shock, a short-term norepinephrine infusion may be required to generate a sufficient pressure head to per-

---

Drug:	**Phenylephrine hydrochloride (Neo-Synephrine)** (alpha agonist)
Mixture:	Direct IV: 1 mg/9 ml sterile water = 0.1 mg/ml
	Infusion: 10 mg/250 ml D_5W = 40 μg/ml = 40 μg/60 μgtt
Dose:	Direct IV: 0.1-0.5 mg initially. Repeated every 10 to 15 minutes. Do not exceed 0.5 mg in single dose. *Highly individualized.*
	Infusion: To raise blood pressure rapidly begin with 50-90 μgtt/minute. When blood pressure is stabilized at low normal level, a maintenance dose of 20-30 μgtt/minute usually suffices. *Highly individualized.*
Protocol:	To treat hypotension associated with paroxysmal supraventricular tachycardia; to manage drug-induced hypotension; to manage shock-like states secondary to anesthesia and hypersensitive reactions; potent long-lasting vasoconstrictor; should not be used when afterload reduction is an objective of therapy.
Precautions:	Use with caution in the elderly, and those patients with bradycardia, heart block, myocardial disease, or severe atheriosclerosis; use with caution when digitalis is being given to avoid cardiotoxic reactions; deliver with infusion pump; requires continuous monitoring of electrocardiogram, blood pressure

Phenylephrine hydrochloride diluent chart: 40 μg/60 μgtt
Titrate to increase blood pressure

$$10 \ \mu\text{gtt} = 7 \ \mu\text{g/min}$$
$$20 \ \mu\text{gtt} = 14 \ \mu\text{g/min}$$
$$30 \ \mu\text{gtt} = 20 \ \mu\text{g/min}$$
$$40 \ \mu\text{gtt} = 27 \ \mu\text{g/min}$$
$$50 \ \mu\text{gtt} = 34 \ \mu\text{g/min}$$
$$60 \ \mu\text{gtt} = 40 \ \mu\text{g/min}$$
$$70 \ \mu\text{gtt} = 47 \ \mu\text{g/min}$$
$$80 \ \mu\text{gtt} = 54 \ \mu\text{g/min}$$
$$90 \ \mu\text{gtt} = 61 \ \mu\text{g/min}$$

fuse the cerebral and coronary circulations. It is possible this agent may increase myocardial oxygen consumption; however, in the setting of life-threatening hypotension, priority dictates use of the drug to maintain viability until mechanical therapy may be instituted. (See box below.)

Chronic heart failure. Currently there are no federally approved oral sympathomimetic agents used to treat chronic heart failure. Oral beta$_1$ agonists often produce the side effects of increased heart rate, increased automaticity, and consequent elevated myocardial oxygen consumption. Furthermore, long-term use is associated with a progressive decreased drug response referred to as tachyphylaxis. These effects must be minimized in order to produce a more effective drug; hence, the efforts to develop a product that will selectively increase cardiac contractility without the side effects. Pharmacological research and clinical investigation is directed toward this goal with prenalterol being one of the agents that is currently under clinical investigation.

Prenalterol. Prenalterol is a new selective beta$_1$ agonist that is available in parenteral and oral preparations. In a study by Awan, prenalterol was found to have salutary effects on cardiac index and left ventricular ejection fraction and to considerably decrease systemic vascular resistance.[3] It did not affect heart rate, mean arterial pressure, arrhythmia production, or myocardial ischemia.

Drug:	**Norepinephrine (Levophed)** (alpha agonist—potent vasopressor)
Mixture:	4 mg/250 ml-16 μg/ml-16 μg/μgtt
Dose:	1-10 μg/minute
Protocol:	Use in severe hypotensive states refractory to beta agonists and volume infusion; continuously monitor arterial pressure or blood pressure if invasive monitoring is not available; deliver with infusion pump
Precautions:	Causes severe tissue necrosis, sloughing, and gangrene; therefore infusion should be through a large vein or central catheter; use a catheter at least 3 inches or more in length if possible; do not mix with other drugs; do not administer bolus medication through the infusion line

Norepinephrine (Levophed) diluent chart: 16 μg/μgtt
Titrate to increase blood pressure

4 μgtt =	1 μg/min	49 μgtt =	13 μg/min
8 μgtt =	2 μg/min	53 μgtt =	14 μg/min
11 μgtt =	3 μg/min	57 μgtt =	15 μg/min
15 μgtt =	4 μg/min	60 μgtt =	16 μg/min
19 μgtt =	5 μg/min	64 μgtt =	17 μg/min
23 μgtt =	6 μg/min	68 μgtt =	18 μg/min
26 μgtt =	7 μg/min	72 μgtt =	19 μg/min
30 μgtt =	8 μg/min	75 μgtt =	20 μg/min
34 μgtt =	9 μg/min	79 μgtt =	21 μg/min
38 μgtt =	10 μg/min	83 μgtt =	22 μg/min
42 μgtt =	11 μg/min	87 μgtt =	23 μg/min
45 μgtt =	12 μg/min	90 μgtt =	24 μg/min

These effects were noted in patients categorized as NYHA Class IIIs and IVs who required 0.25 mg of digoxin daily, 120 to 480 mg of furosemide daily, and/or spironolactone or triamterene daily.[3] The improvement in cardiac failure was noted for several hours after a single bolus injection intravenously. The lowered arrhythmic potential of this beta$_1$ agonist seemed to offer important advantages over other beta agonists, especially in patients with ischemic cardiac failure. The investigators concluded that further intravenous trials were required to evaluate the drug's full potential.[3] Recent results are favorable with oral trials as well.[38,54] Consequently, when further clinical trials are completed, patients with severe congestive heart failure may benefit from this inotropic agent in terms of sustained, effective ambulatory therapy.

Concurrent drug effects. Generally, dobutamine and dopamine have shown evidence of no drug interaction or altered sensitivity with major agents used to treat heart failure. These agents include furosemide, spironolactone, morphine, potassium chloride, nitroprusside, nitroglycerin, isosorbide dinitrate, hydralazine, and digitalis preparations. Isoproterenol is not recommended when digitalis-induced arrhythmias are present. Dobutamine and dopamine are not compatible with alkaline solutions and should not be mixed with products such as a 5% sodium bicarbonate solution.

Relative contraindications. Major sympathomimetics that significantly increase myocardial contractility and heart rate are contraindicated in the setting of subvalvular and valvular stenosis. Under these conditions, a marked increase in contractility generates excessive intramyocardial wall tension, increases ventricular systolic and diastolic pressure, elevates myocardial oxygen consumption, and suppresses intramyocardial blood flow. Coronary blood supply is further depressed in the setting of tachycardia as a result of decreased diastolic filling time. As a result, altered myocardial supply/demand ratio puts these patients at risk for developing myocardial ischemia, infarction, ventricular aneurysm, and rupture. Toxic effects of tachycardia and hyperdynamic contractility may be

counteracted first by stopping drug administration. Since drug metabolism is very rapid it would be unusual to have to administer a beta-blocking agent such as propranolol.

Health care implications
Assessment
1. Identify the underlying cause and the precipitating factors of heart failure by patient interview and review of documented historical data.
2. Determine by physical examination the clinical indicators and degree of acute heart failure.
3. Substantiate suspected problem areas by obtaining further diagnostic data:
   a. Baseline and current hemodynamic parameters
   b. Serum electrolytes and chemistries
   c. Cardiac enzymes
   d. Electrocardiographic studies
   e. Noninvasive cardiac studies when indicated
   f. Chest roentgenograms
4. Identify the primary goal of therapy.
5. Be familiar with each major sympathomimetic agent, actions, prescriptives for use, dose, administration, concurrent drug effects, and relative contraindications and management of toxic response.

Intervention
1. Based on the primary therapeutic objectives, select, carefully calculate dose, and administer the agent of choice as delineated by the health care role.
2. Document the dose, diluent, and route of administration.
3. Observe and record all physical changes and hemodynamic responses to therapy.
4. Communicate therapeutic goal, intervention, and response to therapy to all health care professionals prescribing, treating, and caring for the patient.
5. Explain to the patient and family the rationale for therapy, agents used, side effects, desired therapeutic response, and importance

of reporting subjective response to therapy.

6. Upon discharge, apprise patient and family that major over-the-counter decongestants, and appetite suppressants contain sympathomimetic agents that may elevate heart rate and blood pressure, adding to cardiac work.

7. Stress the need for routine professional health care supervision.

VASODILATOR AGENTS

"The principle of vasodilator therapy is exquisitely simple. If the sick heart works less then it should get better."

Robert Zelis, M.D., 1979[64]

Benefits in heart failure

The current trend in the treatment of congestive heart failure is the addition of vasodilators to the therapeutic armamentarium.[18,33] The therapeutic goal is to optimize cardiac performance by controlling and/or adjusting preload, afterload, myocardial contractility, and oxygen consumption.

The clinical picture of congestive heart failure is characterized by hemodynamic alterations of intense sympathoadrenergic mediated venous and arteriolar constriction and renal mediated neurohumoral mechanisms that result in marked systemic vascular resistance and retention of salt and water.[1,3] These compensatory alterations are activated to restore normal pump function, at the expense of elevating diastolic filling pressures and increasing afterload. This increases heart size and elevates myocardial oxygen requirements.

Definitive vasodilator therapy is predicated on altering peripheral vascular tone. Arteriolar and venous tone is a function of vascular smooth muscle control of resistance and storage in regional arterial beds. When cardiac output drops, blood flow is diverted from renal, mesenteric, integumentary beds to the cerebral and coronary circulation. As a result, the net increase in peripheral vascular resistance elevates afterload, decreases systolic function, and raises myocardial oxygen requirements. Concurrently, autonomic-mediated venoconstriction occurs. This, in turn, augments venous blood return to the heart, increases cardiac filling, and by the Frank-Starling response enhances cardiac contractility.

In the regional capillary beds, the net capillary filtration pressure rises as a result of arteriolar constriction and increased resistance to flow. This is also influenced by local venous pooling, a function of regional vascular storage. As a result intravascular fluid extravasates into the interstitium and appears clinically as pulmonary congestion and peripheral edema. This is a direct result of abnormal vascular storage related to vasoconstriction in heart failure. Thus, based on the physical and biological function of peripheral circulation, vasodilator therapy is directed toward altering preload and afterload with the ultimate goal being a marked improvement in peripheral perfusion.

Preload is a reflection of venous tone, venous capacitance, and blood volume. Patients with heart failure demonstrate intense venoconstriction and expanded blood volume as a result of inappropriate salt and water retention. This contributes substantially to pulmonary venous congestion. Since a small reduction in venous tone may result in marked redistribution of blood volume from the central to peripheral circulation, the administration of venodilating agents may be effective in relieving pulmonary congestion in heart failure. This has particular clinical value to the patient with pulmonary congestion secondary to elevated left ventricular filling pressure (preload). However, it may be contraindicated when cardiac output is depressed. In this setting, a further reduction in preload will contribute to the low-output hypotensive state and will impair myocardial perfusion. Furthermore, patients in whom preload or filling pressure has been normalized by diuretic and/or dietary restriction of sodium would not be candidates for venodilator therapy. Generally, it is initiated in normotensive acute left ventricular failure accompanied by pulmonary edema and in chronic severe heart failure refractory to digitalis and diuretic therapy.

Afterload is a measure of intramyocardial wall tension and is altered by arteriolar tone, elasticity of the large arteries, and condition of the aortic valve. In heart failure, elevated ventricular afterload is a reflection of high systemic vascular resistance and is a function of the following compensatory adjustments:[12]

1. Increased sympathetic vasoconstrictor tone
2. Elevated concentration of circulating catecholamines
3. Activation of the renin-angiotensin system with subsequent production of angiotensin II
4. Decreased elasticity of artery walls as a result of accumulation of extracellular sodium and water

In heart failure, elevated afterload represents a physiological adjustment to depressed cardiac output; however, the inappropriate vasoconstriction of the arteriolar beds may set up a positive feedback loop, leading to progressive deterioration of cardiac function. This occurs in the following manner. Elevated afterload decreases left ventricular stroke volume and increases end-systolic and end-diastolic volume, which leads to diminished cardiac output and/or pulmonary congestion.[13]

The objective of administering arteriolar dilators is to decrease the external forces opposing myocardial fiber shortening and ventricular ejection, ultimately decreasing intramyocardial wall tension and elevating stroke volume, cardiac output, and peripheral perfusion. If the net effect of afterload reduction is a significant rise in stroke volume, then blood pressure may fall only slightly or remain unchanged. This response reflects an increase in pump function.

In patients with depressed myocardial contractility and normal preload, arteriolar dilation may produce only a small increase in cardiac output and a mild drop in blood pressure, while in the patient with depressed contractility and elevated filling pressure, afterload reduction may cause a more effective ejection of volume with a subsequent drop in preload. By the Frank-Starling response, lower filling pressure will diminish contractility in the noncompliant ventricle. Therefore these individuals may benefit from combined therapy; inotropic support to enhance contractility and afterload reduction to reduce ejection impedance.

Myocardial oxygen requirements increase in proportion to activated compensatory mechanisms. Oxygen demand is a function of intramyocardial wall tension (heart size), heart rate, and contractility. The combined effects of elevated preload and afterload may alter the myocardial supply/demand ratio, eventually leading to ischemia and decreased ventricular performance. Elevated afterload increases intramyocardial wall tension, and elevated diastolic filling pressure may interfere with subendocardial blood flow. Recall that the left ventricular muscle receives its major blood supply during diastole. Increased afterload requires the ventricle to contract more forcefully, raising oxygen requirements and interfering with coronary perfusion, particularly in the setting of tachycardia. Administration of agents capable of limiting venous return (preload) and decreasing ventricular impedance (afterload) while maintaining or improving cardiac output and controlling heart rate will have the beneficial effects of reducing myocardial oxygen consumption (demand) and increasing coronary artery perfusion (supply), hence the rationale for vasodilator and inotropic therapy in heart failure.

Overview of agents

Vasodilators are widely used in the therapy of heart failure. The major indication for afterload reduction is still hypertension, for which all vasodilators have been used except nitrates, which are primarily reducers of preload, and the beta agonists, which have a direct inotropic effect.[13] Vasodilators are classified according to their principal sites of action on the peripheral vascular beds (Table 8-9). Drugs that reduce cardiac filling are classified as venous dilators, drugs that increase cardiac output are arteriolar dilators, and drugs with both effects are combined agents. Drugs currently being used for their vasodilating effects in the treatment of heart failure may be divided into the following categories:

1. Direct-acting agents: nitrates, nitroprussides, hydralazine, minoxidil, and isosorbide dinitrate

Table 8-9. Classification and therapeutic benefit of vasodilating agents in heart failure

Agent	Dominant peripheral vascular effect	Hemodynamic effect	Clinical use
Nitroglycerin	Venodilators	Decreased pulmonary and venous pressure	Preload reduction in acute left ventricular failure with marked pulmonary congestion
Isosorbide dinitrate		Little or no increase in cardiac output	Coronary artery dilation in myocardial ischemia, infarction, and angina
Hydralazine	Arteriolar dilators	Increased stroke volume and cardiac output	Afterload reduction in chronic severe heart failure accompanied by low cardiac output and refractory to conventional digitalis and potent diuretic therapy
Minoxidil			
Nifedipine		Slight decrease in systemic and pulmonary venous pressure	Useful in setting of acute myocardial infarction and heart failure
Nitroprusside	Combined venous and arteriolar dilators	Increased stroke volume and cardiac output	Preload and afterload reduction acute left ventricular failure with high pulmonary venous pressures, low cardiac output, and marked peripheral vascular resistance
Phentolamine		Decreased systemic and pulmonary venous pressures	
*Prazosin			
*Captopril			

*Agents used in chronic refractor failure with above characteristics.

2. Alpha antagonists: prazosin and phentolamine
3. Calcium channel blocker: nifedipine
4. Angiotensin-converting enzyme inhibitor: captopril
5. Narcotic analgesic: morphine

Table 8-10 summarizes the dose and the action of specific agents.

Direct-acting agents. Direct-acting agents decrease vascular tone by an undefined direct effect on the smooth muscle. Response to these agents are dose dependent, and effective therapy requires delivery of a sufficient quantity of active drug to peripheral vascular tissue.[48] (See the box on p. 278.)

Intravenous nitroprusside is the direct-acting intravenous agent of choice to reduce afterload in left ventricular failure because it acts rapidly and has a combined effect, dilating arterioles and veins. It is also indicated for management of mechanical lesions that precipitate acute volume overload. Other uses are control of dissecting aortic aneurysms and hypertensive crises associated with acute left ventricular failure.

Nitrates. Nitrates such as nitroglycerin and isosorbide dinitrate are direct-acting agents that primarily dilate coronary vessels and systemic venous beds. They are administered to patients with elevated diastolic filling pressure, pulmonary capillary wedge pressure, and clinical indicators of marked pulmonary congestion. They are less effective in the control of severe chronic heart failure than prazosine or hydralazine but may be used with these agents if patients suffer from intractable pulmonary congestion. They may be beneficial and more benign than other vasodilators in patients with active ischemia and heart failure.

Table 8-10. Pharmacological characteristics of selected vasodilator agents

Drug	Action	Half-life	Route of excretion	Dosage
Nitroglycerin	Direct effect to relax arterial and venous smooth muscle (predominant effect on venous bed with low concentrations of nitroglycerin); venodilation decreases right and left ventricular EDP; arteriolar dilation decreases afterload; redistribution of coronary blood flow to ischemic subendocardium; reduces myocardial oxygen demand	IV: 1-5 min Sublingual: 1-5 min Duration of action Sublingual: 30 min Oral: 3-4 hr Ointment: 5 hr	Hepatic	Sublingual: 0.3-0.6 mg dissolved under the tongue Oral: 1 sustained-release capsule every 2-8 hr Transderm-nitro system: 1 5 mg/24 hr OR 10 mg/24 hr. Optimal dosage based on clinical response Parenteral: See p. 279 for drip preparation and dosage administration
Isosorbide dinitrate (Isordil)	Direct relaxation of vascular smooth muscle	Onset of action Sublingual: 2-3 min Chewable: 3-4 min Oral: 20-40 min Duration of action Sublingual: 45-60 min Chewable: 3-4 hr Oral: 4-6 hr	Hepatic	Sublingual: 2.5, 5, and 10 mg tablets; 1 tablet every 2-3 hr Chewable: 10 mg tablets; ½ to 1 tablet every 2-3 hr Oral titradose: 5, 10, 20, and 30 mg tablets; 10-20 mg qid AC and HS
Sodium nitroprusside	Direct-acting dilator of arteriolar and venous smooth muscle; decreases afterload; decreases preload	2-5 min	Renal	Average adult dose: 3 μg/kg/min (about 200 μg/min), do not exceed 800 μg/min; compound decomposes in light, therefore cover IV bottle with opaque wrapping; solution must be changed every 4 hr; see Table 8-3 for drip preparation and dosage administration
Hydralazine (Apresoline)	Direct inotropic effect; direct effect to relax vascular smooth muscle; the effect is greater on arterioles than veins; decreases blood pressure and systemic vascular resistance; increases cardiac output, stroke volume, and heart rate; secondary increase in renin activity	2-8 hr (average 3 hr)	Hepatic/renal (in severe renal failure reduce dose)	Oral: Initially, 25 mg qid; increase to 50 mg qid; do not exceed 400 mg/day, take drug with meals IV: 10-20 mg slowly and repeat as necessary q 4-6 hr

Table 8-10. Pharmacological characteristics of selected vasodilator agents—cont'd

Drug	Action	Half-life	Route of excretion	Dosage
Minoxidil (Loniten)	Direct-acting dilator of vascular smooth muscle (predominantly arteriolar); reflex-mediated tachycardia; sodium and water retention	4.2 hr; (duration of action much longer)	Renal; (renal insufficiency may require smaller doses)	Oral: 5-40 mg/day
Prazosin Hydrochloride (Minipress)	Receptor-dependent alpha, blocking agent; reduces vascular tone in resistance and capacitance vessels; decreases peripheral vascular resistance without secondary reflex tachycardia or increase in Renin activity	3 hr; half-life prolonged when congestive heart failure present	Hepatic	Initial dose: oral 1-2 mg bid or tid; maintenance dose-dosage slowly increased to a total daily dose of 20 mg in divided doses
Phentolamine (Regitine)	Alpha adrenergic blocker; direct action on vascular smooth muscle[15 p. 183]	Not established	Route of metabolism not known	Oral: 50-100 mg, 4-6 times daily IV: 5 mg for hypertensive crisis continuous intravenous infusion of 0.1-0.2 mg/min
Nifedipine (Procardia)	Calcium channel blocker; direct action on smooth muscle of certain arteries producing vasodilation: (1) strong coronary vasodilating action; (2) decreases pulmonary arterial pressure; (3) decreases systemic arterial pressure Minor negative inotropic effect; decreases myocardial oxygen demand, no depressant effect on SA and AV node	2 hr (therapeutic effect is evident for up to 6 hr)[19]	Renal 75% Hepatic 20-30% Feces 15% use cautiously with impaired liver function	Oral: 10-20 mg every 6-8 hr Sublingual: Investigational dose same as oral IV: Investigational 5-15 μg/kg; (light sensitive)
Captopril (Capoten)	Receptor dependent; angiotensin-converting enzyme inhibitor; decreased angiotensin II formation; decreased aldosterone secretion; decreased peripheral vascular resistance; increased plasma renin	6 hr	Partially renal; dosage adjustment necessary in renal failure	Oral: initially 6.25-12.5 mg tid; may gradually increase over a period of weeks to a maximum dose of 150 mg tid; take 1 hour AC

Continued.

Table 8-10. Pharmacological characteristics of selected vasodilator agents—cont'd

Drug	Action	Half-life	Route of excretion	Dosage
Morphine sulfate	Central nervous system depressant; decrease level of consciousness; relief of pain; decrease respiratory drive. Venodilator; venous pooling decreases preload. Arteriolar dilator; decreased arterial resistance decreases afterload	2.5 to 3 hr	Renal	IV: 2.5 to 15 mg every 1-4 hr to treat pain related to acute MI or acute pulmonary edema

Drug: **Sodium nitroprusside (Nipride)** (Potent arteriolar dilator and venodilator)

Mixture: 50 mg/250 ml D_5W—200 μg/ml—200 μg/60 μgtt

Dose: 0.5-10 μg/kg/minute

Protocol: Monitor and document arterial pressure and hemodynamic parameters continuously until stabilized; protect solution from light; discard solution after 2 hours; do not use as an additive with any other drugs; deliver with infusion pump

Precautions: Overdose may precipitate profound hypotension; prolonged therapy may cause cyanide intoxication and requires daily blood thiocyanate levels; should not exceed 10 mg/100 ml.

Nitroprusside diluent chart: 50 mg/250 ml = 200 μg/ml = 200 μg/60 μgtt

lb	kg	.5	1	1.5	2	2.5	3	3.5	4	4.5	5	5.5	6	6.5	7	7.5	8	8.5	9	9.5	10
88	40	6	12	18	24	30	36	42	48	54	60	66	72	78	84	90	96	102	108	114	120
99	45	7	14	20	27	34	41	47	54	61	68	74	81	88	95	101	108	115	122	128	135
110	50	8	15	23	30	38	45	53	60	68	75	83	90	98	105	113	120	128	135	143	150
121	55	8	17	25	33	41	50	58	66	74	83	91	99	107	116	124	132	140	149	157	165
132	60	9	18	27	36	45	54	63	72	81	90	99	108	117	126	135	144	153	162	171	180
143	65	10	20	29	39	49	59	68	78	88	98	107	117	127	137	146	156	166	176	185	195
154	70	11	21	32	42	53	63	74	84	95	105	116	126	137	147	158	168	179	189	200	210
165	75	11	23	34	45	56	68	79	90	101	113	124	135	146	158	169	180	191	203	214	225
176	80	12	24	36	48	60	72	84	96	108	120	132	144	156	168	180	192	204	216	228	240
187	85	13	26	38	51	64	77	89	102	115	128	140	153	166	179	191	204	217	230	242	255
198	90	14	27	41	54	68	81	95	108	122	135	149	162	176	189	203	216	230	243	257	270
209	95	14	29	43	57	71	86	100	114	128	143	157	171	185	200	214	228	242	257	271	285
220	100	15	30	45	60	75	90	105	120	135	150	165	180	195	210	225	240	255	270	285	300
242	110	17	33	50	66	83	99	116	132	149	165	182	198	215	231	248	264	281	297	314	330

Weight (lb, kg); Dosage: μg/kg/minute

μgtt/minute

Drug: **Nitroglycerin infusion** (Potent venodilator)

Mixture: Tridil ampule = 50 mg IV nitroglycerin. Use glass bottle and special IV tubing

50 mg/250 ml D_5W—200 μg/ml—200 μg/60 μgtt

Dose: Start infusion at 5 μg/minute and titrate in 5 μg increments with increases every 5 minutes until a fall in systemic or left ventricular filling pressure or relief of chest pain or resolution of ischemic ECG changes occur.

Protocol: Monitor blood pressure closely; if available, use hemodynamic data to determine preload status, cardiac index, and peripheral vascular resistance; deliver with infusion pump.

Precaution: May cause severe hypotension if administered to individuals who are hypovolemic.

Nitroglycerin infusion diluent chart: 200 μg/60 μgtt

2 μgtt = 5 μg/min	33 μgtt = 110 μg/min
3 μgtt = 10 μg/min	36 μgtt = 120 μg/min
5 μgtt = 15 μg/min	39 μgtt = 130 μg/min
6 μgtt = 20 μg/min	42 μgtt = 140 μg/min
9 μgtt = 30 μg/min	45 μgtt = 150 μg/min
12 μgtt = 40 μg/min	48 μgtt = 160 μg/min
15 μgtt = 50 μg/min	51 μgtt = 170 μg/min
18 μgtt = 60 μg/min	54 μgtt = 180 μg/min
21 μgtt = 70 μg/min	57 μgtt = 190 μg/min
24 μgtt = 80 μg/min	60 μgtt = 200 μg/min
27 μgtt = 90 μg/min	72 μgtt = 240 μg/min
30 μgtt = 100 μg/min	96 μgtt = 320 μg/min

Nitroglycerin. (See the box above.) Nitroglycerin is the most widely used nitrate in the setting of coronary artery insufficiency and angina. For short-term action, it is administered sublingually and is used topically and transdermally for prolonged hemodynamic effects. For the treatment of acute heart failure, it may be given intravenously at an initial dose of 5 to 10 μg/minute. This may be increased to achieve the desired hemodynamic response. Intravenous nitroglycerin appears to have potent dilating effects on the venous bed and marked reduction in right atrial and pulmonary capillary pressure. It does not directly affect stroke volume and cardiac output; however, it has the potential to suddenly reduce venous return, resulting in acute hypotension.[4] In chronic heart failure, transdermal nitroglycerin may be used to achieve prolonged preload reduction and relief of coronary artery spasm.[23]

Isosorbide dinitrate. Isosorbide dinitrate is a long-acting oral nitrate used to relieve coronary artery spasm and to effect mild peripheral venodilating effects. It may be used in left ventricular failure accompanied by pulmonary congestion, especially when preload reduction and coronary vasodilation are needed. However, in large doses it may cause flushing, headaches, and tachycardia. On occasion, individuals exhibit hypotensive episodes characterized by nausea, vomiting, diaphoresis, dizziness, and syncope. These side effects may be precipitated by alcohol ingestion and may predispose to myocardial ischemia and infarction.

Hydralazine. Hydralazine has dual effects. It is principally an arteriolar dilator and probably has some small direct inotropic effect. In normal subjects, it causes reflex tachycardia as a result of vasodilation, but in heart failure it does not usually significantly affect heart rate. In chronic severe heart failure, a hydralazine-nitrate combination may work well for most patients, with more emphasis on the nitrate if the predominant symptoms are pulmonary congestion and more emphasis on hydralazine if low-output symptoms, such as weakness and oliguria, predominate.[18]

Minoxidil. Minoxidil is also a direct-acting oral arteriolar dilator, but it has potent side effects that limit its use in chronic heart failure. It may precipitate tachycardia and predispose to sodium and water retention. For this reason, it is often administered with beta blockers to control heart rate and diuretics to control fluid retention. It is most frequently used for control of hypertension.[11]

Alpha-adrenergic blocking agents. Alpha-adrenergic blocking agents bind selectively to alpha-adrenergic receptors and interfere with the capacity of sympathomimetic amines to initiate activity at these sites.[15] There are two types of alpha receptors, the presynaptic alpha$_2$ receptors and the postsynaptic alpha$_1$ vascular receptors. Prolonged alpha blockade can lead to tolerance, which may limit the use of these agents in chronic heart failure.

Prazosin. Prazosin exerts combined effects, dilating both peripheral arterioles and veins. It may decrease blood pressure and increase cardiac output. Recent studies have indicated tolerance with the use of prazosin as an oral unloading agent in severe chronic heart failure.[24]

Phentolamine. Phentolamine has a nonspecific vasodilator effect. Although it is primarily an alpha-blocking agent, it may also activate release of norepinephrine. This may account for its inotropic and chronotropic effects. It has been used as an intravenous arteriolar vasodilator in low-output left ventricular failure; however, because large doses are required to sustain vasodilation and because of its tendency to elevate heart rate, it is not considered a major unloading agent in acute left ventricular failure.

Calcium channel blockers. Calcium channel blockers have vasodilator properties that may be important in reducing afterload in heart failure. Furthermore, they also relieve coronary vasospasm, which may extend their use in heart failure secondary to acute myocardial infarction and coronary artery insufficiency.

Nifedipine. Nifedipine is a calcium channel blocker that is indicated in the treatment of ischemic heart disease secondary to coronary artery spasm and characterized by exertional angina.[41] It decreases peripheral resistance and afterload and increases myocardial blood flow by reducing coronary resistance.[37] The drug may be used in combination with nitrates and propranolol to provide a more beneficial effect in relieving angina. Furthermore, nifedipine may have a more therapeutic benefit than verapamil in patients with ischemic heart disease who have concurrent conduction system disease. This is because nifedipine does not lengthen the AV nodal refractory period.[5] The use of this agent as a primary afterload reducer in acute and chronic heart failure requires further clinical trials.

Angiotensin-converting enzyme inhibitors. Angiotensin-converting enzyme inhibitors block conversion of inactive angiotensin I to the potent vasoconstrictor, angiotensin II. This enzyme is also responsible for degradation of the vasodilator bradykinin. Angiotensin converting enzyme inhibitor produces the following changes:
1. Decreased production of angiotensin II
2. Decreased aldosterone secretion
3. Decreased renal-mediated vasoconstriction
4. Increased renin production

Hemodynamic response to these agents may vary directly with the degree of plasma renin activity.

Captopril. Captopril is a relatively new drug in this classification. It is indicated for treatment of hypertensive patients who have failed to respond to conventional drug therapy or who have developed unacceptable side effects. It is most effective when plasma renin is high, as in hypertension secondary to renal artery stenosis. Captopril has also improved cardiac function in patients with chronic refractory heart failure, suggesting it may be a useful therapeutic adjunct in this setting.[26] It has recently been approved as the first vasodilator for adjunctive treatment of chronic heart failure. This judgment was based on a substantial body of favorable subjective and objective evidence. Currently it is gaining popularity as an agent to manage chronic severe heart failure.

Narcotic analgesic agents. Narcotic analgesic agents, specifically morphine, are well recognized therapeutic agents used to treat acute heart failure.

Morphine. Morphine's effect on the circulation appears to be a result of its interaction with opiate receptors in the central nervous system.[65] Opiates decrease the firing of specific receptors in the nucleus ceruleus, probably by blocking neuronal release of norepinephrine.[65] This results in a withdrawal of neurogenic sympathetic vasomotor tone, leading to peripheral vasodilation. In patients with heart failure, the venodilator effect of morphine contributes to the fall in pulmonary capillary wedge pressure. Low doses of morphine used in the treatment of pulmonary edema produce arteriolar dilation, which reduces afterload, resulting in improved cardiac output. Morphine's ability to decrease anxiety also diminishes sympathetic stimulation and its deleterious effects on cardiocirculatory function.

Prescriptives for use

Acute heart failure. Vasodilator therapy in acute heart failure has become an accepted mode of treatment and is administered by intravenous infusion for rapid delivery and meticulous control of dosage. Bedside hemodynamic monitoring of cardiac output, ventricular filling pressure, pulmonary and systemic pressure, and resistance are required to most accurately assess response to therapy. The selected agent, dose, duration, and use of concurrent inotropic and diuretic therapy is determined by underlying cause and precipitating factors of cardiac decompensation.

Acute myocardial infarction. Acute myocardial infarction is the most common cause of acute left ventricular failure. Regional loss of contractile ac-

tivity reduces stroke volume and elevates left ventricular end-diastolic volume and pressure. Clinical indicators usually reflect the hemodynamic abnormalities. The patient may exhibit mild dyspnea, orthopnea, a left ventricular gallop, basilar rales, weakness, and fatigue. The lungs and heart sounds may be normal on occasion, even when filling pressure is markedly elevated. Conversely, if the individual sustained an acute loss of 40% or more of left ventricular muscle, cardiogenic shock generally results.

Therapeutic interventions are directed toward relieving pulmonary congestion by reducing pulmonary capillary pressure and left ventricular filling pressure, correcting peripheral hypoperfusion by increasing cardiac output, and accomplishing these objectives without further increasing the disparity between myocardial oxygen supply and demand.[28] (See Fig. 8-3.) Nitroprusside is the agent of choice when the patient demonstrates low cardiac output associated with elevated left ventricular filling pressure, high peripheral vascular resistance, and normal or elevated blood pressure. This drug dilates the arterioles, lowers vascular resistance, and reduces impedance to ejection, thereby improving cardiac output and lowering myocardial oxygen requirements. Arterial pressure may fall slightly, but it is offset by increased cardiac output.

To preserve the myocardium in the ischemic setting, it is vital to maintain mean arterial pressure at 80 to 100 mm Hg. If the use of nitroprusside cannot significantly reduce filling pressure without causing a marked decrease in arterial pressure, it is necessary to introduce an inotropic agent such as dopamine or dobutamine.

If cardiac output is only minimally decreased and if it is accompanied by elevated left ventricular filling pressure and normal or only slightly elevated systemic vascular resistance, a preload reducer such as intravenous nitroglycerin may be cautiously administered. This agent produces a reduction in filling pressure and relief of pulmonary congestion. However, it also must be closely monitored for its indirect effects on arterial pressure. This may occur as a result of elevated ven-

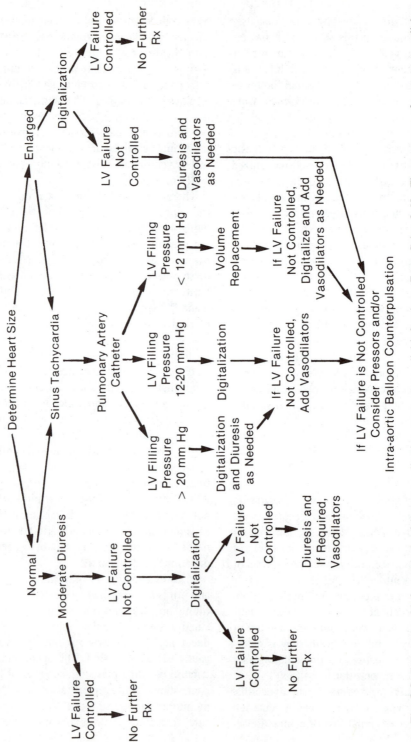

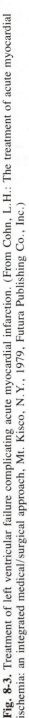

Fig. 8-3. Treatment of left ventricular failure complicating acute myocardial ischemia: an integrated medical/surgical approach, Mt. Kisco, N.Y., 1979, Futura Publishing Co., Inc.)

tricular compliance (a function of the ischemic myocardium), which requires higher filling pressure to effect adequate contractility. If preload is markedly reduced by the venodilating effects of nitroglycerin, hypotension will result, causing reduced coronary perfusion and increased myocardial ischemia. Infusion of volume may be necessary to offset pronounced reduction of preload.[30]

Morphine is also used in the setting of acute heart failure secondary to myocardial infarction. It is administered as an analgesic, but it also has arterial and venous dilating effects that may improve hemodynamics. Again, careful monitoring of circulatory parameters is essential to document drug action. Rapid intravenous administration of morphine may potentiate the dilator effects of nitroprusside and nitroglycerin, resulting in hypotension.

Acute pulmonary edema. Acute pulmonary edema is an emergency that commonly attends acute left ventricular failure. Left ventricular end-diastolic pressure is strikingly increased, leading to a rise in pulmonary capillary wedge pressure, which precipitates fluid extravasation into lung tissue. The resultant hypoxemia and respiratory failure is life-threatening. (For pathophysiology see Chapter 2, p. 79.) The major therapeutic objective is prompt reduction of left ventricular filling pressure and reduction in pulmonary capillary wedge pressure. This is accomplished by administration of rapid-acting diuretics, morphine, and occasionally the use of phlebotomy and rotating tourniquets. These interventions are effective in reducing pulmonary congestion but do little to improve left ventricular function. Furthermore, by the Frank-Starling response, as preload falls contractility may be reduced. In patients whose cardiac output was low to begin with, a further reduction may activate the sympathoadrenergic system, elevating systemic vascular resistance and afterload. Such a response increases the work of the heart and may precipitate cardiogenic shock.

Vasodilators play an important role in preventing this complication. Nitroprusside can reduce pulmonary and ventricular pressures and increase cardiac output, promptly relieving symptoms of acute pulmonary edema. Because the onset of action is immediate, it rapidly reduces systemic vascular resistance. It may be used alone, but it is generally part of a therapeutic regimen that includes rapid-acting diuretics, morphine, and inotropic agents. In patients with left ventricular failure and pulmonary edema secondary to hypertensive crises, nitroprusside is clearly the drug of choice.

The duration of treatment is dictated by clinical and hemodynamic parameters. However, in the setting of pulmonary edema where hypoxemia is a complicating factor, P_{O_2} may fall slightly during nitroprusside therapy as a result of pulmonary shunting. This fall of P_{O_2} should not exceed 10 mm Hg. If this becomes a problem, further assessment of respiratory function and consideration of alternative therapy becomes necessary.

Mechanical lesions. Mechanical lesions of the heart may place a sudden burden on ventricular performance and precipitate acute heart failure. Examples of such lesions are acute mitral insufficiency (from myocardial infarction, ruptured chordae, or infective endocarditis), acute ventricular septal defect (from myocardial infarction), and acute aortic insufficiency (from aortic dissection, infective endocarditis, or chest trauma). The abrupt volume overload results in pulmonary congestion and reduced cardiac output. Reduction of impedance to left ventricular ejection by nitroprusside not only increases the forward stroke volume, but it also reduces the regurgitant volume and the degree of shunting.[24] These mechanisms work to relieve pulmonary congestion and stabilize hemodynamics until surgical treatment can be instituted.

Acute therapy for refractory heart failure. Acute therapy for refractory heart failure is required when patients with chronic severe heart failure are no longer responsive to digitalis and diuretic therapy. These individuals are admitted to critical care units with severe low-output congestive heart failure. They exhibit high pulmonary and left ventricular filling pressures, borderline blood pressure, and low cardiac output. The major clinical indicators include dyspnea, oliguria, weakness, fatigue, and marked peripheral vasoconstriction. In this setting, use of a nitroprusside infusion is effective in reducing systemic vascular resistance and in improving left ventricular function. It is usually administered with an inotropic agent, such as dobutamine, and may be required for an extended period while diuretic and digitalis dosages are adjusted. Frequently, institution of oral vasodilators is required to maintain cardiac function at a level where the patient will again become *relatively* compensated and symptom free.

Postoperative pump failure. Postoperative pump failure and low-output state are serious surgical sequelae. With marked depression of left ventricular function characterized by a cardiac index of 1.5 and 1 L/minute/M^2, mortality may be as high as 40%.[15] Vasodilator therapy may be indicated. Nitroprusside is the agent most frequently used and is generally administered with dobutamine to support contractility. Combined vasodilator and inotropic therapy may also be accompanied by mechanical support such as aortic counterpulsation and left ventricular assist devices. See Chapters 10 and 14 for more detailed information.

Chronic heart failure. Chronic heart failure that does not respond to conventional therapy with digitalis and diuretics is a major clinical problem. It results most commonly from ischemic, valvular, cardiomyopathic, and hypertensive heart disease. Ventricular hypertrophy and dilation are characteristic compensatory mechanisms that alter the myocardial oxygen supply/demand ratio and interfere with intrinsic contractility.

In most patients with severe chronic heart failure, the addition of oral vasodilator agents to the therapeutic regime is indicated if clinical indicators persist, despite adequate digitalization, use of potent diuretics, dietary salt and water restriction, limited physical activity, and correction of underlying causes and precipitating factors of failure. Selection of the appropriate drug is based on clinical symptoms, desired hemodynamic effects, consideration that drug benefits will outweigh potential side effects, and a dosing schedule that will optimize patient compliance.

Nonparenteral forms of nitroglycerin and ni-

trates are widely used in chronic heart failure and in underlying ischemic heart disease. They effectively reduce pulmonary and systemic venous pressure and are useful in relieving pulmonary and systemic congestion. However, they do not significantly elevate cardiac output. Sublingual nitroglycerin has a short duration of action (20 to 30 minutes), which limits its clinical value in chronic heart failure. Topical agents have a longer action of 3 to 5 hours, and they may be useful at night to control episodes of paroxysmal nocturnal dyspnea.[21] Patients with severe ischemic disease may benefit by combining nitrate therapy with a beta blocker or calcium channel blocker to relax smooth muscle and to improve coronary artery perfusion.

Isosorbide dinitrate, a long-acting nitrate, has a similar hemodynamic effect to nitroglycerin; therefore it is used to reduce pulmonary and systemic venous pressure. This agent may be administered sublingually, orally, or in a chewable form, depending on the desired onset and duration of action (see Table 8-11). The side effects of all nitrates include headaches and hypotension, but these are more prominent in patients with mild rather than severe heart failure. Methemoglobinemia is an extremely rare complication that may appear with protracted use of large doses.

Hydralazine is an agent used in severe chronic heart failure characterized by low cardiac output. It is an orally effective potent arteriolar dilator. Oral hydralazine administered in doses of 200 to 400 mg/day produces a significant increase in cardiac output along with a decrease in systemic vascular resistance.[14,15] Furthermore, this agent does not raise heart rate in patients with heart failure.

Prazosin has hemodynamic effects similar to hydralazine and has been studied recently for its unloading effects in chronic severe heart failure. It reduces pulmonary and systemic congestion and raises cardiac output. However, there is evidence that tolerance develops with long-term use.[24]

Currently, there is no single vasodilator agent available that will satisfactorily alter all hemodynamic parameters in chronic severe heart failure. Therefore it is necessary to selectively identify the major therapeutic objectives and administer several agents to satisfy them. Combination therapy with nitrates and hydralazine is being used to reduce congestion and augment cardiac output. Nitrates can be administered at intervals of up to 4 hours, and hydralazine may be given every 6 to 8 hours.[15] Combining these drugs results in hemodynamic effects similar to nitroprusside. Therefore it may be possible to adjust oral vasodilator therapy to relieve pulmonary congestion, elevate cardiac output, or both. Further clinical trials of long-term effects of combined therapy are necessary to establish definitive therapeutic benefit.

Relative contraindications

Use of vasodilators in ischemic heart disease may be effective in decreasing ventricular work, but caution must be exercised to avoid hypotensive episodes. This side effect may impair coronary artery perfusion, worsen myocardial ischemia, and extend infarction.

Vasodilators are generally not indicated to manage stenotic valve lesions, such as mitral and aortic stenosis. The major hemodynamic problem in mitral stenosis is a filling disorder of the left ventricle, producing elevated left atrial and pulmonary venous pressures. Generally, it does not reduce left ventricular function (see Chapter 3, p. 103). Afterload reduction has little effect on left ventricular contractility or on the degree of valvular obstruction.

Aortic stenosis also produces a mechanical filling disorder but, as a result of hypertrophy, left ventricular function is usually impaired. If severe obstruction exists at the valvular level, vasodilators would have limited benefit since they do not affect this site. However, in mild to moderate aortic stenosis that is accompanied by depressed left ventricular function, it is possible that afterload reduction may augment cardiac output. This therapy has a high risk of reducing coronary perfusion because of vasodilator-induced hypotension. For this reason, it is generally contraindicated except when severe left ventricular dysfunction is suspected and hemodynamic monitoring is available.[18]

The clinical benefit of vasodilator therapy in right ventricular failure secondary to pulmonary hypertension, as seen in patients with chronic obstructive pulmonary disease and primary pulmonary hypertension, is marginal. Reduction of right ventricular outflow resistance by lowering pulmonary capillary and left ventricular filling pressure may theoretically reduce pulmonary hypertension. However, vasodilators have a greater effect on systemic rather than pulmonary vascular beds, and to effect the desired results requires high doses. In this setting, hypotension becomes the limiting factor.

Therapeutic guidelines

Care of the patient during oral vasodilator therapy requires astute clinical monitoring and physical assessment since centrally placed catheters for cardiovascular measurement are not maintained in an ambulatory setting. Hypotension is the most limiting hemodynamic effect; therefore close monitoring of blood pressure is essential. To document this, it may be necessary to instruct the patient or family members to do this at home when hypotensive symptoms occur. Decreased exercise tolerance, complaints of fatigue, or shortness of breath may indicate progressive heart failure and the need to adjust drug dosage. Therapeutic guidelines for the outpatient's use of oral vasodilator therapy in severe chronic heart failure include[13]:

1. Vasodilators should not be used if systolic blood pressure is below 90 mm Hg when inotropic agents are first given.
2. Vasodilator therapy in congestive heart failure should not reduce the systolic pressure by more than 5 to 10 mm Hg.
3. Excessive preload reduction must be avoided to prevent hypotension and a consequent drop in myocardial, renal, and cerebral perfusion.

Health care implications
Assessment
1. Establish major clinical indicators of heart failure.

2. Identify underlying causes and precipitating factors in heart failure.
3. Measure all available hemodynamic parameters and correlate with baseline data and clinical indicators.
4. Obtain detailed drug history to determine current therapeutic agents and dosage being used.
5. Establish and set priorities for major therapeutic goals with the entire health care team:
   a. Optimize myocardial supply/demand ratio.
   b. Reduce systemic and pulmonary pressures.
   c. Alleviate systemic and pulmonary congestion.
   d. Augment cardiac output.
   e. Increase peripheral perfusion.
6. Identify the setting in which these goals are to be achieved:
   a. Acute left ventricular failure
      1. With/without pulmonary venous congestion
      2. With/without systemic venous congestion
      3. With/without depressed cardiac output
      4. With/without hypotension
      5. With/without myocardial infarction
      6. With/without mechanical lesions
   b. Chronic severe heart failure
      1. With/without pulmonary venous congestion
      2. With/without systemic venous congestion
      3. With/without depressed cardiac output
      4. With/without hypotension
      5. With/without myocardial infarction
      6. With/without mechanical lesions

Interventions

1. Carefully monitor and document hemodynamic parameters.
2. Continuously assess clinical status.
3. Administer selected vasodilator agents based on the clinical setting and therapeutic goals.
4. Observe for indications of hypotension.
5. Inform patient of therapeutic goals, rationale for drug use, dosage, frequency, and route of administration.
6. Adjust the dose, frequency, and route of administration to optimize compliance and therapeutic benefit.
7. Inform the patient of possible side effects of specific vasodilator agents:
   a. Headache
   b. Dizziness
   c. Muscle weakness
   d. Postural hypotension
8. Advise the patient regarding storage and potency of nitrates such as nitroglycerin.
9. Educate the patient and family to recognize the positive and negative responses to vasodilator therapy:
   a. Positive (increased cardiac reserve)
      1. Decreased dyspnea
      2. Decreased fatigue and weakness
      3. Increased exercise tolerance
      4. Decreased nocturia
      5. Moderate diuresis
   b. Negative (decreased cardiac output and hypotension)
      1. Increased dyspnea
      2. Nocturnal dyspnea
      3. Insomnia
      4. Dizziness
      5. Syncope
      6. Marked weakness and fatigue
      7. Marked decrease in exercise tolerance
      8. Postural hypotension
10. Educate the patient who has severe heart failure and who is receiving vasodilator therapy to avoid conditions that may aggravate a delicately balanced cardiovascular function:
    a. Excessive temperatures
    b. Emotional distress
    c. Excessive or increased exercise

d. Noncompliance to drug therapy
e. Smoking
f. Heavy meals
g. Excessive caffeine
h. Excessive alcohol

DIURETIC AGENTS

The kidney contributes significantly to the pathogenesis and clinical presentation of heart failure. Renal conservation of sodium causes dependent peripheral edema and pulmonary congestion as well as elevated ventricular filling pressures and cardiac dilation. Thus renal compensatory mechanisms will ultimately increase cardiac work and worsen heart failure.

Diuretic therapy is required to effectively manage most patients with heart failure. It is administered to reduce the effects of inappropriate renal conservation of sodium and water (see Chapter 2, p. 65). At the onset of heart failure the kidney responds to depressed renal perfusion by enhanced proximal tubular reabsorption of sodium. The consequent expansion of blood volume may be sufficient to restore normal cardiac output; however, if ventricular function and effective arterial blood volume remain low, the renin-angiotensin-aldosterone axis is activated, which, by hemodynamic and humoral mechanisms, promotes both proximal and distal tubular reabsorption of sodium and elevates peripheral vascular resistance. This results in inappropriate fluid retention, further contributing to hemodynamic overload and precipitating severe refractory heart failure. At this stage, renal circulation is compromised to the point where glomerular filtration rate and filtration fraction drop, prerenal azotemia develops, and renal failure results.

Benefit in heart failure

Diuretic agents are administered to patients in heart failure to achieve the following therapeutic objectives:

1. Enhanced renal excretion of sodium and water
2. Decreased preload
3. Reduced blood volume

4. Lower ventricular filling pressures
5. Resolution of systemic and pulmonary congestion

However, they must be used with caution to prevent the following harmful effects. First, diuretics produce mild to severe electrolyte depletion, including potassium loss, which produces weakness and precipitates cardiac arrhythmias. Second, selected agents may produce vigorous diureses, resulting in hypovolemia and hypotension severely jeopardizing cardiac function. Third, drugs that act at different sites on the nephron or at the same site by different mechanisms have additive effects; and fourth, the action of one diuretic may counteract the effect of another. To maximize the effectiveness and minimize complications, clinicians must carefully assess patients for circulatory status, select and administer the most effective agent, closely monitor diuresis, and recognize and alleviate major complicating factors.

Overview of agents (Tables 8-11 and 8-12)

Diuretic agents commonly used in heart failure may be divided into the following groups: thiazide and thiazide-type agents, loop diuretics, potassium-sparing drugs, carbonic anhydrase inhibitors, and osmotic compounds. The diuretic properties are related to drug action at sites on the nephron (Fig. 8-4).

Thiazide diuretics. Thiazide diuretics act by inhibiting sodium reabsorption at the ascending loop of Henle and distal convoluted tubule, producing an increase in urinary excretion of sodium, potassium, chloride, and water. These agents are absorbed from the gastrointestinal tract and produce diuresis within 2 hours following oral administration. Peak effect may occur in 3 to 6 hours, depending on the agent (see Table 8-12). For this reason, they have replaced mercurial compounds as the oral diuretic of choice in both heart failure and essential hypertension.

By virtue of their ability to rapidly excrete sodium and water, they are the diuretics of choice in right ventricular heart failure characterized by peripheral edema and in mild to moderate left ven-

Table 8-11. Pharmacological characteristics of selected diuretic agents

Generic name	Trade name	Usual dosage and administration	Onset of effect	Peak effect	Duration
Chlorothiazide	Diuril	500-1000 mg OD 500 mg IV, OD	1 hr 15 min	4 hr 30 min	6-12 hr 2 hr
Hydrochlorothiazide	Hydro-diuril	50-100 mg OD	2 hr	4 hr	12 hr or more
Chlorthalidone	Hygroton	100 mg OD	2 hr	6 hr	24 hr or more
Metolazone	Zaroxolyn	5-10 mg OD	1 hr	2-4 hr	24-48 hr
Acetazolamide	Diamox	250-375 mg OD 250-375 mg IV OD	1 hr 2 min	2-4 hr 15 min	8 hr 4-5 hr
Spironolactone	Aldactone	25 mg 4 times/day	24-48 hours	3-5 days after start of therapy	Up to 14 days after cessation of therapy
Triamterene	Dyrenium	100-300 mg OD	2 hr	6-8 hr	12-16 hr
Amiloride	Midamor	5-10 mg OD	2 hr	6-10 hr	24 hr
Furosemide	Lasix	40-120 mg OD, PO, or IV	PO:1 hr IV:5 min	PO:1-2 hr IV:30 min	PO:6 hr IV:2 hr
Ethacrynic acid	Edecrin	50-100 mg OD, PO, or IV	PO:30 min IV:15 min	PO:2 hr IV:45 min	PO:6-8 hr IV:3 hr
Mannitol	Osmitrol	5-10-20-25% concentration prn IV infusion	1-3 hr	Duration of the diuresis	Dependent on medullary tonicity

Table 8-12. Electrolyte and acid-base disturbances with diuretic agents

Classification and generic name	Brand name	Hypo-natremia ($\downarrow$Na)	Hypo-kalemia ($\downarrow$K$^+$)	Metabolic alkalosis ($\uparrow$pH)	Hyper-kalemia ($\uparrow$K$^+$)	Metabolic acidosis ($\downarrow$pH)	Hyper-uricemia
THIAZIDES: THIAZIDE TYPES		+	+	+	–	–	+
Chlorothiazide	Diuril			(does not inhibit effectiveness of these agents)			
Hydrochlorothiazide	Hydro-diuril						
Chlorthalidone	Hygroton						
Metolazone	Zaroxolyn						
CARBONIC ANHYDRASE INHIBITOR		+	+	–	–	+	Unknown
Acetazolamide	Diamox					(inhibits effectiveness of this agent)	
POTASSIUM-SPARING COMPOUNDS		+	–	–	+		–
Spironolactone	Aldactone					–	
Triamterene	Dyrenium					+	
Amiloride	Midamor					+	

+ indicates it is a side effect of agent.

– indicates it is *not* a side effect of agent.

Table 8-12. Electrolyte and acid-base disturbances with diuretic agents—cont'd

Classification and generic name	Brand name	Hypo-natremia ($\downarrow$Na)	Hypo-kalemia ($\downarrow$K$^+$)	Metabolic alkalosis ($\uparrow$pH)	Hyper-kalemia ($\uparrow$K$^+$)	Metabolic acidosis ($\downarrow$pH)	Hyper-uricemia
RAPID-ACTING POTENT LOOP AGENTS		+	+	+	−	−	+
Furosemide	Lasix			(does not inhibit effectiveness of these agents)			
Ethacrynic acid	Edecrin						
OSMOTIC AGENT		+	+	+ (volume contraction)	−	−	−
Mannitol	Osmitrol						

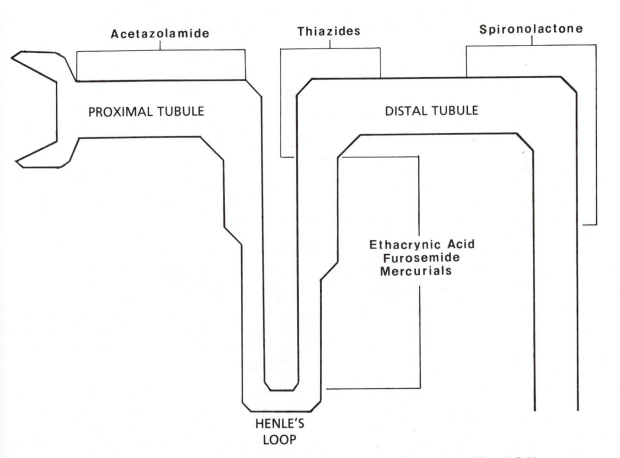

Fig. 8-4. Major sites of action of commonly used diuretics. (Adapted from Augus, Z., and Goldberg, M.: Renal functions in congestive heart failure. In Levine, H.J., editor: Clinical cardiovascular physiology, New York, 1976, Grune & Stratton, Inc., p. 428.)

tricular heart failure. Thiazides are less effective in patients with glomerular filtration rates below 30 ml/minute, which may explain their refractoriness in severe heart failure.[10]

The major complications result primarily from potassium loss. In the setting of heart failure, when patients are receiving digitalis, hypokalemia may induce a cardiotoxic response. Therefore these individuals should be monitored closely for abnormal serum electrolyte concentrations and should be advised to eat potassium-containing foods such as orange juice or bananas. If this is not sufficient, then supplementation with oral potassium chloride is required. It must be noted that potassium supplements or aldosterone antagonists should not be given to patients with impaired renal function. Furthermore, if potassium-sparing compounds such as spironolactone are being used with thiazides, potassium supplements should be discontinued to avoid hyperkalemia.[56]

Loop diuretics. Loop diuretics are potent, rapid-acting agents, so called because they exert their action on the ascending loop of Henle. The most widely used agents are furosemide and ethacrynic acid. Although these drugs are structurally dissimilar, they have similar functional characteristics. They are more potent than thiazides, with the potential of increasing fractional sodium excretion by more than 20% to 25%. Both agents have a rapid onset and a short duration of action and may be administered orally and intravenously. Intravenous administration causes diuresis within 5 minutes, with a peak response occurring at 15 to 20 minutes and a duration of action of less than 3 hours. For this reason, these agents are used to reduce preload and filling pressure in acute left ventricular failure characterized by cardiogenic pulmonary edema.

Furosemide is a particularly versatile agent. When administered intravenously, it exhibits systemic and renal vasodilating effects, resulting in decreased peripheral vascular resistance and in increased renal blood flow. Furthermore, in severe renal dysfunction it can convert to liver metabolism and excretion, which makes it quite useful

when renal failure accompanies heart failure.[36] This agent is also administered orally with thiazides to control fluid retention in patients with chronic severe heart failure; however, like thiazides, it is a sulfonamide derivative and is not recommended for use in individuals allergic to sulfa.

Because loop diuretics exhibit their major effect by inhibiting active transport of chloride in the ascending loop, they can cause marked potassium depletion, alkalosis secondary to hydrogen and chloride loss, and, most importantly, severe hypovolemia. This requires close monitoring for diuretic effect, serum electrolyte concentrations, acid-base balance, and hypotension. Most patients with normal renal function receiving thiazides and loop diuretic agents are required to take potassium chloride supplements.

Sulfamyl diuretics. Sulfamyl diuretics include metolazone (Zaroxolyn). The action of metolazone results in an interference with the renal tubular mechanism of electrolyte absorption. This agent acts primarily to inhibit sodium at the cortical diluting site and in the proximal convoluted tubule. Sodium and chloride are excreted in approximately equivalent amounts. The increased delivery of sodium to the distal tubular exchange site may account for the increase in potassium excretion. The mechanism of this entire action is unknown.

Generally metolazone has achieved modest use in the setting of chronic severe congestive heart failure based largely on its synergistic action with the loop diuretics, in particular furosemide.[4a] Patients who develop furosemide-resistant cardiac edema often achieve an effective diuresis after administration of a furosemide-metolazone combination. However, both agents precipitate marked electrolyte loss. Consequently, it is recommended that individuals initially receiving this treatment be hospitalized for close monitoring of electrolyte loss in order to safely establish proper dosage regimens and concurrent electrolyte replacement.

Dosage should be individualized according to each patient's response. Metolazone has a longer duration than furosemide, from 12 to 24 hours. For those individuals in severe chronic heart failure who experience a sudden weight gain, 2.5 to 5.0 mg of metolazone may be administered daily as an adjunct to furosemide until the desired fluid loss has been achieved. This drug combination acts as a potent saluretic and kaluretic that limits its long-term use for chronic severe heart failure.

Potassium-sparing compounds. Potassium-sparing compounds are distal tubule diuretics. Triamterene acts directly to depress renal tubular transport of sodium, while spironolactone antagonizes the effect of aldosterone by competitively binding to protein that permits potassium secretion at the distal tubule.[36] Generally, these agents are more effective when combined with other diuretics. Spironolactone must be converted into its active metabolite in the liver and has a long onset of action of 24 to 48 hours with a peak effect of up to 3 to 5 days. These factors severely limit its effectiveness in acute congestive heart failure.

Triamterene is not an aldosterone antagonist. It is rapidly absorbed and metabolized in the liver and excreted in the kidneys, producing a diuresis in 2 to 4 hours with a maximal duration of 12 to 16 hours. Although it is more potent than spironolactone, as a single agent it is a mild diuretic. Both triamterene and spironolactone inhibit the exchange of potassium, not only for sodium but also for hydrogen, and may induce metabolic acidosis as well as hyperkalemia. These drugs are not agents of choice for patients with concomitant heart failure and renal dysfunction, but they are most effective in those with marked secondary aldosteronism.[56]

Carbonic anhydrase inhibitors. Carbonic anhydrase inhibitors are diuretics acting in the proximal tubule. Acetazolamide is a potent inhibitor of carbonic anhydrase, the enzyme responsible for hydrogen ion secretion. It also inhibits proximal tubular reabsorption of sodium and chloride. Generally, this agent is able to effect only a 3% to 4% increase in fractional sodium excretion. This results because of the ability of the more distal sites on the nephron to reabsorb a large portion of the proximally rejected sodium. These agents promote

potassium loss and are inactivated in the presence of acidosis. In heart failure, they have a limited effect. They can be used to potentiate the action of the more distally acting diuretics and in the treatment of hyponatremia associated with enhanced proximal reabsorption.[2]

Osmotic agents. Osmotic agents such as mannitol effect diuresis by adding solute to renal tubular fluid. With a higher concentration of solute present, sodium and water are not reabsorbed and are excreted in the urine. In heart failure, these agents may produce cardiocirculatory overload by increasing plasma volume; consequently, they are *not* used to correct cardiac edema.

Prescriptives for use

Acute heart failure. Administration of rapid-acting loop diuretics is a major therapeutic intervention in the setting of acute left ventricular failure characterized by elevated pulmonary venous and ventricular filling pressures and marked lung congestion. Reduction of blood volume and venous return by enhanced urine production is the main objective of diuretic therapy. In addition, preload is also reduced by the action of agents such as furosemide, which increase venous capacitance by approximately 50%.[29] Following bolus infusion, this effect is reflected by an almost immediate decrease in pulmonary capillary wedge pressure, which precedes diuresis. This rapid diuretic therapy is extremely beneficial in improving hemodynamics and in decreasing myocardial oxygen demand.

Extreme caution must be exercised to avoid over-diuresis because the effects will severely limit ventricular function. Because of elevated filling pressures, these patients are functioning on the flat portion of the Frank-Starling curve. As blood volume drops, filling pressure is also lowered. If this compensatory mechanism is removed by over-diuresis, cardiac output and tissue perfusion will become compromised, predisposing to myocardial ischemia and circulatory collapse. In this hypovolemic, hypotensive situation, the initial clinical indicator is elevated heart rate followed by complaints of weakness, confusion, oliguria, and marked peripheral vasoconstriction. Hemodynamic parameters reflect low right atrial pressure, depressed pulmonary capillary wedge pressure, and a marked reduction in cardiac index and mean arterial pressure. Intervention requires immediate termination of diuretic therapy, volume infusion, and the use of pressor agents until functional hemodynamic status is restored. Because of these most serious side effects, it is advised that clinicians be conservative when using potent loop diuretics.

When assessing for therapeutic benefits, it is important to remember that a phase lag may exist between reduced pulmonary capillary wedge pressure and resolution of lung congestion. This may be documented when rapid diuresis does not produce immediate physical and roentgenographic findings consistent with decreased pulmonary pressures. In this situation, further administration of diuretics will most certainly precipitate a hypovolemic, hypotensive episode.

The administration of loop diuretics in acute heart failure secondary to acute inferior or right ventricular myocardial infarction may have grave consequences. In this setting, reduced right ventricular function causes systemic venous congestion and low cardiac output. This is reflected by marked elevation of right atrial and central venous pressures—pulmonary congestion generally is not a classic finding. When cardiac output requires augmentation, therapeutic benefits are derived by volume infusion to elevate left ventricular filling pressures. If diuretics are given to relieve systemic congestion, the subsequent volume depletion and preload reduction will further reduce cardiac output and impair myocardial function. Therefore careful assessment is required to determine the underlying cause of acute heart failure before loop diuretics are prescribed.

Chronic heart failure. The initial treatment of chronic heart failure is correction of underlying causes and precipitating factors followed by improvement of cardiac function with digitalis. When this has been achieved, the next objective is to prevent a positive sodium balance. This may be

accomplished by dietary sodium restriction. In early mild heart failure, it is generally accepted that patients with minimal pitting edema without pulmonary congestion can be adequately maintained on digitalis and a 2-g sodium diet.[31] If further dietary restriction is necessary to control fluid retention, the chance of noncompliance increases. For this reason, initiation of diuretic therapy is a more realistic therapeutic approach.

Sodium retention in heart failure is based on a progression of disturbances and diuretic therapy must change as the renal compensatory mechanisms change. (See Chapter 2, p. 65.) Therapy is directed toward producing sodium balance with the least harmful effects, beginning with thiazides, progressing to aldosterone antagonists, then moving to loop diuretics, and finally moving to proximal tubule agents as diuretic refractoriness and hyponatremia become evident.[2] It is advisable to administer diuretics on alternative-day regimen to allow equilibrium of plasma volume with edema fluid, thereby minimizing diuretic-induced hypovolemia.[2]

Monitoring of diuretic effect is achieved by accurate daily weight determination. Since each liter of lost fluid weighs 1 kg and since daily weight changes in excess of 0.25 kg are the result of loss or gain of water, this parameter may be indispensable.[56] A weight gain of 1 to 2 kg in a few days may indicate that additional diuresis is required. Many diuretics produce electrolyte depletion, so it is necessary to monitor serum electrolytes and supplement potassium-wasting diuretics. It is also necessary to monitor creatinine and blood urea nitrogen levels to determine renal function. During initiation of diuretic therapy, accurate measurement of intake and output, body weight, and daily hematocrit are advised to determine the effects of fluid loss. Patients are also assessed for hemodynamic effects of diuresis. This is done by frequently documenting pulse rate, by monitoring lying and standing blood pressure, and by observing for cardiac arrhythmias, which may be precipitated by both postural hypotensive episodes or electrolyte disorders. Patients are also interviewed regarding symptoms of dizziness, thirst, fatigue, and weakness as well as relief of dyspnea.

As chronic heart failure progresses to the severe refractory state, renal perfusion becomes depressed and glomerular filtration rate (GFR) drops. Other complications that interfere with diuretic effect are acid-base disorders, which may inactivate specific agents (see Table 8-12), and the progression of cardiovascular disease to an advanced stage, causing physiological changes in the kidney that alter diuretic responsiveness.[2] Patients at this stage of failure are usually treated with furosemide and ethacrynic acid, agents that are effective when GFR is below 20% to 25%. If this does not achieve the therapeutic objective, then a potassium-sparing agent may be added. If this combination does not work, a thiazide may be necessary; however, when three diuretics, each with a different primary site of nephron action, are required to produce diuresis, the patient is at higher risk for developing complications such as progressive renal failure and circulatory collapse.[56] At this stage of heart failure, therapy is very complex. Diuretics are administered concurrently with inotropic, sympathomimetic, vasodilator, and antiarrhythmic agents. This requires close monitoring, meticulous assessment, and definitive intervention.

Complicating factors

Generally, the major contraindication of diuretic therapy is anuric renal failure. In most other clinical settings, diuretic agents are essential components of heart failure therapy and are limited by agent-specific side effects. There are, however, several complicating factors that attend therapy. They arise primarily from electrolyte and acid-base imbalance and biochemical disorders.

Potassium depletion. Potassium depletion is a major complicating factor of diuretic therapy for heart failure. In the normal nephron, potassium is filtered at the glomerulus, almost completely absorbed in the proximal tubule, and excreted in exchange for sodium in the distal tubule. The rate of distal tubular excretion is affected by aldosterone activity, rate of sodium delivery to the distal exchange site, carbonic anhydrase inhibition, acid-base status, availability of chloride.[57] In heart failure, these first four factors may be altered by circulatory status, compensatory mechanisms, and diuretic action. Chloride deficit may result from dietary salt restriction, concurrent diuretic therapy, or protracted vomiting.

Patients in severe heart failure are at great risk for potassium depletion since they are generally under intensive diuretic therapy accompanied by sodium restriction and suffer from rapid potassium excretion as a result of secondary hyperaldosteronism. These individuals undergo rapid diuresis with loop diuretics such as furosemide or large diuresis (4 to 5 pounds in 2 to 3 days) with thiazide agents and will exhibit a fall in serum potassium levels.[56] For this reason, they should receive a potassium supplement and be monitored and informed regarding the clinical manifestation of potassium depletion. These include profound skeletal muscle weakness, impaired smooth muscle function reflected by hypomotility of the gastrointestinal tract, and electrocardiographic changes such as ST segment depression and U wave and T wave flattening, depression or inversion. Because these patients are often on concurrent digitalis therapy, they must also be observed for toxic arrhythmias, which may be precipitated by potassium depletion.

Potassium intolerance. Potassium intolerance is unusual in patients with heart failure. However, it has been observed that individuals with severe congestive failure may develop hyperkalemia more easily than those with chronic renal insufficiency.[57] This may be explained by the high rate of proximal tubular sodium removal, which decreases the amount of sodium available at the distal exchange site, thus retarding potassium excretion and causing serum concentrations to rise. Potassium intolerance may also result from misdirected therapy. It may occur when potassium-sparing diuretics such as triamterene or spironolactone are used in conjunction with either potassium supplements or low-sodium diets, particularly when potassium-containing salt substitutes are used. It has also been observed when patients are receiving both diuretics and potassium supplements, but the diuretics are not effective. To avoid these complications, clinicians must be conversant with the action of diuretic agents and must closely assess patients for therapeutic compliance. Furthermore, they must monitor individuals for clinical indicators of potassium intolerance. These include an initial increase in T wave amplitude, followed by development of AV block or sinus arrest. If the patients are receiving digitalis, high serum potassium levels may decrease sensitivity. If the digitalis dose is increased before detecting potassium intolerance, then the individual is at risk for toxic arrhythmias when potassium levels are corrected.

Sodium depletion. Sodium depletion is an important complication and a perplexing problem in heart failure. It results from an imbalance between water ingestion and renal diluting capacity. The loop diuretics and thiazides will decrease the ability of the kidney to dilute urine and excrete solute-free water. This may be potentiated by stimulation of antidiuretic hormone as a result of decreased extracellular fluid volume and by hypokalemia, which causes sodium to move into the cells to displace lost potassium. The clinical indicators will reflect either sodium depletion or water intoxication. (See Table 8-13.) Intervention in the sodium-depleted state requires temporary interruption of diuretic therapy and addition of small amounts of salt to the diet until sodium balance is restored. Patients who manifest water intoxication are treated either by simple water restriction or by extremely cautious administration of small amounts of hypertonic saline if severe neurological involvement (coma, stupor, seizures) exists.

Acid-base imbalance. Acid-base imbalance in patients with mild heart failure usually reflects aberrations caused by diuretic agents. Metabolic acidosis may occur as a complication of treatment with acetazolamide, which causes sodium bicarbonate diuresis. Spironolactone may also precipitate acidosis by antagonizing aldosterone. This triggers potassium and chloride retention, resulting in hyperchloremic metabolic acidosis. Metabolic alkalosis is a complicating factor of thiazide and loop diuretics that accelerates potassium and chloride loss and markedly reduces extracellular fluid volume, producing the condition "contraction alkalosis." In general, metabolic alkalosis is corrected by reexpansion of extracellular volume and potassium supplementation, while acidosis may be corrected by withholding the diuretic agent and administering small amounts of bicarbonate.

When renal insufficiency accompanies severe heart failure, metabolic acidosis presents a serious therapeutic problem. The increased work of the heart associated with acidosis together with the depressant effect on myocardial contractility contribute to cardiac decompensation. In this situation, administration of sodium bicarbonate carries the risk of sodium retention, but it may be used if accompanied by rigid salt restriction.[57] Adminis-

Table 8-13. Clinical indicators of hyponatremia in heart failure

Sodium depletion		Water intoxication	
Causes:	Vigorous diuretic therapy with loop and thiazide agents	Causes:	Excessive water ingestion, progressive heart failure, perioperative state
Effects:	Thirst Orthostatic hypotension Narrow pulse pressure Anorexia Weakness Reduced skin turgor Reduced body weight Elevated BUN Low urine sodium Low serum sodium	Effects:	Elevated pulmonary venous pressure Venous engorgement and interstitial edema Increased body weight Peripheral edema Normal or increased BUN Low urine sodium Low serum sodium Stupor Seizure Coma

tration of an inotrope such as calcium may be indicated to improve cardiac contraction, as well as use of respiratory support devices to decrease the work of breathing.

Hyperuricemia. Hyperuricemia is a complication of long-term diuretic therapy with thiazides, furosemide, and ethacrynic acid. It is postulated that the agents produce urate retention by interfering with uric acid secretion. Most patients tolerate this condition and require no specific treatment. However, in susceptible individuals, hyperuricemia may be associated with attacks of gout, requiring administration of allopurinol.[2,10]

Carbohydrate intolerance. Carbohydrate intolerance may occur in patients with latent diabetes mellitus, especially if they are receiving thiazides. This group of agents has an insulin-suppressive effect thought to be independent of hypokalemia.[16] For this reason, Type II diabetic patients are at risk for developing hyperglycemic events. These individuals must be closely monitored for blood sugar concentrations and should be apprised of the importance of complying with potassium supplementation during thiazide therapy.

Ototoxicity. Ototoxicity is caused by ethacrynic acid and rarely by furosemide. It occurs most frequently when high doses are administered to individuals with renal insufficiency. Hearing loss is usually, but not always, reversible.

Endocrine dysfunction. Endocrine dysfunction is reflected by gynecomastia, impotence, decreased libido, and irregular menses. It occurs secondary to long-term administration of spironolactone, which may interfere with androgen secretion. The problems of sexual dysfunction may also occur if patients are on concurrent beta-blocking therapy. It is most important to assess for these complications and explain the agent-related effects, to avoid serious psychological and interactional problems.

Health care implications
Assessment
1. Identify the cardiac cause of fluid retention.
2. Determine accurate daily body weight as baseline parameter.
3. Measure serum and urine electrolytes, blood

urea nitrogen, creatinine, glucose and uric acid levels to establish baseline data.
4. Evaluate for renal function and presence or absence of endocrine disorders.
5. Measure hemodynamic parameters and vital signs.
6. Obtain a drug history.
7. Assess physical manifestations of expanded extracellular fluid volume and elevated pulmonary and systemic venous pressures.
   a. Weight gain
   b. Peripheral edema
   c. Shortness of breath
   d. Dyspnea on exertion
   e. Rales
   f. Jugular venous distention
   g. Hepatomegaly
8. Establish the major therapeutic objectives:
   a. Reduction of preload and venous pressure
   b. Resolution of pulmonary congestion
   c. Reduction of blood volume
   d. Reduction of peripheral edema

Intervention
1. Select and administer the agent or agents of choice to optimize diuretic effect and compliance:
   a. In collaboration with the patients arrange a dosage schedule that will minimize interruption of meaningful activities and avoid sleep disturbance.
   b. In moderate to severe heart failure, to ensure optimal diuretic effect, administer agent when patients are at rest.
2. Monitor fluid status:
   a. Daily weight
   b. Dependent edema
   c. Hemodynamic parameters
   d. Lung auscultation
   e. Chest roentgenogram
   f. Patient history of weight; fit of clothes; evidence of dependent peripheral edema
3. Monitor electrolyte and biochemical status; correct abnormalities with appropriate supplements:
   a. Laboratory analysis—urine and serum electrolytes, BUN, creatinine, uric acid, glucose

b. Physical indicators—anorexia, nausea, vomiting, thirst, weakness, dizziness, postural hypotension, joint pain, drowsiness, confusion

4. Tailor patient instruction to emphasize the importance of recognizing and reporting symptoms of electrolyte disorders, agent-specific side effects, and clinical manifestations of circulatory status.

5. To optimize the diuretic effect, reinforce the importance of complying with all aspects of the treatment regime:
    a. Diet
    b. Activity restriction
    c. Digitalis
    d. Vasodilators
    e. Potassium supplements

6. Identify the primary health care clinician for the patient and arrange and encourage periodic follow-up and examination.

SUMMARY

The successful management of heart failure depends on accurate determination of underlying cause, effective clinical therapeutics, continuous assessment, and compliance with the treatment regime. Accomplishment of these objectives requires the cooperation of a knowledgeable and collegial health care team. This chapter has presented the key concepts and rationale that are essential to both nursing- and physician-directed management of the pharmacological component of therapy. The major treatment modalities of inotropic, vasodilator, and diuretic therapy were discussed in detail and related to the varied clinical settings of heart failure. It is requisite for all advanced health care clinicians to have a complete understanding of this material and to keep abreast of new developments in the field. This will expedite treatment, minimize complications, and maximize successful health care. It is well recognized that cardiac rhythm disturbances may both precipitate and complicate heart failure. Consequently most patients with heart failure are periodically treated with antiarrhythmic agents. It is beyond the scope of this text to address the topics of dysrhythmia recognition and therapy; however, we strongly urge all involved in the care of these patients to retrieve pertinent information on these topics. There are many excellent references available that address these subjects.

REFERENCES

1. Akera, T., and Brody, T.M.: The role of Na$^+$,K$^+$-ATPase in the inotropic action of digitalis, Pharmacol. Rev. **29:** 187, 1977.
2. Argus, Z.S., and Goldberg, M.: Renal function in congestive heart failure. In Levine, H., editor: Clinical cardiovascular physiology, New York, 1976, Grune & Stratton, Inc., p. 403-439.
3. Awan, N.A., and others: Hemodynamic actions of prenalteral in severe congestive heart failure due to chronic coronary disease, Am. Heart J. **101**(2):158, 1981.
4. Baaske, D.M., and others: Intravenous nitroglycerin: a review, Am. Pharm. **NS22**(2), 1982.
4a. Bamford, J.M.: Synergistic action of metolazone with loop diuretics, Br. Med. J. **282:**1432, May 2, 1981.
5. Barletta, M.: Procardia (Nifedipine): a review, Pfizer Laboratories, New York, 1982.
6. Becker, D.J., and others: Effect of isoproterenol in digitalis cardiotoxicity, Am. J. Cardiol. **10:**242, 1962.
7. Benotti, J.R., and others: Effects of Amrinone on myocardial metabolism and hemodynamics in patients with congestive heart failure due to coronary artery disease, (Abstract) #894, Circulation **60**(4, part 2):II-229, 1979.
8. Berk, J.L., and Sampliner, J.E.: Handbook of critical care, ed. 2, Boston, 1982, Little, Brown & Co.
9. Binnion, P.F.: Drug interactions with digitalis glycosides, Drugs **15:**369, 1978.
10. Braunwald, E.: The management of heart failure. In Braunwald, E., editor: Heart disease, a textbook of cardiovascular medicine, Philadelphia, 1980, W.B. Saunders Co., pp. 510-558.
11. Case, D.B.: Minoxidil, Cardiovasc. Rev. Rep. **1**(6):482, 1980.
12. Chatterjee, K., and Parmley, W.W.: The role of vasodilator therapy in heart failure, Prog. Cardiovasc. Dis. **19:**301, 1977.
13. Chatterjee, K., Doyle, B., and Avakian, D.: Vasodilator therapy for heart failure, Crit. Care Q. **4**(3):13, 1981.
14. Chatterjee, K., and others: Oral hydralazine therapy for chronic refractory heart failure, Circulation **54:**879, 1976.

15. Chatterjee, K., and others: Benefits and limitations of impedance reduction for congestive heart failure in clinical strategies. In Corday, E., and Swan, H.J.C., editors: Ischemic heart disease: new concepts and current controversies, Baltimore, 1979, The Williams & Wilkins Co.

16. Christlieb, A.R.: Diabetes and hypertension, Cardiovasc. Rev. Rep. 1(8):609, 1980.

17. Cogan, J.J., and others: Acute vasodilator therapy increases renal clearance of digoxin in patients with congestive heart failure, Circulation 64(5):973, 1981.

18. Cohn, J.N., and Franciosa, M.A.: Vasodilator therapy for cardiac failure (parts 1 and 2), N. Engl. J. Med. 297:27, 254, 1977.

19. Comer, J.B.: Drugs that affect the autonomic nervous system. In Pharmacology in critical care, Bethany, Connecticut, 1981. Fleschner Publishing Co., pp. 15-31.

20. Croxson, M.S., and Ibbertson, H.K.: Serum digoxin in patients with thyroid disease, Br. Med. J. 3:566, 1975.

21. Dasta, J.F., and Feraets, D.R.: Topical nitroglycerin: a new twist to an old standby, Am. Pharm. NS22(2):28, 1982.

22. Dowdy, E.G., and Fabian, L.W.: Ventricular arrhythmias induced by succinylcholine in digitalized patients, Anesth. Analg. 42:501, 1963.

23. Elbaum, N.: Detecting and correcting magnesium imbalance, Nursing '77, 7:34, August, 1977.

24. Elkayam, U., and others: Marked early attentuation of hemodynamic effects of oral prazosin in chronic congestive heart failure, Am. J. Cardiol. 44:540, 1979.

25. Engel, H.J., and Lichtlen, P.R.: Beneficial enhancement of coronary blood flow by nifedipine: comparison-nitroglycerine and beta-blocking agents, Am. J. Med. 71:658, 1981.

26. Faxon, D.P., and others: Angiotensin inhibition in severe heart failure: acute central and limb hemodynamic effects of captropril with observations on sustained oral therapy, Am. Heart J. 101(5):548, 1981.

27. Fenster, P.E., Hager, W.D., and Ewy, G.A.: Clinical implications of the digitalis-quinidine interaction, Cardiovasc. Rev. Rep. 2(9):921, 1981.

28. Forrester, J.S., and others: Medical therapy of acute myocardial infarction by application of hemodynamic subsets (part 1), N. Engl. J. Med. 295:1356, 1976.

29. Forrester, J.S., and others: Medical therapy of acute myocardial infarction by application of hemodynamic subsets (part 2), N. Engl. J. Med. 295(25):1404, 1976.

30. Franciosa, J.A.: Nitroglycerin and nitrates in congestive heart failure, Heart Lung 9(5):873, 1980.

31. Francisco, L.L., and Ferris, T.F.: The use and abuse of diuretics, Arch. Intern. Med. 142(1):28, 1982.

32. Frishman, W.H.: Clinical considerations in the digoxin loading dose, Pract. Cardiol. 5(5):55, 1979.

33. Giles, T.: Principles of vasodilator therapy for left ventricular congestive heart failure, Heart Lung 9(2):271, 1980.

34. Gilman, A.G., Goodman, L.S., and Gilman, A., editors: Goodman and Gilman's the pharmacological basis of therapeutics, ed. 6, New York, 1980, Macmillan Inc., p. 748.

35. Goodman, L.S., and Gilman, A.: Goodman and Gilman's the pharmacological basis of therapeutics, ed. 5, New York, 1975, Macmillan Inc.

36. Hahn, A.B., Barkin, R.L., and Oestrich, S.J.K.: Pharmacology in nursing, ed. 15, St. Louis, 1982, The C.V. Mosby Co.

37. Iqbal, M., and Liebson, P.: Counterpulsation and dobutamine—their use in treatment of cardiogenic shock due to right ventricular infarction, Arch. Intern. Med. 141:247, Feb. 1981.

38. Lambertz, H., and others: Long term treatment of severe congestive heart failure with the β-agonist prenalterol, Circulation (suppl.) 66:11-20, 1982.

39. Kumpuris, A.G., and others: The role of serum digitalis levels in clinical practice, Heart Lung 8(4):711, 1979.

40. Lee, D.C.S., and others: Heart failure in outpatients: a randomized trial of digoxin versus placebo, N. Engl. J. Med. 306(12):699, 1982.

41. Leonard, R.G., and Tablert, R.L.: Calcium-channel blocking agents, Clin. Pharm. Vol. 1, No. 1, Jan./Feb. 1982.

42. Lown, B., and others: Effects of alteration of body potassium on digitalis toxicity, J. Clin. Invest. 31:648, 1952.

43. Maskin, C.S., and others: Long-term amrinone therapy in patients with severe heart failure: drug-dependent hemodynamic benefits despite progression of the disease, Am. J. Med. 72(1):113, 1982.

44. McDougal, W.S., and Danielson, R.A.: Renal dysfunction. In Berk, J.L., and Sampliner, J.E., editors: Handbook of critical care, ed. 2, Boston, 1982, Little, Brown & Co., pp. 501-530.

45. Morrow, D.H., and Townley, N.T.: Anesthesia and digitalis toxicity: an experimental study, Anesth. Analg. 43: 510, 1964.

46. Opie, L.H.: Drugs and the heart—digitalis and sympathomimetic stimulants, Lancet 1:912, April 26, 1980.

47. Opie, L.H.: Vasodilator drugs, Lancet 1:966, May 3, 1980.

48. Packer, M., and Jemtel, T.: Physiologic and pharmacologic determinants of vasodilator response: a conceptual framework for rational drug therapy for chronic heart failure, Prog. Cardiovasc. Dis. 24(4):275, 1982.

49. Parker, S., and others: Dopamine administration in oliguria and oliguric renal failure, Crit. Care Med. 9(9):630, Sept. 1981.

50. Rubin, S., and Swan, H.: Vasodilator therapy for heart failure: concepts, applications and challenges, JAMA 245(7):761, Feb. 1981.

51. Seltzer, A.: Digitalis: how to use in chronic cardiac failure, Prim. Cardiol. **50**(1):102, 1979.

52. Seltzer, A.: Digitalis in cardiac failure: do the benefits justify the risk? (editorial), Arch. Intern. Med. **141**(1):18, 1981.

53. Shapiro, W.: Digitalis update, (editorial), Arch. Intern. Med. **141**(1):17, 1981.

54. Sharpe, N., and others: Oral prenalterol in chronic heart failure, Circulation (suppl.) **66**:11-20, 1982.

55. Siegel, L.A., and others: Beneficial effect of amrinone-hydralazine combination on resting hemodynamics and exercise in patients with severe congestive heart failure, Circulation **63**(4):838, 1981.

56. Spann, J.F., and Hurst, J.W.: The recognition and management of heart failure. In Hurst, J.W., editor: The heart, ed. 5, New York, 1982, McGraw-Hill Book Co., p. 407.

57. Surawicz, B.: The interrelationship of electrolyte abnormalities and arrhythmias. In Mandel, W., editor: Cardiac arrhythmias, their mechanisms, diagnosis and management, Philadelphia, 1982, J.B. Lippincott Co., p. 83.

58. Vrobel, T.R., Taylor, N.B., and Cohn, J.N.: Comparative effects of nitroprusside and converting enzyme inhibition in patients with congestive heart failure, Circulation **58** (suppl. 2):11-178, 1978.

59. Waters, W.C.: Disturbances in inorganic metabolism in heart failure. In Hurst, J.W., editor: The heart, arteries and veins, ed. 4, New York, 1978, McGraw-Hill Book Co.

60. Weber, K.T., and others: Amrinone and exercise performance in patients with chronic heart failure, Am. J. Cardiol. **49**(1):164, 1981.

61. Williams, J.F., Klocke, F.J., and Braunwald, E.: Studies on digitalis. XIII. A comparison of the effects of potassium on the inotropic and arrhythmic producing actions of ouabain, J. Clin. Invest. **45**:346, 1966.

62. Wilson, R.F., (editor-in-chief): Cardiac failure, critical care manual—principles and techniques of critical care, vol. 1, Kalamazoo, Mich., 1977, The Upjohn Co., pp. 1-21.

63. Withering, W.: An account of the foxglove and some of its medicinal uses: with practical remarks on dropsy and other diseases, London, 1785, C.G. & J. Robinson (reprinted in Medical Classics **2**:305, 1937).

64. Zelis, R., and others: How much can we expect from vasodilator therapy? Circulation **59**(6):1092, 1979.

65. Zelis, R., and Falim, S.: Alterations in vasomotor tone in congestive heart failure, Prog. Cardiovasc. Dis. **24**(6):137, 1982.

CHAPTER 9

Oxygen therapy in heart failure

LORA E. BURKE
JANE FREIN

The use of supplemental oxygen is a therapeutic modality common to many cardiopulmonary disease states. Although oxygen is not a pharmacological agent, it must be considered a medication and its use controlled and monitored as carefully as any drug. As with all medications the use of oxygen should be guided by careful assessment of the clinical indicators and by determination of the optimal amount and method of delivery for each patient. Since oxygen is not always harmless, the health care team must be alert to its possible complications and toxic effects and monitor the patient closely to gain optimal benefit and minimal risk from the therapy.

In the case of the patient with congestive heart failure, several forms of oxygen therapy are utilized, with the method of administration and desired effects dependent upon the severity of the disease. In milder cases the use of oxygen plays a role in the prevention or control of symptoms related to hypoxia. In patients experiencing severe disruptions of cardiopulmonary function, the use of oxygen, in combination with mechanical ventilatory support, may prove to be a lifesaving intervention. In any case appropriate clinical interventions play a key role in gaining optimal benefit from the therapy.

This chapter will present the physiological concepts, assessment parameters, and intervention techniques relevant to the hypoxic patient with congestive heart failure.

PHYSIOLOGICAL CONCEPTS OF HYPOXIA

The term *hypoxemia* refers to a decrease of oxygen in the arterial blood (Pao_2) that is less than adequate. This is generally defined as a Pao_2 less than 80 mm Hg in a person under 60 years of age.[32] The term hypoxia refers to a relative lack of oxygen available at the cellular level. Normal cellular processes are dependent upon adequate oxygenation to provide the energy necessary for chemical reactions. When tissue oxygen tension falls below the critical level necessary for the maintenance of normal cellular function, tissue hypoxia results. Evaluation of the state of tissue oxygenation is purely a clinical assessment, including evaluation of the cardiac status, the state of peripheral perfusion, and the blood oxygen transport mechanism.[32]

Hypoxia may be divided into four types, each indicating a different cause.[32]

1. Hypoxemic hypoxia is caused by inadequate arterial oxygen tension. This is hypoxia caused by hypoxemia, as seen in pulmonary edema, atelectasis, and pneumonia.
2. Anemic hypoxia is caused by a reduction in the oxygen-carrying capacity of the blood, as seen in carbon monoxide poisoning.
3. Circulatory hypoxia involves perfusion to body tissues that is so low that an inadequate amount of oxygen is delivered despite normal arterial oxygen tensions, as seen in

shock. This has also been termed ischemic hypoxia.

4. Histotoxic hypoxia results from failure of the cells to properly utilize the oxygen delivered to them, as seen in cyanide poisoning.

The hypoxemic and circulatory mechanisms are the primary means by which the hypoxic state develops in the patient with congestive heart failure. Pulmonary edema, caused by an increase in the pulmonary capillary hydrostatic pressures secondary to left ventricular failure, causes transudation of fluid into the interstitial and alveolar spaces of the lung. This impedes the normal diffusion of gases and decreases lung compliance. For these reasons arterial oxygen tensions fall, and hypoxia may occur secondary to hypoxemia. Simultaneously, the low cardiac output state in heart failure leads to low tissue perfusion pressures, resulting in a circulatory component of the tissue hypoxia. Although compensatory mechanisms do exist to shift the oxygen-hemoglobin dissociation curve to the right, facilitating the release of oxygen in underperfused tissues, gas exchange is eventually limited by an inadequate blood-tissue oxygen pressure gradient. As tissue metabolism continues in the face of inadequate circulation, tissue hypoxia results.[32]

A combination of these two mechanisms leads to the clinical indicators of hypoxia in the patient with congestive heart failure. Whereas the anemic and histotoxic types of hypoxia may be superimposed in selected patients because of an underlying pathological condition, they are not a direct result of the heart failure.

Oxygen-hemoglobin dissociation curve

Oxygen is carried in the blood in two forms: dissolved in plasma and combined with hemoglobin. The amount of dissolved oxygen is very small—only about 0.3 ml/100 ml of blood. This is about 3% of the total oxygen content. The amount that can be combined with hemoglobin is 1.34 ml of oxygen per gram of hemoglobin. This represents a seventy-fold increase in the oxygen-carrying capacity of the blood above the amount dissolved in plasma.[7]

The percent of hemoglobin that is bound to oxygen is a function of the partial pressure of oxygen in the blood, the Po_2. This is expressed as the percent saturation of the hemoglobin. The relationship of the Po_2 to the O_2 saturation is illustrated in the oxygen-hemoglobin dissociation curve, seen in Fig. 9-1. The upper portion of the curve is flat. At a normal arterial Po_2, from 100 to 70 mm Hg results in very little change in the hemoglobin saturation. The lower part of the curve is steeper. As arterial oxygen tensions fall below 70 mm Hg, the decrease in saturation is rapid and relatively small changes in Po_2 result in large decreases in O_2 saturation. For example, a drop in Po_2 from 60 to 40 mm Hg is associated with a significant reduction in the oxygen carried by hemoglobin.

The position of the oxygen in Fig. 9-1, *A,* assumes a normal pH, carbon dioxide tension (Pco_2), and body temperature. Fig. 9-1, *B,* shows the effect of altered pH levels on the curve. Note that a fall in pH shifts the curve to the right, meaning that for any given Po_2 there is decreased hemoglobin saturation relative to the normal state. A rise in Pco_2 or body temperature similarly shifts the curve to the right. A rise in pH or a decrease in Pco_2 or body temperature shifts the curve to the left. In this case hemoglobin saturation is greater than normal for any given Po_2 level.

It is important to realize that the Po_2 or O_2 saturation alone does not indicate the total amount of oxygen actually being carried by the blood. One must consider both the O_2 saturation and the hemoglobin level to evaluate total oxygen content. For example, the oxygen content resulting from 15 g of hemoglobin, which is 100% saturated, is significantly different from that resulting from 10 g of fully saturated hemoglobin. This example illustrates that in the anemic patient, who has a decreased amount of hemoglobin and therefore a decreased oxygen-carrying capacity, a normal Po_2 and O_2 saturation do not necessarily indicate adequate tissue oxygenation.

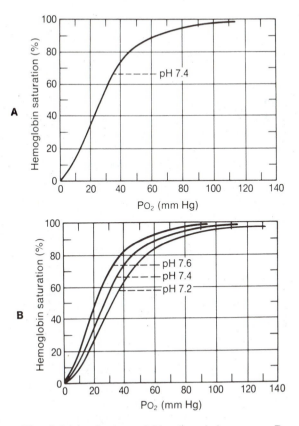

A, Oxyhemoglobin saturation (%) vs PO$_2$ (mm Hg), pH 7.4

B, Hemoglobin saturation (%) vs PO$_2$ (mm Hg), pH 7.6, pH 7.4, pH 7.2

Fig. 9-1. A, Oxyhemoglobin dissociation curve. **B,** Shifts in oxyhemoglobin dissociation curve at varous pH levels. (From Groër, M., and Shekleton, M.: Basic pathophysiology: a conceptual approach, ed. 2, St. Louis, 1983. The C.V. Mosby Co.)

Effects of hypoxia on the myocardium and pulmonary circulation

Oxygen is the most important metabolic substrate for the heart.[30] Without adequate supplies of oxygen, the contractility of the myocardium decreases within a few minutes. This is caused by the change from the normal aerobic to the less efficient anaerobic metabolism, resulting in a net decrease in energy production in the myocardial cell. The loss of vital cellular processes results in a decreased development of intramyocardial tension and, therefore, impairment of normal contractility.[36]

Although increased oxygen extraction is an important mechanism by which peripheral tissues can increase delivery of oxygen to hypoxic cells, this is of much less value to the myocardium, which normally extracts up to 75% of the oxygen presented to it via the coronary arteries.[13]

An important physiological effect of hypoxia is the resultant pulmonary hypertension. When alveolar oxygen tensions fall, the adjacent blood vessels slowly constrict over the following 5 to 10 minutes. The pulmonary vascular resistance can increase to as much as double normal.[19] When left ventricular failure is superimposed on this situation, pulmonary vascular congestion may further elevate pulmonary pressures. This rise in pulmonary artery pressure increases the afterload of the right ventricle and may contribute to increasing right ventricular failure. It is important to note that the hypoxic pulmonary hypertension is a local and reversible phenomenon. Increasing the oxygen tension in the alveoli by the use of appropriate oxygen therapy can relieve pulmonary vasoconstriction resulting from hypoxia and lower pulmonary artery pressures.

Physiological effects of hypoxia

The physical effects of hypoxia are dependent upon the severity of the hypoxic state. Generally accepted arterial oxygen tensions for the various levels of hypoxemia are as follows[32]:

Mild	Pao$_2$ 60-80 mm Hg
Moderate	Pao$_2$ 40-60 mm Hg
Severe	Pao$_2$ <40 mm Hg

Mild hypoxemia has few effects, other than a slight decrease in mental and visual acuity and mild hypertension. In this range, with the PO$_2$ between 60 and 80 mm Hg, the O$_2$ saturation of hemoglobin remains above 90%, generally indicating adequate oxygen availability to all but the most sensitive tissues of the central nervous system. As the hypoxemia worsens and the PO$_2$ falls below 60 mm Hg, physical effects occur that classically manifest themselves in the cardiovascular, respiratory, and central nervous systems.[38]

The body responds to hypoxemia with an increase in sympathetic discharge. This triggers the release of catecholamines, causing the tachycardia characteristic of early hypoxia and heart failure. Cardiac output will increase, provided the individual has an intact sympathetic nervous system and an adequately functioning myocardium. However, if the sympathetic response is inadequate, or if contractility of the heart is severely impaired, bradycardia and hypotension develop. Another cardiac effect of hypoxia is the cardiac arrhythmia, ranging from benign to life-threatening rhythm and conduction disturbances.

The respiratory rate increases as a compensatory mechanism to increase total ventilation and therefore the amount of oxygen available for gas exchange. This mechanism may be inadequate, however, since tachypnea increases the work of breathing and oxygen demand. This increased work of breathing may accentuate the subjective feelings of shortness of breath, particularly in the patient with altered pulmonary compliance, such as that which occurs in pulmonary edema.

As hypoxemia worsens, the early central nervous system signs may be characterized by decreased mental status, drowsiness, disorientation, headache, poor judgment, confusion, or excitement.

ASSESSMENT
Subjective data—the clinical history

An accurate and relevant history may shed a great deal of light on the clinical picture being presented. The amount of information obtained and its accuracy depend on the sensitivity and expertise of the interviewer as well as the ability of the patient to accurately describe and report symptoms and incidences. It is frequently the development of symptoms that stimulates an individual to seek medical attention. Symptoms that are most frequently seen in the context of congestive heart failure are dyspnea, palpitations, and increasing fatigability. These and other less frequently reported symptoms and their significance in assessing the patient with congestive heart failure are reviewed in the following discussion.

Dyspnea. Dyspnea may be described as a subjective sensation of breathlessness related to feelings of ventilatory inadequacy.[9] The conscious awareness of breathing may not always be associated with signs of labored breathing. Dyspnea may be a normal occurrence such as when associated with heavy physical exertion and caused by increased ventilatory demands. It may be abnormal for several reasons, such as anemia, pulmonary disease, or reduced compliance, as occurs with pleural effusion. In the patient with cardiac disease the dyspnea is caused by salt and fluid retention and elevated pulmonary pressures. Because there are many causes of dyspnea, the history must elicit factors that precipitate the onset and relief of symptoms. These include the speed of onset, activity, and body position at the time.

Acute pulmonary edema, caused by a paroxysmal tachyarrhythmia or bradyarrhythmia, acute myocardial infarction, valve rupture, or significant dietary indiscretion, may occur rapidly. Chronic left ventricular failure usually produces a gradual onset unless one of the aforementioned situations arises and precipitates a sudden attack. Asking questions relevant to these conditions and associated symptoms may help identify the specific underlying cause of dyspnea and fatigue.

The level of exertion at which dyspnea develops is important information to help quantitate the severity. Comparing dyspnea that occurs with briskly walking up two flights of stairs with dyspnea that occurs with a short walk on flat ground reflects a different level of impairment. Asking the patient to describe the specific activities that precipitate symptoms and the severity of these symptoms should elicit this information.

Another important variable to cover in the history is the position assumed during the occurrence of dyspnea. Orthopnea is the development of breathlessness while in the recumbent position and usually relieved by assuming an upright position.

If the congestive heart failure progresses, the individual may be unable to lie down to sleep. This symptom may be graded according to the number of pillows needed to sleep, for example, two-pillow orthopnea.

The development of orthopnea is caused by a shift in circulating blood volume during recumbency with a resultant increase in pulmonary blood volume by as much as 500 ml. The augmentation of intrathoracic blood volume combined with decreased pulmonary compliance results in a reduction of vital capacity by as much as 25% to 35%. Changing to an erect position results in a decreased pulmonary engorgement, increased pulmonary compliance and vital capacity, and consequent relief of distressing symptoms.[37]

Severe orthopnea occurring during the night is called paroxysmal nocturnal dyspnea, also known as "cardiac asthma." Patients awaken with a feeling of suffocation often associated with a cough and wheezing. After sitting upright, coughing and working to catch their breath, they frequently experience relief of symptoms. The physiological basis for the development of the syndrome is similar to orthopnea. The important factor in this syndrome is the spontaneous relief that occurs with the change in position. The older patient may exhibit some mental confusion resulting from cerebral hypoxia, which may occur with this acute episode.[25] A few hours in the recumbent position result in a reabsorption of fluid from portions of the body that are usually dependent during the waking hours. This increased intravascular volume combined with the horizontal position results in increased venous return to the right side of the heart and results in pulmonary congestion in the presence of left ventricular dysfunction.[37]

If this acute episode is not terminated by a change to the erect position, a more serious situation occurs. This is referred to as acute pulmonary edema, and the patient is in an emergency. Because of the elevated pulmonary pressure and presence of fluid in the alveolar space, oxygenation is acutely compromised in this situation. Eliciting information from the patient about recent changes in diet, medication adherence, activity, and associated symptoms may give clues to the precipitating factors of the acute event.

Chest pain or discomfort. This symptom is not always associated with congestive heart failure unless coronary atherosclerosis with myocardial ischemia is present. In this context angina may occur with or be precipitated by an episode of dyspnea. Markedly elevated pulmonary pressures may cause chest discomfort in the absence of coronary atherosclerosis. Reduction of these pressures results in relief of symptoms. This is seen more frequently in the patient with severe valvular dysfunction. For these reasons it is important to question the patient about the presence of chest discomfort and the conditions that aggravate or relieve it.

Palpitations. Palpitations refer to the sensation of a pounding or thumping over the precordial area or in the throat. This may signal the occurrence of paroxysmal tachycardia, the leading cause of an acute episode of dyspnea. Asking the patient about the occurrence of such symptoms may give insight into the cause of congestive heart failure or the effectiveness of treatment.

Dizziness. The value of questioning the patient about lightheadedness is that it may also reflect a cause of an acute episode of congestive heart failure, which may be precipitated by bradyarrhythmia or heart block resulting in markedly reduced cardiac output and failure. An excessively rapid tachyarrhythmia may present the same symptoms.

Fatigability. Decreased capacity to carry on activities of daily living is frequently the symptom that precipitates seeking medical attention in the patient with mild heart failure. The sense of increasing fatigability is a reflection of the reduced cardiac output and ability to adequately deliver oxygen to meet the tissue demands. Discussing this symptom when taking a history will frequently provide information about the onset and course of the illness.

While it is important to collect subjective data regarding the events that lead to the acute situation, it is also crucial to assess the subjective response to the interventions and their effectiveness. Questioning the individual about the reduced dyspnea or associated symptoms, comfort in breathing, and present level of anxiety may provide information helpful in evaluating effectiveness of treatment.[1]

Objective data

Objective data to be collected from the patient with congestive heart failure experiencing or at risk for hypoxia include physical, hemodynamic, and laboratory data. By careful assessment and integration of this information, the clinician is able to detect changes in the patient's condition early, intervene promptly, and evaluate the effectiveness of interventions.

Physical examination

Chest examination. Auscultation of the chest of a patient with pulmonary edema will reveal rales and in some cases rhonchi, indicating fluid in the alveoli and airways. Less severe cases may be associated with moist rales at the lung bases. These sounds have been attributed to poor ventilation or transudation of small amounts of fluid into the alveoli. During pulmonary edema, chest expansion may be limited because of a decrease in lung compliance.

Color. Observation of the color of the patient's skin and mucous membranes should be included in the assessment, because they may give some indication of the state of oxygenation. Cyanosis may be present in the hypoxic patient, but it generally occurs quite late in the development of hypoxemia and should not be relied upon as an early indication of changes in oxygenation. Cyanosis occurs when there is greater than 5 g of unsaturated hemoglobin per 100 ml of blood. This will not occur until O_2 saturation falls below approximately 85% or at a Po_2 less than 50 mm Hg. If the patient is anemic, the Po_2 and O_2 saturation will be even lower before cyanosis occurs. In the polycythemic patient, cyanosis may be apparent with relatively mild hypoxia resulting from the high level of hemoglobin. Therefore it is apparent that cyanosis is not a reliable indication of oxygenation in all patients.

Cyanosis that appears on the warm mucous membranes, is known as central cyanosis and is a more accurate indication of blood oxygenation than peripheral cyanosis, which appears on the extremities. The latter may be a result of circulatory disturbances resulting in localized tissue hypoxia despite an adequate Pao_2. The detection of cyanosis depends upon many factors, including the patient's skin thickness, pigmentation, density of capillaries, and the effect of external lighting. In dark-skinned individuals cyanosis may be apparent only in mucous membranes or nail beds.

Heart rate and rhythm. Hypoxia results in tachycardia caused by stimulation of the sympathetic nervous system. Hypoxia may also precipitate dangerous arrhythmias caused by myocardial irritability or damage to the conduction system. When this occurs continuous ECG monitoring should be employed, along with frequent assessment and documentation of heart rate and rhythm.

Systemic and pulmonary pressures. Pulmonary vasoconstriction is known to result from alveolar hypoxia. This will cause an increase in pulmonary artery pressures as measured by an indwelling Swan-Ganz pulmonary artery catheter. In the patient with congestive heart failure, the pulmonary vascular effects of hypoxia may be difficult to distinguish from the elevations in pressure caused by left ventricular failure or the effects of positive pressure ventilation. Frequent determinations of pulmonary arterial pressures may, however, reveal early evolution of pulmonary congestion that, if left untreated, may progress and precipitate further reduction in blood and tissue oxygenation.

The systemic arterial blood pressure can be expected to increase early in hypoxia as a result of sympathetic nervous system stimulation. However, blood pressure may decrease in profound pump failure. As the blood pressure requires close monitoring during hypoxia, an intra-arterial catheter may be appropriate to allow continuous arterial pressure monitoring and frequent arterial blood gas sampling.

Central nervous system. The hypoxic patient

may exhibit an array of central nervous system clinical indicators. Assessment of these patients should include a mental status examination and evaluation of restlessness, excitement, confusion, lethargy, drowsiness, disorientation, headache, and visual disturbances. Although these may be the first indications of changes in oxygenation, they are very nonspecific, and their association with hypoxia should be confirmed by arterial blood gas analysis.

A summary of the physical assessment of the hypoxic patient appears in Table 9-1.

Laboratory data. Two laboratory tests that are important to evaluate in the patient at risk for hypoxia are the tests for arterial blood gases and the hemoglobin concentration. Although these tests are nonspecific for heart failure, they can be of value in determining the patient's need for supplemental oxygen or ventilatory support and in evaluating the effectiveness of therapy.

Arterial blood gases. Arterial blood gases (ABGs) are used to obtain information about the patient's level of oxygenation, ventilation, and acid-base status.[5,15] Blood gas evaluation generally include measurement of the pH, Pa_{O_2}, Pa_{CO_2}, bicarbonate, base excess, and O_2 saturation. The normal values are as follows:

pH	7.40 (7.35-7.45)
Pa_{O_2}	80-100 mm Hg
Pa_{CO_2}	35-45 mm Hg
HCO_3	22-26 mEq/L
Base excess (BE)	-2-$+2$
O_2 saturation	95% or greater

A brief discussion of the meaning of each of these values follows.

pH. The pH is a direct measurement of the acidity or alkalinity of the blood in terms of the hydrogen ion concentration. A pH of 7.40 is normal, and the blood pH value must be maintained within the narrow range of 7.35 to 7.45 to assure optimal cellular functioning. By definition, a pH lower than 7.35 indicates an acidotic state, whereas a pH greater than 7.45 defines an alkaline state. The pH, therefore, indicates the overall acid-base status of the body.

Table 9-1. Physical findings related to hypoxia

Examination	Findings
Chest examination	Rales, rhonchi, ↓ chest expansion
Color	Cyanosis
Vital signs	Heart rate— ↑ or ↓ Blood pressure— ↑ or ↓ Respiratory rate— ↑ with dyspnea Cardiac arrhythmias
Central nervous system	Restlessness, excitement, confusion, lethargy, drowsiness, disorientation, headache, visual disturbances
Hemodynamics	↑ Pulmonary artery pressures, CO ↑ or ↓

Pa_{O_2}. The Pa_{O_2} is a direct measure of the partial pressure of oxygen in arterial blood. The normal value for Pa_{O_2} of a patient breathing room air ranges from 80 to 100 mm Hg. These values vary in the newborn, in whom a normal Pa_{O_2} may be as low as 40 to 60 mm Hg, and in the elderly population. A normal Pa_{O_2} for an elderly patient breathing room air can be estimated by use of the following formula: $80 - 1$ for each year of age over 60.[31] For example, in a 72-year-old individual breathing room air, a normal Pa_{O_2} should be: $80 - 12$, or 68 mm Hg.

Pa_{CO_2}. Pa_{CO_2} is a direct measure of partial pressure of carbon dioxide in arterial blood and an indicator of the efficiency of ventilation. A Pa_{CO_2} greater than 45 mm Hg defines a state of hypoventilation; a Pa_{CO_2} less than 35 mm Hg is definitive of hyperventilation. The Pa_{CO_2} evaluates the respiratory component of the body's acid-base balance.

HCO_3. Bicarbonate is an ion in solution rather than a gas. It is one of the body's main bases and represents the renal-regulated or metabolic component of the acid-base balance. When reported in a blood gas, the HCO_3 is not a directly measured value but is calculated with the use of a standardized nomogram. An HCO_3 lower than 22 mEq/L indicates a metabolic acidosis, whereas a value over 26 mEq/L indicates metabolic alkalosis or bicarbonate excess.

BASE EXCESS (BE). Base excess is the total concentration of base in the blood, measured in mEq/L. It represents the influence of bicarbonate and all other alkaline substances in the blood. Therefore it is a reflection of the total nonrespiratory acid-base status. It is reported as mEq/L of base above or below the normal buffer base range. Thus in metabolic alkalosis in which an excess of base is present, there would be a *positive* base excess. In metabolic acidosis, with a decrease in the normal concentration of alkaline substances, a *negative* base excess would be reported. This is frequently called base *deficit*. These are calculated values, and their reliability depends upon the accuracy of the pH and Pa_{CO_2} measurements.

O_2 SATURATION. Most of the oxygen in the blood is carried by the hemoglobin and is measured or calculated as the O_2 saturation, which is a measure of the percentage of oxygen carried by hemoglobin compared to the total amount of oxygen that the hemoglobin could carry. This is 95% in arterial blood and 70% to 75% in mixed venous blood. The relationship of O_2 saturation to Pa_{O_2} is affected by factors such as temperature, pH, and carbon dioxide tensions, as reflected on the oxyhemoglobin dissociation curve. For example, a shift to the left will increase hemoglobin affinity for oxygen and increase O_2 saturation for a given Pa_{O_2}, whereas a shift to the right will decrease hemoglobin affinity for oxygen and decrease O_2 saturation for a given Pa_{O_2} (Fig. 9-1).

Arterial blood gases in congestive heart failure. Although nonspecific for congestive heart failure, ABGs will provide data for the evaluation of ventilation, oxygenation, and acid-base balance, which may be directly or indirectly altered by the disease process. The blood gas values of the patient with heart failure varies greatly with the stage and severity of the disease. In the patient with chronic congestive heart failure who is receiving long-term diuretic therapy, the usual state is mild metabolic alkalosis.[27] This is thought to be caused

largely by the effects of the diuretics and potassium loss. Since it is rare for metabolic alkalosis to cause a significant decrease in alveolar ventilation, there is a tendency for the alkalemia to remain uncompensated. Typical blood gases in this state are pH 7.56, Pa_{O_2} 100 mm Hg, Pa_{CO_2} 32 mm Hg, HCO_3 28 mEq/L, and BE +6.[32]

In acute heart failure the ABGs will depend upon the specific pathological condition. In early stages patients may have pulmonary congestion but normal tissue perfusion. Mild arterial hypoxemia results, primarily because of the inability of gases to diffuse through the fluid in the interstitial spaces. To compensate for this, ventilation increases, leading to respiratory alkalosis. Typical ABGs in this state are pH 7.51, Pa_{CO_2} 29 mm Hg, Pa_{O_2} 64 mm Hg, HCO_3 23 mEq/L, and BE 0 mEq/L. The response to supplemental oxygen at this stage is usually dramatic.[32] If the fluid accumulation increases and gross pulmonary edema occurs, the hypoxemia may become severe.

In patients with a low cardiac output and impaired tissue oxygenation but without pulmonary congestion, the ABGs will represent metabolic acidosis without hypoxemia. An example of this state is pH 7.27, Pa_{CO_2} 25 mm Hg, Pa_{O_2} 92 mm Hg, HCO_3 11 mEq/L, and BE 14 mEq/L.[28] In this case the Pa_{CO_2} of 25 indicates an attempted respiratory compensation.

In the clinical setting the picture of severe left ventricular failure is frequently a combination of pulmonary edema and low cardiac output with inadequate tissue perfusion. If the lung compliance is markedly decreased because of severe pulmonary edema, the work of breathing greatly increases. As the patient fatigues, decreasing the rate and/or depth of respirations, ventilatory compensation fails and the Pa_{CO_2} rises. This, in combination with metabolic acidosis secondary to inadequate perfusion, will result in a severely acidotic state. An example of these blood gases are pH 7.16, Pa_{O_2} 48 mm Hg, Pa_{CO_2} 52 mm Hg, HCO_3 17.5 mEq/L.[18]

Arterial blood gases should be drawn to evaluate the patient upon admission. Subsequent sampling will be determined by the patient's condition and therapy. ABGs should be drawn 15 to 30 minutes after each change in oxygen therapy or in ventilator settings to evaluate the effect of the change. They should also be evaluated immediately upon any change in the patient's clinical status.

Hemoglobin. The concentration of hemoglobin should be assessed in all patients at risk for hypoxia. Hemoglobin is the main component of the red blood cell and is responsible for the transportation of almost all of the oxygen carried in the blood. Therefore a low hemoglobin concentration would indicate a decreased oxygen-carrying capacity of the blood and may cause or complicate an existing tissue hypoxia. Anemic patients should receive enough supplemental oxygen to keep their hemoglobin saturation near 100%.[10] If this requires toxic concentrations of oxygen, transfusion may be necessary.

Polycythemia is an increased number of red blood cells and is commonly associated with increased hemoglobin concentrations. Chronic hypoxemia frequently results in polycythemia as a compensatory mechanism to increase the oxygen-carrying capacity of the blood.

INTERVENTIONS—METHODS OF OXYGEN DELIVERY

A wide variety of delivery systems for oxygen therapy exist. Ideally, the system selected should deliver both an appropriate fractional concentration of inspired oxygen ($F_{I_{O_2}}$) and a level of humidity at a flow rate needed to provide the desired increase in tracheal $F_{I_{O_2}}$.[29] The $F_{I_{O_2}}$ of the therapy system is not the same as the tracheal $F_{I_{O_2}}$ resulting from oxygen dilution during delivery by entrainment of room air in the airway. The balance between the patient's inspiratory flow rate and the flow rate of oxygen supplied by the system determine the amount of room air entrained. This can only be grossly estimated if a nebulizer is used. The value of humidifying the gas to reduce water loss from the mucous membrane in the nonintubated well-hydrated patient has been questioned. For the patient who is intubated, a humidification device is essential. Another important factor to consider when selecting a method of oxygen delivery is the appropriate alveolar $F_{I_{O_2}}$. Excessive alveolar $F_{I_{O_2}}$ may result in toxic effects on the lung parenchyma particularly when the $F_{I_{O_2}}$ exceeds 40%. The objective of oxygen therapy is maintaining the Pa_{O_2} in the range of 60 to 100 mm Hg (90% to 98% saturation).

It would seem clear that more than one method of oxygen therapy could provide an adequate $F_{I_{O_2}}$, flow, or humidity, particularly for the individual who does not have a special need. Two important determinations to consider when selecting a supplemental oxygen system are the individual's oxygen requirements and willingness or ability to cooperate.

The most common methods of oxygen delivery are the nasal cannula and face masks. The nasal catheter is infrequently used.

Nasal cannula

The nasal cannula is inserted beneath the naris with the flared tips inserted in the naris. It is suitable when small amounts of supplemental oxygen will suffice. If individuals are mouth breathers, they still receive the oxygen but the percentage is reduced by 3% to 5%. The cannula seems to be the most comfortable delivery method and also allows for greater humidification. It is almost as easy to misplace the cannula as it is to keep in good position. Caregivers need to remind patients to keep it on in the proper position.

Face mask

The oxygen mask is used when higher oxygen concentrations are desired. It is placed over the face with an adjustable metal clip at the nose to assist in maintaining proper positioning on the face while allowing for maximum comfort and minimum leakage. All masks may stimulate a feeling of claustrophobia or suffocation and cause patients to remove them frequently. This may be a very important factor in the individual acutely ill with congestive heart failure, particularly when the severe dyspnea is already causing the sensation of suffocation.

There are several types of masks available, depending on the specific needs of the individual. More detailed information on the various types of face masks available is presented in Table 9-2. Important considerations for caring for the person using a face mask are the amount of time the mask is off the person's face for eating or speaking purposes and the maintenance of good skin integrity around the face so that pressure sores do not develop.

Intermittent positive pressure breathing

Intermittent positive pressure breathing (IPPB) is a therapy in which a series of positive pressure inspirations is delivered via a tight-fitting face mask, mouthpiece, or artificial airway with the use of a pressure-limited ventilator. The treatment is used in many cardiopulmonary diseases to increase ventilation and deliver nebulized medications directly to the respiratory tract. The major effects of IPPB are an increase in tidal volume, which serves

Table 9-2. Oxygen therapy

Mode of delivery	Liter flow	% O$_2$ concentration delivered	Advantages	Disadvantages
Nasal cannula or prongs	2-3 L/minute 3-5 L/minute	24%-28% 28%	Allows for uninterrupted flow Is most comfortable Direct O$_2$ through turbinates to allow for greater humidification Inexpensive	Final F$_{IO_2}$ is determined by the proportionate mixing of O$_2$ flow and amount of ambient air (21% O$_2$) moved in and out of lungs Flow greater than 6 L/minute causes drying and irritation of nasal mucosa May become displaced
Nasal catheter	4-6 L/minute	30%-40%	Allows for continuous flow Easily inserted if well lubricated with water-soluble jelly (measure from nose to tip of earlobe; insert with O$_2$ on; should end at uvula) Inexpensive	Requires changing every 8 hours and alternating nares May cause drying of nasal-pharyngeal mucosa, increasing the risk of infection Is less well tolerated than cannula Cannot deliver O$_2$ within a narrow fixed range of F$_{IO_2}$ Complications include gastric distension and rupture and nasal necrosis

Table 9-2. Oxygen therapy—cont'd

Mode of delivery	Liter flow	% O_2 concentration delivery	Advantages	Disadvantages
Oxygen mask	6-8 L/minute 10 L/minute	35%-45% 45%-65%	Allows for slightly higher O_2 concentrations without causing nasal mucosa drying	Interferes with talking, eating, drinking, expectorating One size only Often hot and may have unpleasant odor May cause panic in a patient because of a closed-in feeling Can create pressure sores on face Dangerous in patient who tends to vomit, expecially in those with a decreased level of consciousness whose arms are in restraints Adds dead space to patient's airway, which may be considerable with some appliances Difficult to deliver exact amount of O_2 to patient
Partial rebreathing mask	8-10 L/minute Oxygen flow should be sufficient to keep reservoir bag partially inflated during inspiration	60%	Able to deliver high concentrations of O_2	There are no means of humidifying the gas adequately Dangerous if liter flow decreased—the patient may rebreathe CO_2
Nonbreathing mask	10-12 L/minute	80-90%	No exhaled air rebreathed because of the one-way valve Most precise method of administering a specific gas concentration because the patient inhales the gas present in the bag only Allows for humidification of the gas Some reservoir bags have drain plugs for removal of accumulated moisture	Tight seal needed Often hot May cause panic because of a closed-in feeling Can create pressure sores on the face Is dangerous in a patient who tends to vomit Interferes with talking, eating, drinking, expectorating

Continued.

Table 9-2. Oxygen therapy—cont'd

Mode of delivery	Liter flow	% O_2 concentration delivered	Advantages	Disadvantages
Venturi mask (Venti-mask, air-mix or dilution mask)	4-6 L/minute 4-6 L/minute 8-10 L/minute 8-10 L/minute	24% 28% 35% 40%	Allows for precise concentration of O_2 at low flow $F_{I_{O_2}}$ relatively independent of the O_2 flow rate as long as it exceeds the stated minimum	Uncomfortable and inconvenient Same as for nonrebreathing mask Not always as reliable as claimed Relatively inexpensive
Face tent or trach mask	6-10 L/minute	30-65%	Provides high humidity, allowing wetting of secretions	Appliance attached to face may be a nuisance
Mechanical ventilators	21-100 L/minute	21-100%	Allows for precise $F_{I_{O_2}}$ Allows for the addition of other techniques, such as increased tidal volume or positive end-expiratory pressure (PEEP) to increase oxygenation	Overoxygenation can occur
Intermittent positive pressure breathing (IPPB)	"Air-mix" 100%	40%-90% 100%	Treatment for acute pulmonary edema Allows for administration of medications through nebulizer	Overoxygenation can readily occur

to increase the P_{O_2} and decrease the P_{CO_2}, and a decrease in the airway resistance.[39]

IPPB has been used for many years in the treatment of pulmonary edema. It was thought that the increased pulmonary interstitial pressures generated during positive pressure inspiration served to decrease the filtration of fluid from the pulmonary capillary to the interstitial and alveolar spaces. However, recently the value of this mechanism has been questioned. In fact some studies indicate that positive pressure respirations actually increase the amount of lung water in the pulmonary tissues rather than decrease it.[33]

Another use of IPPB treatments in pulmonary edema has been for the nebulization of alcohol directly into the airways. This was thought to be of value if the airways were filled with foaming edema fluid. It was postulated that the alcohol lowered the surface tension of the fluid enough to reduce the bubbles. The value of this treatment is also questionable, since if the bubbles disperse and are replaced by fluid in the airways and alveoli, gas diffusion may be further impaired.[34]

Much controversy remains over the use of IPPB in pulmonary edema of cardiac origin. Although most of the effects of the treatment are on the lungs and respiratory tract, changes also occur during treatments in the cardiovascular hemodynamics secondary to intrathoracic pressure changes. During pressure inspiration venous return is decreased, which may result in a drop in cardiac output and blood pressure and in further reduction in tissue oxygenation. It is clear that in the hemodynamically compromised patient, IPPB must be used only with great caution. A fall in blood pressure of greater than 30 mm Hg or greater than 15% below baseline is an absolute contraindication for IPPB treatments in this group of patients.[4]

It is imperative that any patient receiving IPPB treatment be sufficiently calm and cooperative to gain the most benefit from the treatment. The nursing and respiratory therapy staff must carefully explain the procedure and purpose of the treatment. The frightened and dyspneic patient can be reassured by the deliberately calm actions of the nurse during a stressful treatment. The patient should never be left alone during the treatment, and careful pre- and posttreatment evaluation of the patient's status must be made as well as continuous monitoring of his cardiac condition during therapy.

Mechanical ventilation

In severe cases of heart failure associated with respiratory failure, mechanical ventilation may be necessary to raise the Pa_{O_2} and control the Pa_{CO_2}. This intervention will also serve to decrease the work of breathing and therefore decrease oxygen demand. Although intubation and the use of mechanical ventilators is not without complications, it can prove to be a life-saving procedure for the severely hypoxic patient.

Many mechanical ventilators in use today are of the positive pressure type, which ventilate the patient through an artificial airway by using greater than atmospheric pressure to introduce air into the lungs. There are presently two types of positive pressure ventilators in common use: pressure-cycled ventilators and volume-cycled ventilators. The two types differ in the parameter by which the inspiratory phase of the respiratory cycle is termi-

nated. The expiratory phase is passive with both types of ventilators.

In pressure-cycled ventilation the inspiratory phase of the cycle is terminated when a predetermined pressure is reached in the airway. In this type of ventilation, peak airway pressures are held constant, but the volume of air delivered to the patient will vary depending upon the airway resistance and pulmonary compliance. For this reason, consistent tidal volumes and minute volumes cannot be assured. Therefore the use of continuous pressure-cycled ventilation is generally limited to short-term, closely monitored clinical situations.

In volume-cycled ventilation the inspiratory phase of the cycle ends when a predetermined volume of gas is delivered through the ventilator circuit. In this case tidal volumes remain constant whereas the peak airway pressure generated in each respiratory cycle may vary. However, volume ventilators are built with a pressure-limiting valve to prevent excessive pressures from developing within the system and the airways. Without this safety system, airway pressures would be allowed to increase indefinitely with the possibility of producing pulmonary barotrauma. Volume-cycled ventilators are commonly used for long-term ventilatory support in the intensive care unit setting, and because of the altered pulmonary compliance occurring in pulmonary edema, they are the preferred machine for these patients.[22]

Cardiovascular effects of positive pressure ventilation. Positive pressure ventilation has characteristic hemodynamic effects because of an alteration in normal respiratory mechanics. During normal spontaneous breathing, inspiration generates negative intrathoracic pressure that augments venous return to the heart. In mechanical positive pressure ventilation, intrathoracic pressure is increased during the inspiratory phase, compressing the great vessels and atria and decreasing venous return. Therefore right ventricular volume decreases. At the same time, increased pressure on the pulmonary vasculature augments left atrial filling. Consequently, cardiac output is transiently increased slightly at the onset of mechanical ventilation. During positive pressure ventilation, however, pulmonary blood flow is decreased because of a limited venous return, with a net effect being an increase in pulmonary vascular pressures and a decrease in cardiac output.[12] The degree to which this occurs depends upon the amount of positive pressure applied. It is known that this effect is exaggerated if the patient is hypovolemic.[2,16,38]

Positive end-expiratory pressure. Positive end-expiratory pressure (PEEP) is an accessory mode available for use with positive pressure ventilation in which a positive airway pressure is maintained at the end of expiration. The purpose of PEEP is to prevent alveolar and airway collapse and to increase the Pa_{O_2}.[38] It does this by increasing the functional residual capacity (FRC) or the amount of gas left in the lungs at the end of a passive expiration. It thereby provides for a larger surface area available for gas exchange across the alveolar-capillary membrane. PEEP should be considered for patients requiring an FI_{O_2} greater than 0.5 to maintain a Pa_{O_2} of at least 60 mm Hg.[34]

Since the use of PEEP increases intrathoracic pressure throughout the entire respiratory cycle, a severe reduction in venous return may occur. Patients requiring PEEP to maintain adequate oxygenation must be monitored closely for signs of hemodynamic compromise, such as a drop in blood pressure or cardiac output. These considerations are especially important in the hemodynamically unstable patient with congestive heart failure. The amount of PEEP used and its positive effect on oxygenation must be evaluated in light of the entire clinical picture of cardiopulmonary dysfunction.

Complications of mechanical ventilation (Table 9-3). Although the use of positive pressure ventilation is a necessary component of therapy for the critically ill cardiopulmonary patient, its use is not without risk. The clinician must be acutely aware of these potential problems and include assessment for them in daily care. One major complication of all oxygen therapy, oxygen toxicity, is discussed in depth elsewhere in this chapter. This

Table 9-3. Complications of mechanical ventilation

Types	Clinical indicators
Pulmonary barotrauma	Pneumothorax Tracheal shift Subcutaneous emphysema Hyperresonant percussion over affected area Asymmetrical chest movement
Pulmonary infection	Fever Increased secretions Change in quality, color, odor of secretions
Hypotension	Low arterial pressure Pallor Weak thready pulse Cool extremities Diaphoresis Peripheral cyanosis Obtundation
Fluid retention	Increased weight gain Increased peripheral edema Increased systemic venous pressure and organ congestion Jugular venous distension Hepatojugular reflux Hepatomegaly
Gastrointestinal distress	Abdominal distention Increased abdominal girth Decreased to absent bowel sounds Generalized abdominal tympany Nausea Bloody nasogastric drainage

section will outline other complications of mechanical ventilation.

Pulmonary barotrauma. Barotrauma refers to tissue injury resulting from pressure. In positive pressure ventilation the lung tissues are subjected to abnormal pressures for the duration of the therapy. It has been reported that the incidence of barotrauma with mechanical ventilation is 10% to

20% in the adult population.[23] Most of these injuries are in the form of tension pneumothorax. In this condition positive-pressure ventilation disrupts the integrity of the visceral pleura of the lung, allowing air to enter the intrapleural space. This results in a rapid rise in intrapleural pressure, collapsing the lung, compressing the great vessels, and shifting the mediastinum to the opposite side. The resultant drop in cardiac output may cause hypotension and even cardiac arrest. In a patient on a volume ventilator, pneumothorax can be detected by a sudden increase in peak airway pressure without a change in tidal volume. Other signs include severe dyspnea and restlessness, decreased blood pressure, tachycardia, weak pulses, decreased breath sounds over the affected lung, tracheal deviation, hyperresonance to percussion, and a sudden decrease in the Pao_2.[11] If this occurs the patient should be disconnected from the ventilator and hand-ventilated with a self-inflating bag until a chest tube is inserted.

Less common complications related to barotrauma include pneumo-mediastinum, pneumo-pericardium, and subcutaneous emphysema.

Pulmonary infection. Patients dependent upon artificial ventilation are unable to clear their airways of secretions. They also lose the ability to filter, warm, and humidify inspired gas. These factors, combined with frequent tracheal aspiration and the possibility of contamination of the ventilator equipment, lead to an increased incidence of pulmonary infection in the ventilator-dependent patient. Retention of secretions may also obstruct airways and cause areas of atelectasis.

Hypotension. As discussed earlier, positive pressure ventilation causes a decrease in venous return, pulmonary blood flow, and cardiac output. The severity of this effect is related to the amount of positive pressure applied and the duration of exposure. That is, the greater the positive pressure applied to the thoracic structures, the greater the possibility of hemodynamic consequences. Also, the longer the inspiratory phase (when the positive pressure is exerted), the greater the hemodynamic effects. This effect can be minimized if the expiratory time is at least 30% greater than the inspiratory time to allow for adequate venous return. The hemodynamic effects are exaggerated with the use of PEEP, or if the patient is hypovolemic.[16]

Fluid retention. Positive pressure ventilation seems to promote fluid retention, which may prove especially problematic for the congestive heart failure patient. The exact cause of this is not known, but it is thought that it may result from an increased secretion of antidiuretic hormone (ADH) by the posterior lobe of the pituitary gland. Adding to this may be the fluid input delivered through the ventilator humidification and nebulization systems. Patients may gain as much as 300 to 500 ml of water per 24 hours via the ventilatory system.[11] Daily weights, adherence to prescribed fluid restrictions, and careful and accurate monitoring of the intake and output are important clinical measures in the care of these patients.

Gastrointestinal distress. Mechanical ventilation is associated with an increased incidence of gastrointestinal complications.[11] A decrease in gastrointestinal motility in combination with air swallowing around the endotracheal tube may cause gastric distention and paralytic ileus. This can be detected by an increasing abdominal girth and a decrease or absence of bowel sounds. Nasogastric suction may be applied to relieve the distention. In addition there is an increased incidence of gastric ulceration and bleeding in the mechanically ventilated patient. This has been attributed to stress, hypersecretion of gastric acid, steroid therapy, and lack of antacid therapy or gastric feedings. The incidence of gastric bleeding may be decreased in this population by aggressive use of antacids, titrating the gastric pH to greater than 3.5 with hourly doses via the nasogastric tube.

Weaning. Weaning from mechanical ventilation should begin as soon as possible. All care delivered to mechanically ventilated patients should be directed toward preparing them for the time they will once again breathe without assistance. Along with the general condition and the status of the primary problem, the following ventilation parameters should be considered in the assessment of a patient's readiness for weaning.

Vital capacity. A vital capacity of greater than 10 to 15 ml/kg of body weight is necessary to maintain adequate alveolar ventilation. This is tested during maximal effort spontaneous respiration.

Inspiratory force. This measurement is used as an index of neuromuscular strength. The normal individual can generate −80 to −100 cm H_2O during inspiration. An inspiratory force of at least −20 cm H_2O is necessary to indicate adequate muscular strength for weaning.

AaDo₂. The alveolar-arterial oxygen tension difference ($AaDo_2$) is a measurement that provides information about intrapulmonary shunting. The degree of shunting determines a patient's ability to maintain adequate arterial oxygenation during spontaneous respiration.[12] This test should be performed serially from the onset of ventilatory therapy. An $AaDo_2$ of less than 300 to 500 mm Hg or a Pao_2 greater than 300 mm Hg on 100% oxygen indicates adequate oxygenation ability for weaning.[3] If PEEP has been used as part of the ventilatory therapy, the patient should be weaned to a PEEP of 5 to 8 cm H_2O and be able to maintain an adequate $AaDo_2$ at this level. These pulmonary weaning parameters are as follows:

Vital capacity	10-15 ml/kg
Inspiratory force	−20 cm H_2O
$AaDo_2$	300-350 mm Hg
Pao_2 on 100% O_2	300 mm Hg

It is clear that for the patient in congestive heart failure, the circulatory and hemodynamic status must be considered before weaning. To date, little if any work has been done to determine adequate cardiac output or left ventricular filling pressures for institution of the weaning process. It has been stated, however, that development of a pulmonary capillary wedge or left atrial pressure above 20 mm Hg or a cardiac index less than 1.9 L/minute/m₂ during weaning is an indication to terminate the weaning attempt.[26] Therefore it may be said that it is inappropriate to attempt to wean patients in whom these values are exceeded. However, op-

timal hemodynamic status remains an individual clinical determination. The critical hemodynamic factor is the patient's ability to maintain or increase cardiac output without developing further left ventricular failure or pulmonary hypertension when breathing off the ventilator. For this reason monitoring of pulmonary pressures and cardiac outputs is vital during weaning of these patients.[26]

Several other aspects of the patient's condition should be evaluated before weaning.

Anemia. Anemia results in a decreased oxygen-carrying capacity of the blood. A hemoglobin of at least 10 g/100 ml of blood is the preferred level before institution of weaning measures.[3] In addition, a hematocrit of 38% to 42% should be established before weaning. An optimal hematocrit and hemoglobin will minimize the demands for increased cardiac output during weaning. This is particularly important for the patient with heart failure who has compromised myocardial performance.[26]

Fluid balance. Hypervolemia or hypovolemia may limit the success of weaning. As stated earlier, fluid retention is a frequent complication of positive pressure ventilation. Hypovolemia may occur for many reasons, including the overuse of diuretics. Careful attention must be given to the patient's fluid balance before weaning. This may be especially important in the patient with congestive heart failure when relatively small alterations in fluid levels have significant hemodynamic effects.

Fever. Oxygen consumption and carbon dioxide production are both increased in the febrile state. It may also indicate infection or sepsis. Ideally, the patients should be normothermic during the weaning process.

Provision for adequate rest. Sleep deprivation is common in critical care settings, particularly for mechanically ventilated patients requiring attention to their airway 24 hours a day. The period of weaning should commence when the patient is adequately rested and has the energy required for spontaneous breathing. This is usually during the daytime.

Medications. Sedatives and paralyzing agents

should be held before weaning, and narcotics should be used cautiously because of their respiratory depressant effects. However, patients with severe pain usually do not tolerate weaning well, and judicious use of analgesics may be indicated in this case.

Acid-base balance. Both metabolic alkalemia and acidemia can compromise weaning by the ventilatory effort to achieve respiratory compensation. Metabolic alkalemia may cause hypoventilation, and metabolic acidemia may cause hyperventilation as compensatory mechanisms. Correction of any underlying metabolic abnormalities is important before an attempt at weaning.

Monitoring the weaning process. The weaning process should be guided by arterial blood gases. ABG samples should be obtained after the first 15 to 20 minutes or sooner if indicated. If weaning must be terminated because of patient distress, this should be documented by ABGs just before placing the patient back on the ventilator.

The F_{IO_2} requirement is generally increased by 10% during weaning because of the usual drop in tidal volume. In general, weaning should not begin until the patient is able to adequately oxygenate with an F_{IO_2} of 0.4 or below while on the ventilator.[3] If the patient was on PEEP, he or she should be weaned to 5 to 8 cm before weaning from the ventilator. This is done by decreasing the PEEP 2 cm at a time and checking blood gases after each adjustment.

During weaning the ECG should be monitored continuously to detect early myocardial irritability. The most common cause of arrhythmias during weaning is transient bouts of hypoxia.[20] Vital signs and hemodynamic parameters should be recorded every 5 to 10 minutes until stable, with frequent checks throughout the weaning period.

The following factors have been identified as indications for termination of weaning and resuming ventilatory support:

1. A rise or fall in blood pressure of 20 mm Hg systolic or 10 mm Hg diastolic
2. An increase in pulse rate of 20 beats per minute or greater
3. An increase in respiratory rate of 10 respirations per minute or greater or a rate greater than 30 respirations per minute
4. A tidal volume less than 250 to 300 ml
5. Significant ECG changes
6. Pao_2 less than 60 mm Hg
7. $Paco_2$ greater than 55 mm Hg
8. pH less than 7.35
9. $AaDo_2$ greater than 400 mm Hg
10. Pulmonary capillary wedge or left atrial pressure above 20 mm Hg
11. Cardiac index less than 1.9 L/minute/m²

Patient consideration during weaning. Confidence and cooperation on the part of the patient are imperative in the weaning process. The purpose and methods of weaning must be carefully explained to the individual. It may be wise to explain to the patient that the weaning is a "trial" for breathing alone so he or she will not become unnecessarily frustrated should the first attempt fail. The patient should be in the upright position if possible to allow for maximal chest expansion and diaphragmatic excursions. Deep breaths should be encouraged frequently. The nurse's presence and encouragement can be a factor in decreasing the apprehension and doubt experienced by the patient and may add to the success of the weaning process.

Care of the intubated patient. Since all patients receiving mechanical ventilation are intubated or have a tracheostomy, much of the care of these individuals is devoted to the maintenance of the artificial airway. This includes maintenance of patency, removal of secretions, and prevention of infection.

Careful attention must be paid to positioning of the patient and the ventilator circuit to avoid kinking of the tubing and occlusion of the airway. Ventilator high-pressure limit alarms must be on at all times to alert the clinician to increasing airway pressures that may be associated with kinking of the tube or accumulation of secretions.

Since intubated patients are unable to clear their airways of secretions, the clinician must suction these secretions intermittently. This should be done observing strict aseptic technique and only when secretions are present, in order to minimize tracheal trauma and infection. In addition to clearing the airway of secretions, suctioning removes gases from the airways and alveoli. For this reason arterial oxygen tension may drop precipitously during suctioning because of the removal of alveolar oxygen. To prevent this hypoxemia from occurring, the patient's airways should be hyperoxygenated before the procedure with either an Ambu bag connected to an oxygen source or extra breaths or signs delivered by the ventilator with an increased F_{IO_2}. Suction should never be applied for more than 10 seconds at a time. The hyperoxygenation procedure should be repeated after each suction aspiration and before replacing the patient on the ventilator. Adherence to these guidelines will aid in the reduction of hypoxemia and tracheal trauma associated with suctioning.

While intubated, patients are denied their normal protective mechanisms of air filtration and therefore are susceptible to pulmonary infections. To prevent this complication, adherence to strict sterile technique during suctioning or handling of the airway or ventilator circuit is essential. The ventilator tubing should be changed daily. In addition, frequent changes of the patient's position and chest physiotherapy will aid in mobilization of secretions and prevention of pulmonary infection.

A very important factor in the care of the intubated person involves psychological support and assistance in communication. These areas are dealt with in depth later in this chapter.

ADVERSE EFFECTS OF OXYGEN THERAPY—TOXICITY

Oxygen is frequently classified as a drug and, like other pharmacological agents, has potential side effects.[6] There is a limited range for effective dosage and if the amount delivered falls below or exceeds this range, the therapy will be ineffective or may cause adverse effects. The patient with congestive heart failure is hypoxic and thereby requires oxygen in a sufficient amount to correct the deficit. Because the individual often is acutely ill and in dire need of oxygen therapy, there is a greater potential for delivery of excess amounts.

Oxygen toxicity could be described as a syndrome that results from prolonged exposure to high tensions of oxygen and affects the lung, central nervous system, retina, hematopoietic system, and endocrine organs. The effects of excess exposure to oxygen on the pulmonary structures and function have been most thoroughly studied.[17,27] Most of the studies have been conducted on animal models.

Factors affecting the development of oxygen toxicity

There are three factors that affect the toxicity of oxygen: (1) host tolerance, (2) effective dose, and (3) duration of exposure.[27]

Host tolerance could be defined as the susceptibility of the individual to develop oxygen toxicity. This can be influenced by some of the modifying factors discussed in the following paragraphs.

Effective dose refers to the F_{IO_2} required to raise and maintain the PaO_2 to the level safe for the patient.

Duration of exposure is the length of time the patient is receiving an F_{IO_2} of 50% to 60% or above. An F_{IO_2} above 90% is frequently lethal within 3 to 4 days.[35]

There is some evidence that suggests that the use of steroids may accelerate the development of oxygen toxicity. Other factors that have been implicated in increasing the chance of oxygen toxicity are hypothermia and the use of epinephrine and thyroid hormones. Factors that may decrease oxygen toxicity are hypothermia, antioxidants, anesthesia, and intermittent exposure. The method of intermittent exposure may prove to be a very practical approach to extending the length of oxygen tolerance. Gradually increasing the F_{IO_2} over several days or intermittently administering a much lower F_{IO_2} will allow the lungs to acclimatize or adapt to the toxic effects of oxygen.[27,40]

Another very important modifier is the preexposure state of the lung. Oxygen toxicity is observed less frequently in individuals with severe pulmonary disease. It has been postulated that this may be caused by the earlier removal of Type I alveolar cells, the cells that are most sensitive to oxygen. With the loss of Type I cells in the lining of the alveolus, there is a proliferation of Type II cells, which appear to be relatively resistant to high oxygen concentrations. Therefore these individuals may be more resistant to the development of oxygen toxicity during excess exposure to oxygen.[14,27]

The other two factors that are under clinical control are the dosage level of oxygen and the duration of exposure.[21] High-dosage levels for a brief period can produce toxicity; low levels for a prolonged period can also be toxic. If possible, oxygen therapy should be administered with levels of less than 60% to 100% and should be maintained for less than 2 days.[35,40]

Clinical picture

The development of oxygen toxicity can be divided into two clinical stages: the early phase affects the larger airways and is called the exudative stage, the later phase affects the alveoli and is referred to as the proliferation stage.[8,14,27,40] The exudative changes of the first stage are reversible if corrections are made in the high level of oxygen exposure. If the proliferative stage has been reached, it is unlikely that complete recovery will occur and permanent scarring of the lung will be present. Few survive once interstitial fibrosis has occurred (Table 9-4).[14]

PSYCHOSOCIAL IMPLICATIONS OF REQUIRED OXYGEN THERAPY

The patient who requires supplemental oxygen may have one or several problems dependent upon such variables as the method of oxygen delivery being used, severity of clinical conditions, and physical environment of the patient. The patient problems can fit into five general categories: noncompliance with therapy because of physical discomfort or lack of understanding of its rationale, alteration in communication and isolation, fear and anxiety, powerlessness and dependency, and sensory alteration. These potential problems will be reviewed along with a discussion of clinical interventions.

Noncompliance with therapy because of physical discomfort or insufficient understanding of treatment rationale

Noncompliance with therapy may occur with the patient who is utilizing a nasal cannula or face mask as well as with the intubated person. Long-term use of the nasal cannula may produce pressure sores about the nares. The discomfort of a face mask is compounded by the accumulation of moisture and increased sense of heat about the face as well as a sense of suffocation that many individuals experience. As a result, patients may refuse to wear the cannula or mask. Patients who are in

Table 9-4. Clinical indicators of pulmonary oxygen toxicity

Site	Exudative (early) stage*	Proliferative (late) stage†
Airways	Tracheal irritation in area of carina, cough, nasal stuffiness, substernal discomfort, pain on inspiration	Tracheobronchitis Bronchopneumonia
Pulmonary function	Reduced vital capacity, functional residual capacity and compliance; shunting, no change in alveolar-arterial O_2 gradient ($AaDo_2$)	Decreased expiratory flow rate and diffusing capacity; increased P_{AaO_2}
Chest radiogram	No change seen	Diffuse patchy infiltrates bilaterally progressing to complete opacification (end stage)

*Occurs after 1 to 4 days.
†Occurs after 4 days, most marked on twelfth day of exposure.

heart failure and early pulmonary edema may already be experiencing significant dyspnea and a sense of suffocation, and adding the mask to their face magnifies the problem. It is a real challenge to enlist the cooperation of the patient in keeping the face mask in place. Obviously, reassuring the individuals and informing them of the benefits of the mask, particularly its ability to deliver higher concentrations of oxygen, should be a primary consideration. Similar but more serious problems may occur with the patient who is intubated. Discomfort caused by the presence of the tube in the throat may be sufficient cause for individuals to make several attempts to extubate themselves. When possible, explaining to the individuals the necessity of the tube and the problems that may occur as a result of excessive movement of the neck or from attempts at extubating themselves helps in gaining cooperation. Restraining the person, which may cause further agitation, or sedation, which may lead to respiratory depression, are measures that should be used as a last resort.

Alteration in communication and isolation

The individual requiring oxygen therapy, with the exception of the patient using a nasal cannula, will experience some obstacle to verbal communication. The person utilizing a mask will need to speak very loudly and clearly to overcome the muffling effect that occurs when speaking through a mask. This may be difficult for the individual, who is undoubtedly working harder to obtain adequate oxygen. It is important for caregivers to acknowledge the individuals difficulty in communicating and exhibit patience in dealing with their expressions of needs. It is also advisable to instruct visitors of the importance of the patient keeping the mask in place.

Offering individuals who are intubated various methods of communication will assist them in coping with the illness and will maintain contact with others and reality. There are several methods that may be used to assist the person in communicating: written communication, hand or sign language, visual aids, and lip-reading.[24]

For written communication the caregiver provides the patient with a means for writing, for example, a clipboard with a felt-tip pen attached by string or a Magic-Slate board. The felt-tip pen requires less pressure to write. Securing the pen to the board with a string prevents loss in a busy environment. In order for both devices to be used, the individual must have freedom of hand movement and have sufficient strength, coordination, vision, and mental alertness. If the person is too weak to write, an alternative method is tracing the letters with a finger on the palm of another's hand.

Other techniques for communcating include the use of hand or sign language or visual aids such as the alphabet printed on a cardboard, language cards, or lists of common requests and needs. An important consideration with the use of visual aids is adequate vision and providing eyeglasses if indicated.

A more difficult and sometimes frustrating technique is having the person form the words with his lips. This has the advantage of not requiring any extra devices and therefore is a method always usable. Unfortunately, it cannot be easily used by the individual who has an oral endotracheal tube. The weak person will be less likely to form words as clearly since this method does involve the use of facial and throat muscles. The following suggestions enhance one's ability to lip-read:

Make sure adequate light is focused on the person's mouth and face.

Be attentive to gestures and facial expressions.

Have the person mouth the complete sentence so the words are received in context.

Ask patients to identify the category of their request or statement, such as something to do with their endotracheal tube, a particular part of their body, or bed position.[24]

The individual may experience a sense of isolation because of the significantly reduced communication abilities. Spending time with the person, particularly when care is not being administered, may lessen this feeling. Individuals will be reassured that sufficient time is being given to them rather than to the mechanical devices. The mere presence of a person at the bedside and the frequent use of touch will lessen the sense of isolation. Making sure that the call bell or some other signaling device is within reach at all times is very important and easily overlooked in a critical care environment.

Fear and anxiety

Anxiety resulting from a sense of one's life being dependent on a machine can be reduced by first making sure that the ventilator is functioning adequately and thus reducing the sounding of alarms and any breathing difficulty the individual experiences. Instructing individuals as soon as they are able to receive information about placement of the endotracheal tube, the functioning of the ventilator, and the role it is playing in assisting breathing may help decrease anxiety and gain cooperation. The use of diagrams to illustrate placement of the endotracheal tube and the explanation of why it interferes with speech and why it is necessary to remain quiet may also be useful. Keeping the patients informed of their progress, particularly if they are beginning to assist the ventilator when arterial blood gases are improving, may lessen the feeling of dependence and associated anxiety.

Powerlessness and dependency

There are additional concerns for the psychological well-being of individuals who are intubated. These people frequently feel that their lives are dependent on the ventilator and have difficulty expressing concern. They are dependent on others to meet basic physical needs and are also hampered by vocal difficulty expressing those needs. The expression of fear, anxiety, anger, and frustration is particularly difficult. Emotional expressions are usually communicated by nonverbal methods. Anger may be expressed by uncooperative behavior and refusal of treatment. Anxiety may appear as restlessness, tachycardia, and tremors. To reduce the sense of powerlessness that intubated patients may experience, several choices may be offered to allow them situational and environ-

mental control; for example, patients may be allowed to decide when to bathe or perform other personal hygiene activities, where to place personal effects, or, if feasible, when to receive sedation or pain medication.

Sensory alteration

Disorientation or misperception of reality may occur as a consequence of the increased amount of abnormal stimuli and the reduction in normal sensory input characteristic of a critical care setting. Sleep is frequently interrupted by such noxious stimuli as suctioning, equipment alarms, or the sounds of other patients. It is well within the realm of nursing's jurisdiction to provide a more therapeutic milieu by reducing these annoying interruptions. At the same time, activities that increase the patient's reality orientation should be encouraged and supported. Some methods include allowing visitors to spend time at the bedside and encouraging them to keep the patients informed of activities and events in their lives outside of the hospital, providing music or the use of a television, and allowing them to use familiar personal items such as their own toilet articles.

Health Care Plan—An Application of Concepts

A discussion of oxygen therapy for the patient with congestive heart failure would be incomplete without addressing the topic of hypoxia and its ramifications on the health care and management of this patient population. It is important to have a good grasp of the pathophysiology of heart failure and the role oxygen therapy plays in its treatment. Interpreting arterial blood gas results accurately is but one part of therapy. Understanding the potential physiological and psychological adverse effects of oxygen is also important. Because oxygen can be administered in many ways, it presents a variety of potential problems. It is vital to understand how to approach and manage oxygen therapy and these attendant problems when delivering care to the patient in heart failure. The following care plans summarize the salient points.

Text continued on p. 324.

HEALTH CARE PLAN—OXYGEN THERAPY FOR ACUTE HEART FAILURE

A 62-year-old male with a history of chronic congestive heart failure came to the emergency room in acute pulmonary edema with signs of myocardial infarction. He was intubated in the emergency room for severe hypoxemia and hypercapnia. He was admitted to the cardiac care unit. Ventilatory support was provided by an MA-I volume ventilator with an Fi_{O_2} of 60%. His blood gases on admission were the following: pH 7.24, P_{CO_2} 60, P_{O_2} 50, HCO_3 26, BE −2, O_2 saturation 82%. He is now in sinus tachycardia at a rate of 130 with frequent ventricular ectopic beats. Blood pressure is 92/64, respiratory rate is 30. Color is ashen with cool and clammy skin. Auscultation reveals rales bilaterally over lower half of both lung fields. He is alert and appears extremely anxious, requiring soft restraints on both arms to prevent self-extubation.

Potential problem	Nursing diagnosis	Interventions
1. Persistent hypoxia	Impaired gas exchange Ineffective airway clearance Ineffective breathing pattern	Maintain patent airway by appropriate suctioning. Hyperoxygenate before and after suctioning. Maintain proper position of tubing to prevent kinking. Maintain proper body positioning to allow for adequate expansion. Turn patient every 1 to 2 hours. Monitor ABGs and breath sounds. Check ventilator for proper settings.

2. Tissue trauma secondary to excessive movement of the endotracheal tube.	Same as above	Explain to patient (with use of diagrams if appropriate):
		    Placement of tube
		    Purpose and necessity of tube
		    Necessity of minimizing excessive neck movement
		Support tubing and maintain in proper alignment.
		Use soft restraints as indicated.
		Administer minimal sedation if necessary.

HEALTH CARE PLAN—OXYGEN THERAPY FOR ACUTE HEART FAILURE—cont'd

Potential problem	Nursing diagnosis	Interventions
3. Pulmonary infection	Same as above	Use sterile suctioning technique.
		Change ventilator tubing daily.
		Administer frequent oral hygiene.
		Reposition every 1 to 2 hours to mobilize secretions.
		Monitor characteristics of secretions. Note change in color, amount, consistency, and odor.
4. Oxygen toxicity	Same as above	Administer aggressive pulmonary care to ensure optimal benefits of $F_{I_{O_2}}$.
		Keep Pa_{O_2} level within patient's normal limits.
		Measure actual inspired oxygen content.
		Reduce $F_{I_{O_2}}$ to 0.5 or less as early as possible.
		Consider use of PEEP to obtain adequate oxygenation.
5. Unable to verbally communicate; unable to express needs	Impaired verbal communication	Use alternative methods of communication, e.g., magic-slate board, pen and paper, lip reading, sign language, visual aids.
		Provide patient time for expression of needs and emotions.
6. Limited visitors; limited communication with significant others	Social isolation	Spend time at bedside in addition to administering physical care.
		Encourage visitors to spend time at bedside.

Continued.

HEALTH CARE PLAN—OXYGEN THERAPY FOR ACUTE HEART FAILURE—cont'd

Potential problem	Nursing diagnosis	Interventions
7. Frequent physiological monitoring; frequent repositioning; frequent treatments; frequent physical exams; noisy, unfamiliar environment; periodic use of narcotics; hypoxia	Sensory perceptual alteration Sleep pattern disturbance	Plan care to allow for periods of uninterrupted rest. Orient patient to surroundings frequently. Reduce environmental noise as much as possible, particularly during periods of sleep. Establish patterns of usual day-night routine. Provide pleasant sensory input when possible, e.g., familiar objects from homes, music, or TV. Allow visitors at bedside as appropriate.
8. Inability to control environment; physical dependence; loss of control of respiratory function; altered cognitive process secondary to hypoxia	Powerlessness Anxiety	Provide explanations to patient and family about acute condition, procedures, and therapy. Include patient in planning of care. Reassure patient that the endotracheal tube placement is temporary and that he will be able to speak after its removal. Spend time with patient when not administering care; provide emotional support.

HEALTH CARE PLAN—OXYGEN THERAPY FOR CHRONIC CONGESTIVE HEART FAILURE

Mr. X was treated with diuretics and nitrates in the CCU. His ventilatory status improved, and he was extubated on the second hospital day. His blood gases on room air are the following: pH 7.48, P_{CO_2} 33, P_{O_2} 50, HCO_3 24, BE +1, O_2 saturation 82%. Discharge is anticipated with indications that home oxygen will be necessary, in addition to pharmacological and diet therapy. This will be part of the treatment regimen because of this patient's cardiac status, which reflects chronic severe heart failure.

Potential problem	Nursing diagnosis	Interventions
1. Insufficient understanding of home oxygen use	Home maintenance management: potential for knowledge deficit: Oxygen administration Safety precautions Side effects	Assess patient's and family's level of knowledge. Instruct patient according to identified needs. Assess need for follow-up home care and make referral if indicated. Refer to physical therapy for breathing training. Refer to occupational therapy for instruction in energy conservation to minimize dependency.
2. Skin breakdown because of cannula and elastic strap	Potential for impairment of skin injury	Instruct patient to pad pressure areas with cotton. Apply lubricant to cannula to decrease irritation of nares.
3. Inability to administer oxygen according to therapeutic directives	Potential for noncompliance with oxygen therapy	Instruct patient and family about importance of oxygen. Assist patient and family in coping with emotional reactions to long-term oxygen use. Provide written directions regarding administration, safety measures, and side effects of oxygen. Provide outside resource to reinforce information and answer questions.

SUMMARY

This chapter has presented a view of the general physiological effects of hypoxia and the specific effects on pulmonary vasculature and myocardium. It discusses oxygen as a primary drug in the treatment of heart failure and elaborates on the route of administration, indications for use, monitoring techniques, dosage, side effects, and complications.

This material delineates the essentials in patient assessment of oxygen need in the setting of heart failure, addresses the major psychological problems associated with oxygen therapy, and discusses rationale and specific clinical interventions. In closing, a health care plan is presented to operationalize the major concepts set forth in the chapter.

REFERENCES

1. Allen, C.B.: Just breathing, Nursing '74 **4:**23, 1974.
2. Biddle, T.L.: Hemodynamic concepts in treating acute pulmonary edema, South. Med. J., **70**(11):415, 1977.
3. Bowser, M.H., Hodgkin, J.E., and Burton, G.G.: Techniques of ventilator weaning. In Burton, G.G., and others, editors: Respiratory care, Philadelphia, 1977, J.B. Lippincott Co.
4. Brooks, R.A.: Mechanical ventilation. In Morrison, M.L., editor: Respiratory intensive care nursing, ed. 2, Boston, 1979, Little, Brown & Co.
5. Broughton, J.O.: Understanding blood gases, Rep. No. 456, 1971, Ohio Medical Products.
6. Burke, L.E.: Drugs commonly used in the cardiac care unit. In Underhill, S., and others, editors: Cardiac nursing, Philadelphia, 1982, J.B. Lippincott Co.
7. Bushnell, L.S.: Physiology of the respiratory system. In Morrison, M.L., editor: Respiratory intensive care nursing, ed. 2, Boston, 1979, Little, Brown & Co.
8. Bushnell, L.S., and Brooks, R.A.: Oxygen therapy. In Morrison, M.L., editor: Respiratory intensive care nursing, ed. 2, Boston, 1979, Little, Brown & Co.
9. Butler, E.K.: Dyspnea in the patient with cardiopulmonary disease, Heart Lung **4**(4):599, 1975.
10. Caldwell, S.L., and Sullivan, K.N.: Important interpersonal and interprofessional relationships in the delivery of successful patient care. In Burton, G.G., and others, editors: Respiratory care, Philadelphia, 1977, J.B. Lippincott Co.
11. Caprio, G.S., and Riley, M.A.: The mechanically ventilated patient. In Morrison, M.L., editor: Respiratory intensive care nursing, ed. 2, Boston, 1979, Little, Brown & Co.
12. Caprio G.S., and Riley, M.A.: Weaning from mechanical ventilation. In Morrison, M.L., editor: Respiratory intensive care nursing, ed. 2, Boston, 1979, Little, Brown & Co.
13. Coglman, M.M.: Effects of oxygen on ischemic myocardium, Heart Lung **7**(4):635, 1978.
14. Egan, D.F.: Fundamentals of respiratory therapy, ed. 3, St. Louis, 1977, The C.V. Mosby Co.
15. Englberg, S.: Understanding blood gases, Crit. Care Update **6**(7):39, 1979.
16. Fitzgerald, L.M.: Mechanical ventilation, Heart Lung **5**(6):939, 1976.
17. Frank, L., and Massare, D.: The lung and oxygen toxicity, Arch. Intern. Med. **139:**347, 1979.
18. Fulop, M., and others: Lactic acidosis in pulmonary edema due to left ventricular failure, Ann. Intern. Med. **79**(2):173, 1972.
19. Guyton, A.C.: Textbook of medical physiology, ed. 3, Philadelphia, 1971, W.B. Saunders Co., p. 265.
20. Hodgkin, J.E., Bowser, M.S., and Burton, G.G.: Techniques of weaning in respiratory care: a guide to clinical practice. In Burton, G.G., Gee, G.N., and Hodgkin, J.E., editors: Respiratory care: a guide to clinical practice, Philadelphia, 1977, J.B. Lippincott Co.
21. Holloway, N.M.: Nursing the critically ill adult, Menlo Park, Calif., 1979, Addison-Wesley Publishing Co., Inc.
22. Johnson, R.A.: Heart failure. In Johnson, R.A., and others, editors: The practice of cardiology, Boston, 1980, Little, Brown & Co.
23. Kirby, R.R., and others: Mechanical ventilation. In Burton, G.G., and others, editors: Respiratory care: a guide to clinical practice, Philadelphia, 1977, J.B. Lippincott Co.
24. Lawless, C.A.: Helping patients with endotracheal and tracheostomy tubes communicate, Am. J. Nurs. **75**(12):2151, 1975.
25. McGurn, W.C.: Congestive heart failure. In McGurn, W.L., editor: Nursing concepts, Philadelphia, 1981, J.B. Lippincott Co.
26. McNabb, T.G., and Hall, S.V.: Weaning from respiratory support, Int. Anesthesiol. Clin. **14:**1, 214, 1976.
27. Menn, S.J., and Tisi, G.M.: Oxygen as a drug: chemical properties, benefits, and hazards of administration. In Burton, G.G., and others, editors: Respiratory care: a guide to clinical practice, Philadelphia, 1977, J.B. Lippincott Co.
28. Michaelson, C.R.: Bedside assessment and diagnosis of acute left ventricular failure, Crit. Care Q. **4**(3):1, 1981.
29. Powner, D.J., and Eross, B.: O_2 therapy for the adult patient, Postgrad. Med. **70**(4):223, 1981.
30. Schlant, R.C.: Metabolism of the heart. In Hurst, J.W., and others, editors: The heart, ed. 4, New York, 1978, McGraw-Hill, Inc.

31. Schrake, K.: The ABC's of ABG's, Nursing '79 **9**(9):26, 1979.

32. Shapiro, B.A., Harrison, R.A., and Walton, J.R.L.: Clinical application of blood gases, ed. 2, Chicago, 1977, Year Book Medical Publishers, Inc.

33. Staub, N.C.: Pulmonary edema—physiologic approaches to management, Chest **74**(5):559, 1978.

34. Sylversten, W.A., and McNalley, M.: Acute myocardial infarction and congestive heart failure. In Burton, G.G., and others, editors: Respiratory care: a guide to clinical practice, Philadelphia, 1977, J.B. Lippincott Co.

35. Tierney, D.F.: Oxygen toxicity, West Med. **190**(3):227, 1979.

36. Walters, W.C.: Disturbances of inorganic metabolism in heart failure. In Hurst, J.W., and others, editors: The heart, ed. 4, New York, 1978, McGraw-Hill, Inc.

37. Wenger, N.K., Hurst, J.W., and McIntyre, M.G.: Cardiology for nurses, New York, 1980, McGraw-Hill Inc.

38. West, J.B.: Pulmonary pathophysiology—the essentials, Baltimore, 1977, The Williams & Wilkins Co.

39. Ziment, I.: Intermittent positive pressure breathing. In Burton, G.G., and others, editors: Respiratory care: a guide to clinical practice, Philadelphia, 1977, J.B. Lippincott Co.

40. Ziment, I.: Respiratory gases. In Burton, G.G., and others, editors: Respiratory care: a guide to clinical practice, Philadelphia, 1977, J.B. Lippincott Co.

CHAPTER 10

Mechanical support of the failing heart

LESLIE FLICKINGER KERN

ROLE OF MECHANICAL DEVICES IN CONGESTIVE HEART FAILURE

Braunwald has described three approaches to the treatment of the patient with heart failure: (1) remove the underlying cause with medical or surgical treatment, (2) remove the precipitating cause by treating any anemia, arrhythmias, or other medical problems, and (3) control the heart failure state by improving pumping performance, reducing the heart's workload, and controlling excessive salt and water retention.[2]

The use of mechanical devices to aid in the treatment of heart failure falls under the third approach, because all devices reduce the cardiac afterload work of the heart. This reduces the pressure against which the heart must pump. Relief of pressure ultimately decreases myocardial wall tension and myocardial oxygen consumption.

Mechanical devices are usually tried as treatment for the patient with intractable heart failure, after all medical approaches have been exhausted. They are viewed as special, life-support measures that are used selectively in patients who have hope for sufficient recovery or improvement in the quality of life.

Devices and indications

The *intra-aortic balloon pump* (IABP) is a counterpulsation device that assists the failing heart by decreasing afterload and increasing coronary artery perfusion.

The IAPB consists of a sausage-shaped balloon that is passed through the common femoral artery into the descending aorta (Figs. 10-1 and 10-2). It is positioned so that it lies inferior to the left subclavian artery and superior to the renal arteries. The balloon itself is made of polyurethane and comes in various sizes, from 10 cc volumes up to 40 cc volumes. Externally it is attached to a power console, which inflates and deflates the balloon with helium or carbon dioxide gas.

The balloon pumping is timed with the electrocardiogram (ECG) or arterial waveform so that it inflates with diastole and deflates with systole. It is commonly used for 24 to 48 hours and then the patient is weaned. On occasion, it has been used for several months.

Although left ventricular failure and cardiogenic shock are the primary indications for the IABP, other indications include mitral regurgitation, unstable angina, postinfarction angina, refractory ventricular arrhythmias, poor preoperative ventricular function, inability to wean from bypass following cardiac surgery, and low cardiac output syndrome following cardiac surgery.[11]

The *left ventricular assist device* (LVAD) is a second mechanical device used to assist the failing heart. It is a grenade-shaped device that diverts the blood from the left ventricle and pumps it into the ascending thoracic aorta (Fig. 10-3). By doing this, the left ventricle is almost totally relieved of its workload. The LVAD closely approximates normal hemodynamic parameters by producing a stroke volume of 85 ml/minute, an ejection fraction of 75%, and a heart rate of 100 beats per minute.[3] It can support circulation for a few days

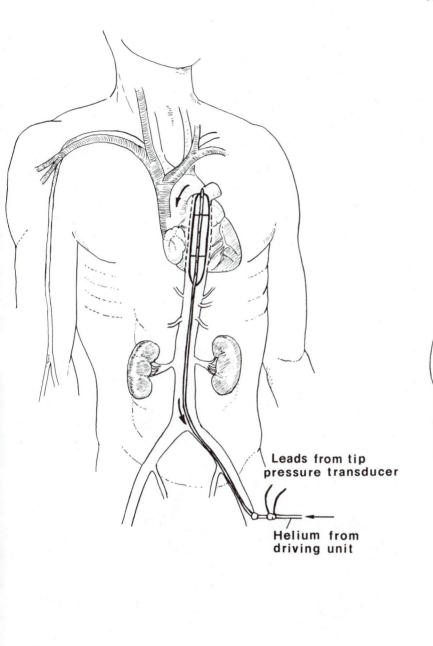

Leads from tip
pressure transducer

Helium from
driving unit

Fig. 10-1. Location of IAPB in body. (Adapted from Lane, C.: Am. J. Nurs. **69:**1655 Aug., 1969.)

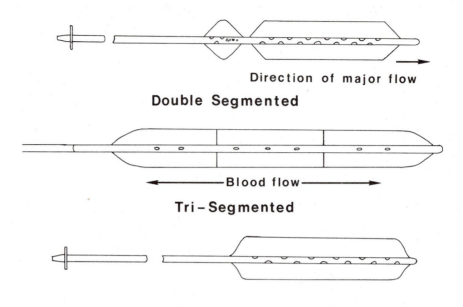

Direction of major flow

Double Segmented

Blood flow

Tri–Segmented

Single Chamber

Fig. 10-2. Schematic representation of three types of balloons used for intra-aortic counterpulsation.

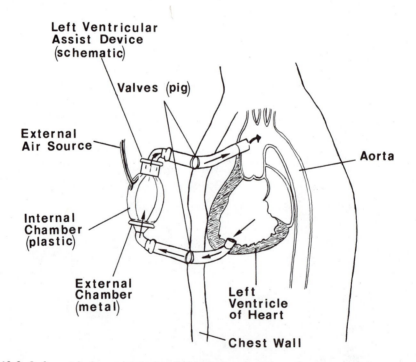

Fig. 10-3. Left ventricular assist device (LVAD) sits on chest wall and pumps blood from left ventricle of heart to aorta, allow heart to mend. (Adapted from McNamara, L.J.: Centerscope Magazine.)

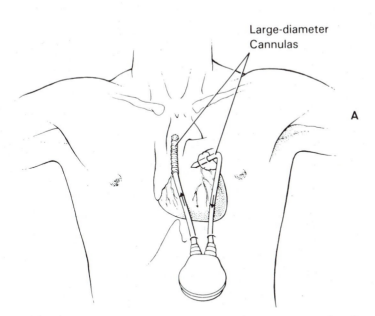

Large-diameter
Cannulas

A

Fig. 10-4. A, ALVAD can be attached to ascending aorta as elliptical device. **B,** Cutaway illustration of interior of left ventricular assist device. (**A** from Pierce, W.S., and Myers, J.L.: J. Cardiovasc. Med. **6**[7]:671, July 1981; **B** from Unger, F.: Assisted circulation, Heidelberg, Germany, 1979, Springer-Verlag.)

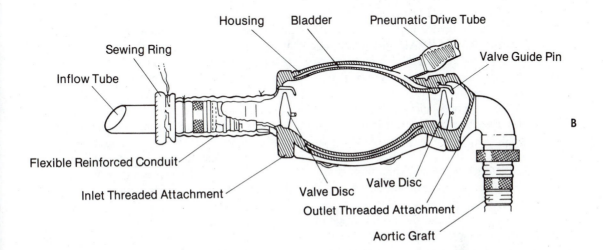

Housing Bladder Pneumatic Drive Tube

Sewing Ring Valve Guide Pin

Inflow Tube

B

Flexible Reinforced Conduit

Inlet Threaded Attachment Valve Disc Valve Disc

Outlet Threaded Attachment

Aortic Graft

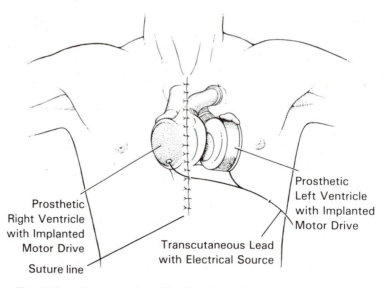

Fig. 10-5. Artist's rendering of implantable totally artificial heart (TAH).

or a few weeks while the damaged left ventricle rests.

Two types of left ventricular assist devices are available: a short-term, external device and a long-term, implantable device. The latter is also known as the abdominal left-ventricular assist device (ALVAD) and requires surgical insertion (Fig. 10-4). In addition to the left ventricular assist devices, there is also a right ventricular assist device (RVAD) and a biventricular assist device (BVAD). The RVAD and BVAD are utilized less often than the LVAD but have been found to be beneficial in the patient with right ventricular or biventricular failure.[3]

The LVAD is a pneumatically (air) powered pump. A cannula in the ventricular apex diverts the blood to the device, which may be inside or outside the body (Figs. 10-3 and 10-4, *B*). Blood is then pumped into the ascending aorta through the inflow cannula. The major portion of the pump is a smooth polyurethane sac that is enclosed in a hard case. The air is pumped into the case, outside of the sac, where it compresses the blood in the distended sac. A pneumatic power unit, similar to an IABP console, is used to drive the air in and out of the assist device.

The ALVAD, which is used for long-term therapy, is somewhat different in concept compared with the LVAD. The abdominal device must be implanted surgically. Blood is received from the left ventricular apex and pumped into the abdominal aorta below the renal arteries. Its placement in the abdomen prevents pulmonary complications that could occur with thoracic placement, and it provides easy access for removal. It is a true intracorporeal blood pump—one within the body. It is also pneumatically driven and has a small tube that passes through the skin to the power source.

Heart assist devices are used primarily for the patient who has undergone cardiac surgery and has severe postoperative heart failure. In these cases standard methods of treatment are usually tried first: correction of metabolic derangements, longer time on cardiopulmonary bypass, use of inotropic agents, use of afterload reducing agents, and use of the IABP.[11] Other indications for use include postinfarction cardiogenic shock, irreversible cardiomyopathies, acute toxic myocarditis with cardiogenic shock, severe left ventricular failure associated with rheumatic valve disease, and bacterial endocarditis. Whatever the use, the goal is to maintain a cardiac index at 2.5 L/minute/m² or

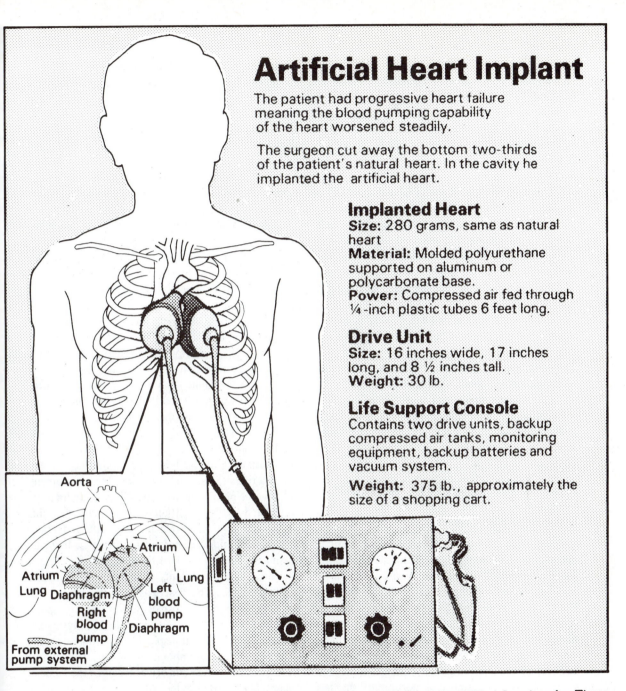

Artificial Heart Implant

The patient had progressive heart failure meaning the blood pumping capability of the heart worsened steadily.

The surgeon cut away the bottom two-thirds of the patient's natural heart. In the cavity he implanted the artificial heart.

Implanted Heart

Size: 280 grams, same as natural heart
Material: Molded polyurethane supported on aluminum or polycarbonate base.
Power: Compressed air fed through ¼-inch plastic tubes 6 feet long.

Drive Unit

Size: 16 inches wide, 17 inches long, and 8 ½ inches tall.
Weight: 30 lb.

Life Support Console

Contains two drive units, backup compressed air tanks, monitoring equipment, backup batteries and vacuum system.

Weight: 375 lb., approximately the size of a shopping cart.

Aorta
Atrium
Atrium
Lung
Lung
Diaphragm
Left blood pump
Right blood pump
Diaphragm
From external pump system

BOZENA SYSKA and GEORGE CAREY / Los Angeles Times

Fig. 10-6. Jarvik-7 artificial heart implant. The two ventricles are cut away as surgeons remove about two thirds of the heart. Two polyurethane cuffs are sewn into the atria, which serve as natural blood reservoirs—they no longer contract rhythmically. The ventricles are replaced with a two-chamber pump that is snapped onto the cuffs. The left chamber is attached to the aorta and the right chamber to the pulmonary artery. Two thin plastic tubes are brought out through the abdominal wall and are attached to an external air-pump driving system. (From Los Angeles Times, Dec. 3, 1982, part 1, p. 3.)

greater and a mean left atrial or pulmonary wedge pressure below 20 mm Hg. These values will ensure that there is adequate body tissue perfusion with the least amount of work being done by the heart. Studies have demonstrated that there is a definite need for heart assist devices. However, they continue to be under experimental investigation.

The *totally artificial heart* (TAH) (Fig. 10-5) is one of the more recent developments in mechanical devices for heart failure.[9,10] It is a man-made pump that is implanted in place of the heart. The TAH is typically made out of silicon, rubber, and Teflon. The majority of these hearts are air powered. However, some nuclear-powered hearts have been developed.

The TAH has been tested extensively in animal models and has recently been inserted in two human subjects. The first recent trial in 1981 was done as a temporary measure in a heart transplant candidate until a donor heart was available.[13] The second trial was performed in 1982 on a patient with refractory heart failure who was not a transplant candidate. In this subject the TAH was intended as a permanent implantable device (Fig. 10-6).

PHYSIOLOGICAL AND THEORETICAL CONCEPTS
Historical perspectives

Death from cardiogenic shock and low cardiac output following heart surgery prompted the search for a mechanical device that would temporarily assist the heart's pumping capabilities. In 1953 Kantrowitz discovered the benefits of counterpulsation and found that coronary artery blood flow could be enhanced by retarding systolic pressure and augmenting arterial diastolic pressure.[1] In 1958 McKinnon followed this concept in his dog experiments. He wrapped a portion of the left hemidiaphragm around the thoracic aorta, stimulated the phrenic nerve, and was able to augment aortic diastolic pressure. Clauss used a somewhat different approach in 1961. He synchronized blood withdrawal and infusion to reduce systolic pressure and augment diastolic pressure in dogs.[1]

It was in 1962 that the first intra-aortic balloon pump was used. Moulopoulos, Topaz, and Kolff developed a carbon dioxide–driven balloon that was prototype for the ones in use today.[1,6] Throughout the 1960s the device was limited to animal experiments, and in 1969 Kantrowitz reported his success with the device in 27 patients with cardiogenic shock.[2] Bregman and others quickly followed with studies to support its use, and by the early 1970s it became an accepted treatment modality for the patient with shock refractory to medical therapy. Since this time it has been used for the treatment and prevention of heart failure caused by myocardial infarction, cardiac surgery, cardiomyopathy, congenital heart disease, and valvular disease.

The development of an artificial heart was alluded to in a science fiction story of the early 1900s. In 1937, however, a Russian developed the first truly artificial heart which he implanted in dogs.[13] In the United States the value of an artificial heart was presented by Dr. Peter Salisbury in 1957 at a national heart conference in Los Angeles.[8] The following year Drs. Akutsu and Kolff reported on their experiments in dogs with their totally artificial heart. This prompted others to experiment, and the 1960s saw the development of several promising models. Clinical findings in dogs and calves in 1969 demonstrated that the TAH was clinically valuable and safe and associated with improved cardiac performance that can result in total recovery of the patient.

Three human implants have been done in the United States. The first was in 1969 before the FDA regulations on these devices were developed. The patient survived 3 days with the device but died 36 hours after transplant with a donor heart. The second human implant was in July 1981 when a 36-year-old Dutch bus driver received the Akutsu heart. This heart kept the patient alive for 30 hours while surgeons awaited a donor heart. The patient did receive the donor heart, but died 1 week later of renal and pulmonary failure.[13] The third implant of a federally approved device occurred on December 2, 1982 when a team of surgeons headed by Dr. William C. DeVries inserted the Jarvik-7 heart into a 61-year-old male subject with refractory heart failure. The 112-day survival of this individual with a TAH is the longest to date; however, the complicated course of this subject will require future reevaluation of these devices.

Principles of counterpulsation

The goal of balloon-pumping or counterpulsation is the interruption of those mechanisms that contribute to intractable heart failure. Ultimately the physician attempts to reverse the heart failure, but this is only possible when there is viable myocardial tissue. Fig. 10-7 reviews the positive feedback mechanisms that aggravate existing left ventricular failure and cardiogenic shock.

Decreased myocardial contractility is the initiating problem for the syndrome of heart failure. This decreased contractility may be caused by myocardial infarction, subendocardial ischemia during heart surgery, or other heart disease that diminishes the available contractile units. (see Chapter 3.) Contributing to the decreased contractility is a decreased coronary blood flow and an increased myocardial wall tension. The end result is decreased body and organ blood perfusion, anaerobic metabolism, and hypoxia. All of these feed back to cause further decreased contractility and increase heart failure. The intra-aortic balloon attempts to interrupt this feedback loop through the physiological mechanisms of diastolic augmentation and systolic unloading.

Diastolic augmentation is the first phase of balloon pumping (Fig. 10-8 *A*).[12] The balloon inflates just after aortic valve closure and remains inflated through diastole. It then deflates just before the beginning of systole. By inflating in diastole, the blood left in the aorta after ventricular ejection is displaced retrograde into the aortic root and brain

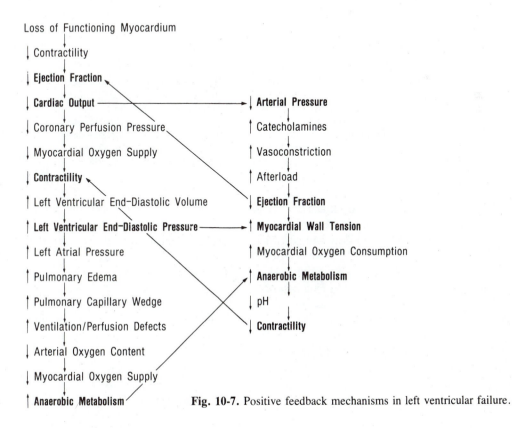

Fig. 10-7. Positive feedback mechanisms in left ventricular failure.

Diastolic Augmentation   Systolic Unloading

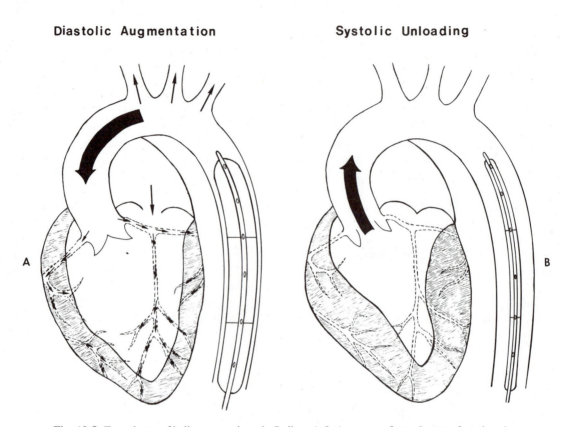

Fig. 10-8. Two phases of balloon pumping. **A,** *Balloon inflation* occurs from closure of aortic valve to end of diastole. Inflation causes retrograde flow of blood in aorta, increasing coronary perfusion pressure without an increase in myocardial work or oxygen demand. Inflation also causes antegrade flow, increasing mean arterial pressure, renal flow, and cerebral flow. **B,** *Balloon deflation* occurs from just before opening of aortic valve to closure of aortic valve. Deflation encourages antegrade flow, decreasing afterload or resistance to left ventricular ejection. Deflation also decreases oxygen required by left ventricle, shortens systolic ejection, and increases stroke volume.

and displaced antegrade to the renal arteries and body. The increased blood in the aortic root causes an increase in coronary blood flow and perfusion. In addition, it has been shown that this causes an increase in collateral coronary circulation.

The second phase of balloon pumping is systolic unloading. The balloon deflates just before the opening of the aortic valve and remains deflated during the ejection of blood into the aorta (Fig. 10-8, *B*). With deflation of the balloon, there is a potential space created in the aorta.[12] It has been suggested that this space created by balloon deflation produces a vacuum that encourages the for-

ward flow of blood out of the left ventricle. This allows the aortic valve to open at a lower pressure and the ventricle can then empty more efficiently against a decreased resistance or afterload. The effects of systolic unloading on the heart are decreased myocardial wall tension and decreased oxygen consumption.

In Fig. 10-7 it can be seen that the IABP interrupts the positive feedback loop at several points. With diastolic augmentation the myocardium receives increased blood flow and oxygen supply. Ischemic tissue is now supplied with oxygen, anaerobic metabolism is reversed, and this tissue

---

SUMMARY OF PHYSIOLOGICAL EFFECTS OF INTRA-AORTIC COUNTERPULSATION

↑ cardiac output

↓ left ventricular end-diastolic pressure

↓ mean right atrial pressure

↓ pulmonary artery pressure

↓ pulmonary vascular resistance

↓ systemic vascular resistance

↑ mean arterial pressure

↑ urinary output

↑ mental alertness

↑ peripheral perfusion

Table 10-1. Problems of timing the intra-aortic balloon

Problem	Consequences
Early inflation	Left ventricle contracts against balloon; causes a severe increase in afterload
Early deflation	Balloon deflates before end of diastole; coronary arteries do not receive full benefit of diastolic augmentation
Late inflation	Coronary arteries are deprived of full benefits of balloon inflation
Late deflation	Balloon remains inflated into ventricular systole and aortic valve cannot open, causes a severe increase in afterload

regains its contractility. The increase in functioning contractile units will contribute to an overall improvement in contraction and increased cardiac output.

Systolic unloading allows the heart to empty more efficiently with less myocardial wall tension. There is increased stroke volume, increased ejection fraction, and an increased cardiac output. This decreases the amount of blood left in the ventricle and results in decreased left ventricular end-diastolic volume and pressure. Pulmonary edema is diminished, arterial oxygenation is improved, and aerobic metabolism can resume in the myocardial and body tissues.

The combination of these therapeutic effects results in the clinical signs of increased mean arterial pressure (MAP), increased urine output, increased mental alertness, warm extremities with adequate perfusion, and improved breath sounds. The box above summarizes the physiological effects of intra-aortic counterpulsation.

The beneficial physiological effects have just been described. However, there can be four situations where the balloon timing is inaccurate and counterpulsation less than beneficial (Table 10-1). These four situations are early deflation, late deflation, early inflation, late inflation. In early deflation, the heart is in diastole, the balloon has inflated on time but deflates early. The effect of this is that the coronary arteries will not receive the full benefit of the diastolic augmentation. In addition, by deflating early the full impact of systolic unloading will not be received. The aortic space will begin to fill with blood and the "vacuum effect" removed. Some unloading will occur, but not as powerfully as would occur with correct timing.

In late deflation the balloon remains inflated into the beginning of systole (isovolumetric contraction phase) and exerts such a high pressure that the aortic valve is unable to open. This causes a substantial increase in myocardial wall tension and oxygen consumption as the heart tries to force blood out and open the aortic valve. This is a very dangerous situation that can lead to further myocardial failure.

Early inflation is another dangerous situation for the heart. If the balloon inflates too soon, the heart is in systole and the ventricle attempts to pump blood into the blocked aorta against a high pressure. This puts a tremendous workload on the heart and can lead to total heart failure or myocardial rupture.

Late inflation is yet another dangerous situation for the heart. The balloon inflates in the middle instead of the beginning of diastole. The result is that inflation time is diminished; the heart does not receive full benefits of diastolic augmentation. It is not a dangerous situation but presents less than optimal unloading effects from the balloon.

Physiological effects of left ventricular assist devices

The LVAD works primarily by reducing left ventricular preload and by reducing the impedance to flow out of the left ventricle (afterload). Reduction of preload is achieved as the blood is diverted from the left ventricle to the device. The diversion of blood away from the left ventricle causes a reduction in myocardial wall tension and a resultant decrease in myocardial oxygen consumption. The decreased volume also results in a decreased left atrial pressure and decreased pulmonary congestion. Fig. 10-7 shows how these effects interrupt the positive feedback cycle.

Reduction of afterload results from the mechanical pumping of the blood into the aorta. By taking over this function, the assist device allows the left ventricle to completely "rest." It no longer has to develop the wall tension or increased contractility to deliver the blood to the body. Because "pressure work" utilizes more oxygen than "volume work," there is a substantial decrease in myocardial oxygen consumption along with the decrease in wall tension. These effects combine to make oxygen more available to ischemic tissue. In comparison with the IABP, the LVAD has been shown to decrease left ventricular work by 90%, whereas the IABP only decreased it by 10%. It also decreased myocardial oxygen consumption (MVO_2) by 40% compared to 10% in the IABP.[8]

An increased cardiac output is achieved artificially with the assist device. It has been found that cardiac outputs of 6 to 8 L/minute can be provided. This is a substantial increase over the IABP, which can only improve the patient's underlying cardiac output by 500 to 800 ml/minute.[8]

Other benefits of the LVAD include (1) provision of partial or total support of the circulation, (2) improved myocardial function within 48 to 96 hours of initiation, (3) ability to measure several hemodynamic parameters while in use, and (4) support of circulation in the presence of atrial and ventricular arrhythmias. The physiological and clinical effects of the LVAD are as follows:

↑ peripheral perfusion
↓ use of IABP
↓ inotropic-vasopressor drugs
↑ cardiac output
  relief of pulmonary congestion
  reversal of myocardial ischemia
↓ heart rate
↓ pulmonary capillary wedge pressure
↑ mean arterial pressure

ASSESSMENT AND INTERVENTION
Preinsertion assessment for the IABP

Assessment prior to insertion of the intra-aortic balloon pump plays a major role in the safe care of the patient on the device. This is necessary to establish baseline data from which a comparative

PRE-IABP INSERTION ASSESSMENT

1. Hemodynamic data
   a. Blood pressure: systolic, diastolic, mean
   b. Pulmonary artery pressure: systolic, diastolic, mean, wedge
   c. Systemic vascular resistance (SVR)
   d. Cardiac output (CO)
   e. Pulmonary vascular resistance (PVR)
   f. Endocardial viability ratio (EVR)

2. Electrocardiogram (ECG)
   a. Heart rate
   b. Rhythm
   c. Ischemic changes

3. Pulses
   a. Left brachial and radial pulses
   b. Balloon leg popliteal, dorsalis pedis, and posterior tibial pulses

4. Urine output

5. Mentation

6. General color

7. Peripheral color, skin temperature, capillary filling

8. Condition of skin

9. Laboratory data
   a. CBC
   b. Clotting studies
   c. Platelets

Formulas for the calculation of hemodynamic data include:

$$SVR = \frac{(MAP - RAP)\ 80}{CO}$$

$$PVR = \frac{(Mean\ PAP - PCWP)\ 80}{CO}$$

$$EVR = \frac{(\overline{DP} - \overline{LAP}) \times DT}{\overline{SP} \times ST} = \frac{O_2\ supply}{O_2\ demand}$$

where

$\overline{DP}$ = mean diastolic pressure
$\overline{LAP}$ = mean left arterial pressure
DT = diastolic time in milliseconds
$\overline{SP}$ = mean systolic pressure
ST = systolic time in milliseconds
MAP = mean arterial pressure
RAP = mean right atrial pressure

assessment can be made after insertion. A summary of preinsertion assessment is presented in the box on p. 337.

The objective data should focus on hemodynamic and circulatory information. Blood pressure, mean arterial pressure (MAP), pulmonary artery pressure (PAP), systemic vascular resistance (SVR), and other hemodynamic values are recorded. Heart rate and rhythm are documented. Location of the S-T segment is noted with thorough documentation of depression or elevation in the 12 leads. Pedal, posterior tibial, radial, and brachial pulses are palpated and noted. A Foley catheter with urinometer should be inserted if not already present and preballoon insertion output recorded. The patient's mentation and alertness are important indicators of brain perfusion. Warmth, color, pulses, and motor activity of arms and legs give clues about peripheral circulation. Overall skin integrity is evaluated, especially areas prone to breakdown. With the patient on prolonged bedrest and minimal nutrition, skin breakdown may easily occur. The physician should require preinsertion laboratory work such as clotting studies, hemoglobin (Hgb), hematocrit (Hct), white blood count (WBC), and platelets.

A critical care unit flow sheet serves to organize this data so that trends can be followed. If balloon insertion is performed outside of the critical care area, in surgery or a special procedure room, then the critical care specialist should arrange to visit the patient beforehand. If this is not possible, then it is imperative that the persons who see the patient before insertion communicate their assessment to the critical care clinicians.

Subjective data to be recorded includes (1) patient-family understanding of the procedure and the underlying disease process, (2) patient's anxiety level before the procedure, and (3) patient's mental status and general orientation to surroundings.

Preinsertion teaching

The patient who requires an IABP is critically ill and in a compromised physiological state. Because of this the family will have many questions and concerns about the use of this extraordinary measure.

Explanations should always be tailored to the needs of the individual. Some people may want to know the details of how the pump works and others may not. In most instances the patient is going to be so weak and fatigued that he may not be receptive to any information that is presented. In these circumstances the family will need and benefit from the teaching. For the person(s) who wish(es) to learn about this machine, topics to be covered are presented in the following list. All or parts of these topics may be covered; it is important to individualize teaching.

Insertion procedure
Location of incision
Use of local anesthetic
Size of balloon
Location of balloon inside aorta
How the balloon assists the heart
Duration of balloon assistance
How long the balloon is kept in place (after assistance is terminated)
How the physician determines termination
Explanation of balloon pump noise and alarms
Explanation of console (lights, moving parts alarms, noise, waveforms)
Emphasis on fact that heart does not stop when balloon does

Preinsertion preparations

A signed surgical consent is required for balloon insertion. Several pieces of equipment must be ready for use before insertion of the IABP. The patient must have a secure and accurate arterial line and tracing. This is used for continuous assessment of arterial pressure, for withdrawal of blood specimens, and for fine-tuning the balloon sequence. A clear ECG tracing is necessary to set the initial timing of the balloon, to trigger balloon pumping, and to detect any arrhythmias that may interfere with regular balloon pumping. An operating room lamp allows the physician to perform the cutdown with optimal illumination. Surgical gowns, gloves, and masks will also be needed, since insertion is performed using sterile techniques. The skin is prepared in the groin area down to the knees. An egg crate or similar pressure relieving mattress is placed under the patient.

Assisting with insertion

A special balloon tray with the equipment for insertion is available at most hospitals. The balloon console must be set up according to the manufacturer's recommendations and often involves the following: (1) plugging in the machine to an emergency outlet, (2) attaching ECG and arterial line tracing to the console, (3) securing all connections between the console lines and the balloon, (4) set-

ting machine alarms, (5) setting preliminary timing (inflation-deflation marker), and (6) setting the augmentation ratio (1:1, 1:2, 1:4, 1:8). The balloon augmentation can be adjusted to pump with every heartbeat (1:1 ratio), with every other heartbeat (1:2 ratio), with every fourth heartbeat 1:4 ratio), and with every eighth heartbeat (1:8 ratio). Ideally, one person should be responsible for console adjustments while another person assists the physician with balloon insertion.

There are now two methods for balloon insertion: the original cutdown method and the new percutaneous insertion. The cutdown method is via the femoral artery with anastomosis of a Teflon graft side arm to the vessel (Fig. 10-9). The more recently developed percutaneous method allows a

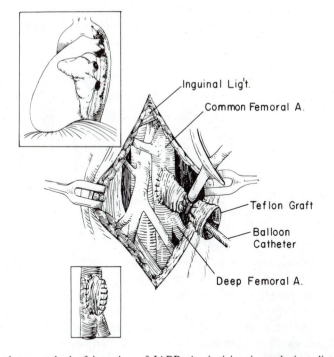

Inguinal Lig't.

Common Femoral A.

Teflon Graft

Balloon Catheter

Deep Femoral A.

Fig. 10-9. Cutdown method of insertion of IABP. An incision is made just distal to inguinal ligament. Tightly woven ⅜ inch Teflon graft is sewn end to side to the common femoral artery. The balloon is then inserted through graft into aorta and positioned in thoracic aorta, with tip below left subclavian artery. It is then sutured in with heavy ligature around graft. Wound is closed, burying graft in subcutaneous tissues with skin closed tightly around shaft of balloon catheter. When balloon is removed, graft is trimmed and oversewn and serves as patch to close femoral artery. (From Behrendt, D.M.: Patient care in cardiac surgery, Boston, 1980, Little, Brown & Co.)

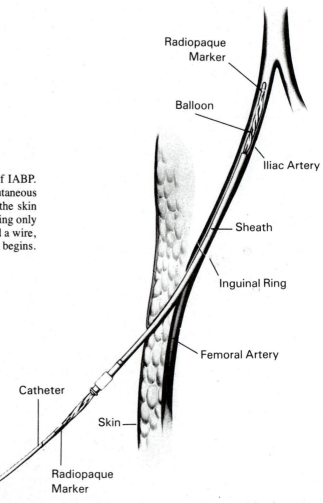

Radiopaque Marker

Balloon

Iliac Artery

Sheath

Inguinal Ring

Femoral Artery

Catheter

Skin

Radiopaque Marker

Fig. 10-10. Percutaneous method of insertion of IABP. No arterial cutdown is needed to insert percutaneous intra-aortic balloon. Balloon is passed through the skin into femoral artery via an introducer sheath, leaving only a small puncture wound. Wrapped tightly around a wire, balloon unwraps and inflates when pumping begins. (From Bricker, P.L.: RN **43:**23, July 1980.)

direct insertion of the balloon through an introducer. The advantage of this method is that it can be done rapidly when the patient requires emergency insertion (Fig. 10-10).

With the cutdown method, the skin is prepared with an antiseptic solution such as povidone-iodine and a local anesthetic infused subcutaneously. Sterile conditions are used with the physicians and assistants gowned, gloved, and masked. The patient may be heparinized before the procedure, but this depends on the individual coagulation status and the physician's preference. A ⅜ inch

woven Teflon graft is anastomosed to the femoral artery. Bleeding is controlled with heavy ties around the graft. The balloon is aspirated with a 50 cc syringe to ensure total deflation as it is passed into the femoral artery and aorta. It is positioned so that the tip lies just distal to the left subclavian artery in the descending aorta. Position is verified by a postinsertion radiogram. Hemostasis is achieved with the use of cautery and the wound is closed with silk or nylon suture.

Certain precautions should be observed during insertion. Examples of this are:

1. The balloon should never come in contact with metal instruments or needles that could perforate or mar the surface.
2. The balloon should not come in contact with powder from gloves.
3. If the balloon is removed from the aorta during the procedure, it must be deluged with heparinized saline until clean.
4. Contact with the balloon should be minimized.

During insertion all vital signs and hemodynamic parameters should be monitored closely. The patient should be observed for complications of insertion, which include dissection of the aorta, arterial perforation, and arterial embolization. These complications would be evidenced by the acute onset of pain, hypotension, and loss of peripheral pulses to the affected limb. The importance of close observation cannot be overemphasized, since one study found that 60% of the complications associated with the IABP occurred with insertion.[6]

CLINICAL RESPONSIBILITIES
Care of the patient on the IABP

The patient with an intra-aortic balloon is usually monitored in a critical care unit until the balloon is removed. The same cardiovascular and hemodynamic data collected during the preinsertion phase are assessed in the postinsertion phase. With improvement of heart failure, clinicians will see a decrease in PAP, pulmonary capillary wedge pressure (PCWP), and SVR. They will also see an increase in MAP, an increase in urine output, and increased cardiac output, and an increase in the patient's mental alertness (Table 10-1). The need for inotropic and vasoconstrictive drug support should decrease.

A decrease in pulse volume and contour on the affected leg is expected, but the development of numbness, pallor, pain, or coolness of the extremity should be reported immediately. Irreversible damage to the limb can occur within 8 hours of arterial occlusion.

Daily chest radiograms are imperative to assess balloon location. They are also valuable in determining the status of pulmonary fluid and infiltrates.

Daily platelet counts are done because of the possibility of the patient developing thrombocytopenia. It has been suggested that balloon inflation causes mechanical destruction of platelets. If heparin therapy is used, there adds an increased risk of the patient bleeding. Therefore clotting studies should also be monitored on a daily basis.

Arterial blood gases are checked as needed to evaluate acid-base and oxygen levels. Arteriovenous oxygen differences are also done to evaluate cardiac output and tissue oxygenation. An A-Vo_2 difference of greater than 30% saturation is associated with low cardiac output and severely decreased tissue perfusion.

In addition to physiological data, patients should be evaluated for their mental status and coping mechanisms. Questions the clinician may ask are: Do they know where they are and why? How are the patients feeling? What are major concerns this time? Do the patients know what all the noises are; what the alarms mean? Do they feel like they will get well or are they feeling hopeless about their condition? The patients' ability to answer these questions will provide information about their mental status, whereas their answers may indicate their level of coping.

These patients require maximum physical care and support. Basic health care of turning, range of motion, oral hygiene, skin care, and attention to nutritional needs is imperative. It is not unusual for these patients to require two clinicians to care for their many needs and staffing patterns should make allowances for this.

Responsibilities for machine maintenance

There are a number of balloon pumps that are now manufactured. Each of these machines is very different and, therefore, clinicians must become familiar with the operation of the machine.

All machines consist of a console and the aortic balloon. The console contains the electronic septum and pump to trigger the balloon, an intricate

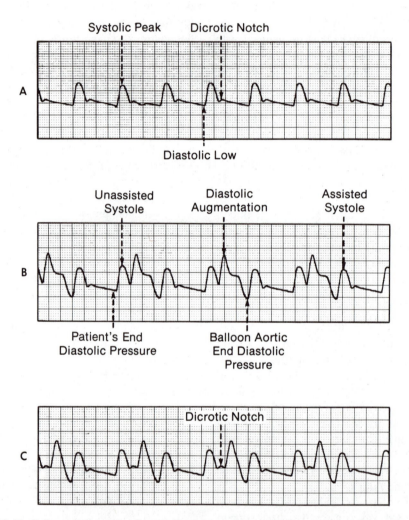

Fig. 10-11. Balloon timing. Waveform **A** illustrates a normal arterial waveform. **B** shows balloon augmentation with 1:2 timing—balloon pumping every other beat. This example demonstrates proper timing of balloon. Waveform **C** is an example of late inflation. Dicrotic notch is quite visible. On a radial line waveform, dicrotic notch should not be visible.

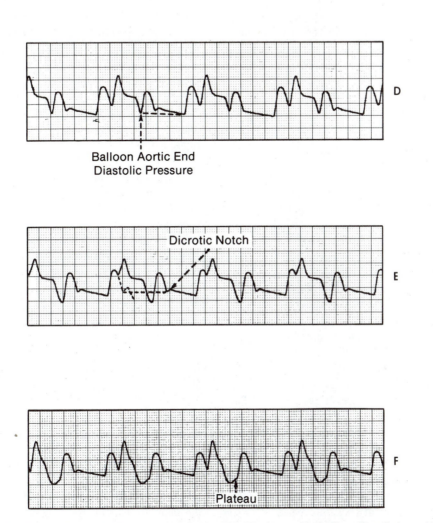

Fig. 10-11, cont'd. Sample **D** shows late deflation. This is evidenced by balloon diastolic low which is higher than patient's diastolic low. Normally, balloon diastolic low should be at least 10 mm lower than patient's diastolic low. Waveform **E** illustrates early inflation. Balloon augmentation is encroaching upon patient's systole. This is an extremely dangerous situation and must be corrected immediately. The last waveform, **F,** demonstrates early deflation. One clue to this abnormal timing is presence of a plateau on upstroke of patient's systole.

alarm system, a display for ECG and arterial tracings, a gas tank, a control panel, plug-in sites for ECG and arterial tracings, a balloon plug-in site, and, in some models, cardiac output computation capabilities. Continuous observation and maintenance are necessary to maintain console function. Some of the components needed to be checked are:

1. Helium or carbon dioxide levels in gas tank
2. Accumulation of water vapor in trap
3. Balloon pressure waveform or slave balloon inflation
4. Balloon volume
5. Alarm system

The hospital biomedical engineering department usually plays a major part in machine maintenance.

Timing the balloon

Proper timing of the IABP will allow the patient to receive the maximum benefits of the balloon and will prevent life-threatening complications. Table 10-1 summarizes the consequences of improper timing. Ideally, the clinician controls timing to achieve maximum diastolic augmentation and maximum systolic unloading.

The effects of the balloon and the timing can be observed on the arterial pressure waveform. Timing is done with the balloon in a 1:2 mode. Fig. 10-11, *A,* shows a normal arterial waveform with each component labeled. Fig. 10-11, *B,* shows an arterial trace with the balloon pumping every other beat (1:2 augmentation). With proper timing the diastolic augmentation peak should be greater than or equal to the patient's systolic peak. Between these two peaks should be a sharp V rather than a U shape (Fig. 10-11, *B*). The dicrotic notch should not be visible (on a radial line trace). The presence of the dicrotic notch, a U shape between, or the patient's systolic peak higher than balloon augmentation would indicate *late inflation* (Fig. 10-11, *C*).

In Fig. 10-11, *B,* it can be seen that the balloon end-diastolic dip is lower than the patient's low and, if it is not, this is indicative of *late deflation* (Fig. 10-11, *D*) and should be corrected immediately.

Two other conditions of improper timing may occur. These are early inflation and early deflation. When early inflation occurs, the balloon diastolic augmentation waveform encroaches upon the patient's systolic waveform (Fig. 10-11, *E*). This is a dangerous situation because the balloon is inflating during ventricular systole, causing a sudden increase in aortic resistance (afterload) and creating a massive strain on the heart, which will try to pump against the inflated balloon. This will lead to rapid increased heart failure and possible myocardial rupture if not corrected immediately. Early deflation (Fig. 10-11, *F*) is not life-threatening; however, by deflating early the patient does not receive the full benefits of diastolic augmentation, and therefore the clinician would want to correct this situation.

The final landmarks to be evaluated when examining balloon timing are the assisted and unassisted systoles. Looking at Fig. 10-11, *B,* one can see that the balloon-assisted systole is lower than the patient's (unassisted) systole. This is the graphic representation that maximum left ventricular unloading is taking place.

Once the clinician has evaluated these landmarks and adjusted the timing, the balloon can be switched back to 1:1 augmentation if desired. All alarms should be set and the timing reevaluated if the patient: (1) changes position in bed, (2) is moved for a procedure, such as a chest radiogram (3) displays a change in arterial waveform configuration, (4) requires a change in the augmentation ratio, (5) develops arrhythmias or has a significant increase or decrease in heart rate, or (6) if the balloon becomes disconnected from the console or the console is turned off for greater than 1 minute.

Evaluating the effectiveness of the IABP

The effectiveness of the IABP is judged by the patient's clinical response. Often the patient will be on numerous intravenous medications along with the IABP. These medications are administered to increase contractility and decrease afterload and preload and may include dopamine, nitroprusside, nitroglycerin, dobutamine, and isoproterenol. Chapter 8 contains specific drug information.

The immediate hemodynamic response to the IABP should be reflected by the following changes in clinical and physiological parameters: increased cardiac output, increased urine output, increased MAP, decreased PCWP, increased level of consciousness, and signs of increased peripheral perfusion. As balloon pumping continues, there should be gradual improvement in the hemodynamic parameters and the clinician should be able to begin to wean the patient off supporting inotropic medications. Ideally, by the time the balloon is removed, the patient should be on little or no pharmacological support when the balloon is removed. The rationale for this is, should the patient decompensate after the balloon is out, the physician has the option of reinitiating drug support rather than taking a chance on the patient not responding to high doses of these drugs. In addition, reinsertion of a balloon is very difficult and not desirable. Therefore upon initiation of balloon pumping, the clinician should see immediate improvement in the patient's clinical status, and the patient should not be weaned from mechanical

support until he or she no longer needs inotropic and other drug therapy.

Complications of the IABP

Recent studies have indicated that a number of complications occur with balloon insertion and frequently are not recognized. In one study the rate of these complications was 36%.[6] Autopsies have demonstrated the presence of dissection of the aorta and its branches and arterial perforation. Other complications not related to insertion include arterial emboli, arterial thrombus formation, ischemic limb, local sepsis, local hematoma, thrombocytopenia, and increased myocardial failure related to improper timing. The clinical indicators of these are presented in Table 10-2. Prevention of these complications cannot be overemphasized, since they all occur with relatively high frequency in the clinical setting.

Care of the patient with a LVAD

In general, the caregiver should see similar clinical signs of improvement in the patient with a LVAD as would be seen in the patient with an IABP. Fig. 10-12 demonstrates a case study of a

Table 10-2. Complications of intra-aortic balloon with clinical indicators

Complication	Clinical indicators
Arterial emboli	Absent pulses; cool, numb, pale, and occasionally painful extremity; pallor of extremity upon elevation
Aortic dissection	Upper abdominal, palpable, pulsating mass, possible back or leg pain
Aortic perforation	Sudden onset of sharp, severe, abdominal and back pain; sudden drop in blood pressure with tachycardia developing; decreased Hct and syncope
Limb ischemia	Diminished pulses to extremity; cool and slightly mottled, cyanotic digits
Local sepsis	Fever; local swelling, pain, tenderness; purulent drainage
Local hematoma	Local swelling, ecchymosis; a swollen hard area under skin near incision
Thrombocytopenia	Platelet count of less than 150,000/ml; tendency toward bleeding
Increased myocardial failure	Decreased cardiac output; increased PCWP, diminished urine output, decreased blood pressure

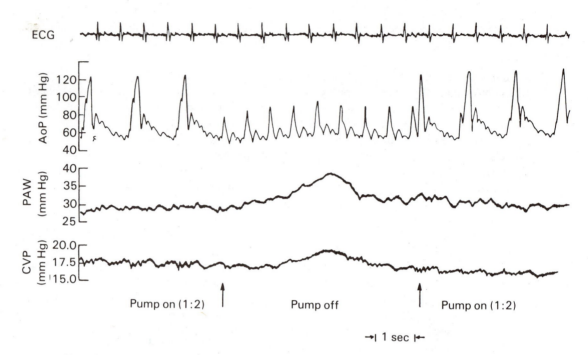

Fig. 10-12. Hemodynamic effects of LVAD in patient. In this patient, on day 6 following pump implantation, one can see what happened when the device was off. There is a dramatic drop in blood pressure. However, before this time patient had been unable to maintain any blood pressure when LVAD was stopped. Increase in wedge and venous pressures was caused by respirator. *AoP,* Aortic pressure; *PAW,* pulmonary artery wedge pressure; *CVP,* central venous pressure. (From Pierce, W.S., and others: Prolonged mechanical support of left ventricle, [Suppl. I], Circulation **58**(3):141, Sept. 1978. By permission of the American Heart Association, Inc.)

patient who was on the LVAD and its effects on hemodynamic data. The complications of the device vary with location and the type of device used. Three of these complications have been cited repeatedly in the literature—bleeding disorders, emboli or thrombus formation, and local infection.

Bleeding disorders are related to the use of heparin with the device. Overuse of heparin has led to fatal hemorrhage in studies on necropsy.[6] Clinicians should therefore be especially alert to this possible complication in their patients and observe daily clotting values.

Thrombus formation is related to the type of device used. In some early trials, thromboembolic complications were high because of the type of material used in the lining of the device. Fortunately, these problems were discovered in animal studies and the incidence has decreased dramatically. However, with any mechanical man-made device, clot formation is a potential problem.

Local infection can be a problem with the external device where cannulas enter and exit through the skin. Daily dressing change with use of an antiseptic ointment should be done.

Little is known about the long-term complications of the device. Care should focus on assessment of the physical and hemodynamic status of the patient and the prevention of complications of the device. The patient with a heart assist device has the major problem of diminished cardiac output and therefore health care will also focus on interventions for this shock state. Special attention will need to be given to patient and family education about the device. The family will especially need much emotional support because of the patient's critical status and the increased risk of death from heart failure.

HEALTH CARE IMPLICATIONS
Patient problems

Many of the problems that can occur with someone on the IABP also occur in the patient with a LVAD. Several major physiological problems appear simultaneously.[4] The patient is critically ill and has little energy to cope with the threat to life the disease presents. The family is hopeful but anxious about the possible outcomes. The practitioner who cares for this patient is faced with a variety of major patient-family problems and must act quickly to prioritize these many problems and develop a plan with workable interventions.

The most common problems that will be encountered when caring for patients with these devices are as follows:

Fear and anxiety

Impaired physical mobility

Potential for alteration in tissue perfusion to affected extremity

Potential for bleeding

Potential for alteration in tissue perfusion to left arm

Potential for alteration in tissue perfusion to brain

Potential for impaired renal tissue perfusion

Arrhythmias

Alteration in cardiac output

There should be a standardized care plan for these patients that addresses these common problems but that also allows for individualization of the interventions.[7]

Fear and anxiety. Fear and anxiety always accompany life-threatening illness. Fear is seen as a stress response to a threat that is known and recognized, and anxiety is a stress response to an unknown threat. They both create an uneasy, panicky feeling in the patient that leads to increased secretion of catecholamines.

Patients on the balloon pump are usually aware there is something seriously wrong with their hearts and they may be afraid to ask questions and hear additional "bad news" about their conditions. They also may be half awake and half unconscious because of drug effect and decreased brain perfusion. Whatever their mental state, they need continual, frequent reassurance and explanations. A daily report of progress and improvement will give them the hope they need to cope with this life-threatening situation.

Impaired physical mobility. This can create other complications such as skin breakdown, atelectasis, peripheral emboli, and muscle atrophy. Supportive interventions should include the following: (1) use of the egg crate mattress, (2) regular turning schedule, (3) range of motion to extremities (except hip flexion on balloon leg), (4) regular skin care with emphasis on keeping skin clean and dry, and (5) good pulmonary and oral hygiene.

Potential for alteration in tissue perfusion to affected extremity. Some degree of decreased leg perfusion is expected on the extremity where the balloon was inserted. The pedal and posterior tibial pulses should be present if they were present before insertion. These pulses may be weak but should be palpable or heard easily by Doppler ultrasound. The foot should be warm and pink with rapid capillary filling. Any changes in these physical findings or the development of numbness, pain, pallor, cyanosis, or decreased temperature of the foot should be reported immediately. These signs indicate arterial occlusion, and an embolectomy or removal of the balloon will need to be done. Measures that can be utilized with decreased peripheral perfusion include (1) use of a sheepskin or heel protectors under feet to prevent pressure sores, (2) use of lamb's wool between the toes of the balloon leg, (3) use of a foot cradle, (4) frequent range of motion to the affected leg, and (5) skin care to the affected foot three times a day. The skin care should include washing of the foot with lukewarm water, a thorough drying of the foot, and massage of the foot with lotion.

Potential for bleeding. Potential for bleeding results from the decrease in platelets related to mechanical destruction by the balloon and the use of low-dose heparin infusion with the balloon. Heparin is often not infused after cardiac surgery but will be used after myocardial infarction to maintain prothrombin time approximately two times normal. The balloon insertion site is a common place for bleeding and hematoma formation and therefore is observed frequently the first 24 hours. After initiation, other sites observed for bleeding are the gastrointestinal tract, oral and upper airway mucosa, and intramuscular injection sites. Daily prothrombin times are done, as well as daily platelet counts. Any patient with a history of gastric ulcers or other gastrointestinal disturbances should be placed on prophylactic antacids either orally or via a nasogastric tube. Should bleeding develop, heparin would have to be discontinued and appropriate therapy initiated.

Potential for alteration in tissue perfusion to left arm. Decreased perfusion to the left arm can result from migration of the balloon and occlusion of the left subclavian artery. Assessment of the left radial and brachial pulses on a regular basis is the best method of detection. Movement of the balloon upward can be prevented by keeping the head of bed below 30 degrees. A sign may be posted if necessary to remind others (x-ray technicians, respiratory therapists, and medical residents) not to raise the head of the bed.

Potential for alteration in tissue perfusion to brain. Decreased perfusion to the brain may occur because of a deterioration in the patients' hemodynamic state or result from positioning the balloon high in the aortic arch. Prevention is directed toward (1) maintaining head of bed below 30 degrees, (2) trouble-shooting machine problems immediately to prevent emboli development on an immobile balloon, and (3) monitoring hemodynamic and physical data to immediately correct any deficiencies.

Potential for impaired renal tissue perfusion. Decreased urinary output may occur if the balloon is pulled down into the descending aorta, blocking the renal arteries. Any sudden decrease in urine output or the development of hematuria should be immediately reported to the physician, because the balloon will most likely have to be removed.

Arrhythmias. Arrhythmias can lead to an extremely dangerous situation if they interfere with balloon pumping. In the presence of arrhythmias, most machines have a range in which they can maintain pumping. For example, one type of balloon pump will normally function at heart rates of 30 to 130 beats per minute. Heart rates outside of this range, irregular rhythms, and change in the QRS configuration can cause cessation of balloon pumping. Prevention is important in the patient on the IABP. Hypoxia, acid-base, and electrolyte abnormalities should be promptly corrected. Antiarrhythmic medications should be administered. If the rhythm is very irregular, pacing may be necessary to maintain balloon pumping. Changes that can be made with the machine that will aid pumping include (1) decreasing the augmentation ratio from 1:1 to 1:2, (2) slightly reducing the pumping volume for fast rates so the balloon can inflate and deflate more rapidly, and (3) changing to a bigeminal mode of pumping (for premature ventricular contractions).

Alteration in cardiac output. The last major health care problem is continuation of an inadequate cardiac output. The nurse should check balloon timing and pumping every 1 to 2 hours. Daily chest radiograms should be done to ensure that the balloon remains in proper position. All intravenous medications should be replaced with fresh solutions at least every 24 hours to ensure their effectiveness. Infusion pump alarms should be on. All of these measures are to ensure that the patient is receiving proper and safe therapy.

If equipment, medications, and other measures are properly applied and cardiac output remains low, then a reassessment of the patient's hemodynamic status is in order. Intracardiac pressures, ECG, echocardiogram, multigated nuclear cardiac scintography (MUGA), blood pressure, systemic vascular resistance, chest radiogram, and physical findings should be reevaluated in order to pinpoint the cause of continued cardiac failure. The four determinants of cardiac output—preload, afterload, contractility, and heart rate—should be manipulated to provide maximum pumping with minimal work and myocardial oxygen consumption.

WEANING THE PATIENT OFF THE IABP

Weaning off the balloon pump should be done gradually over a period of 8 to 24 hours.[5] As discussed earlier, the patient should be off vasopressor, vasodilator, and inotropic support before weaning. The balloon assistance is then decreased from 1:1 to 1:2, 1:4, 1:8, and then removed. Once the IABP is on 1:8, the balloon should be inflated on a 1:1 mode for 5 minutes each hour to prevent clot formation on the balloon folds. The clinical indicators of intolerance are presented in the following list:

Decreased cardiac output
Increased pulmonary wedge pressure
Hypotension
Decreased urine output
Clouding sensorium
S-T changes on ECG
Angina
Decreased peripheral perfusion
Increased heart rate
Arrhythmias

Hemodynamic data should be recorded every 5 minutes $\times$ 2, every 15 minutes $\times$ 2, then every 1° as the condition stabilizes. Any signs of intolerance are immediately reported since alterations in therapy will be required.

At the time of removal, a surgical tray with necessary equipment and operating light should be available. Emergency drugs and volume expanders should be available. The clinician fully assesses the patient before removal, then does a complete assessment after removal. The insertion site should continue to be vigilantly observed for bleeding or hematoma formation for the first 8 hours.

POTENTIAL MACHINE PROBLEMS

Every clinician directly caring for a patient on the IABP must have a working knowledge of the machine functioning and possible problems that can occur. Some of the more general problems are outlined in Table 10-3.

The most important thing for the nurse and physician to remember is, when in doubt, ask someone else. The nurse and physician who are uncomfortable or unsure about a problem with the balloon should ask for help. The machine is a complex instrument, and, as with any machine, one will not feel comfortable with it unless one uses it frequently.

CASE STUDY

The case study on p. 352 illustrates a course of therapy with a mechanical assist device in the setting of congestive heart failure. A health care plan on p. 350 is based on the case history and outlines an approach to major health care problems related

Table 10-3. Machine problems

Problem	Interventions
Improper Timing	Fine tune with A-line in 1:2 mode.
Malposition of balloon	Prevent. Keep head of bed below 30°. Keep balloon leg straight. Daily chest x-ray. Notify physician of malposition.
Balloon kink	Prevent. Keep head of bed below 30°. Keep balloon leg straight. Daily chest radiogram. Notify physician of malposition. Keep all lines free of kinking.
Leak in system	Locate leak. If external, repair. If internal, notify physician for immediate balloon removal.
Disconnect	Locate and correct.
Balloon rupture	Call physician immediately.

HEALTH CARE PLAN

Potential problem	Nursing diagnosis	Goals	Interventions

1. Loss of left leg	Inadequate tissue perfusion to left leg related to presence of intra-aortic balloon	Mrs. M will demonstrate adequate left leg perfusion:
		  Warm left foot
		  Normal capillary filling time for left toes
		  Palpable dorsalis pedis pulse
		  Ability to move left foot upon request
		  Pink coloring of left foot
			Monitor left leg for signs of diminishing peripheral perfusion every 1-2 hours. Notify physician immediately of any changes.
			Place a sheepskin or heel protector under left foot and lamb's wool between toes.
			Provide a foot cradle for left foot.
			Give active range of motion to left lower leg every 4 hours. Ensure that leg is not flexed during exercises.
			Assist physician in the correction of hypovolemia, if this develops. This will ensure adequate blood flow to extremity.
			Regulate heparin drip per physician's order to maintain prothrombin time at 2 times normal. For Mrs. M this must be carefully evaluated in lieu of her hematoma.

2. Arterial occlusion and/or significant blood loss	Potential for inadequate (L) leg tissue perfusion related to arterial occlusion by hematoma	Mrs. M will demonstrate adequate (L) leg perfusion and resolution of hematoma.	Apply sandbag weight to balloon insertion site and/or pressure dressing. Observe site every hour for 4 hours for the development of increased swelling.

HEALTH CARE PLAN—cont'd

Potential problem	Nursing diagnosis	Goals	Interventions
			Monitor prothrombin time to assure that it is maintained at 2 times normal values. Monitor peripheral circulation every 1-2 hours for changes. Assist physician with evacuation of hematoma.
3. Inadequate coronary artery perfusion and further extension of myocardial infarction	Arrhythmia: supraventricular tachycardia	Mrs. M will have regular sinus rhythm.	Treat any PACs immediately to ward off the development of an SVT. Correct hypoxia, acid-base disturbances, and electrolyte imbalances—all of which can contribute to development of arrhythmias. For SVT, treat intravenously with digoxin or verapamil per physician's order. Decrease frequency of balloon augmentation to 1:2 when SVT occurs. Use pacing if necessary to override arrhythmias. Decrease balloon inflation time slightly to allow balloon to inflate and deflate more rapidly. Use cardioversion to convert SVT if Mrs. M becomes symptomatic.

Continued.

HEALTH CARE PLAN—cont'd

Potential problem	Nursing diagnosis	Goals	Interventions
4. Potential for complications of immobility: pneumonia, decubitus ulcers, muscle atrophy, decreased peripheral circulation	Impaired physical mobility related to presence of IABP	Mrs. M will not develop the complications of immobility.	Turn Mrs. M every 2 hours. While IABP is present, do not flex leg that balloon is inserted in. Have Mrs. M breathe deeply and cough every 2 hours. Active range of motion exercises to all extremities 3 times a day. Skin care to coccyx, back, perineum, and other skin folds every 6-8 hours. Monitor peripheral perfusion every 1-2 hours. Egg crate or air mattress, sheepskin or Clinitron therapy should be used. Log-roll patient onto side every 2 hours.

to mechanical therapy and underlying disease. The outcome of the history does not reflect the course of all patients who require mechanical support of the failing heart.

CASE STUDY: MRS. M

Mrs. M is a 63-year-old chronic heavy smoker with a history of hypertension who sustained an inferior wall myocardial infarction 3 years before admission. Two years later, she sustained a second infarction involving the lateral wall. Eight months before admission, Mrs. M began to have symptoms of progressive congestive heart failure. Until the time of her present admission, her condition had been stable on medical therapy including digoxin, diuretics, and nitrates.

The patient was admitted with recurrent chest pain

unrelieved by nitroglycerin. She admitted to increasing dyspnea on exertion and to increasing orthopnea for the last 2 days before admission and had two episodes of paroxysmal nocturnal dyspnea the previous night.

An admission ECG demonstrated S-T segment elevations in leads V_1 through V_4. Creatinine phosphokinase on admission was 478. Mrs. M was assessed to have sustained an anterior myocardial infarction and was admitted to the cardiac care unit. Over the initial 6 hours her course was uncomplicated but her blood pressure subsequently dropped to 80/50 and it was noted that urine output had markedly decreased and the patient was no longer mentally alert.

On further physical examination, Mrs. M had bilateral rales involving the lower lung fields and a summation gallop (S_3 and S_4). She was administered furosemide

(Lasix) intravenously and oxygen by mask and a dopamine infusion was begun. A Swan-Ganz catheter was inserted as an emergency procedure and revealed a PCWP of 28 mm Hg. The cardiac index was calculated to be 1.9 L/minute/M². The patient was clearly in cardiogenic shock and low-dose nitroprusside was initiated.

Mrs. M's condition stabilized on this therapeutic regimen and a mean blood pressure of 60 mm Hg was maintained. Urine output gradually increased and mental status improved. However, by the following morning, Mrs. M's condition again deteriorated. Her blood pressure again fell and she complained of more chest pain, which was minimally responsive to infusion nitrates. An intra-aortic balloon pump was placed at this time percutaneously via the left femoral artery.

Her condition again stabilized and chest pain was controlled. Her subsequent course was complicated by a falling hematocrit and a large hematoma was noted at the insertion site. Furthermore, on examination many hours later, the left foot was noted to be cool and cyanotic. A dorsalis pedis pulse, previously palpable, was no longer present. While arrangements with a vascular surgeon were being made, the patient developed a supraventricular tachycardia. Her blood pressure dropped, necessitating emergency direct current cardioversion. Sinus rhythm was restored, but the patient's rhythm again degenerated into a supraventricular tachycardia and subsequently into ventricular tachycardia. Despite vigorous attempts at resuscitation, the patient died 1 hour later.

SUMMARY

Mechanical devices are used in the patient with heart failure refractory to medical treatment and when the physician believes there is sufficient viable myocardial tissue present to sustain life. The three major classes of devices currently being utilized are (1) the counterpulsation devices such as the intra-aortic balloon pump, (2) the heart assist devices such as the left-ventricular assist device, and (3) the artificial heart. These devices have major mechanical and functional differences, but their goal is the same—to relieve the left ventricle of its workload and to improve cardiac output.

Skilled nurse clinicians play a major role in the outcome and patient response to therapy. They must not only be adept at caring for the critically ill patient but also have knowledge of the mechanical function of these devices and be able to handle any problems that arise.

The health care problems that occur with these devices are related to changes in hemodynamic status and to physical and emotional needs. In addition, prevention of complications of these devices becomes an additional focus for health care. The relatives of these patients are in great need of emotional support and play an integral part in reorienting the patient to reality.

REFERENCES

1. Adams, D., and Thomson, N.B.: Intra-aortic balloon counterpulsation, Roslyn, N.Y., 1981, St. Francis Hospital.
2. Braunwald, E., editor: Heart disease: a textbook of cardiovascular medicine, Philadelphia, 1980, W.B. Saunders Co., p. 557.
3. Bregman, D., and Cohen, S.R.: Mechanical support of circulation: current status, Contemp. Surg. **18**:71, 1981.
4. Chrzanowski, A.L.: Intra-aortic balloon pumping: concepts and patient care, Nurs. Clin. North Am. **13**:513, 1978.
5. Frazee, S.: New challenge in cardiac surgery: the intra-aortic balloon, Heart Lung **2**:526, 1973.
6. Isner, J.M., and others: Complications of the intra-aortic balloon counterpulsation device: clinical and morphologic observations in 45 necropsy patients, Am. J. Cardiol. **45**:260, 1980.
7. Johanson, B.C., and others: Standards of critical care, St. Louis, 1981, The C.V. Mosby Co.
8. Norman, J.C.: The role of assist devices in managing low cardiac output, Cardiovasc. Dis. Bull. Texas Heart Inst. **8**:119, 1981.
9. Pierce, W.S., and Myers, J.L.: Left ventricular assist pumps and the artificial heart, J. Cardiovasc. Med. **6**(7):667, 1981.
10. Shinn, J.A.: Cardiac transplantation and the artificial heart, New York, 1980, Appleton-Century-Crofts.
11. Sturn, J.T., and others: Treatment of postoperative low output syndrome with intra-aortic balloon pumping: experience with 419 patients, Am. J. Cardiol. **45**:1033, 1980.
12. Whitman, G.: Intra-aortic balloon pumping and cardiac mechanics: a programmed lesson, Heart Lung **7**:1034, 1978.
13. Wren, M.: The artificial heart is here, Life, p. 28, Sept. 1981.

ADDITIONAL READINGS

Bricker, P.L.: The intense nursing demands of the intra-aortic balloon pump, RN, p. 23, July, 1980.
Unger, F.: Assisted circulation, ed. 1, Heidelberg, Germany, 1979, Springer-Verlag.

CHAPTER 11

Diet therapy in heart failure

ANNA GAWLINSKI

Congestive heart failure is a physiologic state in which the heart is unable to eject an amount of blood sufficient to meet the metabolic needs of the body.[1] It results from many underlying processes and is not actually a disease in itself. Despite many advances in technology and in therapeutic modalities, dietary restriction of salt remains a basic ingredient in a program for treating congestive heart failure. In whatever setting the clinician is working, whether a critical care area or medical or surgical unit, the clinician will invariably care for patients in some phase of congestive heart failure. Therefore it is imperative that clinicians develop a thorough knowledge of diet therapy in treatment of congestive heart failure.

The purpose of this chapter is to identify the physiological basis for sodium-restricted diets as a treatment for patients in heart failure; to present the objectives of diet therapy; to identify foods low and high in sodium content; and to define the clinician's role in operationalizing and evaluating diet therapy.

HISTORY OF DIET THERAPY IN TREATING CONGESTIVE HEART FAILURE

The historic studies of the effects of sodium chloride and water retention began in 1901.[2] By 1904 research demonstrated the usefulness of dietary salt restriction in patients with cardiovascular disease.[3] In the 1940s and 1950s medical journals published several articles describing manipulation of dietary salt intake to either precipitate or prevent an episode of congestive heart failure.[4,5]

Today the therapeutic and prophylactic value of diet therapy in congestive heart failure is an accepted doctrine. This intervention alone may restore cardiac compensation in patients with mild congestive heart failure. Along with diuretics and vasodilators, diet therapy continues to be an important adjunct to treatment in patients with more advanced forms of congestive heart failure.

EFFECTS OF SODIUM AND FLUID RETENTION IN CONGESTIVE HEART FAILURE: A PHYSIOLOGICAL BASIS FOR SODIUM-RESTRICTED DIETS

Congestive heart failure is associated with an increase in total sodium chloride in both extracellular and intracellular fluid. In advanced congestive heart failure, the body can retain as much as 10 L of extra fluid and 80 g of sodium. This retention of sodium and water results in tissue edema.[6]

The exact mechanism of edema is caused by many factors. It has been attributed to venous congestion secondary to a failing left ventricle. This results in an increased intravascular pressure within all capillary beds that is greater than the intrinsic colloid osmotic pressure within the capillaries. Transudation of fluid occurs from the intravascular (capillaries) to the interstitial space (tissues).[7]

Within the chambers of the heart increased pressures in the left atrium result in an increased pressure in the pulmonary capillaries. Transudation of fluid in the lungs occurs, and a condition called pulmonary edema results. In the right atrium, increased pressures cause rising systemic capillary pressures. This causes edema of the lower extremities, peritoneal cavity, liver, and other organs.

Finally, the renal response to low cardiac output further contributes to the dynamics of congestion in the patient with heart failure. Normally the kidney receives approximately 25% of the cardiac output. In patients with congestive heart failure, this amount is decreased to as low as 8% to 10%. This decrease in renal blood flow reduces glomerular filtration rate and results in greater reabsorption of sodium at the level of the proximal tubule. This reduced blood flow in the kidneys causes an increase in renin secretion by the juxtaglomerular apparatus. Renin in turn acts on circulating angiotensinogen to produce angiotensin I. This is then converted to angiotensin II. Angiotensin II acts directly on the zona glomerulosa of the adrenal gland to increase aldosterone secretion (Fig. 11-1).

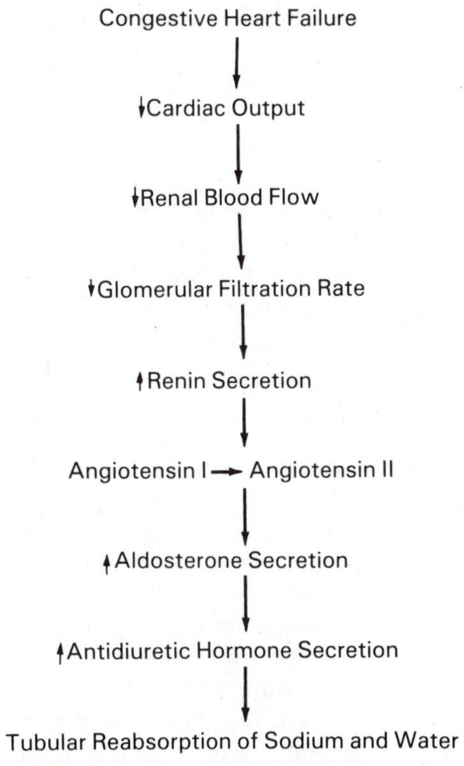

Congestive Heart Failure

↓

↓Cardiac Output

↓

↓Renal Blood Flow

↓

↓Glomerular Filtration Rate

↓

↑Renin Secretion

↓

Angiotensin I → Angiotensin II

↓

↑Aldosterone Secretion

↓

↑Antidiuretic Hormone Secretion

↓

Tubular Reabsorption of Sodium and Water

Fig. 11-1. Pathophysiology of congestive heart failure.

Aldosterone in turn acts on the distal renal tubule to increase absorption of sodium and water. The reabsorbed sodium and water stimulate antidiuretic hormone secretion. This results in increased tubular reabsorption of water.[8] The amount of sodium and water retained by the body, as a result of the effects of congestive heart failure, can be altered by decreasing the amount of salt ingested in the diet. This is the physiological basis for the sodium-restricted diet. A low-sodium diet may be used alone or in combination with drugs as a therapeutic treatment for patients with congestive heart failure.

OBJECTIVES FOR DIET THERAPY

The objectives for diet therapy in treating patients with congestive heart failure include the following:

1. To prevent and reduce formation of edema
2. To decrease oxygen demands on the heart and circulatory system
3. To maintain adequate nutritional status of the patient
4. To develop a dietary regimen that is mutually acceptable to the patient and health care provider

GUIDELINES FOR SODIUM-RESTRICTED DIETS

The average unrestricted American diet contains 6 to 15 g of salt, which has a sodium content of 2.4 to 6 g. The usual patient with congestive heart failure does not require rigid sodium restriction. By omitting use of table salt after food is served, dietary sodium initially can be reduced to 4 to 7 g of salt a day (1.6 to 2.8 g of sodium). However, if failure is not controlled with this regimen, it may be necessary to eliminate all salt in cooking. This will reduce salt content to 3 to 4 g (1.2 to 1.4 g sodium). A strict low-sodium diet would require patients to buy foods with low sodium content. This would reduce daily salt to 0.5 to 2.5 g (0.2 to 1 g sodium). This is usually recommended for patients with end-stage congestive heart failure.[9]

General guidelines for patients on a sodium-restricted diet include the following:

1. Do not add salt to foods at the table.
2. Purchase more fresh foods: meats, vegetables, and fruits. These are generally free of flavorings and preservatives, which contain sodium.
3. Use seasonings such as lemons, oranges, fresh or dried herbs, garlic, or onions.
4. Avoid all condiments marked "salts" or "powders" (garlic, onion, or seasoned salts).
5. Read all labels for "bicarbonate of soda," "salt," "sodium," "Na," "MSG," or "NaCl." These are all a form of salt.
6. Avoid convenience foods such as TV dinners, deli foods, canned meats and soups, bacon, and sausage.
7. Take medications such as Alka-Seltzer, laxatives, and antacids only with the doctor's permission. These contain salt.
8. Check your weight daily. Sudden weight gain can be a sign of water retention resulting from too much salt.[10]

The patient should be given a list of foods low in sodium (Table 11-1) and a list of foods moderately high in sodium (Table 11-2).

TYPES OF SODIUM-RESTRICTED DIETS

The 4 g sodium diet is the "no added salt" diet. This diet is basically a regular diet that excludes foods high in sodium. General recommendations for this diet include:

1. Use no salt at the table.
2. Use only half the amount of salt requested in the recipe.
3. Concentrate on foods listed under "Foods Relatively Low in Sodium" (see Table 11-1).
4. Use only minimal portions of "Foods Moderately High in Sodium" (see Table 11-2).
5. Avoid foods high in sodium such as sauerkraut, olives, dill pickles, soy sauce, pretzels, and other snack foods, as well as cheese, canned fish, meats, and vegetables.

The 2 g sodium diet is a much stricter low-sodium diet. No salt in any form is permitted. The guidelines for this diet include:

1. No TV dinners permitted.
2. Milk limited to no more than 1 quart daily.
3. Eggs cooked any way without salt.
4. Avoid all foods high in sodium.
5. Use foods listed in Table 11-2 with the following restrictions:
   a. Vegetables—fresh, cooked, or frozen. Canned preparations limited to two servings a day.
   b. Breads—limited to six slices a day.
   c. Fats—unsalted salad dressing and peanut butter.
   d. Cheese—cottage and cream cheese only. No hard cheeses.
   e. Desserts—limit baked products to one serving a day.

POTASSIUM SUPPLEMENT

The patient with congestive heart failure may also be taking diuretics in conjunction with a low-sodium diet. These patients may require a potassium supplement or foods high in potassium. Foods such as bananas, oranges, cranberries, tomatoes, lettuce, and other green vegetables are high in potassium. In most patients with heart failure, food alone is not sufficient to replace the amount of potassium required. Nevertheless, patients should be informed about high-potassium foods so that they can make a knowledgeable choice of appropriate foods.

LOW-FAT–LOW-CHOLESTEROL DIET

Studies have demonstrated the relationship between serum cholesterol levels and cardiovascular disease. The development, progression, and regression of atherosclerosis are closely associated with the plasma cholesterol level. Risk of coronary heart disease, which includes congestive heart failure, has increased for subjects with plasma cholesterol levels above 250 mg/ml. The level of plasma cholesterol is determined partly by dietary intake of cholesterol, saturated and polyunsat-

Table 11-1. Foods low in sodium (approximately 500 mg or less)

Food groups	Food items
Milk and dairy products	Milk, eggs, cottage cheese, ice cream, cream cheese
Meats	Fresh fish, turkey, lean beef, tuna packed in water, chicken, veal, lamb, liver
Fruits and vegetables	Any fresh vegetable or canned fruit
Juices	Any juice except tomato or V-8
Desserts	Almost any, Jello or fresh fruit are best
Seasonings	Allspice, marjoram, almond and vanilla extract, bay leaves, caraway, cinnamon, sage, thyme, fresh dried herbs
Fats	Regular butter, margarine, oils, shortening, cream, unsalted salad dressings
Miscellaneous	Vinegar, Jello, unsalted nuts, popcorn, tea, coffee

Table 11-2. Foods moderately high in sodium (approximately 1 g)

Food groups	Food items
Milk and dairy products	Processed cheese, buttermilk
Breads	Commercial pancake mix, pizza, macaroni and cheese
Fruits and vegetables	All canned vegetables, dill pickles, olives
Juices	Tomato juice and V-8
Baked goods	Cake, doughnuts, fruit pies, chocolate
Sauces and seasonings	Steak sauce, catsup, chili sauce, soy sauce, mustard, canned soups, meat tenderizer (MSG)
Fats, oils	Peanut butter, dips and party spreads, commercial salad dressing
Miscellaneous	Baking soda, baking powder

urated fats, and total calories. Dietary saturated fatty acids tend to increase plasma cholesterol levels, and polyunsaturated fatty acids tend to decrease them.[11]

To reduce the risk of coronary artery disease in the patient with congestive heart failure, a diet low in saturated fat and cholesterol is usually prescribed. The following are guidelines for the low-fat–low-cholesterol diet.

1. Eat no more than three egg yolks per week.
2. Limit the use of organ meats and shellfish.
3. Eat only 6 ounces of lean meat, fish, poultry, or vegetable protein a day.
4. Choose lean cuts of meat. Trim off all visible fat.
5. Avoid fried foods. Broil, bake, or boil them.
6. Restrict the use of luncheon meats.
7. Use margarine and other liquid vegetable oils. Do not use butter.
8. Use skin or low-fat milk or milk products.

LOW-CALORIE DIET

The indirect benefit of a low-calorie diet for the patient with congestive heart failure results from its reduction of the workload of the heart. Obesity increases the workload of the heart by increasing the requirement for oxygen as a result of the expanded tissue mass. In addition, there is an increased heart size and blood volume. This results in left ventricular hypertrophy. This can cause an increase in left ventricular end-diastolic pressure. Therefore congestive heart failure may occur in markedly obese patients, and it is a common cause of death in these patients. Weight reduction may help reverse some of these pathological changes.

A reducing diet in an older adult should restrict calories by 250 per day. Average patients with congestive heart failure who are restricted to complete bed rest require approximately 1500 calories per day. Daily basal caloric requirement for normal, healthy adults is estimated at 6 to 10 calories per pound of ideal body weight. A low-calorie diet should be divided into three or more meals per day. In addition, some form of exercise, such as walking, is an important adjunct to weight reduction.

THE NURSE CLINICIAN'S ROLE IN DIET THERAPY

Learning to eliminate salt from the diet is not an easy task. Education regarding the prescribed diet is imperative for the patient with congestive heart failure. The teaching process for inpatients and outpatients is the same. Initially, individualized instruction and counseling should occur. The use of teaching materials such as booklets or pamphlets is an essential adjunct to this instruction. When teaching patients on a salt-restricted diet, it is especially important to assess the cultural background, food preferences, and home situation. Questions used in taking a dietary assessment of these patients would include:

1. What is your understanding of your medical condition?
2. What effect does salt intake have on your condition?
3. What foods do you like?
4. What foods do you dislike?
5. Who takes care of food preparation in the household?
6. Do you limit food selections because of financial restraints?
7. How often do you eat out?

Both patient and spouse should be taught about the necessary dietary restrictions. The nurse clinician should inform and consult with the dietitian to share the assessment and progress for the patient education that is occurring.

How to teach patients

1. Become knowledgeable about the patient's food preferences and eating habits.
2. Include this information in planning the patient's individualized diet.
3. Reinforce information provided, ask the patient for feedback, and allow time for questions.
4. Use family members in the teaching sessions so that they are aware of the diet regimen of the patient.
5. Provide the patient with resource material for reinforcement of information.[12]

Content of patient teaching

The content area for sodium-restricted diets should include:

1. A discussion of salt, sodium chloride, and other sodium-containing compounds
2. An explanation of the relationship of sodium to fluid retention and congestive heart failure and the rationale for eliminating sodium from the diet
3. Identification of foods allowed, foods limited, and foods to be avoided
4. A discussion of salt substitutes and other seasoning for foods
5. Identification of medications that are to be avoided because they are high in sodium content
6. A discussion of special considerations for the elderly

7. A discussion of restaurant food selection
8. A summary of information
9. A question and answer period

Evaluating the teaching-learning process

Methods used to measure comprehension and effectiveness of teaching require the teacher to obtain feedback from the patient. This would include asking the patient to:

1. State the purpose of sodium in the body.
2. Discuss the rationale for following a low-sodium diet.
3. List foods high in sodium that should be avoided.
4. List foods low in sodium that are acceptable in the diet regimen.
5. Describe menu selection when eating out.

In addition, the nurse clinician can have labels of products and have the patient place them in order of salt content. Use of both of these techniques is an excellent method for evaluating the learning experience.

Problems that the nurse clinician may encounter when teaching patients include:

1. Lack of knowledge regarding disease process
2. Difficulty learning as a result of shortness of breath and general discomfort
3. Noncompliance with diet because of financial limitations
4. Anger and frustration because of the dietary restrictions prescribed

One can see that the approach to the patient must be physiological, psychological, and sociological in nature. Therefore the nurse clinician must be astute in diagnosing barriers to learning. Once the problem is accurately identified, strategies can then be developed and implemented.

SUMMARY

This chapter has stressed the importance of diet therapy in treating the patient with congestive heart failure. Diet therapy is an integral part of the total treatment. The nurse clinician must be knowledgeable about factors that may affect the patient's ability to learn. Problems regarding compliance should be anticipated and support given to assist the patient with this change. Finally, communication with other health team members is imperative to facilitate a team approach to these challenging patients.

REFERENCES

1. Achard, C., and Loeper, M.: Compt. Rend. Soc. Biol. **53**:346, 1901; quoted Wheeler, et al. J.A.M.A. **133**:16, 1947.
2. Ambard and Beujard: Arch. Gen. Med. **1**:520, 1904; quoted by Leiter, L.: Modern nutrition in health and disease, ed. 4, Philadelphia, Lea & Febiger, 1968, p. 864.
3. Cooper, L.F., and others: Nutrition in health and disease, Philadelphia, 1963, J.B. Lippincott Co.
4. Feldman, E.B.: Does nutrition play a role in cardiovascular disease? Geriatrics, **35**(7):65, 1980.
5. Guyton, A.C.: Textbook of medical physiology, Philadelphia, 1976, W.B. Saunders Co.
6. Hill, M.: Helping the hypertensive patient control sodium intake, Am. J. Nurs. **5**:906, 1979.
7. Hurst, W.J., and Logue, R.B.: The heart, New York, 1974, McGraw-Hill Book Co.
8. McIntosh, H.D., Gotto, A.M., and Scott, L.W.: Diet and heart disease, medical communications, 1978.
9. Sidd, J.J., Congestive heart failure, Orthop. Clin. North Am. **9**(3):745, July, 1978.
10. Slater, G.: Nutrition and the M.D., P.M. **2**(9):86, 1976.
11. UCLA Hospital and Clinics: Diet therapy for the cardiac patient, 1981.
12. Uthaman, C.B., and Cherian, G.: Dietotherapy of congestive heart failure, Indian J. Chest Dis. Allied Sci. **22**:47, 1980.
13. Warren, J.V., and Stead, E.A.: Fluid dynmics in chronic congestive heart failure, Arch. Intern. Med. **73**:138, 1944.

ADDITIONAL READINGS

Karliner, J.S., and Gregoratos, G.: Coronary care, New York, 1981, Churchill Livingstone.
Purcell, J.A., and Johnston, B.: A stronger pump (a patient consumer manual on heart failure), Pritchett and Hull Associates, Inc. 1980.
Wallis, C.: Salt: a new villain? Time, p. 64, March 1982.

CHAPTER 12

Education and rehabilitation of the patient with heart failure

LORA E. BURKE

In reviewing the literature on cardiac rehabilitation, the reader will consistently find congestive heart failure listed as a contraindication to participation in a cardiac rehabilitation program.[8,11,18,26] When cardiac rehabilitation is viewed in a more narrow sense with the major emphasis of the program being physical conditioning exercises, this is more easily understood. The functional consequences of left ventricular failure are pulmonary congestion and low cardiac output. The congestion results in dyspnea, and low cardiac output limits skeletal muscle performance. The patient with advanced or decompensated congestive heart failure experiences significant limitation in functional capacity.

One study recently reported that well-managed, carefully selected individuals can safely participate in a conditioning program and achieve cardiovascular training effects. These results must be considered preliminary because the sample size was only 10. This is the only published study concerning the exercise response and conditioning effects in the individual with a severely depressed left ventricle, and it points out the need for further study in this area.[11] Currently, the entrance criteria in a majority of cardiac rehabilitation programs would still exclude these individuals from exercise.

In addition to physical training, a cardiac rehabilitation program provides education and counseling regarding living with heart disease and risk factor modification. These treatment modalities will be the focus of this chapter. There will also be a discussion of the implications of exercise in this group of individuals and incorporation of this topic into their education and counseling program.

Cardiac rehabilitation is traditionally defined as the process by which an individual is restored to optimal physical, social, emotional, psychological, and vocational status. H. Hellerstein has said that, "Successful rehabilitation is the complete development of a pattern of living that will enable the individual to enjoy the fullest physical and mental capacities with due allowances for impairments, and included vigorous efforts to reverse or to prevent the progression of the underlying disease process."[16]

Like any individual with a chronic illness, it is important that the patients with congestive heart failure understand the underlying disease that is causing their symptoms and the limitations on their life-style. The individual needs to adhere to the program in order to maximize the therapeutic benefits of the prescribed therapy.

The goals in educating patients are to increase their understanding of the prescribed regimen concerning medications, diet, and activity so that they may be more cooperative in adhering to the program and assume increasing responsibility for their own health. Research has shown that teaching individuals while they are in the hospital can reduce anxiety, thereby allowing them to better cope with the illness and with the crisis of being hospitalized, increase the likelihood of cooperation with health care management, and consequently, experience fewer complications. Inclusion of family members in the teaching sessions has also been shown to reduce anxiety, and it allows them to be more supportive when they have an increased understanding of the disease and its management.[20] A study concerning individuals with long-term congestive heart failure showed that through a continuing education program it is possible for the patient to improve adherence to the regimen, achieve a higher level of functioning, and decrease the number of hospital readmissions.[31]

Teaching can no longer be considered an option in the management of patients with acute or chronic illness. It is a very necessary and important component of total care. The growing importance of this activity is reflected in its inclusion in a growing number of policy statements. The Joint Commission for the Accreditation of Hospitals reviews and evaluates patient education activity in making its decision to grant accreditation. The Patients' Bill of Rights, developed by the American Hospital Association, states that it is a patient's right to know pertinent aspects of disease and treatment.[3] The Standards of Cardiovascular Nursing Practice[12] and Rehabilitation[34] specialties as well as the Social Policy Statement[5] developed by the American Nurses Association have included patient education as an important component of the nursing practice.

The purpose of this chapter is to discuss the role of education in the rehabilitation of patients with congestive heart failure and to identify the essential teaching principles, important assessment data, pertinent content, evaluation criteria, and available resources and material.

REVIEW OF THEORETICAL CONCEPTS

An individual's background of physical and mental skills, attitudes, and beliefs regarding health are important as he or she experiences a health crisis. When the illness becomes chronic, such as congestive heart failure, and when it includes an impairment of bodily function over a period of time, individuals are faced with adjustments, long-term conflicts, and psychosocial situations to which they must adapt. For further discussion of this subject, refer to Chapter 13.

Teaching-learning process

The teacher's role centers on activities that promote learning and on the assessment of the patient's current knowledge. The learner's responsibility is to participate in activities that result in learning or in desired behavior change.[26]

Learning is influenced by several factors, probably the most important being the patient's desire to learn or lack thereof. Difficulty in adapting to the illness or a difference in value systems or health beliefs between the patient and the health professional may result in an absence of motivation. The special concerns precipitated by an illness will also alter the patient's interest and emotional stability.[26] For these reasons objectives or goals must be suited for the individual.

There are several principles one can use in the teaching-learning process.

1. *Learning is more effective when the patient is ready to learn.* Readiness to learn is comprised of motivation and previous experiences.[8,26,30] Readiness will frequently come with time as the patient adapts to the illness. Motivation can be enhanced if the instructional material is organized so that it is meaningful to the individual and so that new material is related to previously learned ideas or skills. The provision of information may result in clarification of misconceptions the patient has about the illness or the threat it poses and this may also stimulate readiness.[26,30]

2. *Incentives motivate learning.* Providing positive reinforcement will often result in increased willingness to learn and participate. Affecting an attitude change so that the individual receives internal satisfaction from acquisition of new health behaviors is longer lasting and more self-directive than external motivation.[26]

3. *Individuals vary in their readiness for health learning because of their general educational background, intellectual ability, and attitudes toward acceptance of responsibility.*[26] It should be noted that one's intellectual ability may not

be reflected by his level of education.

4. *Learning is more effective when the content is relevant to the patient's concerns.* Where the individual is in the adaptation process is important in terms of the patient's readiness to receive new information.

5. *Learning is more effective when the patient participates in goal setting.* The health teacher can assist the patient in setting goals and in determining if they are realistic.

6. *Because it requires a change in behaviors and in beliefs, learning usually produces a mild level of anxiety.* A mild level of anxiety can be useful in motivating an individual; however, severe anxiety reduces the individual's perception and interferes with learning.[26]

7. *Learning is enhanced when associations between ideas are strengthened.* This is especially important to keep in mind for the patient who is newly diagnosed, the patient who knows nothing about the concepts that are to be taught, or the less sophisticated learner.[26]

8. *Learning is more effective if carried out over a period of time.* Learning and retention are limited during the acute phase of illness. Retention of information is increased when the teaching is conducted over a period of time (e.g., several visits to the clinic).

9. *Retention of material is increased when the different senses are involved in the learning.*[26]

10. *Active participation is preferable to passive reception.*[22] Having the patient perform the skill, such as counting his or her pulse, will increase the individual's confidence in his ability to perform the skill, as well as increase retention of material.

11. *Distractions reduce the efficiency of teaching and learning.*[32] Adjustments should be made to minimize distractions and provide privacy when teaching personal or sensitive topics.

12. *The environment can be used to focus the patient's attention on what is being learned.*[26] Providing posters, reading material, or cassette tapes for patients to use while waiting in a clinic or hospital is an ideal use of time and an excellent way to implement this principle.

The simultaneous use of several of these principles can significantly enhance learning and retention of information.

ASSESSMENT

One can draw parallels between the teaching and nursing process in that each has the same steps or phases. They are: assessment, diagnosis, planning, intervention, and evaluation.

There are four purposes for assessing the patient and the family before beginning the teaching process: (1) to collect data to individualize the teaching plan, (2) to identify the sequence of topics and the teaching methods, (3) to evaluate the acquisition of information, and (4) to coordinate the teaching with the patient and family's readiness to learn.

The outcome of the assessment process is an individualized teaching plan that includes what will be taught, when the teaching will be done, and which methods will be used. An assessment of the following factors will be the basis of the teaching plan:

1. Assess *demographic variables*. These can be easily obtained from the medical record or through an interview with the patient. Knowledge of the patient's social class, which may be reflected in the occupation or educational background, may provide a clue to health beliefs and related behavior as well as the ability to afford certain dietary recommendations, etc. The composition of the family will provide insight into the home situation and the available support systems. Ethnic and religious background will frequently influence the individual's attitude toward health beliefs and behavior, as well as dietary habits (for example, some ethnic foods have a high salt content). Age may influence the individual's willingness to accept restrictions or to learn new behavior. The educational level is also a factor to consider in terms of selecting appropriate teaching tools. All of these factors need to be considered in relation to the patient's acceptance of the diagnosis, adaptation to the illness, and readiness to learn.[26,30]

2. Assess the patient's *preexisting knowledge*

and misconceptions regarding the illness, treatment, and prognosis. This is particularly important in terms of medications. Previous experiences with illness or hospitalization by the patient or family will frequently influence their current ideas. These can be elicited through an interview. This information will also provide information about past nonadherence to therapy or to its potential in the future.

3. Assess the individual's *life-style and habits,* such as diet, activity pattern, and use of tobacco and alcohol. Of particular importance are habits that may aggravate the illness and therefore need modification, for example, high intake of salty foods by the patient with CHF or the activity pattern in recreation and employment and the environment in which it is performed.

4. Assess the patient's *readiness to learn.* The individual who asks questions concerning the disease process, treatment, prognosis, etc. is indicating readiness. Letting the patient and family know that they are expected to ask questions and providing an atmosphere that is conducive to this may facilitate this behavior. Frequently, the first topics for questions concern dietary change and activity restrictions.

5. Assess the phase that has been reached by the individual in *adapting to the illness* and the behavior or defense mechanisms that are being used. Again, refer to Chapter 13 for further discussion of this subject.

6. The patient's *major concerns* need to be assessed on an ongoing basis so that the sequence of content being presented can be determined. If the patient is concerned about activity and the spouse is interested in the diet, then each of these topics should be covered, whether or not these were the topics on the health teacher's list for that day.

7. The *progress* made by the patient and by the family should be assessed continuously so that their retention of the information can be determined.[30] The teachers should have frequent reviews of prior teaching sessions to evaluate retention and to provide reinforcement of previous learning. This is important for new skills such as taking one's pulse and evaluating one's response to increased activity.

8. It is important to assess the likelihood of *noncompliance* before presenting the patient with the planned therapeutic regimen.[19] There are several reasons why an individual may not adhere to therapy. These may include a misunderstanding of the therapeutic regimen, poor motivation, a belief system that views medications unfavorably, intolerable side effects, and prohibitive costs.[15] Based on a review of past habits or anticipation of one of these non-compliance factors, a need for increased education in one area may become apparent.

DEVELOPMENT OF A PLAN FOR INTERVENTION

Once an assessment has been conducted the data need to be analyzed and learning objectives need to be set for the patient. This will constitute the foundation of the plan. The individual's readiness to learn as well as the goals that can be accomplished by teaching need to be considered. The general goal of health teaching is to assist individuals in developing their optimal health potential. When setting objectives for a patient with a chronic disorder it needs to be remembered that frequently there is no cure and that the patient is not a passive recipient. Rehabilitation focuses on modifying the patient's behavior in order to increase performance within the restrictions of the disease. Teaching is one method used to change patient behavior and/or increase adherence to the therapeutic regimen.

The objectives or goals of health teaching are the desired outcome behaviors. Goals refer to the end point that should be reached, For example, the reduction or minimization of the workload of the heart. Objectives state how we will reach that goal, for example, helping the patient understand activities that place the least demand on the heart.[8] The teaching and learning activities are guided by the objectives. Objectives also serve as a means of evaluating the teaching process; that is, have the objectives been met and can the patient perform as desired? Developing clear, precise goals and objectives will provide clear direction to the patient and to the teacher. These should be written in measurable behavioral terms so that they may be evaluated.

The objectives may be both long- and short-term since many of the things that patients must learn require days, weeks, or even months of practice. It is important to develop a realistic plan that is easily attainable within the time allotment of the teaching program.[1]

The teaching plan should include a description of the program's objectives, the content, and the teaching actions. Frequently the content is presented in a particular sequence. It is best if a certain amount of flexibility is allowed so that teaching a specific topic can take place out of sequence if the situation arises. It is also best if content is planned so that the teaching actions describe how the content should be presented to the patient, for example, methods of instruction and use of audiovisual aids. Content and instructional aids are discussed in detail later in this chapter.

IMPLEMENTATION AND EVALUATION OF THE TEACHING PLAN

Once the preliminary steps have been accomplished, one can begin to implement the teaching plan. Based on an ongoing assessment of each patient as the plan is being implemented, modifications will need to be made to meet the needs of each individual. Changes should also be made as a response to feedback from the participants.

The three basic methods of teaching are lecture, discussion, and demonstration. The two basic approaches are individual and group.

Lecture

Lecture is the presentation of information through a highly structured format, and it is usually used within a group setting. The advantage of the lecture format is that it is an efficient method of providing a great deal of material to a small or large group of people. Depending on the creative ability and skills of the lecturer, it may also be a very interesting way to learn. The disadvantages of the lecture method are that it frequently does not provide for student-teacher exchange, nor does it

guarantee that the student is actively thinking about the material being presented. Learning through the lecture method can be enhanced by adding elements of the other methods, for example, providing time afterward for discussion or questions or following the lecture with a demonstration.

The lecture method could be used with the patient with congestive heart failure in various situations, for example, in an inpatient unit where there is a group of individuals being treated. The individual who is acutely ill, such as one with acute myocardial infarction who has subsequent heart failure, may not do as well with this approach as the chronically ill patient who is in for a reevaluation and/or adjustment of therapy. Individuals who are acutely ill, especially with an acute myocardial infarction, are more apt to be in various stages of adaptation to the illness, and they may also be self-preoccupied so that they do not do well in a group approach. Individuals who have been living with this condition for some time have also been learning by trial and error and will probably appreciate the group approach, frequently learning that they are not the only ones who have been experiencing a particular symptom or fear. Particularly since many of these individuals cannot participate in group exercise sessions in a cardiac rehabilitation program, their only exposure and opportunity to share with others is through group education or support sessions.

In spite of these attractions to this method, teaching the hospitalized patient by way of the classroom lecture is less successful for the following reasons. As previously mentioned, the acutely ill individual is often preoccupied with his or her own illness and concerns. Patients often find excuses for not attending classes when they have to leave their bedside. Brachen and associates used the lecture method with videotape and followed up by nurse visits to each patient so that the material could be clarified and questions answered.[7] This approach proved to be successful and should be considered by others since the method ensures a uniform presentation of content, the teaching can be done by those who are most skilled at it, and several persons can be reached in less time. The lecture method seems to be quite appropriate for teaching patients in a clinic setting, either through group classes or by using the videotape method for groups in the waiting room.

Discussion

Discussion involves an exchange of ideas between persons, it is less structured, and it usually occurs in small groups. There is usually more assurance that the patient understands the material when this method is used. When implementing the discussion method the teacher is able to adapt the material to the person or persons in the group. Examples would be focusing on the risk factor or change in life-style that is important to that patient or focusing on the diuretic therapy used in the treatment of congestive heart failure. Altering the vocabulary for individuals who are not well educated or who are from a different cultural background and providing a less structured environment for learning are also possible through the use of this method. Redman[26] cautions health educators to look at the cultural values of the group members when using this method because discussion is readily accepted by middle-class Americans but not always by other ethnic groups. When the goal is developing or changing a particular attitude, the discussion approach is most useful. As mentioned previously, the acutely ill person is self-preoccupied and therefore does very well in discussions that involve himself, the spouse, or other family members. This allows the individuals to more freely express anxieties or other emotions. It is also the ideal way to teach individuals about sensitive or personal topics, such as resumption of sexual activity. The major disadvantage of the discussion method is that it is time consuming and therefore may be costly and inefficient. This is particularly true if a large number of patients need to be reached.

Demonstration

Demonstration is the third basic teaching method, and it can be defined as an acting out of a procedure accompanied by an oral explanation. This can be an intellectual skill, such as differentiating angina from heartburn, or the demonstration of a motor skill, such as taking a pulse. The selection of the demonstration method is based on the objective of wishing to provide the learner with a clear idea of how to perform a particular skill. Therefore it is essential that the demonstration be clearly visible to the learner and that it be accurate. Learning and retention are enhanced if the patient is provided the opportunity to practice the skill under supervision and in a setting that closely resembles the circumstances under which the activity will be performed. It is also helpful if the individual is given feedback on his performance of the skill or task. Having the patient count his pulse rate in relation to a medication or performance of activity is an example of this. The health teacher would also check the patient's pulse to verify the patient's accuracy.

Selection of a teaching method is determined mainly by the content to be learned, which is based on an assessment of the patient's major concerns. It is the patient and the family's concerns and needs that actually determine the content and its sequence of presentation. Most health teachers use a combination or interchange of the three methods.

Several factors need to be considered when choosing whether to use the individual or group approach. Where the individual is in the adaptation process, adjustment to the illness, and subsequent to this, the person's readiness to learn are important considerations. As discussed previously, teaching a group of acutely ill individuals is less than successful. For the patient who is no longer in the acute phase of congestive heart failure but is now being followed-up in a clinic the group instructional approach may be quite successful. With the use of the group process the patients are able to learn from each other as well as from the health professional.

Another consideration is the number of staff available. If there is only one health teacher available then there may be no other viable choice. When this occurs in the acute care setting, the teaching sessions should be supplemented with handouts of printed material for the patient or family members to refer to later. Because this approach is not ideal and because retention is always limited during the hospital course, the printed material may compensate for deficiencies that may occur in learning. The use of printed material is also indicated in long-term outpatient teaching as a means of reinforcing the oral presentation. Two good examples of such printed material is a simple fold-up sheet printed by the American Heart Association entitled ''Facts about Congestive Heart Failure'' and a more elaborate booklet, ''A Stronger Pump,'' which is published commercially and is available for purchase.[25] Hospital staff can develop their own printed material covering specific aspects of congestive heart failure, such as the signs and symptoms of worsening failure, when to see a physician, activity guidelines, and medications commonly used in the treatment. Depending on the available financial resources, this material can be mimeographed, photocopied, or printed in a very professional manner. Making the information available for later reference is what is important.

The individual approach to teaching can be beneficial at any time and is usually appropriate in most circumstances. It is more highly predictive of success during the acute phase of an illness, and it is the better choice when covering personal or sensitive topics. It is also more effective in certain situations such as teaching a patient with cultural barriers, one who is poorly educated or not fluent in English, or one who is emotionally labile.

Evaluation techniques

Evaluation techniques involve measuring the behavior and interpreting the results in terms of desired behavior change. Evaluation should occur during and at the conclusion of each segment. This ongoing process has several important purposes: (1) to provide a measure of the patient's knowledge and understanding, (2) to provide a time for progress analysis, (3) to provide a basis of direction for future instruction, (4) to provide the health professional with feedback on effectiveness of their teaching, and (5) to reinforce successful behaviors of both learner and teacher.[26,30]

There are various ways to evaluate teaching-learning. Direct observation is more effective in evaluating learning in some areas than others, for example, observing the performance of motor skills as compared to cognitive skills. The method of oral questioning can be expensive in staff time but is valuable in that it provides immediate feedback on the learner's knowledge and understanding. This is more appropriate for use when teaching is done on an individual basis. Individuals who have difficulty expressing themselves may be handicapped by both the oral and the written questioning method. Therefore, the use of a combination method, such as observation of behavior and oral questioning, can provide a more accurate picture.

Skill and tact must be used when presenting questions to learners so that they do not feel like they are being grilled. Facial expression can provide important clues when observing or questioning learners as to whether they understand. Some persons are not able to identify or express what it is they do not understand. Repeating the instruction or demonstration and interspersing questions throughout may be helpful in identifying areas that are unclear. It is advisable to have patients respond to questions at least at the end of each segment rather than conducting a prolonged teaching program and not evaluating where patients are at each step.[26]

An important area for evaluation when doing health teaching is the ability of the patient to transfer knowledge and skills to various situations. Questions should be constructed that deal with situations related to what has been taught to measure transference. A series of questions regarding various hypothetical situations, such as the occurrence of shortness of breath or chest pain, is a way to test this.

The evaluation should be interpreted by both the teacher and the learner. The learner should be asked for his assessment of learning and progress. This should then be discussed, particularly if differences occur in the evaluation results. The limitations of teaching must be considered especially when teaching individuals about adjusting to changes in body image and life-style. Behaviors occurring as a part of the adaptation process can influence the learning process, especially the patient's motivation. Reality factors such as poverty or family crisis may also affect learning or the individual's ability to implement into his life-style what has been learned. Insight may be obtained through inquiry of the patient's perceptions, motives, values, and understanding as well as his current life situation.

Thus the evaluation that is conducted throughout and at the conclusion serves many purposes. It is a summation and interpretation of the measurement results, and it serves to reinforce success and provide information for analysis of the lack of success. When possible, it should be conducted periodically in the period following instruction since one of the teaching goals is aimed at long-term behavior change.

Establishing new goals is part of the ongoing process of periodic reevaluation of patient learning and practice through adherence to therapy. The length of time between meeting with the patient and reassessment is dependent upon the severity of the disorder or problem and the progress made toward resolving it. The Standards of Cardiovascular Nursing Practice identify some patient outcome criteria that can be used to help determine the frequency of follow-up visits as well as the need for additional instructions and reinforcement.[12] A few of these are listed below.

1. The patient demonstrates adequate knowledge for appropriate modification of life-style.
2. The patient participates in planning the altered life-style and shows evidence of accepting these modifications.
3. The patient demonstrates effective coping mechanisms to adapt to the restrictions.
4. The patient maintains the dietary intake, phamacological regimen, and activity pattern that is compatible with therapeutic and personal goals.
5. The patient is free from preventable adverse effects and demonstrates the ability to recognize these effects if they occur.

An effective, comprehensive patient education program is an important part of the overall management program in order to see that these criteria become realized.

TEACHING CONTENT

The severity of the patient's condition will vary, depending upon the underlying cause and where the individual is in the stage of illness. This will also influence how the patient's condition is managed and whether or not hospitalization is required. If heart failure is caused by an acute myocardial infarction or if the individual has pulmonary edema, he or she is faced with the crisis of surviving a critical illness. During this time period the patient will undergo the adaptational process one experiences with an acute illness while also needing to learn about the illness and how to participate in the care. The individual who undergoes a period of hospitalization will be able to receive intensive instruction with frequent follow-up sessions where questions can be asked and material reinforced. The patient will also have several health team members, such as the pharmacist and the dietitian who may not be present and available to teach in an ambulatory care setting. The patient whose condition is well managed on an outpatient basis will need to receive instructions during office or clinic visits that will consequently be influenced by the constraints of limited staff and time. These are important factors in determining the content to be covered, methods to use when teaching, and instructional approach most suitable for the situation. The following section will review this in terms of the patient with congestive heart failure.

For various reasons the patient, whether in an acute care facility or in an office or clinic, will often not receive instruction on all the topics pertinent to participation in the management of his or her illness. As the patient gains independence the need for long-term teaching emerges. During the later hospital period or early in the outpatient treatment phase the topics listed in the box on p. 368 should be presented.

Because the hospitalized individual may not be interested in or be able to deal with learning about his or her condition, priority needs to be given to a

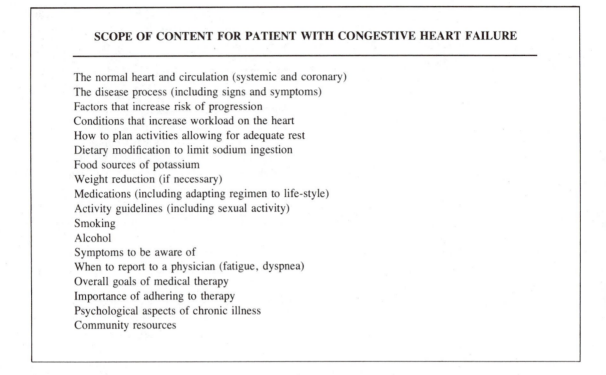

SCOPE OF CONTENT FOR PATIENT WITH CONGESTIVE HEART FAILURE

The normal heart and circulation (systemic and coronary)
The disease process (including signs and symptoms)
Factors that increase risk of progression
Conditions that increase workload on the heart
How to plan activities allowing for adequate rest
Dietary modification to limit sodium ingestion
Food sources of potassium
Weight reduction (if necessary)
Medications (including adapting regimen to life-style)
Activity guidelines (including sexual activity)
Smoking
Alcohol
Symptoms to be aware of
When to report to a physician (fatigue, dyspnea)
Overall goals of medical therapy
Importance of adhering to therapy
Psychological aspects of chronic illness
Community resources

few topics. Topics to be covered before hospital discharge are directed toward (1) reducing the cardiac workload, (2) enhancing myocardial contractility, and (3) controlling excessive fluid retention.[19,21]

Activity planning

An objective in meeting the first goal, and a high priority in teaching, is assisting the patient to plan activities that do not place excessive demands on the cardiac workload. The patient should be instructed about appropriate activities and about an activity plan that allows for adequate rest. The Functional Classification of the New York Heart Association can be used in determining which activities are appropriate, as well as the expected symptoms (see the box on p. 369).

It is essential to include the influence of various environmental factors when instructing a patient about a planned activity program. As body temperatures rise above 98.6° F vasodilation occurs with a subsequent reduction in central blood volume, which results in a reduced stroke volume and a compensatory increase in heart rate. The body's physiological mechanism for dissipation of heat is carried out through skin vasodilation. During exercise 75% of oxygen used in the production of energy is converted into heat. Consequently, as the activity creates a greater metabolic demand, the thermal load added to the body is also greater. Therefore exercising in a hot environment exposes one to both internal and external sources of heat. Two major circulatory functions at this time are the delivery of required oxygen to the exercising muscles and the transport of heat from these muscles to the skin's surface for dissipation. Sweating alone does not cool the body. It is the evaporation of sweat that causes dissipation of heat, which can become a significant problem when one exercises in a climate with a high humidity.[17]

Based on this it is important to relay to the patient information about when to carry out such ac-

FUNCTIONAL CLASSIFICATION OF HEART DISEASE—
NEW YORK HEART ASSOCIATION CLASSIFICATION

I. Patients with cardiac disease but without resulting limitations of physical activity. Ordinary activity does not cause undue fatigue, palpitation, dyspnea, or anginal pain.

II. Patients with cardiac disease resulting in slight limitations of physical activity. Ordinary physical activity may result in fatigue, palpitation, dyspnea, or anginal pain.

III. Patients with cardiac disease resulting in marked limitation of activity. They are fairly comfortable at rest. Less than ordinary activity causes fatigue, palpitation, dyspnea, or anginal pain.

IV. Patients with cardiac disease resulting in inability to carry on any physical activity without discomfort. Symptoms of cardiac insufficiency or of the anginal syndrome may be present even at rest. If any physical activity is undertaken, discomfort is increased.

tivities as walking or doing yard work, appropriate clothing, and adjusted limits to the activity itself since the environment is imposing an increased workload on the heart. The activity itself should be modified in a hot, humid environment and possibly eliminated if it is too taxing. Clothing that allows for heat dissipation should be light, both in color and in weight, loose fitting, and preferably of cotton material. The individual should be advised to curtail outdoor activity during extreme elevation of temperature and/or humidity and preferably do all outdoor activity during the warm seasons in the early morning and late afternoon.[17]

Cold temperatures will precipitate peripheral vasoconstriction and result in reduced tissue oxygenation. Exercising in those conditions results in peripheral tissue and myocardial ischemia as well as in arrhythmias and higher blood pressure. In winter climates adjustments also need to be made for the level of activity, the time of day it is done, and the attire. Clothing needs to be darker and heavier, and activities, which need to be modified when temperatures are low but still above 40° F, should be done during the warmer period of the day such as between 10 AM and 2 PM. If the temperature is below 40° F, activity should be restricted to indoors.[17]

Three other environmental factors that can influence the patient's condition are altitude, terrain, and air pollution. As the level of altitude increases the oxygen saturation of arterial blood decreases. It is advisable that a period of acclimatization be allowed before engaging in physical activity and that activities at elevations of 7000 feet be allowed only after extensive medical evaluation of individuals with cardiac disease and heart failure. Terrain can influence the workload of the heart during exercise if the individual is climbing a steep hill. This obviously increases the intensity of the exercise compared to walking on level ground. Air pollution has more effect on the pulmonary system but may also influence the individual with cardiac disease by affecting the oxygen supply. If the patient lives in an area with air pollution he should be advised about this and instructed to curtail outdoor activity when announcements are made through the media about significant levels of pollution in the air. It should also be pointed out that higher levels of humidity and temperature augment the effects of some pollutants.[17]

Advice concerning the specific activities that are allowed should always be individualized and should take into consideration the extent of the patient's disease, its concomitant limitations, the patient's prior activity pattern, the extent of recovery and stability of current condition, as well as the patient's current living environment. Ideally, the individual will be first evaluated in a monitored situation, if only walking the hallways or up the stairs at the hospital while on telemetry. Under these conditions at least the blood pressure, heart and respiratory rate, as well as subjective response to increased activity can be evaluated and used as a basis for recommended activity.

When instructing a patient about activity it is important to include symptoms that should be recognized as signals to curtail or end the exercise. Endpoints vary for each individual but may include fatigue, a sensation of skipped beats, chest discomfort, or shortness of breath. The patient should be advised not to consume a large meal or alcoholic beverages before increased activity. Timing certain medications with activity may allow exercise without the development of symptoms. For example, the administration of nitrates one half hour before exercise may enhance tolerance, while administration of potent diuretics should be delayed until after the exercise period to enhance action and avoid inconvenience.

The patient should participate in activity planning and identify what types of activities are desirable. Isometric exercises should be discouraged since they do not improve cardiovascular conditioning and result in increased blood pressure and workload on the heart. Aerobic exercises such as walking and bicycling are beneficial and will result in improved cardiovascular conditioning and increased functional capacity. Jogging and swimming are also good but may be too strenuous for the patient with congestive heart failure. The individual should be instructed regarding the activity that best suits his or her limitations and life-style. The patient should be taught how to measure the pulse rate and advised what the upper limit is for exercise. This may be based on an exercise test. If the individual is not at the stage where the physician wishes to do an exercise evaluation, the exercise heart rate should not exceed the resting rate by more than 20 to 25 beats per minute. With all

outdoor activities, particularly walking and cycling, it is important to keep in mind the effects of temperature, humidity, air quality, and terrain. As far as other activities are concerned, such as routine daily activities, the energy expenditure is listed in several sources. When you can quantify the level of activity tolerance allowed for the patient, you can advise what other comparable forms of exercise or chores may be performed.

If the patient's condition is stable and managed well medically, he or she may be a candidate for a cardiac rehabilitation program. If this is the situation, particularly if the person requires medical supervision during exercise, then he or she should be referred to such a program where activity can be increased as tolerated and continued education and counseling can occur.

Pharmacological therapy

The first management goal of reducing the cardiac workload may be achieved through pharmacological therapy, in addition to restricted physical activity. The second goal, enhancing myocardial contractility, is accomplished through drug therapy. The individual's cooperation in taking prescribed medications should result from informing the patient about each drug, its purpose, action, and how and when to take it. Instructions should include symptoms that may indicate the development of a side effect or a drug reaction that needs to be reported to the physician. See Chapter 8 for details on drug therapy.

The use of vasodilators for unloading therapy is a valuable adjunct in the treatment regimen for reducing the workload on the heart, and therefore it is important to have the patient's cooperation in taking it as prescribed. The nitrates are one group of vasodilators that cause severe headaches in some individuals and result in noncompliance. The patient needs to be informed that with continued use the headaches will decrease and then subside. If they are particularly bothersome the dosage may be reduced to the level where headaches do not occur.[9] A simple explanation of how these agents work and their beneficial effects on reducing the workload on the heart should result in better understanding of the rationale for use.

The appropriate use of cardiac glycosides is crucial to proper management of heart failure. Myocardial contractility is enhanced by the administration of digoxin, which is one of the most frequently prescribed medications for heart failure. Patients should be instructed never to increase the dose without physician consultation even if one has missed a dose or is experiencing increased symptoms. The patient should be instructed to recognize symptoms of toxicity such as blurred vision, nausea, or anorexia. Because these individuals are often taking diuretics and potassium supplements, they must be cautioned to closely adhere to the prescribed regimen since hypokalemia predisposes to rhythm disturbances in the setting of concomitant digitalis administration. These individuals should be apprised of the symptoms of palpitations, dizziness, weakness, and fatigue that often accompany potassium depletion and arrhythmias.

When dietary measures are not adequate in controlling excessive fluid retention, further pharmacological therapy needs to be instituted with diuretic therapy. The instruction of administration of these agents should also address the problem of noncompliance along with the usual information of dosage, frequency of administration, and side effects.

Factors that may contribute to noncompliance include the following: (1) diuretics, like many other medications, are frequently expensive, (2) the patient may need to take it more than once a day, and (3) the effects of the drug may be a nuisance, for example, being unable to go somewhere or having to worry about the location of the nearest restroom. It is important for the health teachers to be aware of what they are asking their patient to do. It is also wise for the patients to understand the effects of not taking the medications.[26,27] The individual will be able to see within a few days of stopping diuretic therapy that he or she is retaining fluid, gaining weight, and possibly experiencing some shortness of breath when in the recumbent position. It may prove helpful to explain what effect the increased fluid has on the heart as a pump and how this may affect its ability to meet the demands of increased activity. It must be stressed that the refusal to take potassium, particularly if the individual continues taking the diuretic, will result in electrolyte imbalance, severe leg cramps, and possibly life-threatening rhythm disturbances.

The individual who is taking several medications is more apt to forget taking some of the doses or just decide not to take some or any of the medicines because of feeling overwhelmed, or because he just does not like putting pills into his body. This makes it essential that the patient understand the purpose of each drug, the major goal of combined drug therapy, and the significance of noncompliance. It may also be helpful to allow the patient to express any views concerning the taking of medications and what this means.

Pharmacological therapy also includes administration of other agents. Individuals, particularly those with valvular disorders or those who experience intermittent atrial fibrillation, may require anticoagulation therapy. This requires that the individual understand the importance of periodic monitoring of blood coagulation, regulation of dosage, and drug and food interactions.

Weight control

The prevention of fluid retention may be controlled initially through dietary restriction of sodium (see Chapter 11). However, for some individuals, this type of therapy may be more difficult to manage than diuretic therapy. All progress made in adhering to dietary sodium restrictions requires reinforcement and encouragement to promote continued compliance. This is equally important when calorie restriction is required to control weight (see Chapter 11).

Discharge planning—symptom recognition

The patient who is being discharged from the hospital should be instructed when to contact the physician upon recognition of symptoms of wors-

---

GUIDELINES FOR RECOGNITION OF SYMPTOMS

Notify your physician or clinic if:

1. Your rings begin to feel tighter or shoes become too tight.
2. You begin to gain weight.
3. You find that you can no longer do the same activities you are presently able to do, for example, vacuum the carpet or walk up a flight of stairs, without developing symptoms such as breathlessness or increased fatigue.
4. You lose your appetite or experience a full feeling all the time.
5. You experience palpitations or a sensation of rapid, irregular heart action.
6. You are requiring more pillows to sleep at night or awaken with a sense of air hunger.

---

ening heart failure. These include decreased exercise tolerance, exertional dyspnea, generalized weakness and fatigue, weight gain of more than ½ to 1 pound per day, and increased peripheral edema. Since many individuals may attribute these clinical indicators to other causes, they and their families must be informed of the significance of them as they relate to cardiac function. Providing individuals with an outline of their baseline tolerance will assist them in evaluating the progression of symptoms. (See box above.)

These guidelines should be given to the patient early and reinforced on subsequent visits by reviewing if any of these changes have occurred.

Control of risk factors

The importance of eliminating or controlling the factors that increase the workload on the heart and predispose to the progression of the disease and aggravation of the symptoms is the final area that should receive priority for instruction. These factors include uncontrolled hypertension, obesity, abuse of alcohol, cigarette smoking, and excessive physical or mental stress. Explaining to the patient the effect on the cardiovascular system of these conditions and how they may aggravate the course of the disease may be helpful. Each of the factors listed increase the workload on the heart through

various mechanisms. The amount of alcohol allowed, if any, should be determined by the physician and will be influenced by the degree of left ventricular impairment present since alcohol can have a depressant effect on the myocardium. The nicotine in cigarettes causes vasoconstriction, increased heart rate, and increased blood pressure, and it consequently increases cardiac workload. The carbon monoxide attaches itself to the hemoglobin molecule and therefore reduces its oxygen-carrying capacity. These plus the pulmonary effects are important reasons for the individual with congestive heart failure to discontinue smoking. Excessive stress will stimulate an outpouring of catecholamines and result in an increased myocardial oxygen demand resulting from increased heart rate and blood pressure. If necessary the patient should be referred for additional therapy to a specialist in modifying these risk factors.

When possible, all information in the boxed material above should be presented to the patient and family during the hospital course or early in the outpatient treatment phase if the individual does not require hospitalization. Because of the associated stress and the anxiety caused by the acuteness of an illness requiring hospitalization, there is limited retention of information presented during the acute phase. This reinforces the need for printed material that the patient can take home for use after discharge and for follow-up sessions in the office or clinic.

Instructional aids

Instructional aids for the health professional exist in three formats: printed material, audiovisual aids, and physical objects. When evaluating these materials, vocabulary, sentence length, illustrations, type size, and style of writing as well as readability and correctness of information should be carefully considered. Printed material can be in the form of diagrams or illustrations, flip charts, booklets, pamphlets, or one-page handouts. If the teacher's time is limited this method is useful since learning does not require the presence of an instructor.

Audiovisual aids have the added benefit of combining sight and hearing with other senses such as touch, smell, or taste. The use of these materials ensures a uniform presentation of content that can be supplemented by health care personnel.

Physical objects, such as prosthesis, pacemaker, or pills, or models if the actual object is unavailable can supplement teaching and improve retention by involving several senses in the learning process.

Other resources, such as the American Heart Association, provide materials free or for a nominal charge. Examples would be pamphlets on heart disease, risk factors, angina, pacemakers, heart surgery, and congestive heart failure. Commercially developed aids are also available for purchase. If cost is a prohibiting factor, one can develop one's own instructional material and reproduce it in the most economical fashion. The crucial element is the provision of take-home instructions that are appropriate and accurate.

COMPLIANCE WITH TREATMENT REGIMENS—IMPLICATIONS FOR HEALTH CARE PRACTICE

Wide variations in the extent to which patients default have been reported. Failure to follow the physician's recommendation has been reported to be 30% to 35%. Because of differences in defining and measuring compliance the range is reported from 4% to 100%. Compliance has not been found to be related to such factors as age, sex, race, education, marital, or socioeconomic status.[18,32] However, it has been shown that the family's participation may exert a strong influence on the patient's learning and long-term behavior.[27]

As the complexity of the regimen increases, compliance seems to decrease. This has major implications for the patient with congestive heart failure who has dietary and pharmacological regimens to follow. The patient's perception of the severity of the illness may also influence adherence. Health-seeking behavior is believed to increase as the individual perceives the illness as being more serious. Factors that tend to reduce compliance are chronicity or difficulty of the illness, a complicated treatment regimen, and number of medications prescribed. One study showed that over 50% of the patients were making medication errors, many because they were confused about at least one of the medications. Generally it seems that difficulty with compliance occurs most frequently in regard to medications, dietary restrictions, and activity limitations or progression. Following through on referrals or returning to the physician for follow-up are also potential problem areas for compliance.[18]

Study results imply that medications need to be clearly labeled and the pill itself should be used as a visual aid when instructing the patient. Printed information regarding the purpose, dosage, side effects, storage, and usage of the medication should be provided for the patient to take home. Assisting the individual to set up a schedule for taking the medications may be quite helpful if there are several pills to be taken. The health teacher needs to take extra measures when instructing individuals over 75 years of age, who have less formal education, live alone, or have several illnesses. If the person does not understand how the medication relates to the illness or to a particular symptom or if the drug is expensive, cooperation in taking the medication is reduced.

Dietary and pharmacological therapy are the core of therapeutic management of the patient with congestive heart failure. Therefore it is crucial to obtain the individual's cooperation with the therapeutic regimen. Follow-through behavior does not occur automatically; it needs to be planned. The nurse can do this through patient education.[26]

The following boxed material illustrates the use of teaching in providing care to the patient with congestive heart failure in an inpatient and outpatient setting.

SUMMARY

The role of cardiac rehabilitation and its application in caring for the patient with congestive heart failure was introduced in this chapter. Because

---

TEACHING-LEARNING PROCESS FOR THE PATIENT WITH CONGESTIVE HEART FAILURE

ACUTE PHASE

Teaching objectives

To assess patient's and family's knowledge base and level of understanding in reference to congestive heart failure

To reduce anxiety and increase cooperation through provision of information

To begin instructing the patient and the family about diet, medication, and activity as appropriate for the patient's condition

Instructional content

Orientation to routines, equipment, procedures

Basic information about medications (i.e., name and purpose)

Activity restrictions during acute phase and gradual progression as condition allows

Purpose of activity restrictions (reduce workload on heart)

In-bed exercises and purpose during restricted activity phase

Dietary restrictions and purpose (i.e., salt and fluid limit)

Overview of treatment program (i.e., prepare for transfer out of ACU, liberalized restrictions, prepare for changes in staff, increased activity/independence)

Instructional methods

Individualized instruction with patient and spouse

Instructional aids

Printed materials:

    Booklet to introduce and review congestive heart failure—causes, symptoms, treatment, etc.

    Pamphlet on prescribed diet

    Fact sheet on prescribed medications

    Pictures or diagrams of heart, lungs, and circulation

Expected outcomes

Reduced level of anxiety about environment, treatment, etc. in patient and family members

Increased cooperation with treatment regimen

Patient asks pertinent questions

these individuals are limited in their physical activity, exercise plays a minor role. Education and counseling of the patient and family assume increased importance and are the main components of a rehabilitation program.

The teaching-learning process is reviewed and twelve principles that can guide this process are discussed with examples as they apply to the patient with congestive heart failure. The reasons for and the areas of assessment are also covered. The

---

SUBACUTE PHASE (Convalescent Period)

Teaching objectives

To prepare for changes in routine and increased independence of convalescent unit
To decrease anxiety by responding to expressed concerns of patient and family
To prepare for discharge

Instructional content

Review of basic cardiovascular anatomy and physiology with emphasis on heart's function as a pump
Causes and/or precipitating factors of congestive heart failure
Symptoms to be aware of and when to report to physician and/or clinic
Self monitoring, such as how to take own pulse, daily weight, and signs of fluid retention
Medications that will be prescribed for continued use—name, purpose, dosage, how and when to take, special precautions, storage, administration, and side effects
Prescribed diet—purpose, how to select and prepare foods, label reading, dining out, acceptable substitutions
Activity—schedule for progression, symptoms to monitor in progression (shortness of breath, excessive heart rate increase, fatigue), precautions (environment and terrain)
Follow-up care—clinic appointments, blood test, etc.

Instructional methods

Individualized instruction with patient and family, particularly for personal topics
Small group instruction if patients are similar in disease progression stage and prescribed treatment

Instructional aids

Printed material to cover above content for take home use
Flip charts, diagrams, etc. to cover any of content, particularly in group approach
Audiovisual aids such as films or slides for group approach
Audiocassette tapes for individual use
Physical objects such as heart model

Expected outcomes

Patient is able to identify precipitating factors of congestive heart failure
Patient is able to demonstrate accurate pulse measurement
Patient is able to list symptoms that should be reported to physician/clinic
Patient is able to list medications and identify on paper appropriate schedule for taking medications
Patient is able to discuss diet and demonstrate understanding of restrictions
Patient is able to review activity progression and identify precautions
Patient is able to demonstrate through answers to verbal or written questions an understanding of the content presented

Continued.

TEACHING-LEARNING PROCESS FOR THE PATIENT
WITH CONGESTIVE HEART FAILURE—cont'd

MAINTENANCE PHASE (Following hospital discharge)

Teaching objectives

To keep informed of any changes in treatment regimen

To reinforce previously learned materials

To provide content that the patient did not receive before this time

Instructional content

Same as listed in convalescent phase. Repetition of material can be in greater depth as patient's level of understanding allows. Note: Because of differences in length of convalescent period and availability of staff to teach, the patient may not have received all of the instructional content listed in convalescent phase.

Instructional methods

Individualized instruction with patient and/or spouse, particularly for personal topics

Small group lecture or discussion—may be particularly beneficial to diet or activity-related topics

Instructional aids

Same as listed in convalescent phase

Expected outcomes

Patient is able to demonstrate understanding of new or repeated content through answers to written or verbal questions.

Patient demonstrates understanding though adherence to treatment regimen.

---

educational content for the patient with congestive heart failure and the teaching methods of lecture, discussion, and demonstration are presented. The individual and group approach as well as instructional aids and resources for these are reviewed. Evaluation, the final step in the teaching-learning process, is discussed as well as compliance, particularly as it relates to an individual with congestive heart failure.

During the course of long-term treatment, routine assessment will identify new needs for learning or counseling. These may include new skills for better self-management by the patient. Involving the patient as an active problem solver in his care enhances adherence with long-term regimens required for individuals with congestive heart fail-

ure. Close collaboration of all members of the health care team will assure optimal delivery of rehabilitation and education, important components of care.

REFERENCES

1. Abels, L.F.: Patient teaching in critical care. In Abels, L.F., editor: Mosby's manual of critical care, St. Louis, 1979, The C.V. Mosby Co.
2. Abrahm, H.S.: The psychology of chronic illness, J. Chronic Dis. **25:**659, 1972.
3. American Hospital Association: A patient's bill of rights, Chicago, 1972, The Association.
4. American Nurses Association, Division on Medical-Surgical Nursing Practice and The Association of Rehabilitation Nurses: Standards of rehabilitation nursing practice, Kansas City, The Association, 1977.

5. American Nurses Association: Nursing—a social policy statement, Kansas City, The Association, 1980.
6. Baden, C.A.: Teaching the coronary patient and his family, Nurs. Clin. North Am. **7**:363, 1972.
7. Bracken, M.B., Bracken, M., and Landry, A.B.: Patient education by videotape after myocardial infarction: an empirical evaluation, Arch. Phys. Med. Rehabil. **58**:213, 1977.
8. Burke, L.E.: Learning and retention in the acute care setting, Crit. Care **4**(3):67, 1981.
9. Burke, L.E.: Nitrates. In Underhill, S.L., and others, editors: Cardiac nursing, Philadelphia, 1982, J.B. Lippincott Co.
10. Cardiac Rehabilitation Committee, American Heart Association Greater Los Angeles Affiliate: Guidelines for cardiac rehabilitation centers, Los Angeles, 1978, American Heart Association.
11. Conn, E.H., Sanders, R., and Wallace, A.G.: Exercise responses before and after physical conditioning in patients with severely depressed left ventricular function, Am. J. Cardiol. **49**(2):296, 1982.
12. Council on Cardiovascular Nursing, American Heart Association and American Nurses' Association, Division on Medical-Surgical Nursing Practice: Standards of cardiovascular nursing practice, Kansas City, 1975, American Nurses Association.
13. Crate, M.A.: Nursing functions in adaptation to chronic illness, Am. J. Nurs. **65**:72, 1965.
14. Fardy, P.S., and others: Cardiac rehabilitation; implications for the nurse and other health professionals, St. Louis, 1980, The C.V. Mosby Co.
15. Foster, S.B., and Kousch, D.: Adherence to therapy in hypertensive patients, Nurs. Clin. North Am. **16**(6):331, 1981.
16. Hellerstein, H.K.: Cardiac rehabilitation: a retrospective view. In Pollock, M.I., and Schmidt, D.H., editors: Heart disease and rehabilitation, Boston, 1979, Houghton Mifflin Co., pp. 509-520.
17. Johnston, B.L.: Influence of environmental factors on exercise and activity of cardiac patients, Cardiovasc. Nurs. **18**:7, 1982.
18. Marston, M.V.: Compliance with medical regimens: a review of the literature, Nurs. Res. **19**:312, 1970.
19. McGurn, W.C.: Congestive heart failure. In McGurn, W.C., editor: People with cardiac problems: nursing concepts, Philadelphia, 1981, J.B. Lippincott Co.
20. Nassen, A.M.: Principles of teaching and learning applied to critical care. In Kinney, M.R., editor: AACN's clinical reference for critical care nursing, New York, 1981, McGraw-Hill Book Co.
21. National Institutes of Health, Public Health Service: Fact sheet—congestive heart failure, National Heart and Lung Institute, DHEW Publication No. (NIH) 76-923.
22. Nursing Education Committee: MI: guidelines for patient and family teaching, Seattle, 1974, Washington State Heart Association.
23. Nutter, D.O.: Clinical recognition and management of heart failure. In Wenjer, N., Hurst, W., and McIntyre, M.C.: Cardiology for nurses, New York, 1980, McGraw-Hill Book Co.
24. Pollock, M.L., and Schmidt, D.H.: Heart disease and rehabilitation, Boston, 1979, Houghton Mifflin Co.
25. Purcell, J.A., and Johnston, B.: A stronger pump (a patient consumer manual on heart failure), Atlanta, 1980, Pritchett and Hull Associates, Inc.
26. Redman, B.: The process of patient teaching, ed. 4, St. Louis, 1981, The C.V. Mosby Co.
27. Redman, B.K.: Client education therapy in treatment and prevention of cardiovascular diseases, Colo. Nurse **74**:6, July, 1974.
28. Rosenburg, S.G.: A case for patient education, Hosp. Form. Manag. **6**:1, 1971.
29. Sackett, D.L., and Haynes, R.B.: Compliance with therapeutic regimens, ed. 2, Baltimore, 1979, The Johns Hopkins University Press.
30. Scalzi, C.C., and Burke, L.E.: Patient family education. In Underhill, S.L., and others, editors: Comprehensive cardiac care, Philadelphia, 1982, J.B. Lippincott Co.
31. Simonds, S.K.: The educational care of patients with congestive heart failure, Health Educ. J. **25**:131, 1967.
32. Storlie, F.: Patient teaching in critical care, New York, 1975, Appleton-Century-Crofts.
33. Wenger, N.K., and Hellerstein, H.K.: Rehabilitation of the coronary patient, New York, 1978, John Wiley & Sons, Inc.
34. Winslow, E.H.: The role of the nurse in patient education, Nurs. Clin. North Am. **11**:213, 1976.

ADDITIONAL READINGS

Comoss, P.M., Burke, E.A.S., and Swails, S.H.: Cardiac rehabilitation: a comprehensive nursing approach, Philadelphia, 1979, J.B. Lippincott Co.

Czerwinski, B.S.: Manual of patient education for cardiopulmonary dysfunctions, St. Louis, 1980, The C.V. Mosby Co.

Fournet, Sr. K.M.: Patients discharged on diuretics: prime candidates for individualized teaching by the nurse, Heart Lung, **3**:108, 1974.

Freedman, C.R.: Teaching patients, San Diego, 1978, Coureware, Inc.

Garcia, R.N.: Rehabilitation after myocardial infarction, New York, 1979, Appleton-Century-Crofts.

Zander, K.S., and others: Practical manual for patient teaching, St. Louis, 1978, The C.V. Mosby Co.

Zangari, M.E., and Duffy, P.: Contracting with patients in day-to-day practice, Am. J. Nurs. **80**:451, 1980.

CHAPTER 13

Psychosocial problems in congestive heart failure: health care implications

CARMELA RIZZUTO

The psychosocial problems that frequently accompany the development of congestive heart failure have not been extensively explored in nursing literature. Much has been written about patients' reactions to acute myocardial infarction. Numerous authors have researched the psychological sequelae in persons who have had such attacks. For those who undergo cardiac surgery, clinicians have resources that detail the psychological and teaching needs of this population. However, the needs of the person with congestive heart failure have been lost in the shadows. The purpose of this chapter is to focus attention on the psychosocial problems experienced by those with congestive heart failure resulting from chronic cardiac disease. These problems can be the source of psychological and physiological stress for patients who do not adequatley cope with them. For persons with congestive heart failure, such stress can have negative outcomes. Thus it is imperative that they receive a careful assessment of their psychosocial status and that interventions be instituted to assist them in coping with the problems identified.

According to recent statistics, 30 million people suffer from chronic diseases. Cardiac conditions are the underlying cause of activity restrictions in 16% of persons with chronic ailments.[27] Age is a critical factor in the number of persons with cardiac disease. Almost 200 persons in 1000 over the age of 65 have chronic cardiac conditions that are second only to arthritis in prevalence in that age group.[26] Of the 5 million persons who have chron-

ic cardiac diseases, coronary artery disease is the primary disabler, followed by hypertensive heart disease and disorders of heart rhythm.[28] It is projected that these numbers will increase significantly as the percent of older persons in the population increases to almost 25% during the next 15 years. Congestive heart failure is an outcome of various chronic cardiac diseases, such as coronary artery disease and hypertensive heart disease. The progressive severity of the syndrome necessitates repeated hospitalization and supportive health care in the home. Thus clinicians in a variety of health care settings need to be able to recognize the psychosocial problems that patients face and be able to intervene appropriately.

This chapter will outline the common psychosocial problem areas in congestive heart failure. The specific objectives of the chapter are:

1. To outline the disease trajectory in congestive heart failure resulting from chronic cardiac disease
2. To discuss patient responses along the disease trajectory
3. To provide theoretical bases for assessment and intervention of the psychosocial problems encountered by the patient with congestive heart failure
   a. Changes in life-style related to diagnosis
   b. Adherence to therapeutic management of the disease
   c. Loss of physical integrity, role function, and interdependency

d. Facing death
4. To provide a guideline for application of the concepts discussed by means of a case study

ILLNESS TRAJECTORY IN CONGESTIVE HEART FAILURE
Nature of the trajectory

The majority of chronic diseases are characterized by a trajectory that is relatively predictable.[24] The trajectory is initiated by the onset of disease. This is followed by a period of disease progression that terminates in death. Many cardiac diseases that are the underlying causes of congestive heart failure are chronic. The disease is never "cured," and the person experiences symptoms and/or acute episodes of illness periodically. Therefore one can project the probable course of the disease over a period of time.

What trajectory can be projected for many chronic cardiac disorders, and what factors affect their outcome? First there is the initial onset of disease: an attack of anginal pain, a myocardial infarction, or abnormal electrocardiogram and heart murmur of idiopathic hypertrophic subaortic stenosis (IHSS). The second stage, that of disease progression with increasingly compromised cardiac function, varies according to underlying cause and treatment effectiveness. As the disease worsens and treatment becomes less effective, episodes of disabling congestive heart failure can become more frequent. During this stage mild congestive heart failure progresses to severe heart failure. Dyspnea is produced by lesser degrees of activity until the individual is dyspneic at rest.

During the final stage congestive heart failure persists despite adequate treatment. Clinical indicators of congestion are combined with low cardiac output at rest. This stage culminates in death as a result of the cardiac disease itself and/or multiple organ failure. The trajectory can be applied not only in congestive heart failure, coronary artery disease, and IHSS, as indicated earlier, but also in rheumatic heart disease and the various cardiomyopathies.

Although the disease trajectory for persons with chronic cardiac disease has some common elements, its impact is unique for each individual and family. Thus the problems encountered by them will have both commonalities and differences. The degree of cardiac impairment at the time of initial diagnosis and its resultant functional disability for the individual affects the emotional impact of the disease. In addition, the psychosocial problems with which the person must cope are also related to the exact nature of the disease, its severity, and the resultant disability. Other factors, such as age, presence of other chronic diseases, concomitant life stresses, physical conditioning, and adequacy of medical or surgical treatment can affect not only the disease trajectory but also the nature and type of psychosocial problems encountered by the individual.

Uniqueness of chronic cardiac disease

As a chronic illness, cardiac disease is unique in several ways. First, diseases of the heart carry with them the possibility of sudden death. The role of the heart in maintaining other vital functions as well as its unique circulation and biochemistry are at the basis of this difference. Regardless of treatment, the specter of death occurring at any point in time is an issue that must be dealt with by the individual. This threat of sudden death, while a possibility for everyone, is usually of much less concern for the person with a noncardiac chronic illness, such as arthritis, diabetes, and cancer.

Chronic cardiac disease differs in a second way, in the meaning of the affected organ to the individual. The heart can symbolize not only love or affection but also the center of one's entire being. Thus a threat to the integrity of the heart can be interpreted as a threat to the integrity of the entire person. Such a meaning is not ordinarily attached to other parts of the body.

Finally, cardiac disease differs from other chronic diseases in the cultural myths surrounding it. The person with a cardiac disease is viewed as "different." Cultural misconceptions foster the idea that the individual cannot participate in activities requiring exertion, including sexual activity.

ONSET ————————————————→ DISEASE PROGRESSION ————————————→ DEATH

Characteristics

Mild to Severe

Varied Etiology

Different Meanings to
  Individual and to
  Society

Variable Cardiac
  Functional Capacity

Spectre of Sudden
  Death

Variable Prognosis

Decreased Cardiac Status

Additional Acute Episodes
  of Disease

Increasing Disability

Increasing Symptomatology

Decreasing Treatment Effects

Can Occur at Any
  Time

Fig. 13.1 Trajectory in chronic cardiac disease.

The individual must be "protected" from having to do heavy work and from emotional upheaval as well.

Thus cardiac disease is unique in its trajectory, in its potential for sudden death, and in its meaning to the individual and to those around him. This affects both the initial impact of diagnosis upon the individual and the effectiveness of his coping mechanisms throughout the disease trajectory. The unique characteristics of the trajectory of chronic cardiac disease are presented in Fig. 13-1.

Patient responses along the disease trajectory

The response of the individual to chronic cardiac disease underlying congestive heart failure is variable. However, evidence does exist to support the concept that persons who are diagnosed with a chronic disease, cardiac or otherwise, have similar emotional responses. For the sake of clarity the emotional and behavioral responses to these problems in the person with chronic cardiac disease will be divided into three phases: (1) onset of disease, (2) disease progression, and (3) end-stage or terminal phase (Table 13-1). This does not imply that such responses will occur only during that particular phase. For example, the responses to loss, which usually occur during the onset of the dis-

ease, may appear later in the trajectory or may reappear as additional losses are felt.

Several problems arise during the period of initial onset of the disease. For example, if the symptoms of the disease at this stage are severe enough to require hospitalization, the person is likely to experience anxiety and feelings of loss. Anxiety is aroused as the disease and its prognosis are perceived as a threat to physical and ego integrity. Fear of death may also increase the level of anxiety. Depending upon the degree of apprehension experienced and the person's ability to cope with it, a crisis may develop at this juncture.

Reactions to the perceived loss follow the pattern of the grieving process. The person experiences initial shock, disbelief, anger, denial, and depression. How these feelings are displayed or acted out varies with individuals. Anger may be displaced onto staff or family. Manifestations of anxiety, such as restlessness, tension, impaired decision making or other mental processes, and insomnia, vary with its intensity. Denial may take several forms: (1) total denial of the disease and its symptoms, which may be accompanied by such behavior as signing out of the hospital against medical advice or refusing treatments and medication; (2) major denial of fear or anxiety, but ac-

Table 13-1. Problems and responses along disease trajectory

	Problems	Responses
Onset	Loss Adjustment to medical diagnosis Coping with changes in life-style Coping with changes in self-concept	Grief response—shock, disbelief, anger, depression, resolution Adjustment or maladjustment Anxiety about possibility of death
Disease progression	Additional losses Adjustment to increased physical disability Coping with further changes in self-concept Adjustment to maturational changes	Depression, anger Anxiety Further adjustment
End stage	Facing death	Denial Anger, depression Acceptance

knowledgement of the existence of disease; and (3) minimal denial.

After the initial period of shock and denial, depression often follows as the loss becomes real to the individual. The extent of changes in life-style, self-concept, interdependency, and role behavior will influence the individual's perception of the severity of the losses.

Final phases of the grieving process, if they occur, follow in subsequent weeks and months. If the patient is successful in dealing with his anxiety and feelings of loss, adaptation to the illness may also be positive. However, maladaptation can occur in some instances as evidenced by overdependency and hypochondriasis. The most severe form of the latter displays itself in cardiac invalidism. Thus the outcome of adaptation to the initial stage of illness can affect the patient's ability to handle later stages.

The second phase of the trajectory, disease progression, can result in continued or renewed feelings of anxiety and depression. Increasing symptoms, recurrent hospitalization, and increasing physical disability trigger such feelings. Problems in adjusting to the demands of the therapeutic regimen can arise. The feelings of helplessness, anger, depression, and isolation experienced can lead to the behavior exhibited by the cardiac cripple. Assisting individuals to cope with losses and changes during this period may be critical to successful adaptation.

Those who have not been successful in solving the problems of earlier stages will carry their unresolved feeling into the final stage of the trajectory. As attacks of cardiac failure become more frequent or symptoms of failure become less responsive to treatment, the possibility of death becomes more real. Facing death can be difficult not only for the patient but for the family and caregivers as well. Table 13-1 summarizes the psychosocial problems and patient responses along the disease trajectory.

THEORETICAL BASES OF ACTION

Before proceeding to definitions of psychosocial problems and the clinical interventions applicable in each, an overview of the theoretical bases for action is indicated. The concepts of stress and adaptation provide the clinician who practices in a variety of settings with a scientific foundation for assessing the patient, determining goals, and instituting interventions. These concepts have been the target of much research related to cardiac disease—in particular, coronary artery disease. Thus they provide an appropriate framework in caring for the person with chronic heart failure.

Stress

Historical overview. The concept of stress was introduced by Hans Selye as a nonspecific physiological response of the organism to demands made upon it. The body's reaction to stress was termed the "general adaptation syndrome." This syndrome, as postulated by Selye, has three stages.

1. Alarm reaction—general mobilization of the body's defensive forces occurs.
2. Resistance—the body's defensive responses engage the stressor in an attempt to restore physical equilibrium.
3. Exhaustion—the body's defensive forces are depleted.[23]

This model of stress is essentially a biological one and is concerned with physiological responses. Janis[8] introduced the concept of psychological stress as a response of individuals to traumatic events. Subsequent proliferation of writings on this topic attest to its importance as a framework for understanding certain aspects of human behavior.

However, the multiplicity of research has produced some difficulties for the practitioner interested in formulating guidelines for action. The major problem lies in the lack of a widely accepted definition and model of stress. Certain models, for example, those of Selye, Mechanic, Wolff, and Dohrenwend, are field specific and cannot be extended to include all levels of human reactions.[15] Thus the model that is proposed in the following sections is of necessity an eclectic one. Concepts will be drawn from various researchers in an attempt to provide a comprehensive understanding of stress and its relationship to cardiac disease.

Nature and components. The model of stress used in this chapter emphasizes the interrelationship of physiological and psychosocial processes within the individual. It is generally accepted that tensions and strains that occur at one level of functioning, for example, the physiological, also affect other spheres, such as the intellectual and/or emotional. In general, the individual functions as an integrated whole. Any conceptualization of stress, then, must take into consideration both aspects of human functioning, the physiological and the psychosocial. The model proposed is based on that of Dohrenwend[3] and is supplemented by concepts proposed by Lazarus,[14] Scott and Howard,[22] and Caplan[2] (Fig. 13-2).

What are the components of stress theory? Stress has been variously defined. Caplan's definition includes the following components: demands made upon the individual; the organism's ability to respond; the discrepancy between the two; and consequences that will be detrimental to the person. Other authors include the idea of threat to integrity of the individual as an essential part of defining stress. According to Dohrenwend's model of stress there are four main elements. First is the stressor, the stimulus that impinges upon the individual, disturbing its state of equilibrium. This stressor may be external to the individual or originate from within. If it is external, it may arise from a situation, an event, the action of others, or any number of physical stimuli within the individual's environment. Alternately, stressors can originate from the individual's internal psychological or physical spheres. Physical illness would be considered an internal physiologic stressor.

Factors mediating the effects of the stressor on the individual constitute the second element of the stress concept. Mediating factors are partially dependent upon the nature of the stressor, its se-

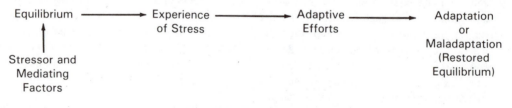

Fig. 13-2. Model of stress.

verity, intensity, and actual or potential consequences. In general, stressors that pose a threat to ego integrity are affected by numerous factors. These include internal mediating factors such as perception of the stressor and perception of ego resources—for example, intellectual ability, knowledge, and problem-solving skills. Success or failure of previous attempts at coping with similar stressors is also of major importance.[19] In addition to internal mediating factors, external ones, such as material resources, and the presence of a supportive social structure of family and friends can mitigate the impact of the stressor upon the individual as well as the duration of its effects.

The third element of the model is the experience of stress that is the result of the interaction between the stressor and the mediating forces. If the threat is purely an internal physical one, the response of the organism may only include physiological sequelae, such as increased metabolism, increase in white blood cells, and increased production of corticosteroids. However, when there exists a concomitant threat to the integrity of the individual from a physical stressor, as in cardiac disease, a psychological response can be expected. Feelings of anxiety arise with its attendant physiological symptoms. If the stressor carries with it the threat of loss or actual loss, a grief reaction can complicate the picture.

The experience of stress is followed by coping behavior, which generally falls into two categories, fight or flight. Flight behavior includes mental mechanisms such as denial, with behavior designed to remove the individual from the perceived threat. Fight behavior includes anger, problem-solving behaviors, and other actions designed to remove or mitigate the source of stress.

The last element in the stress model is adaptation. If coping mechanisms have been successful, internal equilibrium and relationship with the environment will be reestablished. If coping behavior has been unsuccessful, maladaptation occurs. This is evidenced when subjective distress continues, when somatic symptoms emerge, or when the person's behavior deviates from social norms or expected functioning. As was discussed earlier, persons with chronic cardiac disease can adapt positively or develop maladjusted behavior patterns.

Effects of stress and their relationship to cardiac disease. Stress has been implicated in the development of cardiac disease, specifically coronary artery disease, which is a major cause of congestive heart failure, and arrhythmias, both fatal and nonfatal, have been linked to stress. The exact role stress plays in the cause of coronary artery disease is still being investigated. However, authors are beginning to explore possible causal models. Eyer[4] implicates stress as a factor in social causes of coronary artery disease, while Jenkins[11] and others focus on life stresses and behavioral risk factors in the development of coronary artery disease (Fig. 13-3).

Since biological risk factors account for approximately half of the incidence of coronary artery disease, researchers have investigated the influences of personal behavior and emotional factors. Several studies have shown that measures of anxiety, neuroticism, and depression correlate with future development of angina pectoris and possibly of coronary death. In addition, Theorell's

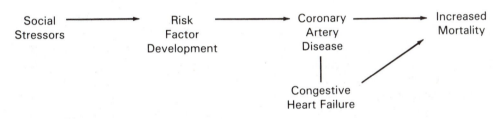

Fig. 13-3. Model of cause of coronary artery disease.

study of Swedish construction workers has linked disturbing emotional conflicts to development of myocardial infarction.[28] Additional behavioral factors that have shown a positive correlation with both future myocardial infarction and angina pectoris have been sleep disturbance and emotional drain or exhaustion.[10] At the present time, exact causal models are lacking to explain these findings, but they suggest the influence of psychological mechanisms upon the cardiovascular system.

The Type A behavior pattern has been widely researched as a risk factor in coronary artery disease. The results of several large-scale prospective studies, the Framingham Heart Study[7] and the Western Collaborative Group Study,[18] have shown that the Type A behavior pattern is unquestionably a risk factor in the development of coronary artery disease. Type A behavior is described as an emotion-action complex that includes extremes of competitiveness, striving for achievement, aggressiveness, haste, impatience, restlessness, intensely alert posture, and feelings of time pressure. Jenkins stresses that it is a *reaction* of a psychologically predisposed person to a challenging situation. It is not a personality trait but a behavior pattern.

While its existence as a risk factor for white middle-class men and women is now uncontested, the mechanisms by which Type A behavior influences the development of coronary artery disease are still debatable. Research points to the possibility of the classic physiological responses to stress as an intermediary between the behavior pattern and the future development of coronary artery disease and of increased risk of myocardial infarction and angina pectoris. In addition to the physiological responses to stress, experimental evidence suggests the possibility of other physiological responses as mediators of coronary artery disease in persons with Type A behavior pattern. Physiological changes that occur during mental work, sensory intake, or vigilant behavior are thought to be mechanisms involved in the development of coronary artery disease.[86] Additional research is required before the link between Type A behavior,

stress reactions, and coronary artery disease can be fully explained. Current studies are exploring these linkages, as well as the psychological underpinnings of coronary prone behavior, but results are too tentative to draw any firm conclusions.

Palpitations and tachycardia are among the most widely recognized physical effects of psychological stress. Studies demonstrate that emotional stress can play a role in the precipitation of premature ventricular arrhythmias in persons with heart disease.[30] As with other findings that connect stress with cardiac disease, the exact mechanism producing these effects is still conjectural. However, there is overwhelming evidence supporting the idea that the stress reactions have a major role in the development of certain cardiac diseases and in the occurrence of complications.

It is evident that the stress concept provides a useful framework from which to assess and intervene in the psychosocial problems faced by the individual with chronic heart failure. The extent to which these problems act as stressors will determine their physiological effects and their possible impact on underlying cardiac dysfunction. There are no long-term studies demonstrating that stress reduction or successful adaptation to stressors positively affect morbidity or mortality in chronic cardiac disease. However, recent reviews have revealed that successful adaptation to myocardial infarction as a major stressor may reduce the possibility of repeated infarction and cardiac death.[5,17] Thus evidence supports assistance in stress reduction and adaptation as goals for those providing care to persons with chronic cardiac disease.

PROBLEM AREAS
Changes in life-style related to diagnosis

The problem areas identified as possible stressors for the person with chronic cardiac disease and resultant congestive heart failure are: (1) changes in life-style related to cardiac disease; (2) compliance; (3) dealing with loss of physical integrity, social roles, or interdependency; and (4) facing death. Although these problems can exist in any combination, they will be discussed individually. This will facilitate identification of problem areas that are most stressful to the patient. It will also simplify the selection of appropriate interventions and the evaluation of their effectiveness.

The overall goals for psychosocial intervention in chronic cardiac disease and in congestive heart failure are (1) to assist the patient to successfully cope with the changes resulting from cardiac disease throughout the illness trajectory and (2) to decrease the effects of stress on the cardiovascular system. With these goals in mind, one of the first areas to be assessed is the effect of the disease and medical management on the individual and the family.

Assessment of life-style changes

1. Identify the cause of the disease and its effects.
   a. When did symptoms first appear?
   b. What factors (persons, situations, emotions, activities) negatively affect symptoms?
   c. What is the extent of the disease?
   d. What was the patient's life-style like before the onset of the disease and subsequent diagnosis including activities (work and recreation) and relationships with others?
   e. What cardiac risk factors exist?
   f. What is the current level of disability related to the diagnosis?
   g. Are there other disabilities or diseases present that would complicate the need for changes in life-style?
2. Determine current medical management.
   a. What medications are prescribed?
   b. What are their potential side effects?
   c. Has the therapeutic regimen been successful in controlling symptoms?
   d. Is surgical intervention being planned in the near or distant future?
3. Determine the stage of emotional adaptation to the diagnosis.
   a. What is (was) the patient's and family's initial reaction to the diagnosis? How did they view it?

   b. What stage in emotional adaptation currently exists?
      (1) Shock and disbelief
      (2) Defensive retreat
      (3) Active coping
      (4) Adaptation or maladaptation
4. Determine the nature of changes in life-style required by the diagnosis or treatment regimen.
   a. Are changes in the type and quantity of food and their preparation required?
   b. What changes in activity are required?
      (1) Work
      (2) Recreation
      (3) Sexual activity
   c. Will reordering time of activities be indicated?
   d. What other adjustment will be necessary as a result of treatment; for example, more frequent urination if diuretics are prescribed?
   e. To what extent will changes impact upon the patient's family?
   f. What are the patient's and family's perceptions and misconceptions regarding necessary changes?
   g. To what extent will patient and family require assistance in adaptation?

Interventions in problems related to life-style changes. Once the initial assessment has been made, the clinician can begin to assist the patient and family in adjusting to the necessary changes. The major goal of intervention is to maintain as much normalcy as feasible in their life-style. Attention should be focused on what the patient can do, prescriptions, rather than on limitations or restrictions. A number of interventions are possible. The major one is active problem solving. This engages the patient and family in resolving the problem identified and in mutual goal setting. By shared problem solving, the patient is assured greater control over his or her life. This increases the possibility that projected changes in life-style will become a reality.

The initial step in active problem solving is to

assist the patient in determining how anticipated changes can be incorporated into the present lifestyle. This involves not only identifying changes but also correcting misconceptions about them. The second step is to provide the patient and family with the resources available to assist them in making the required changes. For example, if diet changes are indicated, helping the patient to modify favorite meals or recipes may be indicated. There are a number of cookbooks now on the market that can be useful to those on low-sodium or low-cholesterol diets. Trying new foods or recipes may be difficult for some; therefore, setting a goal of one or two new ones a week may be a more acceptable solution.

For the patient with functional cardiac impairment who must limit activities, exercise guidelines are indicated. If the patient has undergone exercise testing, the exact level of exercise tolerance is known. Exercise equivalent tables, such as that published by the Colorado Heart Association, list activities according to METS, that is, their metabolic requirements.[6] It provides patients with a concrete list of activities. It is a more useful guide than general instructions to avoid strenuous exercise. For those with decreased cardiac function, assistance may be required in planning rest periods and activities so that favorite activities can continue to be enjoyed.

A major area in which patients require education is that of sexual activity. Myths surrounding this topic have led many patients with cardiac disease into abandoning it needlessly. Some patients have experienced impotence or lack of sexual desire, particularly following a myocardial infarction. However, it can also be a problem for any person with decreased cardiac functional capacity. Several excellent sources are available to the clinician when this difficulty arises for patients and their spouses.[13,21] The boxed material below may be useful as a guideline for teaching patients and their spouses basic information regarding intercourse.

Instructions to the patient should take into account the level of cardiac function, previous history of impotence, and the patient's usual pattern of sexual activity. For those with severe cardiac

---

INSTRUCTIONS REGARDING SEXUAL INTERCOURSE

1. Orgasm itself requires approximately 5 METS, the equivalent of climbing 20 stairs in 10 seconds.
2. Engage in sexual intercourse only when well rested. Postpone intercourse for approximately 3 hours after heavy meals or alcohol consumption.
3. Intercourse should occur in a relaxed unhurried atmosphere, preferably with a usual partner. Assume comfortable positions.
4. Warning signals that intercourse may be too strenuous include: (a) a rapid heart rate that persists for longer than 4 to 5 minutes after orgasm; (b) feeling extremely fatigued the day after intercourse; (c) chest pain during or immediately following intercourse.
5. Nitroglycerin may be prescribed by some physicians to be used prophylactically by those experiencing angina. Such a possibility should be discussed with the physician.
6. Some medications, such as propranolol (Inderal), methyldopa (Aldomet), and chlordiazepoxide (Librium), may affect sexual response.

impairment, engaging in sexual intercourse may not be physically possible. In such instances, the patient and spouse should be encouraged to use alternate means of demonstrating love and affection.

Evaluation. We have focused on two major interventions, providing accurate information and assisting in active problem solving by identifying changes, suggesting alternatives, options, resources, and achieving realistic goal setting. Evaluating the outcome of these interventions is an important aspect of care. Specific outcome criteria can help determine if interventions are successful or if alternative approaches are required. Examples of outcome criteria are:

1. The patient will verbalize how three favorite meals can be altered to comply with dietary restrictions.
2. The patient will identify those activities that may be engaged in from a list of activities that include their MET requirements.
3. The patient and spouse will verbalize satisfaction with sexual intercourse and/or expression of love and affection.

Compliance with therapeutic regimen

The problem of adherence by the patient to the therapeutic management of the disease is a critical one. Failure to adhere may mean increased frequency of symptoms, hospitalization, and possibly death for those with chronic cardiac diseases and congestive heart failure. Literature on the topic of compliance with medical regimens has proliferated since the 1970s, but no generally accepted model for assessment and intervention in the problem area exists. However, there is general agreement that the problem is a complex one involving a multiplicity of factors, including personal ones and those related to treatment.

Personal factors include motivations, beliefs, intentions, values, perception of severity of illness, physician-patient relationship, age, attribution of causality of the illness, perceived control of the illness or its symptoms, and patient satisfaction with caregivers and effects of treatment.[9,20] Variables related to the treatment also affect patient adherence. These include complexity of the treatment, cost, undesirable side effects, and intrusion of treatment into life-style. Exactly how all these variables interact to increase or decrease the likelihood of compliance has not been established.

The following assessment guidelines assume that major denial of illness is not present in the patient. Other barriers such as anxiety and depression can negatively affect compliance, especially in the patient with chronic cardiac disease. These may require intervention in their own right. Considering the state of flux in compliance research, the practitioner should keep in mind that some interventions may not work and alternatives may need to be tried.

The assessment section has been designed so that negative answers indicate that that factor is a hindering force in compliance and that a positive answer is an enabling force. This should assist in identifying negative factors, which may need to be eliminated or decreased, and positive factors, which should be enhanced in an effort to increase compliance to the medical regimen.

Assessment of compliance factors

1. Personal factors
   a. Does the patient have the intellectual ability to understand the medical regimen and its purpose?
   b. Does the patient have the physical energy necessary to carry out the treatment plan?
   c. Does the patient admit the seriousness of the illness?
   d. Does the patient believe that control of the disease and its symptoms is his responsibility?
   e. Is the patient willing to make a commitment to adhering to the medical regimen?
   f. Does the patient have a positive attitude toward maintaining his health?
   g. Does the patient have positive past experiences with the effectiveness of adherence to a therapeutic regimen?
   h. Does the patient trust the medical authority of his physician and other caregivers?

i. Is the patient satisfied with his interaction with his physician and other significant caregivers?

j. Does the proposed regimen minimally interfere with the patient's social roles?

2. External factors
   a. Does the patient have the funds necessary to comply with the regimen?
   b. Does the regimen have a minimal amount of uncomfortable side effects?
   c. Does the regimen have a small number of components?
   d. Are the caregivers interested in the patient? Do they convey this to him?

Interventions for problems in compliance. From the assessment guideline presented, it should be obvious that a patient may face numerous problems that interfere with adherence to a therapeutic regimen. These include such problems as cost, negative health attitudes, lack of knowledge, feelings of helplessness, and unwillingness to take responsibility for self-care related to the disease. Obviously interventions should be appropriate to the problems identified. For example, if cost is a major barrier, assisting the patient to obtain funding is necessary. The cost of medication may vary considerably from one prescription center to another, especially when generic drugs, such as digoxin, are prescribed. Bargain hunting may be indicated to decrease drug treatment costs.

If the problem is lack of information, teaching may be the intervention of choice. Patients often draw inaccurate inferences from the limited knowledge that they have about their illness. Therefore correcting inaccurate information may help the patient to perceive the situation more realistically and facilitate adherence. (See Chapter 12.)

When feelings of helplessness exist, setting realistic goals with the patient may be indicated. This allows as much control as possible in individualizing the therapeutic regimen and in controlling symptoms. Such a plan encourages the patient to take some responsibility for controlling his disease. However, some patients may be resistant to

taking responsibility, since individuals tend not to want to take the blame for failure. It is much more acceptable to blame caregivers if a regimen is unsuccessful. Contracting with the patient may be an alternative means of achieving this objective. It specifies what actions will be taken by the patient, as well as by the caregiver, and both are bound by it.[31]

Changing attitudes and behaviors can be challenging. Techniques for attitude change and behavior modification are presented in an excellent test by Kanfer and Goldstein.[37] Behavior modification techniques, in particular, have been successfully applied to increase compliance with therapeutic regimens in patients with chronic health problems. This intervention maximizes the impact of the clinician-patient relationship. The clinician serves as a source of reinforcement and rewards that are important in helping the patient make the behavioral changes necessary.

Participation in groups with common health problems can also be an important means for behavior change in patients. Groups serve as an additional source of models, reinforcements, and rewards. In addition, groups encourage social contacts and norm setting and provide for peer surveillance. They are also an important means of helping the patient to solve difficulties in complying with a regimen. Finally, groups are a source of emotional support and can reduce the isolation often felt by those with chronic diseases.

Not only is participation in a group having a similar diagnosis helpful, but other types of groups exist that offer similar benefits. For example, patients whose regimen includes weight reduction or stress reduction might better achieve their goal if they join a group with that as its main objective. Such groups have proliferated, especially in urban areas. The family is another important social group that is often ignored as a source of rewards and reinforcement. It can be actively involved in assisting the patient to comply with the therapeutic regimen.

All of the possible interventions discussed require a time commitment by the clinician in finding solutions to the problems of compliance, which are unique to each person. Such an involvement in itself is an important factor in supporting patient compliance.

Evaluation. Evaluation of outcomes depends upon the aspect of compliance identified for intervention. In the case of dietary compliance, the following criteria can be used as guidelines.

1. The patient will identify self-rewards for complying with dietary restrictions.
2. The patient will list three realistic means by which family members can help him to comply with a weight loss program.

Loss: a major problem in chronic cardiac disease

Threats to the self-concept, especially in those areas that are highly valued by the individual—physical integrity, social roles, and interdependent relationships with others—can result from physical illness. Actual or perceived loss in any of these three valued areas can precipitate the grieving process. Such losses can occur or unresolved losses can resurface at any given point along the disease trajectory. Thus coping with loss is a problem to be faced by the person with chronic cardiac disease and congestive heart failure.

Loss has been defined as "the act of losing possession."[29] For the loss to be followed by the grieving process, the object lost, actually or potentially, must be of value to the individual. Psychological processes and emotions that occur subsequent to the actual or potential loss of a valued object is termed mourning, or the grieving process.

The three stages of the grieving process are (1) shock and disbelief, (2) developing awareness, and (3) resolution. During the first stage, shock and disbelief, the person may feel numb, anxious, and tense, and he may deny that the loss has occurred. During the second stage, developing awareness, the reality of the loss and its meaning become apparent to the individual. This stage is accompanied by feelings of anger, sadness, helplessness, empti-

ness, and hopelessness and by behaviors such as crying and withdrawal and detachment from others and the environment. During the final stage, resolution, the person begins to deal with the loss. The individual may want to bring up the topic frequently and may appear to be preoccupied with it. Finally the person begins to relinquish the pain and the loss. This resolution stage usually take place 6 to 12 months after the initial loss. However, for some the grieving process is drawn out over a longer period, or it may never be resolved.

Loss of physical integrity. Losses for the chronically ill can occur in three spheres of the self-concept, physical integrity, role function, and interdependency. The loss of physical integrity can take a variety of forms. Actual anatomical changes occur in the heart itself. These lead to decreased cardiac function, which results in curtailment of activity levels. Changes in life-style as a result of disease and its treatment imply a loss of control over bodily processes. These can be compounded by the maturational changes of aging, such as decreasing eyesight or hearing, and decreasing energy levels. Finally, changes in physical abilities can lead to losses in other areas, such as role function and interdependency.

Loss of social roles. Persons carry out a variety of roles in society—parent, friend, lover, spouse, worker, boss, community leader or supporter. The changes that occur in these roles as a result of chronic cardiac disease can be experienced as losses. Some roles may be disrupted or curtailed. For example, a person may have to retire earlier than expected or may have to change the type and/ or amount of work performed. Certain activities related to one's role as spouse may be taken over by the husband or wife, resulting in a partial role reversal. In addition, decreased libido or inadequate sexual functioning can compound the problems of role alteration.

One's roles in life are usually important sources of self-esteem, arising from feelings of accomplishment, power, and contribution to society. Role changes can be perceived as loss of these important sources of self-esteem and can lead to feelings of worthlessness. These feelings may be compounded, if one is elderly, by societal attitudes toward the aged, attitudes that place a premium on youth and vitality. Concurrent situational changes, such as children leaving home and death of a spouse, can add to the sense of loss that is related to role changes.

Losses related to alterations of interdependency. Interdependence has been defined as a balance between dependence and independence in relationships with others.[16] It includes help-seeking behaviors, attention- and affection-seeking behaviors, initiative taking, as well as task and obstacle mastery. Chronic cardiac disease can precipitate changes in the balance of independent and dependent behaviors. A person may require help carrying out previously independent tasks, thus increasing dependency in relationships with others. Retirement or a job change, as a result of illness, can mean a loss of long-time friends and sources of attention and affection. Social activities, which are often additional avenues of affiliation, may be curtailed or eliminated, especially when physical disability is severe. Concurrent or subsequent deaths of loved ones can complicate the impact of these losses. Powerful feelings of loneliness that result from lack of interpersonal intimacy may accompany such losses. For the chronically ill person, therefore, numerous possibilities for experiencing loss exist.

The role of clinicians when such losses occur is to assist the patient through the grieving process. Clinicians in the acute care facility may find their role limited to assessment and intervention during the initial phases of shock and disbelief and beginning acknowledgment of the loss. For the practitioner in an outpatient or community health setting, assessment and intervention during the final phases of acknowledgment and resolution may be indicated. Since loss for the chronically ill can occur in any one area important to the self-concept, or in a combination of areas, the assessment and intervention presented will include all three areas, physical integrity, role function, and interdependence.

Assessment of losses

1. General assessment
   a. Identify stages of grief process (shock and disbelief, acknowledgment of the loss, resolution).
   b. Determine which is the major area of potential or actual loss as perceived by the patient (physical integrity, role function, interdependency).
   c. Determine if other areas of loss exist.
   d. Determine if losses not related to chronic cardiac disease have occurred in the recent past that increase the impact of the current loss.
   e. Determine if the patient's perception of the loss is realistic or nonrealistic.
   f. Determine adequacy of situational supports (family, friends, social activity groups).
   g. Determine the patient's perception of the adequacy of coping mechanisms during previous losses or crises (problem solving skills, help-seeking behavior).

2. Assessment of loss of physical integrity
   a. What is the cause of the cardiac disease?
   b. What is the current cardiac status?
   c. How well is therapy controlling symptoms?
   d. What physical disability is present?
   e. What does the patient perceive to be losses of physical ability or integrity?
   f. How does the patient perceive these losses as affecting other areas of functioning (role, interdependency)?

3. Assessment of loss of role function
   a. What roles does the patient perceive as being changed, lost, or curtailed as a result of the disease?
   b. What aspects of that role were most important to the patient? Will they be changed or eliminated?
   c. What roles remain unaffected?
   d. What sources of self-esteem exist for the patient?

4. Assessment of losses related to interdependency

a. What independent behaviors does the patient perceive as lost or changed?

b. What will be the extent of dependency on others? Does the patient view these as affecting his feelings of self-worth?

c. What other avenues of achievement and sources of attention and affection are available to the patient?

d. What independent behaviors important to the patient will remain?

Intervention in the grieving process. The goals of intervention for the person experiencing loss are: (1) to assist the person throughout the grieving process and (2) to help the person achieve eventual resolution of the loss while minimizing the stress of the situation. The extent of intervention depends upon the severity of the loss and the adequacy of the patient's personal and situational resources. Some patients may require extensive intervention because they lack the personal and situational resources to deal with the problem. Others may need only minimal intervention for the opposite reason—adequate coping mechanisms and support systems. The interventions will be presented according to the stage in the grief process for which they are appropriate.

Stage I: shock and disbelief. This phase, characterized by denial of the loss, usually lasts only a few hours or days. Intervention measures are related to the denial and feelings of anxiety that are experienced. The clinician's attitude should be one of support and caring. Expression of feelings by the patient should be encouraged. Denial, if it does not interfere with therapy, should be allowed. If denial is major and interfering with therapy, intervention by a mental health professional is indicated.

Anxiety that is usually present may range from mild to severe. Dependent behaviors may increase if the patient feels unable to handle decision making or day-to-day activities. Allowing such dependency on family members or health care staff is indicated at this point in time. Providing accurate information about the disease is important, especially if the patient uses intellectualization as a coping mechanism. This information may need to be repeated later since acute levels of anxiety can interfere with information processing and retention. Finally, one must assist the individual in controlling his anxiety. The nurse can help him identify his usual method of handling anxiety. If these are not effective, focused breathing exercises or other methods of producing the relaxation response may be used. The boxed material on p. 392 outlines one popular way of eliciting the relaxation response that can be taught to patients. Encouraging the patient to engage in activities requiring minimal mental effort can help distract him from the pain of the experience. Occasionally medication to control anxiety may be needed to augment the interventions already described.

Stage II: acknowledgment of the loss. This phase can last for several weeks or months. Once the clinician has assessed the patient's perception of the loss and its impact, the next step is to assist the patient in making a realistic appraisal of the loss or losses. Misconceptions should be corrected and accurate information regarding changes in physical functioning, role functions, and interdependency provided. Active problem solving should be encouraged as the person indicates readiness to deal with the loss. One must allow expression of feelings and accept other grieving behaviors. The patient can be assured of the normalcy of his reactions. Feelings of anger should be dealt with calmly and matter-of-factly. Angry feelings should be acknowledged and the patient helped to recognize their source.

Feelings of sadness and depression usually are self-limiting. However, if other losses compound the problem, or if the patient has a history of depression, it may require psychiatric therapy. The following interventions may be useful in self-limited depression. One must help the patient to realize that his feelings are related to his anger over losses related to his disease. Since negative thoughts play a role in depressive feelings, the patient should be encouraged to become aware of these thoughts and counterbalance them with positive ones. For example, "I won't be able to work full time, but I'll have more time for my favorite hobby, sport, etc." Keeping busy is an effective way to deal with depression. One must help the patient to make plans

---

GUIDELINES FOR PRODUCING THE RELAXATION RESPONSE

---

1. Place yourself in a quiet room, where you will be free from distractions and interruptions. Lighting should be subdued.
2. Assume a comfortable position, lying down or sitting in a chair with head, arms, and legs supported. Loosen or remove constraining clothing.
3. Focus your attention on a pleasant word or sound. Mentally repeat that sound, gently clearing the mind of distracting thoughts or images.
4. Assume a passive attitude. Allow your body to relax; allow tense muscles of face, back, abdomen, arms, and legs to go limp.
5. If distracting thoughts occur, gently begin repeating the selected word.
6. Continue to relax for about 15 to 20 minutes. When the time period is completed, allow yourself several minutes to "awaken." Slowly begin to move arms and legs and to open your eyes.
7. Plan your relaxation sessions so that they will not occur within one hour after eating. Avoid stimulants such as tea, coffee, or other caffeine-containing beverages for several hours before your relaxation sessions.
8. Producing the "relaxation response" takes time to learn. If you allow yourself one to two sessions daily, you should find that you will become relaxed quickly after a week or so.

Adapted from Patricia Carrington, Freedom in meditation, New York, 1978, Anchor Press.

to keep active, even if the activities are solitary ones. The patient should be encouraged to use sources of emotional support, such as close family members and friends.

Interventions suggested for active problem-solving related to changes imposed by the diagnosis and therapy are also indicated. One must assist the patient to adapt to losses related to social roles, achievement, and affiliation. Unfortunately, in many instances the clinician may have limited access to the patient during this phase. However, there is increasing evidence that various patient groups can have positive outcomes both psychologically and physiologically for patients with cardiac disease. Hopefully, these benefits will be made available to the increasing number of patients who suffer losses related to chronic cardiac disease.

Stage III: resolution of the loss. Optimally during this phase memory of the loss decreases in frequency and the person experiences renewed feelings of happiness and enjoyment of life. For some patients with chronic cardiac disease this period may last for a long time. For others it may be short lived as losses related to decreased cardiac function occur. The wounds of old losses may be reopened and grieving renewed. For those with deteriorating cardiac function, acceptance of continued losses may be viewed as the only alternative. Some patients become chronically depressed, others seek to extract as much happiness as possible from life. If the patient has moved successfully through the grieving process, intervention at this point is minimal. The patient should be encouraged to examine how effective problem solving has helped him reach the resolution of the loss. For patients who experience recurrent losses, continued support in dealing with feelings and in problem solving may be required.

Evaluation. The interventions in this section have focused on ways of helping the patient to resolve grief over losses related to chronic cardiac disease. Assessing the success of these actions will be related to the specific stage in which the clinician has the opportunity to intervene. The following outcome criteria are guidelines for evaluation.

1. The patient will verbalize decreased feelings of anxiety after correctly employing the relaxation response.
2. The patient will develop a plan for engaging in activities and implement the plan within the next week.
3. The patient will call a close friend and arrange to spend several hours together during the next week.

Facing death: a special problem in chronic cardiac disease

The final outcome of chronic cardiac disease and chronic congestive heart failure is death. It may occur soon after initial diagnosis, as in a massive myocardial infarction. Or it may occur after years of slowly deteriorating cardiac function. As cardiac failure becomes intractable to management, the possibility of death is difficult to deny. Death has connotations of nullifying not only life itself but also the objectives sought in life. Initial reactions to the possibility of death can range from denial to anger and depression. Theorists compare these reactions to those of the grief process.

The optimal outcome of coping with the fear of death or its imminence is acceptance. However, research indicates that not all those close to death achieve this end. Dying persons may continue to deny or to be alternately angry or depressed. Thus what were once considered stages of coping with impending death actually may be repetitive cycles of emotions and defense mechanisms. Some may verbally deny the possibility of death, but their behavior indicates that death is not far off. Others deny death both in word and in deed. Still others, while acknowledging the closeness of death by putting their affairs in order, also cling to life as avidly as possible. In addition, responses may be related to the various persons with whom the patient interacts. For example, acceptance may be voiced to the clinician but denial may be expressed to a spouse or family member. If the patient has done some preliminary grieving, reactions may be less strong.

Providing care for the chronically ill can be disruptive of daily living for the family. At times spouses will forsake friends and favorite activities in order to care for the patient at home during the final stages of illness. When family members and the patient are willing, care can continue to be provided at home. If necessary, home health agencies can provide the nursing support required to make death at home possible. However, at times the resources of family and community are unable to meet the needs of the terminally ill cardiac patient and hospitalization in an acute or long-term facility is indicated.

The period before death can be one of anticipatory grieving for the family. It can positively affect the subsequent adjustment of the family members to the loss of their loved one. Anticipatory grieving diminishes the shock caused by death and allows time to prepare for its finality.

The role of the clinician in caring for the patient and the family is a supportive one. However, it is one that not all individuals have the emotional energy to undertake. But for some it is fulfilling and at times strengthening.

Determining what care is required means assessing both the patient's and the family's reactions to impending death as well as the patient's physiological needs. Although the problem of facing death can occur at any time along the disease trajectory, consideration will be given primarily to the problem during the terminal phase of illness.

Assessment of the problems related to impending death

1. Determine the patient's and the family's level of awareness of impending death:
   a. Unaware
   b. Aware, but pretending unawareness
   c. Aware
2. Assess the patient's and the family's response(s) to impending death:
   a. Denial
   b. Anger

    c. Sadness, crying, depression or withdrawing
    d. Acceptance, but with feelings of anger and/or sadness
3. Assess the physical care required by the patient:
    a. Oxygen
    b. Medication
    c. Personal hygiene
    d. Nutrition
    e. Preventative measures
    f. Elimination
4. Determine what visitors the patient wishes to have and the length of their stay.
5. Determine what objects or activities can be provided to give pleasure during the terminal period; for example:
    a. Favorite belongings
    b. Music
    c. View of trees and sky
6. Determine what sources of support are available to the patient and the family:
    a. Friends, neighbors
    b. Pastor, rabbi

Interventions for problems related to impending death. Both physical and psychological interventions are important to the dying person with chronic cardiac disease. The patient should continue to receive adequate medical and nursing care. The constant use of oxygen by the patient will cause drying of nasal and oral mucous membranes. Therefore cleansing of the nostrils and mouth will need to be done more frequently. With increased shortness of breath, small, more frequent feedings can replace larger meals. Frequent turning and care of skin over dependent areas is even more important when edema resulting from cardiac failure is present. The anxious patient, fighting for breath, may require sedation. These as well as measures to maintain physical appearance are important in sustaining a dignified self-image.

The psychological support needed by the patient and the family is dependent upon their level of awareness, their responses to impending death, and their ability to cope with the situation. Some patients may need to resolve business, financial, or family matters. Visiting hours should be relaxed to permit family members as much closeness as they desire. The patient who is able should continue to take an active part in decision making related to family matters and personal care. Patients should be encouraged to verbalize feelings to supportive family members, friends, or staff. For those in the intractable stages of congestive heart failure, energy is at a minimum and most of their effort is focused on trying to breathe. Consequently, rather than expecting much verbalization from these patients, words of understanding and empathy may be more appropriate.

Family members, even those who have watched the slow deterioration of a loved one approaching death, may continue to deny its possibility; but frequently family members view death as an end to suffering. The support they require is dependent upon their place in the grieving process and whether family members are mutually supportive. Some may only need a shoulder to cry on or a sympathetic listener. Others may require assistance in problem solving. Whatever their reactions, most require the reassurance that their loved one is receiving the best in health care and is being kept as comfortable as possible.

Evaluation. Determining outcomes of interventions is, of course, dependent upon the problems identified and the interventions required. The goal for the patient is a dignified and peaceful death. However, as an outcome statement it is difficult to measure. Expecting verbalizations from patients regarding acceptance of death is not always realistic, since it is sometimes communicated by a look or even a gesture. Consequently outcome statements may be limited to comfort measures, such as the patient verbalizes a level of comfort commensurate with respiratory and cardiac status. Other expected outcomes will be specific to the situation.

APPLICATION OF CONCEPTS

The central concept of the preceding sections is that the stress of the psychosocial problems that arise as a consequence of chronic cardiac disease create stress for the individual. Therefore, in addition to intervening in the physical problems related to the disease, the clinician should also be concerned with reducing the stress created by psychosocial problems. The following case study applies assessment and intervention techniques outlined in this chapter to a specific patient situation. It is recognized that the patient's physical problems may assume priority at times during the disease trajectory. However, in order to simplify the case presentation, only the patient's psychosocial problems will be covered.

CASE STUDY

Three years ago at the age of 63, Mrs. W had a myocardial infarction. She was hospitalized for 15 days, 4 of which were in a coronary care unit. During that time she had one episode of mild congestive heart failure that responded to therapy. She was placed on a no-added-salt diet. During the first year after the myocardial infarction there were no further episodes of congestive heart failure. Approximately 2 years after her hospitalization her husband died suddenly. Several months later she was admitted to the hospital with mild congestive heart failure. Testing revealed no further infarction. She was sent home taking digoxin, 0.125 mg daily and a no-added-salt diet. She was also told not to do anything strenuous. Her cardiac status was determined to be slightly compromised and her prognosis good with therapy.

Two days ago Mrs. W was again admitted with congestive heart failure. The failure responded to increased digoxin dosage, diuretic therapy, and bed rest. During this initial period of hospitalization one of the nurses, Ms. K, noted that Mrs. W seemed depressed. She spoke only in answer to questions and seemed to have little interest in what was happening to her. A daughter had been in to visit during the first 2 days. However, she lived 200 miles away and had returned home for a few days to take care of family responsibilities, she had promised to return in 2 days time. Today, as Ms. K assisted in her case, she mentioned to Mrs. W that she seemed ''down'' and was wondering what was upsetting her. Mrs. W's eyes filled with tears. She felt her heart ailment was getting worse that she might soon be an invalid. Mrs. W cried for a short time. She then said that she felt better having talked to someone and that she had not wanted to burden her daughter with her concerns.

Later that morning Ms. K spoke with Mrs. W's physician. He said that Mrs. W's cardiac status was un-

changed and her prognosis was good with therapy. However, it seemed that she had not been taking her digoxin regularly and had not been adhering to the sodium-restricted diet. This precipitated her current episode of congestive heart failure. He said he thought that changes in Mrs. W's life since her husband's death was contributing to her dejection. Ms. K suggested that the clinical nurse specialist could assist in obtaining more information and formulating a plan of care for hospitalization and following discharge. The physician thought it was an excellent idea. He also mentioned that he planned to have Mrs. W seen at home for several months after discharge by a public health nurse. He wanted Mrs. W's physical status monitored and hoped the more frequent visits by health care personnel would increase her compliance with the medical plan of care. Ms. K contacted the clinical nurse specialist. She agreed to assist in assessing Mrs. W and in devising a plan of care.

Using the guidelines for assessment presented in this chapter, the following patient problems were identified: (1) failure to comply with the medical treatment plan because of lack of knowledge, fatigue, and feelings of loss of control and (2) moderate feelings of depression because of multiple losses and life changes during the past year. Mrs. W agreed that these two problem areas existed and promised to help in making a realistic plan to help solve them.

The two nursing diagnoses will be discussed individually, and the assessment data that led to each diagnosis will be presented. In addition, the interventions developed by the nurses in conjunction with Mrs. W, as well as outcome criteria, will also be detailed.

Nursing diagnosis: Failure to comply with the medical treatment plan because of lack of knowledge, fatigue, and feelings of loss of control.
Assessment data
1. Positive personal factors affecting compliance
   a. Has the intellectual ability to understand treatment plan
   b. Admits to seriousness of illness
   c. Is willing to try to comply with the medical treatment plan
   d. Has had positive experience during this hospitalization with the effectiveness of the treatment plan
   e. Is trusting of physician and nurses
2. Negative personal factors affecting compliance
   a. Lacks necessary energy to carry out parts of treatment plan (often does not feel like cooking and eats frozen TV dinners high in sodium)

b. Feels that cardiac disease is getting worse and she cannot control it

c. Feels treatment plan will interfere with her life (frequent urination resulting from diuretic therapy)

d. Does not understand dietary restrictions and finds them undesirable

e. Anxious about trying new things

f. Depressive feelings contribute to feelings of fatigue

3. External factors

a. Has necessary funds to carry out treatment plan (has Social Security, annuity funds, owns own home)

b. Has supportive daughter who visits monthly and brings her two children

Interventions	*Outcome criteria*
1. Make referral to dietitian for basic instruction in a 3000 to 4000 g sodium-restricted diet to be followed upon discharge	By discharge the patient will: Identify foods that she likes that are low in sodium
2. Refer to dietitian for initial problem solving regarding implementation of diet: (a) fixing of meals, (b) possible menus, (c) new recipes	Verbalize how two of her favorite recipes can be modified so that they conform to sodium restrictions Select two new recipes from a cookbook for persons on a sodium-restricted diet
3. Assist patient to achieve a more realistic assessment of her physical and cardiac status by (a) pointing out decreasing fatigue once adequate therapy was followed, (b) instructing how drugs and diet work to help her control symptoms, (c) pointing out that stresses and depressive feelings can contribute to feelings of fatigue, (d) remind her that her cardiac status is unchanged according to her physician.	Verbalize an understanding of how the prescribed drugs and diet to be followed at home will control symptoms Verbalize how stresses can contribute to fatigue
4. Involve patient in devising a schedule for drug taking	Assist in devising medication schedule
5. Begin self-administration of medication after obtaining physician's order	Correctly take drugs for 3 to 4 days before discharge

Interventions	*Outcome criteria*
6. Make referral to Public Health Agency for nursing follow-up post discharge	Agree to be visited by public health nurse and verbalize understanding of the reason for referral
7. Begin interventions to decrease depressive feelings that contribute to patient's feelings of fatigue	

Evaluation. The dietitian visited with Mrs. W and determined that 15-minute sessions twice a day would be the best schedule to carry out the teaching needed. Mrs. W read the literature left by the dietitian in between their sessions at her own pace. She carried out her "assignments" and agreed to try one new recipe a week for 4 weeks when she returned home. When her daughter visited again Mrs. W explained her new diet to her. The daughter suggested that they try out a new recipe together when she visited each month. When the need for home visits was explained to Mrs. W, she seemed pleased by the arrangement. She expressed relief that someone would be checking in on her. Her husband, she said, made her feel secure and had been the problem solver. Having someone to help her adjust at home was welcomed by her.

By discharge Mrs. W demonstrated adequate knowledge of the sodium-restricted diet. Her physician agreed that having Mrs. W begin taking her own medication might help and wrote the order. By the discharge date Mrs. W had taken her medication as scheduled. Once she returned home the public health nurse would continue to monitor her adherence to the therapeutic regimen and assist Mrs. W in making necessary adjustments.

Nursing diagnosis: Moderate feelings of depression resulting from multiple losses and life-style changes during the past year.

Assessment data

1. Loss of interdependence

a. Death of husband 1 year ago, which has not been resolved

b. Increased dependence on daughter and friends (she does not drive and various friends take her shopping for food and take her to church)

c. Only daughter lives a distance away and can visit only once a month

d. No longer has vegetable and flower garden (loss of source of self-esteem)

2. Loss of role function
   a. Loss of role of wife since husband's death
   b. Decreased social role (has stopped playing bridge with friends since husband's death)
3. Loss of physical integrity
   a. Has dyspnea with normal exertion
   b. Has stopped gardening activities since husband's death (gardener cares for lawn and shrubs)
   c. Has decreased housekeeping activities (her daughter does heavy cleaning chores once a month)
4. Personal strengths
   a. Intelligent and willing to participate in problem-solving ways to help herself
   b. Has maintained an interest in world affairs (reads newspaper and watches news reports on television)
   c. Handles household and financial affairs capably
5. Support system
   a. Has several friends who visit or call regularly
   b. Has daughter who is concerned and supportive but whose work and family responsibilities prevent her from visiting more frequently

Interventions	*Outcome criteria*
1. Provide opportunities for expression of feelings regarding losses	Patient will express feelings regarding losses
2. Engage patient in problem solving to increase social activities and to participate in activities that will help her to feel useful	Identify several activities she can engage in and make concrete plans to be implemented upon discharge
a. Identify what past activities can be restarted, for example bridge club	Select several books from the patient library to read during hospitalization
b. Stress importance of keeping busy and occupied as a way to combat depressive feeling	Set up possible activity schedules that include periods of rest
c. Develop, in conjunction with patient, possible activity schedules that include periods of rest	

Interventions	*Outcome criteria*
3. Assist patient in realistically assessing her situation	
a. Focus on identifying what she has not lost, for example: financial security; good friends; attentive daughter and grandchildren; expertise as bridge player	Identify five positive aspects of her life
4. Instruct patient in how to use positive thoughts to combat depressive feelings	Identify at least three persistent negative thoughts and three positive thoughts to counterbalance them
5. Begin discharge planning	Employ positive self-thoughts at least three times daily for the duration of hospitalization
a. Discuss patient situation with physician	
b. Make out referral to public health nursing agency for continued health assessment and follow up on plans to increase compliance and decrease depressive feelings	

Evaluation. Although Ms. K provided a number of opportunities for Mrs. W to talk about her feelings regarding the losses and changes of the previous year she declined to do so. However, she did agree to try positive thoughts to counteract her negative ones and found it helpful. As her physical symptoms responded to therapy and she felt less fatigued, Mrs. W did chat more with her hospital roommate. However, she continued to appear dejected at times. It was expected that the public health nurse would reassess Mrs. W's depressive feelings after she had returned home. In addition, the nurse could support Mrs. W's plans to begin playing bridge again and restart other social activities that would help decrease her depressive feelings and the fatigue associated with them.

SUMMARY

In the preceding sections, the problems faced by the patient with chronic cardiac disease and congestive heart failure have been delineated. Assessment and intervention for such problems as adjusting to changes in life-style, compliance with medical regimens, dealing with loss, and facing death have been presented. In addition, a framework for caring for the chronically ill patient was suggested; this included concepts of stress and adaptation. It is expected that the successful resolution of problems will reduce the toll of stress upon the patient. But it should be remembered that not all patients have the same problems to the same degree and that the resilience of human beings is tremendous. Many with chronic cardiac disease have made the necessary changes in their lives and continued to be productive and happy.

Patients and caregivers can draw inspiration and perhaps resolve from the story of Arthur Ashe, professional American tennis player. At the height of a brilliant tennis career, Arthur suffered a massive heart attack on August 1, 1979. As a result his cardiac status was severely compromised and he underwent cardiac surgery for quadruple coronary artery bypass grafts. For Arthur, life could no longer be taken for granted. The possibility of another heart attack always lurked on the fringes of his mind. His physical limitations meant that he had to give up competitive world tennis for a less physically demanding position as captain of the U.S. Davis Cup team. Although such events might have devastated a much less determined person, he looked at his life and made the necessary changes. What is most important about Arthur is his attitude. His words say it all and are a fitting ending to this chapter.

I have had to think about death and this has made life more precious. My task was to grab myself by the shoulders and say, "From this day forward, life is going to be different."

REFERENCES

1. Ashe, A.: Shifting gears, World Tennis **29**(4):117, 1981.
2. Caplan, G.: Mastery of stress: psychosocial aspects, Am. J. Psychiatry **138**(4):413, 1981.
3. Dohrenwend, B.: Class and race as status-related sources of stress. In Levine, S., and Scotch, N.A., editors: Social stress, 1970, Aldine Publishing Co.
4. Eyer, J.: Social causes of coronary heart disease, Psychother. Psychosom. **34**:75, 1980.
5. Frank, K.A., Heller, S.S., and Kornfield, D.S.: Psychological intervention in coronary heart disease, Gen. Hosp. Psychiatry, **1**(1):18, 1979.
6. Hackett, T.P., and Cassem, N.H.: Psychological factors related to exercise, Cardiovasc. Clin. **9**(3):223, 1978.
7. Haynes, S.G., Feinleib, M., and Kannel, W.B.: The relationship of psychosocial factors to coronary heart disease in the Framingham Study. III. Eight year incidence of coronary heart disease, Am. J. Epidemiol. **111**(1):37, 1980.
8. Janis, I.L.: Psychological stress, New York, 1958, John Wiley & Sons, Inc.
9. Janis, I.L., and Rodin, J.: Attribution, control and decision making: social psychology and health care. In Stone, G., Cohen, F., and Adler, N.E., editors: Health psychology, San Francisco, 1979, Jossey-Bass, Inc., Publishers.
10. Jenkins, C.D.: Behavioral risk factors in coronary artery disease, Ann. Rev. Med. **29**:543, 1978.
11. Jenkins, C.D., and Zyzanski, S.J.: Behavioral risk factors and coronary heart disease, Psychother. Psychosom. **34**:147, 1980.
12. Kanfer, F.H., and Goldstein, A.P.: Helping people change, New York, 1975, Pergamon Press, Inc.
13. Krozy, R.: Becoming comfortable with sexual assessment, Am. J. Nurs. **78**:1036, 1978.
14. Lazarus, R.S.: Psychological stress and the coping process, New York, 1966, McGraw-Hill Book Co.
15. Levine, S., and Scotch, N.A.: Social stress, Baltimore, 1970, Aldine Publishing Co.
16. MacIntier, T.M.: Theory of interdependence. In Roy, C., editor: Introduction to nursing: an adaptation model, New Jersey, 1976, Prentice-Hall, Inc.
17. Rahe, R.H., and others: Brief group therapy in myocardial rehabilitation: three to four year follow up, Psychosom. Med. **41**(3):229, 1979.

18. Rosenman, R.H., and others: Coronary heart disease in the Western Collaborative Group Study: final follow up experience of 8½ years, J.A.M.A. **233:**872, 1975.

19. Roskies, E., and Lazarus, R.S.: Coping theory and the teaching of coping skills. In Davidson, P., and Davidson, S.M., editors: Behavioral medicine, New York, 1980, Brunner/Mazel, Inc.

20. Sampson, J.J., and Arbona, C.L.: Causes and effects of noncompliance in cardiac patients, Clin. Cardiol. **3:**207, 1980.

21. Scalzi, C.C., and Dracup, K.: Sexual counseling of cardiac patients. In Gentry, W.D., and Williams, R.B., editors: Psychological aspects of myocardial infarction, ed. 2, St. Louis, 1979, The C.V. Mosby Co.

22. Scott, R., and Howard, A.: Models of stress. In Levine, S., and Scotch, N.A., editors: Social stress, Baltimore, 1970, Aldine Publishing Co.

23. Selye, H.: Stress without distress, Philadelphia, 1974, J.B. Lippincott Co.

24. Strauss, A.L.: Chronic illness and the quality of life, St. Louis, 1975, The C.V. Mosby Co.

25. Theorell, T.: Life events and manifestations of ischemic heart disease, Psychother. Psychosom. **34:**135, 1980.

26. U.S. Department of Commerce, Bureau of the Census: Social indicators III, Washington D.C., 1980, U.S. Government Printing Office.

27. U.S. Department of Commerce: Statistical abstract of the United States, Washington, D.C., 1980, U.S. Government Printing Office.

28. U.S. Department of HEW–Public Health Service: Prevalence of chronic circulatory conditions, Vital Health Statistics Service, vol. 10, no. 94, National Center for Health Statistics, 1974.

29. Webster's new collegiate dictionary, Massachusetts, 1974, G. & C. Merriam Co.

30. Wheeler, E.O., and Sheehan, D.V.: Emotional stress: cardiovascular disease and cardiovascular symptoms. In Hurst, J.W., and Logue, R.B., editors: The heart, New York, 1978, McGraw-Hill Book Co.

31. Zangari, M., and Duffy, P.: Contracting with patients in day to day practice, Am. J. Nurs. **80**(3):451, 1980.

PART IV

SPECIAL HEALTH CARE CONSIDERATIONS

CHAPTER 14

Surgical treatment of underlying heart disease: coronary artery bypass, heart valve replacement, heart transplant

LESLIE FLICKINGER KERN

Throughout this book the reader has been learning about the medical management of the patient with congestive heart failure. It is always desirable to treat the patient medically and avoid the physical and mental stress of surgery. However, there are times when the patient's condition continues to deteriorate despite intensive medical therapy, and the physician must look for other causes of failure and for other alternatives to treatment. When this happens, the heart failure is termed "refractory" and the physician may consider surgical treatment.

Surgery is not always reserved as last in the line of treatment options. Patients who have had mitral stenosis since adolescence or childhood and who become symptomatic may have other medical therapies available but are now ready to have the problem corrected surgically so that they do not develop severe heart failure. On the other hand, patients with coronary artery disease will usually have little choice about the need for surgery in order to prevent significant ventricular dysfunction.

Surgery is therefore done as an elective procedure or as an emergency procedure. If medical therapy, surgical therapy, and all known therapeutic measures have been tried and failed, this is referred to as "intractable" heart failure.[2]

The purpose of this chapter is to present an overview of the major surgical procedures performed to correct heart disease that underlies or precipitates heart failure. The procedures and special techniques required to perform coronary artery bypass

grafts, aortic and mitral valve replacement, and heart transplantation are presented and are accompanied by a comprehensive discussion of the nursing process as it relates to patient management during the preoperative, immediate postoperative, post–intensive care, and discharge phases of recovery.

Emphasis is placed on the physiological problems that may complicate recovery and the appropriate interventions. This is accompanied by a presentation of the psychological and social alterations commonly experienced by patients and families facing these surgical procedures. In conclusion a case history and care plan is presented to operationalize and summarize the major concepts addressed in the chapter.

GOALS FOR SURGERY

The first goal for surgical management is to prevent further injury to myocardial tissue that is already ischemic. This applies primarily to patients who are undergoing coronary artery bypass. In patients with myocardial infarction (MI) there is an ischemic area of heart tissue where cells are viable but have depressed contractility. This depressed area contributes to heart failure. If the blood supply to this area is increased by a bypass graft, blood supply is restored, further death of tissue may be avoided and the depressed contractility reversed.[5]

The second goal for surgery is to improve left ventricular function. By increasing coronary blood supply, coronary artery bypass surgery can lead to an improvement in left ventricular function.[10,11] Patients who have aortic valve disease and heart failure may also demonstrate improved left ventricular function following valve replacement.

The third goal is to prolong life. Current evidence indicates that patients with left main coronary artery disease or triple or double vessel disease have an increased survival when treated surgically. Patients with heart failure who have valvular defects that can be corrected also have an increased survival over nonsurgically managed patients.[13]

Improvement of exercise tolerance is the fourth goal of surgery. This applies to coronary artery bypass surgery and valve surgery. Older patients with severe angina may be unable to walk short distances without incurring pain and dyspnea. The young adult who has had progressive symptoms associated with valve disease may no longer enjoy jogging or other sports. Surgery therefore not only prolongs life but also attempts to improve the quality of life.

The final goal is to relieve the patient of symptoms. It has been said that patients with the most severe symptoms derive the greatest relief from surgery. This is especially true of patients with angina and shortness of breath.[13]

THE CONTROVERSY OF SURGICAL MANAGEMENT

Looking at the goals for surgery, it would seem that the decision for surgery would be an easy one for the physician and patient. Fortunately, though, medicine closely controls new procedures and cardiac surgery is no exception. Because it is only about 12 years old, and because the techniques continue to be improved and modified, there is a continual controversy over the indications for surgery. This is especially true of coronary artery bypass.

To reduce resting blood flow, a lesion in the coronary artery must be very severe—reducing 90% of the vessel's cross-sectional area. A 75% lesion will impair the flow of blood during exercise, and a 50% lesion may cause little problem.[13] The patient may have one to six major vessels with varying degrees of disease, and the severity of disease and the vessels involved must be weighed against the symptoms.

Many studies have been done to evaluate the indications, and the following is a list of some currently accepted criteria for coronary artery bypass surgery:

1. The patient with 50% or more stenosis of the left main coronary artery. The reason for this is that the left main coronary artery supplies half of the left ventricle, if all diagonal branches are included. Therefore this patient is at a higher risk for sudden death.
2. The patient with triple-vessel disease who has 90% stenosis of two or more vessels.
3. The patient with persistent pain and other signs of ischemia unresponsive to medical therapy.
4. The patient who has an MI after a cardiac catheterization or balloon dilation.
5. The patient with double-vessel disease in which there is a significant stenosis and in which the two vessels feed a large portion of the heart.[13,17]
6. The patient with heart failure who has ischemic myocardium with an ejection fraction of 15% or greater (the percentage of the left ventricular end-diastolic volume ejected per beat, normal is 60%).

Valve surgery does not face the scrutiny that coronary artery bypass surgery does because valve replacement or repair is generally reserved for symptomatic patients after all medical treatment has been tried.

Indications for valve replacement are:

1. The patient with mitral stenosis who is symptomatic and whose orifice is less than 1.5 cm.[2]
2. The patient with mitral regurgitation who can no longer perform activities of daily living.
3. The asymptomatic patient with severe aortic stenosis (valve gradient of 50 mm Hg or greater) and left ventricular hypertrophy.

4. The patient with aortic stenosis who has symptoms from pulmonary hypertension, fluid retention, or repeated syncope.
5. The patient with acute, severe aortic regurgitation—there is a high mortality associated with this if surgery is not done immediately.
6. The patient with nonacute aortic regurgitation who is symptomatic.
7. The patient with combined valve and coronary artery disease who has an indication for one or the other should have surgery for both at the same time.[19]

The value of coronary artery bypass or valve replacement in patients with congestive heart failure is another controversial matter. Some think that there is little chance for improvement unless the mechanical problems of the heart can be corrected.[13] Others believe that coronary artery bypass can result in improved ejection fraction, improved symptoms, and improved long-term survival compared with medical therapy.[10,11]

For patients with aortic stenosis, heart failure is the leading cause of death and is best treated with valve replacement before the onset of severe failure. However, left ventricular failure should not be a contraindication for surgery.[19]

RISKS OF SURGERY

It is known that the person with congestive heart failure presents a much higher surgical risk, with a 12% to 30% mortality for coronary artery bypass surgery and a 15% to 30% mortality with valve surgery.[10,19] The majority of patients with failure are also elderly with possible diminished hepatic, renal, or pulmonary function. Their ejection fraction is often less than 40%, which puts them at risk for low cardiac output syndrome following surgery. In addition, the low ejection fraction may cause problems in weaning from bypass and the patient may require an intra-aortic balloon pump (IABP) (see Chapter 10).

If medical therapy has been vigorous, fluid and electrolyte disturbances may be present. Other factors that increase operative risk are a history of smoking, presence of lung disease, obesity, arrhythmias, and a history of multiple myocardial infarctions.

The patient with heart failure who requires cardiac surgery has the advantage of the recent advances that have been made in intraoperative myocardial protection and improved anesthesia. Myocardial protection with cardioplegia and hypothermia has enabled the surgeon to work for a longer period on bypass without causing further myocardial damage. Because of this, many patients who would not have been candidates for surgery in the past are now able to withstand this physiologically trying procedure.

THEORETICAL AND PHYSIOLOGICAL CONCEPTS
Historical perspectives

Coronary artery bypass. The earliest attempts at surgical management of coronary artery disease were aimed at the relief of the severe disabling anginal pain. In the early 1900s, Professor Thomas Jonnesco performed a sympathectomy to treat angina. At first, there was some interest in the procedure as it proved successful in 75% of patients; but the interest quickly diminished as the newer methods of myocardial revascularization came about.

In 1935, Beck and Tichy performed a cardioplexy procedure in which adhesions were induced on the heart surface to stimulate blood flow. Materials used to induce the adhesions included talc, sand, and asbestos. Some physicians tried grafting omentum onto the heart. Even today, there are patients alive who had these procedures and who are now having bypass operations.

Zoja and Bianchi ligated the internal mammary artery to increase blood flow in the heart by way of pericardiophrenic branches and the collateral branches that developed.

Another radical procedure was the Beck I and II procedure. Venous stasis in the coronary arteries was surgically induced with the purpose of reversing coronary blood flow. There was a high mortality associated with this procedure because extracorporeal circulation had not yet been developed.

In 1945 Vinberg advocated the use of an extracoronary supply of blood to feed the myocardium. He suggested the implanting of the mammary artery directly into the myocardium. Unfortunately, his ideas were not taken seriously until 1959 when Sones and Shirley demonstrated the technique of coronary arteriography. Since that time thousands of Vinberg procedures have been done, providing marked relief of angina. The next procedure tried was endarterectomy. The concept was good, but the mortality was high—about 50%.

In 1962 the first coronary artery bypass was attempted by Sabiston. Unfortunately, the patient died 3 days later from a stroke. In 1964 Garrett performed the same procedure using a graft from the leg and was very successful. His patient lived for 7 years.

Since that time, the technique for coronary artery bypass has progressed rapidly. The development of extracorporeal circulation allowed the surgeon to have a bloodless field and a still heart on which to work. Other myocardial preservation techniques such as hypothermia and cardioplegia have prevented fatal complications and improved mortality. Coronary artery bypass is now a safe and accepted procedure, with over 100,000 being done annually in the United States.

Valve surgery. The developments in valve surgery have paralleled coronary artery bypass surgery. Valve surgery received an earlier start with repairs and annuloplasties being performed in the 1940s. The early 1950s saw the development of a Lucite valve to be implanted in the descending aorta, but it was not until Lowell Edwards developed the first implantable artificial valve in 1958 that surgery for valve disease became a recognized therapeutic modality. Albert Starr implanted the first of the Starr-Edwards valves in 1960. Since then thousands have been used around the world.

Lowell Edwards could be called the father of artificial valves. Two of his workers, Don Shiley and Warren Hancock, went on to develop their own valves, the Bjork-Shiley disk valve and the Hancock porcine valve. All three types of valves are widely used today, along with many other models.

Physiological stress response to heart surgery

It is vital that clinicians understand the physiological changes that occur during heart surgery. By understanding these changes, they will be better prepared to evaluate the patient and respond to postoperative complications. The physiological responses that are discussed are summarized in the following outline:

A. Local responses
  1. Heart and lungs
    a. Inflammation
    b. Edema
    c. Blood loss
  2. Wound site
    a. Release of proteins
    b. Release of electrolytes
    c. Release of enzymes that activate the clotting system
B. General responses
  1. Shock state
    a. Epinephrine released
    b. Vasoconstriction
    c. Tachycardia
    d. Increased contractility of heart
    e. Increased metabolism
  2. Cellular level changes
    a. Hypoxia
    b. Anaerobic metabolism
    c. Production of lactic acid
  3. Alterations of blood components
    a. Mechanical destruction of RBCs and platelets by heart-lung machine
    b. Blood anticoagulated with heparin
  4. Electrolyte/acid-base imbalances
    a. Increased extracellular chloride
    b. Sodium and potassium move into cell
    c. Metabolic acidosis associated with shock state
    d. Sudden alkalosis may occur
  5. Diminished pulmonary function
    a. Edema of lung tissue
    b. Development of atelectasis and retained secretions
    c. Increased pulmonary vascular resistance
    d. Hypoventilation

An operation of the magnitude of thoracotomy and cardiotomy precipitates major injury response by the body. Any wound alters the body's homeostasis by a combination of local and general effects. The two local organs most affected are the heart and lungs. Inflammation, edema, plasma or blood loss, and malfunction of organs involved constitute the local changes. In addition, at the site of the wound the products of tissue breakdown—electrolytes, enzymes, and proteins—are released into the blood and body. The enzymes released partially activate the body's clotting system, which may be a source of major problems.

Generally, the body's response is much like its response to shock. The invasion of the body sets off a number of neural-endocrine reactions. Epinephrine is secreted, and it produces vasoconstriction, and increases heart rate, contractility, and metabolism. With increased metabolism, there is increased glucose use and production. Fatty acid levels in the bloodstream also rise. These factors together enable the organism to maintain perfusion to all vital organs in the face of an acute reduction in blood volume and resultant shock state.

The low perfusion state also produces changes at the tissue level. Cellular metabolism must now continue with decreased oxygen. This anaerobic metabolism produces a lactic acidosis and eventually results in a general metabolic acidosis. This, in turn, stimulates a compensatory response by the respiratory center to increase respiratory rate, thereby removing carbon dioxide. In this way, and by other mechanisms, the body attempts to maintain a physiological equilibrium.

The shock response is similar for all surgeries but will be more pronounced in the presence of heart failure, hypoxia, or hypovolemia. Patients undergoing cardiac surgery are especially prone to the shock response because of the lower perfusion that is maintained during extracorporeal circulation.

Anesthesia plays a major role in the physiological changes that take place. Many agents depress the myocardium, and all agents partially inhibit sympathetic activity, especially the barbiturates. Anesthesia induction can be a dangerous period for patients with marginal heart function who are dependent upon sympathetic vasoconstric-

tion to maintain blood flow. If there is any hypoxia present, complete circulatory failure may occur.

Positive pressure breathing through an endotracheal tube can also contribute to a decreased cardiac output. Distention of the lung raises the pulmonary vascular resistance, impeding blood flow out of the right ventricle. This can aggravate failure and even lead to pulmonary edema in the borderline patients.

Cardiopulmonary bypass creates several physiological changes in the body. To maintain adequate circulation to all parts of the body when the heart is not functioning, blood must be pumped from the venous to the arterial system at a rate sufficient to supply the requisite oxygen and meet the other metabolic needs of all tissues. In order to achieve this, a series of lines, pumps, and filters must be used. The blood returning to the vena cava and the right atrium is drained by catheters and is carried to the heart-lung machine. In the machine is an oxygenator that bubbles oxygen into the blood and a series of membranes that allow the carbon dioxide to diffuse out. The blood is then pumped back into a major artery, usually the ascending aorta, where it begins its circulation within the body. The blood undergoes a variety of changes during bypass. It is anticoagulated with heparin and subjected to turbulent flow, frothing, and rapid gas exchange. The trauma to the blood is cumulative and increases with the time on bypass. Red cells are destroyed, platelets adhere to the filters, and frequently sludging of red cells occurs at the tissue level.

At the onset of partial perfusion, there is a period of hypotension that is usually transient. Not only does this decrease the oxygen to the myocardium, but it also may contribute to arrhythmia development, creating a risk particularly for the patient in heart failure.

Electrolyte fluctuations occur throughout the surgery. Extracellular chloride rises, sodium and potassium are reduced, with little change in serum calcium levels. In reduced perfusion, these responses may reverse with the escape of potassium out of the cell.

During hypothermia, unusual patterns of metabolic acidosis are observed. Acidosis is generally most intense during the period of rewarming, suggesting that vascular stasis may have occurred during the hypothermic period. Severe alkalosis may occur suddenly and may produce ventricular fibrillation. Consequently, there are many unpredictable changes that can occur, and the surgical team must be alert to the patient's labile condition.

The last major area of physiological changes is pulmonary function. Patients with chronic heart disease may enter surgery with edema, fibrosis, and thickening of the vascular walls of the lung. Superimposed upon these changes may be lung injury incurred at operation.

Lung tissue becomes edematous because of handling during the surgery. The time on the heart-lung machine, when the lungs are flaccid, may lead to congestion, vasculitis, and focal areas of atelectasis. These tissue changes may result in decreased gas diffusion and in the development of pulmonary hypertension. Because of this, the patient may suddenly develop right ventricular failure in the early postoperative period, which would be evidenced by an increased right atrial pressure, jugular venous distention, and increased liver size.

Surgical anesthesia and analgesic drugs cause depression of the respiratory center leading to hypoventilation the first few postoperative hours. Acidosis may develop with Pco_2 levels rising above 70 mm Hg. The pH may then fall below 7.2. A pH this low can cause ventricular arrhythmias or decreased cardiac output. This situation can be dangerous in a cardiac patient and must be guarded against by the avoidance of depressive narcotics and by the use of assisted ventilation.

Bronchiolar inflammation and retained secretions may also affect the airway resistance. In people with asthmatic manifestations, congestive heart failure, or emphysema, this feature may be prominent. Focal atelectasis plays an important role in alterations of gas diffusions because of the changes in the ventilation-perfusion ratio. In many ways, the lungs of a patient following bypass are very similar to the newborn with hyaline membrane disease. Mechanical ventilation and good pulmonary care are therefore mandatory for patients who have undergone cardiac surgery and cardiopulmonary bypass.

In summary, the physiological response of the body to heart surgery is much like the response to shock. The use of cardiopulmonary bypass further adds to this shock state by creating a low perfusion state. Bypass also causes major derangements in blood-clotting factors, electrolyte balance, and pulmonary function. The clinician who is aware of these physiological changes will be better prepared to intervene and assist the patient to return to homeostasis.

Physiological effects of coronary artery bypass surgery

Bypass surgery is indicated in patients with heart failure when there is viable ischemic myocardium. It is believed that with the placement of the bypass grafts, the flow distal to the obstruction is reestablished, hence providing the oxygen needed by the ischemic myocardium. Theoretically, the ischemic zone would then reverse itself and again become part of the functioning myocardium. Studies of patients after surgery seem to support this hypothesis, for there is an improvement in ejection fraction that could not be possible if some of the myocardium did not again become viable. In addition to an increase in resting blood flow, there is an increase in blood flow with exercise. Part of this can be explained in terms of the new blood supply and part because of the improved ejection and subsequent improved cardiac output.

Physiological effects of valve replacement

Valve replacement produces quite a different physiological response from that produced by coronary artery bypass surgery. In aortic valve replacement for aortic stenosis, the ventricle no longer has to contract against a small opening. Left ventricular hypertrophy will eventually decrease and the pulmonary symptoms will also disappear.

Mitral valve disease presents a more difficult physiological problem to correct. Long-standing left atrial hypertension leads to atrial dilation, fibrillation, and pulmonary vascular changes. All of these conditions continue to present problems after restoration of normal pressures in the left atrium. Grossly dilated atria decrease in size but rarely return to normal. Chronic atrial fibrillation of long duration tends to recur after defibrillation attempts, despite repair of the valve lesion. Advanced changes in pulmonary vascular resistance rarely return to normal, but follow-up catheterization has shown that improvement may occur over a period of years.[14]

ASSESSMENT AND INTERVENTION
Preoperative patient assessment

The patient with congestive heart failure presents a unique challenge for the clinician who must prepare him for surgery. If time allows, all preparations will be directed toward the relief of clinical indicators of the heart failure and the return of the patient to his ''dry'' weight. If the patient is already in cardiogenic shock with no results from medical therapy, the clinician must then act quickly to prepare the patient for the events to come.

Subjective data. A general history should be done for all newly hospitalized patients. In addition to this, specific information that relates to their cardiac disease should be obtained: (1) history of present illness, (2) previous operations, (3) cardiac medications, (4) cardiac risk factors, and (5) cardiopulmonary related symptoms. When a quick assessment must be made, information related to the patient's disease and proposed surgery should be obtained. A sample of this quick assessment guide can be seen in Fig. 14-1. Sources of information for the history include physician's notes, old charts, the family, and the patient.

Objective data. The collection of objective data constitutes the second part of the preoperative assessment. Emphasis is placed on the physical assessment, but concurrently the clinician should be collecting objective data about the patient's psychosocial adjustment. For example, while examining the heart, the clinician will also be watching for all overt signs of anxiety—a tense facial expression,

rapid eye movement, restlessness, wringing motion of the hands, and rapid speech.

In all aspects of health care, there is the ideal way and the realistic way. This is especially true with the assessment. What is presented here is the minimal physical assessment that should be done preoperatively. A systemic approach should be used and include the following.

Cardiovascular assessment. The skin and mucous membranes should be assessed for color and the presence of any ulcers. Pale general coloring and pale palmar skin folds may indicate anemia that should be corrected before surgery. Peripheral cyanosis in nailbeds and earlobes should be noted, especially if this is a normal occurrence in the patient. If peripheral cyanosis is acute in onset, it may indicate hypoxemia, low cardiac output, or arterial emboli—all of which should be corrected before surgery. Cyanotic cheeks will be observed in the patient with mitral valve disease who has a decreased cardiac output and an increased pulmonary vascular resistance.

It is also important to assess the presence of skin ulcers on the leg or foot. There is a high correlation between the presence of peripheral vascular disease and coronary artery disease in adults. New or healed leg ulcers should indicate that this patient will require vigilant vascular precautions.

Palpation of skin and peripheral pulses is also part of the cardiovascular assessment. Cold hands and feet may be the result of preoperative anxiety, but they may also be the result of a low output state. If only the patient's feet are cold it is most likely the result of arteriovascular disease with decreased perfusion to the extremities. While palpating for skin temperature, the clinician should also look for edema in the feet, ankles, or presacral areas. All peripheral pulses should be palpated and their presence and fullness documented. This information will serve as a basis for assessing the complication of postoperative peripheral emboli.

Heart sounds should be auscultated to establish baseline data. If heart sounds are distant, this will be important to document so that it is not mistaken for a sign of tamponade after surgery. The heart

PREOPERATIVE RAPID ASSESSMENT
CARDIAC SURGERY PATIENT

Name_____ Age_____ Surgeon_____

Proposed Surgery_____ Hospital No._____

Height_____ Weight _____

MEDICAL HISTORY: (Current cardiac history, previous surgeries, other contribu-
tory illnesses)_____

_____

_____

_____

SOCIAL HISTORY: (Family members, phone nos., occupation, hobbies, interests)

_____

_____

_____

PHYSIOLOGICAL PROFILE: BP_____ HR_____ RR _____ PAP_____

PCWP_____ C.O._____ B.S.A._____ C.I._____

E.F._____ Hct._____ Smoker?_____

Pulses: D.P. (right)/ (left) P.T._____/_____ Femoral_____/_____

         Radial_____/_____

Cardiac Catheterization:_____

_____

_____

Abnormal Lab Results: _____

_____

ECG and previous arrhythmias: _____

_____

PATIENT ASSESSMENT/PROBLEM LIST:

Fig. 14-1. Preoperative rapid assessment. This rapid assessment form can be used by critical care nurses when they visit the patient before surgery. This gives vital information on the baseline status of the patient and clues to areas for potential postoperative complications. *BP,* Blood pressure; *HR,* heart rate; *RR,* respiration rate; *PAP,* pulmonary artery pressure; *PCWP,* pulmonary capillary wedge pressure; *CO,* cardiac output; *BSA,* body surface area; *CI,* cardiac index; *EF,* ejection fraction; *Hct,* hematocrit; *DP,* dorsalis pedis pulse; *PT,* posterior tibial pulse. Pulses are recorded as palp. (for palpable) or Dop. (for pulses heard with Doppler only). (Adapted with permission from University of California at Los Angeles, Department of Nursing Services.)

rate and rhythm should be documented by an ECG strip.

Results of diagnostic tests are also an important source of information for the clinician. The 12-lead ECG should be examined for signs of ischemia or previous MI. Intraoperative MI is a more serious complication of cardiac surgery that is primarily detected by ECG changes. Cardiac catheterization results should be examined. Knowing that a patient had an area of hypokinesis on ventriculography will alert the clinician that this patient is especially prone to postoperative heart failure and fluid disturbances. The echocardiogram may show ventricular hypertrophy from chronic valve disease. This alerts the clinician that this patient will be at risk for developing subendocardial ischemia and intraoperative MI during surgery.

Finally, recent laboratory results should be reviewed and recorded for postoperative reference. Cardiac enzymes, complete blood count (CBC), platelet count, prothrombin time, and partial thromboplastin time are the most important for the cardiovascular assessment. (See Chapter 5 for normal values.)

Pulmonary assessment. The patient's general color, state of alertness, and state of comfort give the clinician a clue to his oxygenation and acid-base status. The chest wall anatomy should be inspected for any bony abnormalities such as kyphosis, scoliosis, or pectus excavatum that could impair respiration. A barrel chest would most likely indicate that the patient has chronic obstructive pulmonary disease.

Skin color is equally important in the pulmonary assessment as in the cardiac assessment. Cyanosis should be documented and investigated. Hands should be observed for clubbing which indicates possible pulmonary disease, intracardiac shunt, or liver disease.

Patterns of respiration should be noted. Are they regular? Is the rate normal? Is the patient using accessory muscles or does he have supraclavicular or intercostal retractions? These findings may indicate severe air hunger that must be corrected immediately.

Auscultation of breath sounds is an essential part of the assessment. Rales will likely be heard if the patient is in failure, but they also may indicate the presence of pneumonia, bronchitis, or mitral lung disease. Wheezes are heard during bronchospasm and when there is any obstruction to the flow of air. The cause for wheezes should be investigated and treated before surgery. Decreased breath sounds should also be documented. This may be the result of previous pulmonary surgery or may appear with pleural effusion.

Palpation for decreases or increases in vocal fremitus will give clues to the presence of pneumonia, pleural effusion, or atelectasis—all of these could contribute to postoperative respiratory complications.

Percussion is another technique used by skilled clinicians to assess preoperative lung excursion. Postoperatively the clinician can detect any decrease in the depth of respirations or areas of consolidation indicating effusion or atelectasis.

All physical findings should be documented in specific terms. If the patient is in pulmonary edema, an attempt should be made to quantify and detail the extent of rales or rhonchi. For example, the assessment could say, "rales heard in posterior lower third of left lung field and in the lower left lateral area." This would tell the postoperative clinicians that any new sounds above this area could be reflecting an increase in pulmonary congestion. In this case, the clinician would then evaluate the most recent chest roentgenogram to confirm physical findings.

The results of pulmonary function tests should be documented. A maximum breathing capacity (MBC) (an index of the maximum ventilation achievable) of less than 50% of the predicted normal value has been found to be associated with higher postoperative mortality in thoracic surgery.[16] Another indicator would be a FEV_1 (the volume of air expelled in 1 second during a forced expiration, starting at full inspiration) of less than

2.0 L. This would also indicate a high risk for pulmonary problems and death. The patient's tidal volume and vital capacity (VC) should also be recorded for comparison in the postoperative period.

Laboratory tests to evaluate pulmonary function include arterial blood gases and hemoglobin.

Renal assessment. The patient's history is the most important part of the renal assessment. BUN, creatinine, urinalysis, and electrolyte results should be evaluated and any abnormalities recorded and investigated.

Neuromuscular assessment. When examining the patient, the clinician should observe the patient's ability to move the extremities. Any handicaps, motor weaknesses or sensory loss should be written in the assessment. Speech and facial expressions are naturally observed. The patient's mental status is also evaluated. Can he answer simple health questions without difficulty? Is he able to give his age, address, name of spouse correctly? Does he know where he is and why? A more in-depth mental status examination can be done when indicated, but noting that the patient is oriented and answering questions without difficulty should be sufficient for the preoperative assessment.

Gastrointestinal assessment. Ideally, the nurse clinician would do an abdominal examination on every patient, but realistically this may not be possible. For the cardiac surgery patient, the gastrointestinal assessment plays a minor role because it is rare that he will encounter gastrointestinal complications in the postoperative period. It is, however, important to note the last bowel movement before surgery. Patients who have had a recent MI or have congestive heart failure may have been on a regime of bed rest for a number of days and need a laxative or an enema preoperatively. It is also often worrisome to patients if they have not had a recent bowel movement and then go for 2 to 3 days after surgery without one.

Psychosocial assessment. This is one of the most important areas of the preoperative assessment. Subjective data about the patient's adjustment to hospitalization and surgery should include information on:

1. Previous experiences with surgery. Did the patient experience any complications or behavior changes?

2. Previous experiences with pain. Has the patient ever experienced surgical pain or had any problems with chronic pain or pain management? What are the patient's perceptions about the pain that will be experienced after surgery?

3. Knowledge of heart surgery. Does the patient know anyone who has undergone heart surgery?

4. Characteristic ways of coping with stress. Does the patient rely on relaxation techniques (yoga, progressive relaxation), use denial, become angry or become depressed? Does he tend to want to be alone or have others around?

5. Sleep habits. Does the patient rely on sleeping pills or sedatives to help with sleep at night?

6. Psychological assistance. Has the patient ever sought the help of a psychologist or psychiatrist? For what reason(s)? How recently? Is the patient currently taking any medications for diagnosed psychological problems?

7. History of drug or alcohol abuse. If the patient has a history of drug or alcohol abuse, has he or she been in any type of rehabilitation program? What is the current status of the problem? Does the drug abuser require higher doses of pain medications?

8. Mental status. If the patient is having difficulty in constructing thought or in remembering recent events, then a mental status examination should be performed.

9. Support systems. Information about spouse, friends, or relatives who are closest to the patient should be written in a place accessible to everyone.

10. Who does the patient rely on for support? Who should be called in the event of an emergency?

11. Sight or hearing impairments. These are

important to note in the psychosocial assessment because of the problem of sensory deprivation that can occur in the postoperative period.

There is much information to be gained from planned observation of the patient's behavior. Objective data about the patient's psychosocial status should include:

1. The patient's prevailing temperament or mood. Is it private, friendly, depressed, indecisive, optimistic, pessimistic, or anxious?
2. Level of intellectual functioning. Are the patient's thoughts organized and clearly expressed or does he tend to ramble and go off on a tangent?
3. Speech patterns. Is the patient's speech rapid as seen in anxiety or slow and deliberate as seen in organic brain syndrome?

By gathering this subjective and objective data on preoperative psychosocial adaptation, the nurse can develop a plan for prevention of postoperative problems and, in addition, prepare a plan for the health care team so that the patient is approached in a way that meets his or her individual psychological needs.

Family assessment

The final area for assessment is the family assessment. The care plan or problem list that is started on the patient should include the names and phone numbers of close relatives or significant others. The spouse and children are usually the most concerned and in need of much support during the entire surgical experience.

What then should nurse clinicians assess? First they should find out if relatives are alone or if there are other relatives or friends to support them while the patient is in surgery. If the family member is alone, the clinician should find someone who can be a contact person for that relative. This may be the critical care nurse, a clinical nurse specialist, a social worker, or a volunteer. It is ideal if they can also impart information about the status of the patient during surgery.

Second, nurse clinicians assess the family's knowledge about the impending surgery. They may have unfounded fears about anesthesia or the procedure that could be allayed with the proper information.

Third, nurse clinicians observe the family interactions and coping patterns. Who seems to make the decisions? Whom does everyone lean on? Who is quiet? The leader may be the one to go into crisis if the patient develops a complication after surgery. The quiet one may have reconciled that the patient is going to die and be unable to talk about it. How have these individuals coped in the past? Do they rely on God for hope and support? Nurses should encourage use of coping mechanisms that have worked in the past, but most importantly, they should be available to the family. Nurses should encourage family members to come to them before their fears get out of hand. The family should be informed how to contact the nurse for information regarding the progress in surgery. The nurse should also show them around the floor and intensive care unit (ICU) if they have never seen one; this will assist them to feel at home, for the hospital will be their home for the next couple of weeks.

Preoperative teaching

Teaching techniques. The timing of teaching the preoperative patient is very important. Teaching done too soon may be forgotten, teaching done just before surgery will not be retained because of the patient's high anticipatory anxiety. Ideally then, teaching should begin early enough to allow the patient to digest the information and to incorporate it into his self-concept and future plans.

Often the patient is admitted the day before surgery. This does not allow enough time for teaching. Some hospitals have dealt with this problem by sending out booklets to the patient at home, a week or two before surgery. Other hospitals have developed regularly scheduled preoperative teaching programs that patients can attend at the hospital prior to admission. The patient with heart failure presents a challenge because often the decision to perform surgery is made on an emergency basis and allows little time for formal teaching.

Another point regarding timing is that the information presented to the hospitalized patient should be given in three to four short intensive sessions rather than one long session. It has been some educators' experience that preoperative surgical anxiety is generally very high and patients can become overwhelmed with all the information that is presented. Short sessions allow patients time to think about the information, practice breathing exercises, and formulate questions. The coordination of short teaching sessions may sound difficult but may be simplified when there is a teaching flow sheet to follow.

The second technique that should be practiced is the individualization of teaching. Some people want extensive detailed information and some people do not. The nurse must respect the patient's desire for information because this may be reflecting his way of coping with a very stressful situation; conversely, studies have indicated that a patient should not be forced to receive information he does not want.[8]

The patient who is having his second bypass or valve procedure will probably not need as much information and some of the things you try to tell him may conflict with his experience. For the patient who speaks a foreign language, an interpreter will be needed. The patient will gain the most benefit if the clinician has taken the time to individualize his teaching.

Group learning is another teaching technique. Gathering patients together before surgery gives them the opportunity to share concerns and develop confidence by knowing they are not alone in what they are about to encounter. The difficulties with group teaching are: (1) choosing times and days that can service all patients and (2) keeping the group controlled so that one patient or family does not dominate the teaching session to meet their own needs.

The last teaching technique to emphasize is the use of teaching aids during instruction. No matter how well one explains what a Bjork-Shiley valve looks like, nothing can substitute for the patient seeing the real thing. Heart models or drawings are excellent visual aids. There are several booklets, films, and slide presentations available for purchase that can assist in patient education (see the list at the end of this chapter).

Team approach to preparation of the patient. The ideal approach to preoperative preparation of the patient uses a primary care nurse to direct the activities of all resource people. The respiratory therapist, physical therapist, rehabilitation nurse, dietitian, social worker, clinical specialist, staff nurse, critical care nurse, surgery nurse, and physician all have a role in the preparation of the patient and his family. This is the ideal and realistic approach that is currently in use at a number of hospitals. Who can better teach the patient the mechanics' of deep breathing and the use of the incentive spirometer than the respiratory therapist? The physical therapist and rehabilitation nurse can demonstrate leg exercises necessary when the patient will be placed on a regime of bedrest and develop goals for postoperative ambulation. The dietitian begins a diet history and food preference list, then follows the patient after surgery with teaching and low-cholesterol menu planning. The social worker or mental health clinical nurse specialist discusses the normal responses to surgery and assists the patient and family to adapt to the loss of control they experience. The critical care nurse discusses the ICU phase of hospitalization and gives the patient and family a tour of the unit. The surgery nurse describes the operating room for the patient and makes a note of important information, such as a hearing loss or the presence of an artificial eye. The primary care nurse carries the great responsibility of coordinating all of these resources and seeing that the patient has received the best preparation possible.

Another resource for the preoperative education of the patient is the Mended Hearts Association. This is an organization comprised of individuals who have all undergone cardiac surgery. They meet on a regular basis and have lectures of interest on various topics related to their surgery. Members also make visits to patients during hospitalization to answer questions and share experiences. They are located throughout the United States and provide a very valuable service.

Content for teaching. There are many excellent articles that describe the content to be covered in the teaching of cardiac surgery patients. As was mentioned earlier, there are also many teaching aids available to assist the nurse in patient education. Each hospital should develop its own program that is comprehensive and that uses all resource personnel. The content also must reflect the procedures and routines as they are done in that hospital.

To keep track of the teaching that is done and the personnel who have done it, a documentation system must be developed. This may be accomplished by use of a flow sheet or checklist. The flow sheet lists the actual content areas to be covered in teaching and provides columns to record the date, the instructor's initials, and the patient's response to teaching. A sample of such a flow sheet can be seen in Fig. 14-2. This flow sheet assures that the responsibility for teaching is shared by the health care team and at the same time indicates to the primary nurse what teaching the patient has or has not received. This flow sheet stays at the patient's bedside and becomes a permanent part of the chart. It also serves as a method of communicating teaching needs to the rehabilitation nurse or clinical nurse specialist who will see the patient after discharge.

General statements of content are listed on the flow sheet. On a separate sheet are listed the objectives and specific information to be covered (Table 14-1).

In summary, the content for teaching should be individualized for the hospital. A system of documentation should be developed and everyone should be familiar with the teaching protocol. The reader is referred to the literature for further information on the content for teaching.

Preoperative preparations for the patient

The patient with congestive heart failure presents a special challenge to the health care team who must prepare him for surgery. If he has been in active failure, he must be stabilized before surgery. Ideally, he will not have any signs of fluid overload, electrolyte imbalance, or decreased cardiac output, his hemoglobin and hematocrit will be normal, there will be no arrhythmias, and he will be psychologically prepared to undergo an additional stress to his body.

The preoperative laboratory data to be collected on the patient will vary somewhat from hospital to hospital, but there are some basic data that must be collected on all patients. A complete blood count should be done the day before surgery. The patient with congestive heart failure may have a decreased hemoglobin and hematocrit because of hemodilution. A hemoglobin of less than 10 g/100 ml severely decreases the oxygen carrying capacity and therefore should be corrected before surgery. The patient's white blood count (WBC) may be elevated because of the stress response to congestive heart failure but may also indicate sepsis and therefore should be investigated.

Electrolytes are often abnormal in the setting of congestive heart failure, again because of hemodilution, but also because of the excessive use of diuretics. The high or low sodium or potassium must be corrected preoperatively because of the electrolyte fluctuations during surgery.

Renal function is evaluated with urinalysis, BUN, and creatinine. Patients with coronary artery disease often have atherosclerosis of other major organ vessels, including the renal vessels. If the patient has borderline renal function preoperatively, a drop in cardiac output postoperatively could put him in renal failure.

Comprehensive coagulation studies are done. Prothrombin time, partial thromboplastin time, thrombin time, fibrinogen and platelet counts are important to evaluate because of the opportunities for bleeding during and after surgery. Aspirin products must not be taken within 3 weeks of surgery. Warfarin (Coumadin) is discontinued 72 hours before surgery.

Cardiac enzymes, creatine phosphokinase (CPK), serum glutamic-oxaloacetic transaminase

Patient name _____

CARDIAC SURGERY TEACHING FLOWSHEET

I. PREPARATION FOR SURGERY	DATE	INITIALS	N/A	COMMENTS
1. Explain purpose of surgery				
2. Discuss client's feelings about surgery				
3. Routines the day before surgery				
4. Insertion of Swan-Ganz catheter				
5. Morning of surgery				
II. THE ICU EXPERIENCE				
1. Purpose of the ICU				
2. ICU environment				
3. Routine care in ICU				
4. Explain lines/tubes				
5. Pain management/ surgical incision(s)				
6. Postoperative pulmonary care				
7. Postoperative leg exercises				
8. Psychological responses				
9. Family support measures				

Fig. 14-2. Cardiac surgery teaching flowsheet. This flowsheet encompasses the four phases of hospitalization: preoperative phase, ICU phase, post-ICU phase, and discharge preparations. (Courtesy University of California at Los Angeles, Department of Nursing Services.)

III. POST-ICU PHASE	DATE	INITIALS	N/A	COMMENTS
1. Transition from ICU to floor				
2. Need for IV				
3. Diet				
4. Intake and output				
5. Bowel function				
6. Pacing wires				
7. Activity				
IV. PREPARATION FOR DISCHARGE				
1. Medications				
2. Diet				
3. Care of incisions				
4. Activity at home				
5. Sleep and rest				
6. Risk factor modification				
7. Cardiac rehabilitation programs				
8. Instructions for valve patients				

Fig. 14-2, cont'd. For legend see opposite page.

Table 14-1. A sample of learner objectives for the cardiac surgery teaching flowsheet*

Preparation for surgery	Learning objective	Teaching resources	Teaching activity
1. Purpose of surgery	The patient and family will verbalize an understanding of basic anatomy and physiology of the heart, the patient's heart disorder, and the surgical cedure.	Booklet: "Open Heart Surgery at UCLA" Heart model Heart diagrams AHA booklets Staff nurse	Informal nurse/patient discussion. Using visual aids, discuss the following: The heart as a muscle pump Circulation of the blood through the heart Location of coronary arteries and values The patient's disease process Discuss surgical procedure, benefits for the patient, and the approximate time spent in surgery.
2. Discussion of patient's feelings about surgery	The patient and family will verbalize feelings about hospitalization and surgery.	Primary nurse · Clinical nurse specialist	Nurse should use open-ended questions and active listening to facilitate patient and family expression of feelings. Explain how pHisoHex shower will decrease number of skin bacteria and decrease chance of infection.
3. Routines the day before surgery	The patient and family will discuss the purpose of pHisoHex shower, enema, no eating or drinking before surgery, sleeping pill, and skin shave preparation.	Primary nurse	Explain how hair harbors bacteria and that preparation will remove excess hair. Discuss the purpose and procedure for enema. Discuss the availability of sleeping pill and the importance of a good night's sleep. Discuss the rationale and the importance of not eating or drinking anything after midnight.

*The objectives and specific information to be covered are on a separate sheet in the teaching guide. This serves as a reference for the nurse and as a way of informing new personnel what is to be taught. Courtesy University of California at Los Angeles, Department of Nursing Services.

(SGOT) and lactate dehydrogenase (LDH) are measured to establish a baseline for comparison postoperatively. Serum glutamic-pyruvic transaminase (SGPT), alkaline phosphatase, and albumin levels give some clues to liver function in the patient with alcoholism or who has a history of hepatic failure.

Arterial blood gases will give information about the acid-base balance and oxygenation. The goal is for the patient to have values as normal as possible before surgery.

Diagnostic tests are done to determine the extent and location of the cardiac lesion. The cardiac catheterization gives the surgeon information about the location of the lesion or defect, the extent of the lesion, the hemodynamic effects of the lesion on heart functioning, the operability of the lesion, and the heart anatomy. During the catheterization procedure, any one or combination of the following procedures is done: (1) coronary angiography, (2) ventriculography, (3) measurement of heart pressures and pulmonary artery pressure, (4) measurement of valve gradients and areas, (5) cardiac output measurement, and (6) mixed venous blood sampling. All of this information assists in planning the surgical approach and assists in the management of the patient during and after surgery.

Other diagnostic tests that are often done are an echocardiogram, a treadmill test, a multiple-gated acquisition (MUGA) scan, a thallium scan, an exercise thallium scan, and a pulmonary function test. The echocardiogram is required in the evaluation of valve disease. It provides information about left ventricular wall motion, septal wall motion, valve motion, and chamber size. The MUGA scan indicates the ventricular wall motion and ejection fraction. The thallium scan will light up areas of the heart that are without an adequate blood supply.

Another part of the preparation of the patient includes the skin and bowel preparation. The skin is usually shaved the evening before surgery from the neck (below the jaw) down, through the perineum, to the knees for a valve replacement and to the ankles for a coronary artery bypass. The anterior and lateral portion of the chest is shaved and the entire leg surfaces shaved. Following the skin preparation, the patient takes a pHisoHex or Betadine shower and scrubs himself with the antiseptic cleanser.

Bowel preparation protocol varies from surgeon to surgeon. Usually a Fleet enema is given the night before surgery, primarily to assure patient comfort in the postoperative period.

Preoperative medication usually combines a narcotic, a sedative, and an anticholinergic. Ideally, these medications should not cause myocardial depression. Morphine has little myocardial depressing effects and has been thought to enhance coronary blood flow and maintain analgesia over a longer period of time. Meperidine (Demerol) has marked myocardial depressant affect.[15]

A sedative such as diazepam is an excellent agent of choice because it does not depress the myocardium and provides complete amnesia during surgery. Hydroxyzine is also often used, but it causes some myocardial depression and hypotension.

For anticholinergic effects, scopolamine is an agent of choice. It inhibits secretions while providing amnesia and sedation. Atropine is not usually administered because of its vagolytic effects, which predispose to tachycardia.

There is no special preoperative diet for these patients unless they are on sodium or fluid restrictions to control fluid retention resulting from heart failure. All patients refrain from eating and drinking after midnight the day of surgery and should be informed regarding the rationale and specific restrictions.

Special techniques in heart surgery

Hemodynamic monitoring. This has become an integral part of the intraoperative and postoperative phase of cardiac surgery. Several cardiac pressures are monitored simultaneously, allowing continuous regulation of fluids and drugs.

In the operating room an arterial catheter is inserted percutaneously and remains in the patient 2 to 3 days following surgery. This line allows digital and waveform readings of systolic, diastolic, and mean arterial pressures. It is used to detect sudden changes in arterial pressures and respiratory variations on pressure as occurs with pulsus paradoxus, to fine tune intra-aortic balloon pump (IABP) inflation and deflation, and as a port from which to draw blood samples. However, it is not possible to obtain specimens for clotting studies from the arterial line because the heparinized flush solution used to maintain patency will alter test results.

The arterial line is a vital part of hemodynamic monitoring but also a source of complications to the patient. If it comes apart and is not noticed, the patient could lose a significant amount of blood. The stopcock from which blood is drawn is a source of infection if not capped and kept free from old blood. The patient can develop arterial insufficiency of the hand distal to the catheter if ulnar artery circulation is inadequate. Arterial lines can infiltrate and cause severe swelling or hematoma at the insertion site, which also causes inaccurate readings.

Flow-directed balloon-tipped catheters, such as the Swan-Ganz catheter, are often used in patients who undergo cardiac surgery, especially when congestive heart failure is present. It may be inserted preoperatively so that vasodilator drugs (unloading therapy) can be started, or it may be inserted in the operating room at the beginning of surgery. The one time it will not be used is when the patient is having tricuspid valve replacement.

During surgery, the Swan-Ganz catheter provides information about left and right ventricular pressures and cardiac output. From the Swan-Ganz values, other hemodynamic data can be calculated, such as the systemic vascular resistance and pulmonary vascular resistance (see Chapter 7). It also provides information that can be used to make decisions about drug therapy, and response to anesthesia.

Postoperatively, the Swan-Ganz catheter remains in place the first 1 to 2 days while signs of complications are being monitored and drug therapy regulated. Recordings of pulmonary artery pressure, pulmonary capillary wedge pressure, right atrial pressure, cardiac output, cardiac index, systemic vascular resistance, and pulmonary vascular resistance are made hourly, and more often when needed. In addition, the pacing Swan catheter has atrial and ventricular electrodes within it that allows performance of atrial, AV sequential, and ventricular pacing operations (Fig. 14-3). Furthermore, the newest Swan-Ganz catheter, has an extra lumen, a venous infusion port, that has been specially designed for the administration of fluids.

Other lines that may be used for hemodynamic monitoring are the central venous pressure line and the left atrial pressure line. The central venous pressure may be used in the elective candidate for fluid administration but is less often used for hemodynamic monitoring of fluid status in patients with congestive heart failure since the development of flow-directed catheters. The rationale for this is that it does not detect changes in left ven-

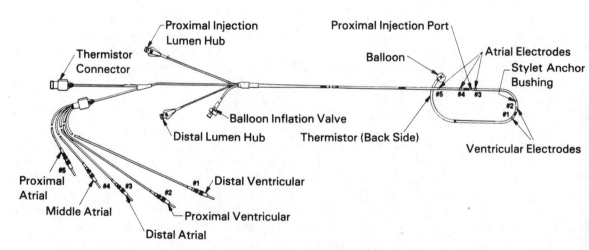

Fig. 14-3. Pacing Swan-Ganz catheter. (Courtesy American Edwards Laboratories, Santa Ana, Ca.)

tricular pressures as early as the flow-directed balloon-tipped catheter. The left atrial pressure line is used in special cases when a pulmonary artery catheter cannot be used and when accurate monitoring of left atrial pressure is indicated. This line is placed directly in the left atrium during surgery and brought out through the chest wall. Although it is very accurate for measuring left ventricular pressures, it carries the risks of air emboli to the brain and/or infection, causing endocarditis.

Anesthesia for heart surgery. Cardiac surgery requires use of special precautions in anesthesia. The majority of general anesthetics lead to myocardial depression, decreased conduction, and decreased contractility. Some anesthetics dilate the vascular bed and cause acute hypotension. Enflurane is used in uncomplicated cases, but in the patient with congestive heart failure, morphine may be the anesthetic agent of choice in a dose of 1 to 3 mg/kg. It does not cause myocardial depression and provides a significant decrease in afterload. During induction and surgery the anesthesiologist attempts to maintain total analgesia, sedation, and muscle relaxation while preventing increases in myocardial oxygen demand and decreases in myocardial oxygen supply. This is done by avoiding hypotension, hypertension, arrhythmias, or changes in contractility.

Other benefits of morphine use for anesthesia are that it provides for a smoother transition of the mechanically ventilated patient from the operating room to the post-anesthesia room, its analgesia effects continue into the postoperative period, and it has no effect on cardiac rhythm.[7]

Intraoperative hypertension, if it occurs, is treated with nitroprusside. It acts on venous smooth muscle for immediate vasodilation. Phentolamine, an alpha blocker, may also be used to control an increased afterload if arterial pressure is normal or low.

Extracorporeal circulation. Basically, blood is diverted from the right atrium, and carried to an oxygenator where it receives oxygen and where carbon dioxide is removed. The machine then pumps the blood back into the ascending aorta

where it continues its circulation through the body.

Cardiopulmonary bypass, or extracorporeal circulation as it is sometimes called, allows work to be done inside and outside the heart and on the great vessels (Fig. 14-4). The bypass can be total or partial. With total bypass, the tapes around the cannula in the venae cavae are tied tight so that all blood is diverted to the machine. By the heart beating in an empty state, the myocardial oxygen requirements are dramatically reduced.

In partial bypass, the tapes are left loose and allow some of the blood to go through the heart and normal circulation. During bypass the lungs are generally left in a partially deflated state and have circulation by way of the bronchial arteries and veins. They are hyperinflated at regular intervals to prevent atelectasis and retention of secretions.

The heart-lung machine must be primed before initiation of bypass. Usually an electrolyte solution and blood is used. The patient must also be anticoagulated for bypass with 2 to 3 units/kg of heparin. During bypass, an attempt is made to maintain a hemoglobin of 7 or greater and a hematocrit of 21 or greater. The flow or cardiac index to be maintained is 2.2 L/minute/M^2. The mean arterial pressure is usually maintained at 50 to 85 mm Hg. As discussed under physiology, the heart-lung machine has many damaging effects on the blood.

Myocardial protection. In the past few years several techniques have been developed to provide protection to the myocardium and to prevent the development of myocardial ischemia or infarction during surgery.

The first of these is hypothermia. It is well known that a reduction in the temperature of a tissue will reduce its metabolism and therefore its oxygen needs. During cardiac surgery, the patient's body is cooled to 25° to 28° C with topical cooling of the heart to a temperature of 10° to 20° C. During bypass, total body cooling is desirable because there is a decreased perfusion and decreased oxygen available to the tissues. Cooling lowers the oxygen needs and prevents the development of local acidosis. Cooling of the heart serves the same

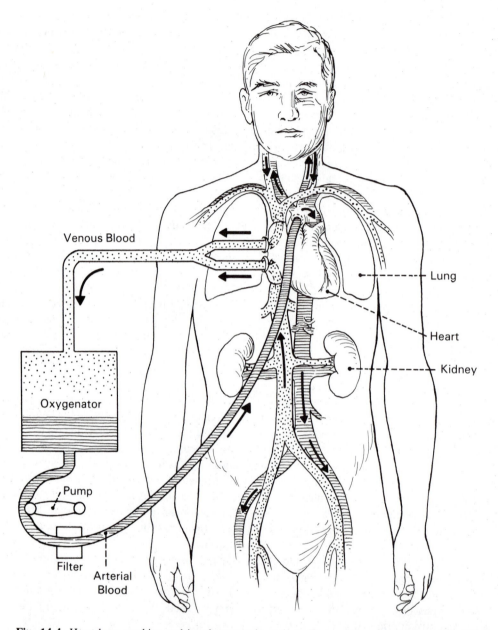

Venous Blood

Lung

Heart

Kidney

Oxygenator

Pump

Filter

Arterial
Blood

Fig. 14-4. Heart-lung machine and its placement in patient. Two venous cannulas are placed in inferior and superior venae cavae. Blood is diverted away from body, through these cannulas to oxygenator where oxygen is bubbled into blood, across a filter. Blood is then pumped back into body by way of arterial cannula, which lies in ascending aorta just distal to aortic root. Oxygenated blood then circulates to body through normal channels. (© Copyright 1969, 1978, CIBA Pharmaceutical Company, Division of CIBA-GEIGY Corporation. Reprinted with permission from The Ciba Collection of Medical Illustrations, illustrated by Frank H. Netter, M.D. All rights reserved.)

purpose. Blood flow through the coronary arteries is slowed or stopped during surgery; therefore cooling of the heart is necessary to lower the metabolic needs and prevent cellular acidosis.

A second technique to prevent ischemia used during bypass is the use of cardioplegia to produce cardiac arrest. This solution consists of potassium, procainamide, and, more recently, blood. It is injected into the aortic root when slowing of the heart is desired. Cardiac arrest occurs rapidly and the solution is reinfused every 20 minutes to maintain arrest. It is a high pH, low-calcium solution that is helpful in combating the deleterious effects of ischemia. Before the development of cardioplegia, anoxic arrest was used to stop the heart; however this was shown to result in higher incidence of intraoperative MI and therefore is not the procedure of choice.[1,4]

Pulsatile assist device. This is a plastic, disposable device that is inserted into the arterial cannula during bypass. It consists of a polyurethane balloon with an opening on either end through which the blood flows. It is connected to an intraaortic balloon pump console that synchronizes the balloon pumping with the ECG. It produces pulsatile bypass, which more closely approximates the natural flow of blood, and simulates the action of an IABP. The results of this pulsatile flow are improved capillary perfusion, decreased metabolic acidosis, increased renal perfusion, decreased systemic vascular resistance, improved cerebral perfusion, improved coronary artery perfusion, and higher mean arterial pressure.[3] It is especially useful in the patient with congestive heart failure and a preoperative ejection fraction of less than 30%. Studies have shown an improved mortality over patients who did not undergo pulsatile flow during bypass.[3]

Intra-aortic balloon pump (IABP). The intra-aortic balloon pump is another life-saving machine that is discussed in detail in Chapter 10 of this text.

Procedure for coronary artery bypass surgery

The patient receives a preoperative medication 1 hour before coming to the operating room. The preoperative injection usually includes morphine, scopolamine, and a sedative. On arrival in the operating room, the patient is asked to lay supine on the operating room table. Usually a cooling blanket is placed underneath him.

Intravenous infusions will be initiated, and the Swan-Ganz catheter and arterial lines will be inserted. The patient may be sedated further for these procedures or intravenous anesthesia started after the procedures are completed.

Once unconscious, the patient is intubated, and anesthesia is begun. The skin is then cleansed with providone-iodine or a similar skin preparation, and the adhesive plastic barrier placed on the dried skin. This plastic adheres to the skin and provides added protection from skin and other body bacteria.

For a coronary artery bypass operation, at best two surgeons must be present: one to open the sternum and prepare the heart and the other to work on the leg to harvest the saphenous vein grafts. The surgeon at the chest almost always requires an assistant.

In addition to the surgeons, there will be the anesthesiologist, often a cardiologist, the pump technician, one scrub nurse, one or two circulating nurses. There may also be present students or residents who are observing the procedure.

Leg inclusion. The condition of the extremity determines which leg is used as a source for the vein graft. If there are signs of trauma, old scars, or vascular disease, a leg will not be used. Rarely will there be problems in both legs that contraindicate vein use. However, in these rare cases, a vein from the arm may be used, or in some institutions, there is a vein bank where fetal vessels are preserved for use in needy patients.

The leg incision is begun 2 cm below the inguinal ligament. The incision is made on the medial aspect of the leg along the saphenous vein. This is usually one continuous incision that makes one stop at the knee but continues down the leg. Blunt dissection is used to locate and remove the vein. Approximately 20 cm is removed for each graft. The vein branches are tied off and the vein

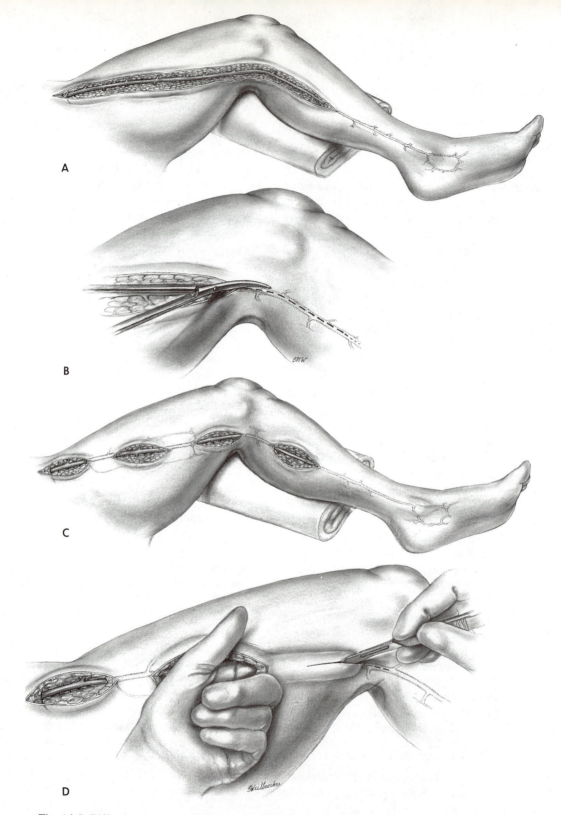

Fig. 14-5. Different types of leg incisions. **A** and **B** illustrate technique for continuous leg incision using Metzenbaum scissors. **C** and **D** show technique for a leg incision using short skin bridges. (From Ochsner, J.L., and Mills, N.L.: Coronary artery surgery, ed. 1, Philadelphia, 1978, Lea & Febiger.)

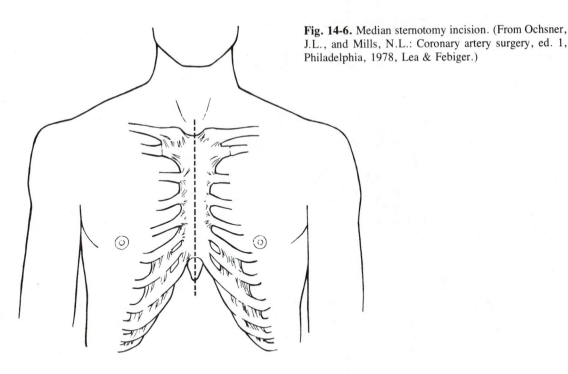

Fig. 14-6. Median sternotomy incision. (From Ochsner, J.L., and Mills, N.L.: Coronary artery surgery, ed. 1, Philadelphia, 1978, Lea & Febiger.)

flushed with heparinized saline. Some physicians think that it is helpful to cut the valves within the graft because it allows for unencumbered blood flow and decreases the incidence of thrombosis, so this may be an additional procedure that is done (Fig. 14-5).

The leg wound is then irrigated with an antibiotic solution. The incision is closed with nylon sutures and Steristrips. Hemovac drains may be placed and removed within 24 hours. With normal wound healing, the sutures can be removed in 7 to 9 days.

Patients often wonder whether or not their circulation will be compromised by the removal of the saphenous vein. The answer is no. The saphenous vein is a superficial vein and therefore plays a minor role in returning blood to the heart. The leg has many additional deep and collateral veins that can make up for the saphenous vein loss; however, it is not unusual for patients to have temporary postoperative edema of the affected extremity.

Chest incision and graft anastomosis. Following skin preparation, a midline sternal incision, referred to as a medial sternotomy, is made from below the sternal notch to just below the tip of the xiphoid (Fig. 14-6). Electrocautery is used to cut through the subcutaneous tissue.

The sternum is divided with an electric saw. Cautery is used to control bleeding and bone wax applied to the edges. The pericardium is then incised and sutured to the wound edges so that the heart is lifted and more easily visualized (Fig. 14-7).

At this time, the cannulas for bypass are placed in the inferior vena cava, superior vena cava, and ascending aorta. A left ventricular vent will also be placed to prevent the distention of the ventricle, and coronary artery catheters are placed for infusion of cardioplegia solution. A clamp is placed on the aorta to stop coronary artery blood flow and to prevent bypass blood from going into the left ventricle. The patient is gradually put on bypass, and the heart is arrested by hypothermia, cardioplegia solution, and aortic clamping.

The saphenous vein is reversed so that blood can flow forward through the valves of the graft. It is

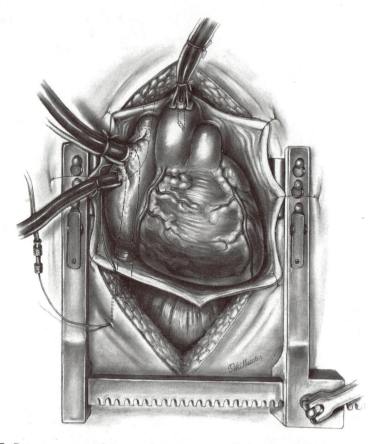

Fig. 14-7. Retractors are used to spread sternum open. Pericardium is incised, then sutured to wound edges so that heart is lifted up out of thoracic cavity. Venous cannulas are seen in superior and inferior venae cavae. The arterial cannula is seen in the aorta. (From Ochsner, J.L., and Mills, N.L.: Coronary artery surgery, ed. 1, Philadelphia, 1978, Lea & Febiger.)

then anastomosed to the coronary artery, distal to the narrowed segment (Fig. 14-8). A continuous suture is used to secure the graft. The proximal end of the graft is then sutured to the ascending aorta. The entire procedure takes approximately 12 minutes per graft. In between grafts, the aortic clamp is released and blood allowed to flow through the coronary arteries.

Single or sequential grafts may be done. A sequential graft is one graft that is supplying two or more vessels (Fig. 14-9). The advantages of sequential grafting are that a shorter graft is needed, fewer anastomoses and consequently less operative

time are required, and the technical aspects of the operation are simplified.[15] Each graft is tagged with radiopaque markers that assist with identification in future roentgenograms. Finally flow through the new grafts is tested with a flowmeter. A flow of 90 ml/minute is considered to be optimal.

Removal from bypass. Before removal from bypass, all anesthesia is discontinued, the lungs are ventilated, and the patient is warmed. Extracorporeal circulation is gradually weaned until the patient is off the pump. Blood samples for hemoglobin, hematocrit, electrolytes, and blood gases

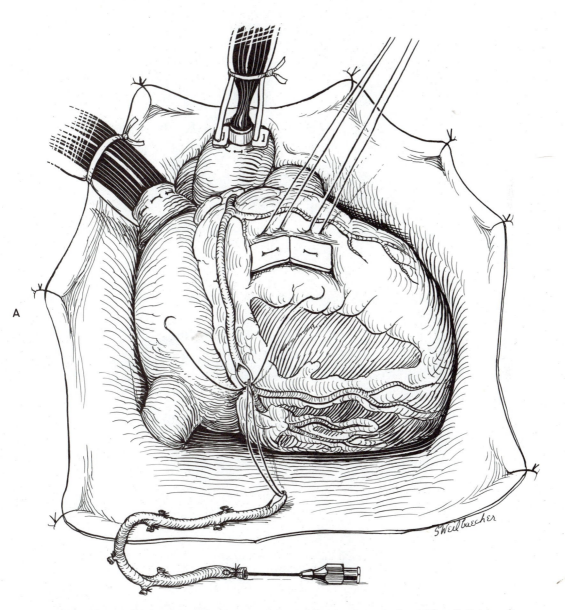

A

Fig. 14-8. The distal graft **(A)** is anastomosed first, while heart is motionless. After all distal grafts are done, then aortic anastomoses **(B)** are made. (From Ochsner, J.L., and Mills, N.L.: Coronary artery surgery, ed. 1, Philadelphia, 1978, Lea & Febiger.)

Continued.

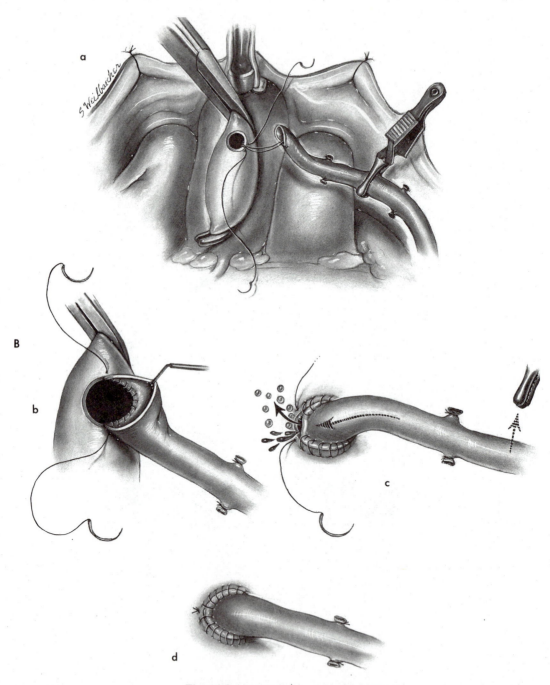

Fig. 14-8, cont'd. For legend see p. 427.

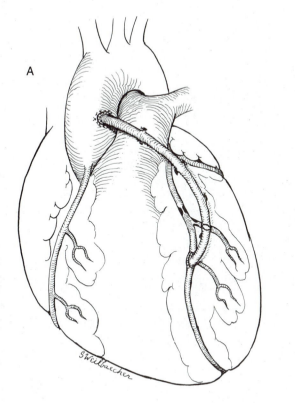

A

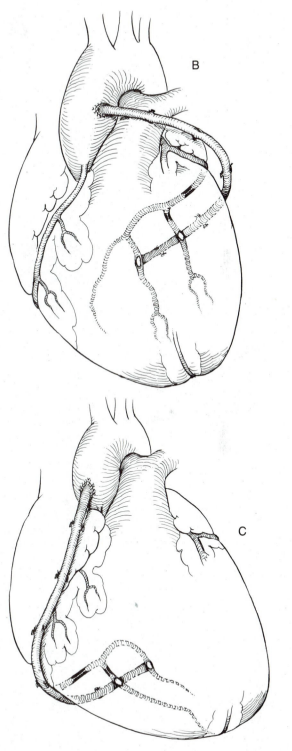

B

C

Fig. 14-9. Single grafts are seen in **A. B** and **C** demonstrate procedure of sequential grafting. (**A** from Stiles, Q.R., and others: Myocardial revascularization: a surgical atlas, ed. 1, Boston, 1976, Little, Brown & Co. **B** and **C** from Ochsner, J.L., and Mills, N.L.: Coronary artery surgery, ed. 1, Philadelphia, 1978, Lea & Febiger.)

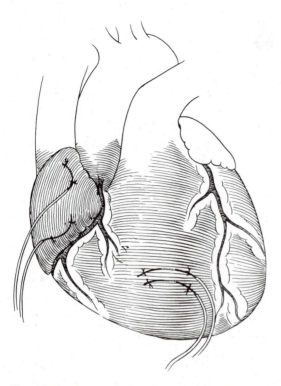

Fig. 14-10. Placement of atrial and ventricular pacing wires in the epicardium. (Reprinted with permission Behrendt, D.M.: Patient care in cardiac surgery, ed. 3, Boston, © Copyright 1980, Little, Brown & Co.)

are obtained. As much as possible of the perfusate is returned to the patient. Any left in the machine is centrifuged into red blood cells and returned to the patient.

At times, patients may not wean off bypass the first time. This may be a serious problem if the preoperative ejection fraction was low (less than 40%) or if the patient sustained prolonged subendocardial ischemia during surgery. Signs of difficulty weaning include increased pulmonary capillary wedge pressure, decreased blood pressure (below 100 mm Hg), and arrhythmias. Bypass may then be reinstituted, or inotropic drugs may be given to support the heart.

Closure. All coronary anastomoses are in-

spected for bleeding. The caval cannulas are removed. Protamine is given to reverse heparinization. The aortic cannula is removed when as much of the blood as possible has been returned to the patient.

Pacing wires, two atrial and one ventricular, are passed through the epicardium with a needle and brought out through the skin (Fig. 14-10). These wires allow the patient to be paced from the atria, ventricles, or in the AV sequential mode if needed. The pericardium is generally left open.

Chest tubes are placed in the anterior and posterior mediastinum. Their primary purpose is to drain and measure blood loss and prevent tamponade. If the pleural space has been entered, a chest tube will also be placed in the pleural space and brought out through the intercostal space.

Incisional edges are brought together and a stainless steel wire placed around the manubrium and twisted together. This wire is permanent and will show up on roentgenograms for the rest of the patient's life. Suture material is used to close fascia, subcutaneous tissue and skin. Steristrips are placed to reinforce the skin incision and usually a light gauze dressing secured that will remain in place for 2 to 3 days after surgery.

Procedure for valve replacement

Mitral valve repair. The early process of rheumatic mitral valve disease consists of thickening and scarring of the leaflets and chordae tendineae with varying degrees of fusion of the commissures. Later in the process, both the valve and the annulus become calcified. Those patients whose disease process is detected in the early stages are candidates for dilation and plastic procedures. The patient with moderate to severe calcification, mixed stenosis and insufficiency, and pure insufficiency will require valve replacement.

Commissurotomy is a dilation procedure that can be performed as a closed procedure without cardiopulmonary bypass or as an open procedure with bypass. In closed commissurotomy, a dilating instrument is passed through an incision in the left ventricle, up through the valve, and opened to break loose the tight valve leaflets. A drawback of this procedure is the high incidence of valve injury.[14]

The open commissurotomy is done through medial sternotomy with the patient on bypass. The left atrium is incised anterior to the right pulmonary veins, and a finger or instrument is used to dilate the tight valve. Commissurotomy is simple and quick; however, it has been associated with a high incidence of recurrent stenosis and therefore is usually not the procedure of choice.

One of the most commonly used procedures for mitral insufficiency is annuloplasty. Special suturing techniques are used to draw up the dilated annulus and reduce the amount of regurgitation (Fig. 14-11).

Mitral valve replacement. The procedure for mitral valve replacement begins similarly to that of the coronary artery bypass with a medial sternotomy incision and use of total cardiopulmonary bypass. Aortic cross-clamping is used to slow the heart. (Fig. 14-12).

The entire valve, including papillary muscle and chordae tendineae, is removed. The annular tissue must be removed carefully because if too much is taken away, the new valve prosthesis may impinge on or injure the aortic valve, which is located nearby. Posteriorly, the AV node can also be affected by prosthesis placement. Interrupted sutures are placed in the annulus of the valve and the skirt of the valve prosthesis. A special valve holder allows the sutures to remain lined up and evenly distributed. The valve is then lowered into place and the sutures tied off. The left atrium is closed and air expelled.

Aortic valve replacement. Significant aortic stenosis is often the result of the presence of calcium deposits on the valve. Rheumatic carditis is the most common cause in adults. When calcification is present and the patient is symptomatic, then valve replacement must be done. Insufficiency of the valve results from rheumatic heart disease, congenital anomalies of the leaflets, or a number of conditions that cause dilation of the aortic root— Marfan's syndrome, syphilis, arteriosclerotic heart disease, and dissection of the ascending aorta for example. If insufficiency is causing symptoms,

then valve replacement must be done. At times, there may also be mitral insufficiency or coronary artery disease in association with aortic valve disease. This presents a special challenge to the surgeon who must do the two procedures at once.

The surgical procedure begins with the medial sternotomy and the placement of the patient on cardiopulmonary bypass (Fig. 14-13). Cardiac arrest takes place. A transverse aortotomy is made 1 to 2 cm above the coronary ostia. It is important to remember that the AV conduction bundle is located in the noncoronary cusp and is subject to injury during debridement and placement of sutures. As many calcium deposits as possible are scraped away. The sutures are placed below the coronary ostia and then through the prosthesis, which is lowered into place. The incision into the aorta is closed. Air in the ventricle and aorta is removed through a needle, and the aortic clamp is released. As blood flows through the coronary arteries, the heart begins beating again.

Tricuspid valve disease. As an isolated entity, this is a rare occurrence, and is usually seen in conjunction with mitral or aortic valve disease. At times, however, this valve may need to be replaced at the same time the mitral and aortic valves are replaced. Technically, there is little difference between the procedures.

Heart transplant

The heart transplant procedure is reserved for the patient with congestive heart failure that is refractory to medical therapy and cannot be helped by traditional cardiac surgery.[9] Ideal candidates are young (under 50) and otherwise healthy with end-stage cardiac disease. They are without other major or chronic diseases, such as peripheral vascular disease, pulmonary disease, or insulin-dependent diabetes. These are individuals who generally have incurred massive myocardial damage as the result of recent disease, such as myocarditis or cardiomyopathies.

The procedure for transplant consists of the recipient being put on bypass with the use of hypothermia. An attempt is made to keep the donor's conduction system intact, but postoperative ar-

Text continued on p. 437.

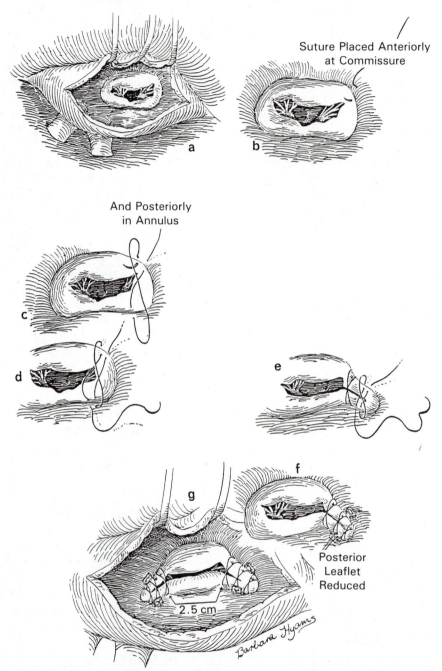

Fig. 14-11. Mitral valve annuloplasty. Mitral valve is exposed through left atriotomy incision. Initial suture is placed at commissure and commissural zone gathered together with continuous running suture. Procedure is repeated on opposite side of valve, and as seen in final drawing, valve orifice is much smaller and tighter, which will hopefully decrease degree of regurgitation. (From Cooley, D.A., and Norman, J.C.: Techniques in cardiac surgery, ed. 1, Houston, 1975, Texas Medical Press, Inc.)

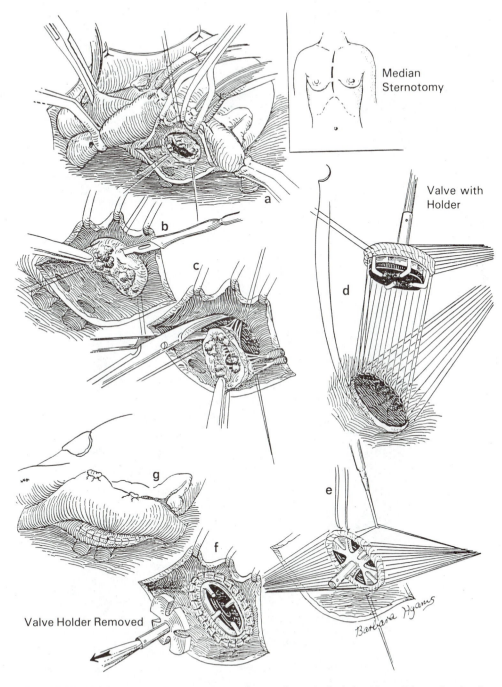

Median
Sternotomy

Valve with
Holder

Valve Holder Removed

Fig. 14-12. Mitral valve replacement. An atriotomy is made in left atrium. Diseased valve is inspected and decision for removal is made. It is then excised with chordae tendineae and apices of papillary muscle. Using interrupted sutures, artificial valve with holder is lowered into position. Sutures are tied off, holder removed, and left atrium closed. (From Cooley, D.A., and Norman, J.C.: Techniques in cardiac surgery, ed. 1, Houston, 1975, Texas Medical Press, Inc.)

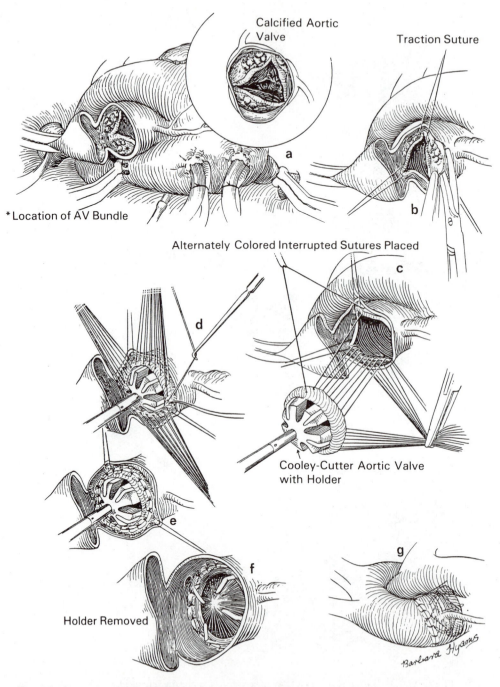

Calcified Aortic Valve

Traction Suture

*Location of AV Bundle

a

b

Alternately Colored Interrupted Sutures Placed

c

d

Cooley-Cutter Aortic Valve with Holder

e

Holder Removed

f

g

Barbara Hyams

Fig. 14-13. Aortic valve replacement. An incision is made into aorta. Diseased valve is removed and new valve is lowered into place with assistance from valve holder. Interrupted sutures are used to secure valve, and aorta is closed. (From Cooley, D.A., and Norman, J.C.: Techniques in cardiac surgery, ed. 1, Houston, 1975, Texas Medical Press, Inc.)

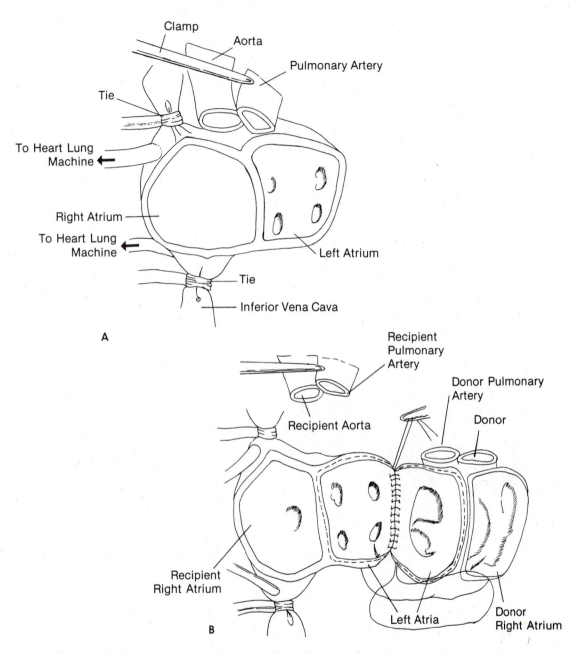

Fig. 14-14. Technique for heart transplant. Operation is performed as conventional open-heart procedure with usual equipment and instrumentation. It does not present any particular mechanical difficulties. Patient is prepared routinely and a median sternotomy is performed. Patient is then connected to cardiopulmonary bypass machine following systemic heparinization. Donor heart is excised following arrest obtained by infusion of cold cardioplegia solution. It is then placed in cold saline for transfer to recipient's operating room. Heart of recipient is excised simultaneously. **A,** Aorta and pulmonary artery are divided immediately above their respective valves. Atrial walls and interatrial septum are divided near atrioventricular groove, leaving two large right and left atrial cuffs. **B,** Orthotopic graft is performed by anastomosing recipient and donor atrial walls and interatrial septum.

Continued.

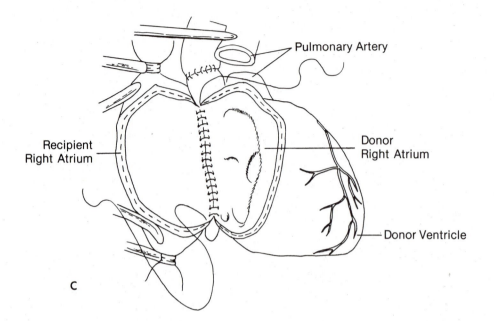

Pulmonary Artery

Recipient
Right Atrium

Donor
Right Atrium

Donor Ventricle

C

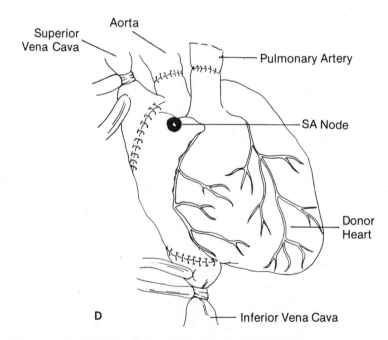

Aorta

Superior
Vena Cava

Pulmonary Artery

SA Node

Donor
Heart

Inferior Vena Cava

D

Fig. 14-14, cont'd. C and **D,** Major vessels of donor and recipient. Aorta and pulmonary artery are trimmed and sutured, reestablishing anatomical continuity. Cardiac transplantation procedure is terminated as any conventional open-heart procedure, taking great care to prevent hemostasis and to eliminate entrapped air in graft. Donor heart often starts beating spontaneously in sinus rhythm when perfusion is reestablished and rewarming is achieved.

rhythmias remain a common complication (Fig. 14-14).

The patient receives immunosuppressive drugs in the early postoperative period. The drugs usually used are prednisone and azathioprine (Imuran). Biopsy of myocardial tissue is done regularly to assist in the detection of rejection.

Although a number of these procedures have been done, there still remain some major complications. Primarily, accelerated coronary atherosclerosis has been observed, limiting long-term survival. Rejection is still a problem. Infection complications have also contributed to the mortality. Advancements in the technique continue, and 3 year survival rates are now at 50%.[20]

CLINICAL FINDINGS
The postoperative cardiac surgery patient

The care of a patient after cardiac surgery is a challenging and satisfying experience. The patient arrives in the postanesthesia room or ICU invaded by tubes, wires, and catheters. Nurses must per-

---

ICU PREPARATIONS FOR THE CARDIAC SURGERY PATIENT

Bedside equipment should be set up before the arrival of the cardiac surgery patient. Monitors must be turned on and given time to warm up. Suction machines should be checked to be sure they are functioning properly. The hemodynamic monitoring lines should be checked by a second nurse to be sure no air is present and to assure the accuracy of calibration. The checking of equipment before patient arrival ensures a smooth admission of the patient to the ICU and a rapid response to any emergencies.

1. Cardiac monitor with electrodes attached
2. Hemodynamic monitoring equipment—transducers and ports for:
   a. Swan-Ganz line
   b. Arterial line
   c. Left atrial pressure line
   d. Central venous pressure line
3. Cardiac output machine and injectate
4. Suction machines
   a. Endotracheal suction
   b. Nasogastric
   c. Chest tube
5. Emergency equipment
   a. Emergency room drugs
   b. Emergency room cart
   c. Defibrillator
   d. External pacing generator
6. Intravenous infusion pumps
7. Hyperthermia blanket
8. Other supplies
   a. Acohol and Betadine swabs
   b. Syringes of various sizes
   c. Needles
   d. Vacuum tubes for blood samples

form a thorough assessment and be prepared to respond to a variety of problems. These clinicians must have experience in care of the critically ill and be familiar with signs of postoperative complications.

Preparations in the ICU. Before the arrival of the patient to the ICU, the bedside environment should be prepared and checked for the proper equipment. The box on p. 437 summarizes the equipment needed. Ideally, clinicians who will care for the patient should set up the equipment so that they are aware of its location and proper functioning.

Admission to ICU. When the patient arrives in the ICU, a minimum of two clinicians are needed, a primary nurse and a secondary or assisting nurse. As outlined in the box on p. 440, the clinician who is assisting will connect the cardiac and hemodynamic monitors. The chest tube is placed at -20 cm H_2O suction, and the patient is connected to a mechanical ventilator if he is still intubated. This clinician can also obtain ECG and hemodynamic waveform strips for mounting in the chart. Necessary laboratory samples are drawn and the bedside chart organized.

The primary clinician caring for the patient must quickly assess the patient's vital signs and heart and pulmonary pressures, make sure all lines are intact and secure, and perform a quick physical assessment. The primary clinician receives reports from the operating room or postanesthesia room clinician, reviews the events of surgery, and reviews the postoperative orders.

At this time, the patient may have some initial changes in vital signs as a result of the movement to the ICU. These are usually transient and subside within 30 minutes.

Once the patient is settled, the family will probably want to visit. If they have not been warned previously, it is important that the staff explain the normalcy of the many tubes that surround the patient. The clinician should also explain that the patient will be very drowsy for several hours and that he cannot communicate with the

endotracheal tube in place. The clinician may also want to have some spirits of ammonia ready. It is not unusual for visitors to become faint when they first enter the ICU.

Hemodynamic assessment. The first 8 to 12 hours after surgery is when the patient must be closely monitored. A flow sheet such as the one in Fig. 14-15 allows the clinicians to evaluate at a glance the trends in the patient's cardiovascular status. Vital signs and other critical data are recorded hourly or more often as needed. The values to record include the heart rate, respiratory rate, blood pressure, mean arterial pressure, pulmonary arterial pressure, pulmonary capillary wedge pressure, cardiac output, cardiac index systemic vascular resistance, and pulmonary vascular resistance. Also included in the cardiovascular assessment is observation of the ECG for arrhythmias or signs of ischemia, auscultation of heart sounds, peripheral vascular examination, and monitoring of cardiac related laboratory data.

Respiratory assessment. The patient is usually intubated for the first 12 to 20 hours following surgery; however, there are some institutions where the patient is extubated before leaving the operating room. Either way, a complete respiratory assessment is done—auscultation of breath sounds, observation of respiratory excursion, observation of general skin and peripheral coloring, assessment of the characteristics and amount of secretions from lungs and airways, and respiratory rate. Mediastinal and chest tubes are checked for drainage and patency. Arterial blood gases are measured on admission to the ICU and within 1 hour of any ventilation changes. A daily chest roentgenogram will show any signs of pulmonary edema, pneumonia, pneumothorax, or tamponade.

The usual ventilatory checks should be done with the goal of maintaining normal values for oxygenation and acid-base balance. It is especially important that these patients not be allowed to become hypoxic. Deep breathing and coughing remain the best way to prevent pulmonary complications. Hypoxemia can also be avoided by pre-

NAME: _____ HOSPITAL NO. _____

DATE: _____ WT.: _____ HT.: _____

	Time:																									

VITAL SIGNS
- BP sys/dias
- MAP
- Pulse
- Respirations
- CVP (RAP)
- PA sys/dias
- PA Mean
- PCWP
- C.O./C.I.
- SVR
- PVR

IV MEDICATIONS

INTAKE
- IV fluids (total)
- P.O. (total)
- Blood products

OUTPUT
- Urine
- Chest tube (total)
- NG
- Other

Fig. 14-15. Sample ICU flowsheet. A good ICU flowsheet allows the clinician to flow trends in vital signs and correlate the patient's pressures with medical treatment or interventions. This is especially important for regulation of intravenous cardiotonic or vasoactive drugs. Continuous assessment of fluid balance and blood loss is also imperative in the cardiac surgery patient.

ICU ADMISSION OF THE CARDIAC SURGERY PATIENT

The primary nurse is the person primarily responsible for the patient's care and the person who assumes full care of the patient when his condition is stable. The secondary nurse assists the primary nurse with the admission of the patient.

PRIMARY NURSE RESPONSIBILITIES

1. Initially assess the patient
   a. Blood pressure, pulse, respirations, temperature
   b. Cardiac and pulmonary pressures
   c. Physical examination
   d. Urinary and chest tube output
2. Regulate intravenous fluids and medications based on assessment
3. Receive report from operating room or post-anesthesia nurses
4. Review postoperative orders

SECONDARY NURSE RESPONSIBILITIES

1. Assist in connection of patient to mechanical ventilator
2. Connect ECG electrodes and establish tracing
3. Connect hemodynamic monitoring lines; level, zero, and calibrate them if needed
4. Connect chest tube(s) to low constant suction
5. Connect nasogastric tube to suction
6. Attach a urinometer to Foley catheter
7. Obtain recorded strips of ECG and pressure waveforms
8. Draw necessary laboratory samples
9. Connect hypothermia blanket
10. Assist primary nurse in taking of physician orders and assembling bedside chart

---

oxygenation before suctioning, maintaining a clear airway, and observing for early signs of hypoxia, which include increased heart rate, increased respiratory rate, and restlessness.

Renal assessment. Renal evaluation is critical in these patients. Hourly intake and output are recorded along with specific gravity and urine color. BUN and creatinine are measured daily.

Neurological assessment. Neurological assessment is necessary to detect any complications of stroke or hypoxia that can occur as a result of the surgery or heart-lung bypass. Immediately postoperatively, a baseline assessment should be done and compared with the preoperative assessment.

The most important areas to assess are the level of consciousness, responsiveness to verbal and tactile stimuli, pupil response, movement of extremities, and when the patient is extubated, speech and thought patterns.

Gastrointestinal assessment. Gastrointestinal assessment includes assessment of the abdomen for distention and the presence or absence of bowel sounds. Nasogastric drainage is inspected for blood.

Fluids and electrolytes. Fluids and electrolytes are monitored because of the changes that occur during bypass and because of the use of diuretics and large amounts of blood products. Ideally the patient is maintained in a negative fluid balance to prevent the development of cardiac failure. The nursing responsibility for this includes accurate documentation of intake and output, daily weights performed in a consistent manner, maintenance of intravenous fluid rates as ordered, observation for elevation of pulmonary capillary wedge pressure, observation for peripheral edema, monitoring of electrolytes, and observing the ECG for signs of hyperkalemia or hypokalemia.

Other observations. Other items to assess are wounds, IV and catheter sites, skin integrity, and oral integrity. Psychological response should be recorded and will be discussed in more detail under the section "Health Care Implications."

ICU care and interventions. The patient who has had congestive heart failure presents a special challenge in the early postoperative period. The primary goals at this time are (1) to decrease the workload of the heart and (2) to maintain adequate peripheral perfusion. Each goal is achieved through various interventions that are dependent upon the underlying disease process and the type of procedure the patient has undergone.

The patient who has undergone coronary artery bypass is most likely to have problems of increased systemic vascular resistance or afterload in the early postoperative period. For reasons that are still unclear, around 60% of patients who have coronary bypass have a transient hypertension lasting the first 24 to 48 hours after surgery. The dangers of sustained hypertension are that it can increase myocardial oxygen demand, increase the workload of the heart, and decrease the stroke volume or cardiac output. The decrease in cardiac output would result in lower coronary artery perfusion, decrease myocardial oxygen supply, and cause further depression of myocardial contractility and subsequent failure. In addition, the hypertension puts a strain on the aortic suture line that could lead to bleeding. Systolic hypertension should therefore be controlled with intravenous nitroprusside. This is especially important when the systemic vascular resistance is greater than 1500 dynes cm^{-5}. Once nitroprusside is started, an increase in cardiac out-

put and stroke volume should be seen almost immediately along with a drop in systolic pressure.

A second challenge in the care of the patient with previous congestive heart failure is the maintenance of an adequate left ventricular filling pressure to augment cardiac output without producing pulmonary congestion. The techniques of the surgery all contribute to depression of ventricular compliance in the early postoperative period. For the patient who has had congestive heart failure, this compounds an already existing problem. The heart has responded to the high filling pressures by increasing the chamber size and now has undergone surgery that further decreases ventricular compliance. Therefore a higher than normal filling pressure (pulmonary capillary wedge pressure) will be needed in order to maintain an adequate cardiac output. The filling pressures or preload can be increased through the administration of blood to elevate the hematocrit to 40 or of plasma protein fraction (Plasmanate) to expand intravascular volume. Ideally, therapy is directed to maintain a cardiac index at 2.5 L/minute/M^2. Concurrently, the patient's pulmonary status must be observed for any signs of congestion.

The patient with mitral valve replacement has similar problems but with a different cause. The goal is to maintain adequate pulmonary circulation by maintaining higher than normal preload. The patient who has had mitral valve disease for a number of years most likely has responded to the obstruction by developing the vasculature of the pulmonary system. Just as the arterioles of the body become thickened and stronger in response to hypertension, the pulmonary arteries and veins respond the same way, and the patient develops mitral lung disease with severe pulmonary hypertension. The pulmonary arterial pressure, pulmonary capillary wedge pressure, and pulmonary vascular resistance may be very high, depending upon the extent of the disease. There may also be right ventricular hypertrophy. In the early postoperative period, although the diseased valve has been replaced, it will take some time for the pulmonary hypertension to improve. Until then, this

Table 14-2. Cardiac surgery activity progression protocol demonstrating the normal progression in activity that the cardiac surgery patient can undergo

Approximate days	Level	Activity	Exercise prescription	METS
Preoperative	0	Activity tolerance assessment. Activity ad lib within functional limitations of existing disease	Teach positioning, mobility in bed, and transfer from bed to chair Teach postop exercises, posture, and body mechanics Orient to the specifics of the cardiac rehabilitation program	
0 to 1 postop	I	Bed rest Bathe assisted by nurse, brushes own teeth, (arms supported as needed) Feed self in bed, nurse prepares tray—as appropriate	Active, assisted exercise to four extremities supine or semi-fowler b.i.d. Diaphragmatic and lateral costal breathing exercises b.i.d.	1.0-1.5
ADVANCE TO LEVEL II FOLLOWING REMOVAL OF LA LINE				
1 to 4 postop	II	Bathe, shave, brush teeth in bed with back and arms supported (optional) Dangle, then sit in cardiac chair 30 min. × 1—progress to sitting 30 min. × 3 q.d. Feed self and prepare own tray Bedside commode	Active ROM exercise in semi-fowler b.i.d. Diaphragmatic and lateral costal breathing exercises b.i.d. Review transfer activities and body mechanics instruction Reorient to specifics of rehab program Transfer to floor in cardiac chair	1.0-2.0
4 to 6 postop	III	Bathe and groom seated at sink or in shower, seated* Sit in chair as tolerated Bathroom privileges	Active ROM sitting Breathing and posture exercises, sitting Ambulation in room, monitored Teach self-monitoring of activity tolerance Job and home assessment	1.5-2.5
6 to 9 postop	IV	Bathe or shower, standing Ambulate in hallway, increasing pace and length of time ad lib with supervision Attend group teaching and exercises	Active exercise sitting to standing Ambulate in hallway, monitored Review physical limitations secondary to cardiac disease/surgery Assess self-monitoring skills	2.0-3.0
9 to discharge	V	Dress in street clothes Ambulate ad lib, self-monitored Attend group teaching and exercise Group dining Self-care protocol	Active exercise standing, incorporating breathing exercise Stair climbing as indicated with supervision and monitoring Home program instruction; review of daily prescription and rest/activity ratio	2.5-3.5

Reprinted from Stuart, E.M., and others: Nursing rounds: care of the patient with a mitral commissurotomy, Am. J. Nurs. p. 1630, Sept. 1980. Copyrighted by the American Journal of Nursing Company.
Criteria for advancement: absence of uncontrolled hypertension, uncontrolled arrhythmias, severe CHF, continued chest pain, shock, or postural hypotension.
1 MET is the energy expended at rest and is equivalent to approx. 3.5 ml/O_2/kg body wt/min.
*Shower if pacing wires are out and incision shows signs of healing.

patient will also need higher than normal filling pressures to keep the pulmonary vessels open. Nurses therefore must monitor the pulmonary capillary wedge pressure and pulmonary vascular resistance closely for signs of increased resistance and/or decreased filling pressures. They should also monitor the right atrial pressure for unusual elevation indicating venous congestion or right ventricular failure.

Normal progression of activities. The normal course of events is presented in Table 14-2. It should be emphasized that this progression will vary from hospital to hospital and from patient to patient. This chart is general and intended to be interpreted as such.

Complications of cardiac surgery

The goal for this section is to describe the cause and assessment of the complications of cardiac surgery. These complications and precipitating factors are summarized in the following outline.

1. Low cardiac output syndrome
   a. Myocardial depressing drugs
   b. Subendocardial ischemia
2. Hypovolemia/hemorrhage
   a. Inadequate fluid replacement
   b. Prolonged pump time with platelet destruction
   c. Inadequate hemostasis in surgery
   d. Inadequate reversal of heparin
3. Arrhythmias
   a. Hypoxia
   b. Hyperkalemia
   c. Acidosis
   d. Suture placement
   e. Pain
   f. Anemia
4. Perioperative myocardial infarction
   a. Ventricular hypertrophy
   b. Arrhythmias
   c. Hypotension
   d. Prolonged pump time
5. Inadequate ventilation/atelectasis
   a. Lung disease
   b. Smoking history
   c. Anesthesia
   d. Sedation
6. Pulmonary embolism
   a. Microemboli
   b. Coagulation abnormalities
   c. Atrial fibrillation
7. Respiratory failure/adult respiratory distress syndrome
   a. Myocardial failure postoperative
   b. Fluid shifts
   c. Prolonged intubation
8. Cerebral infarction
   a. Hypotension
   b. Microemboli
   c. Calcium deposits from valve
   d. Mural thrombus
9. Renal failure
   a. Hypotension
   b. Low cardiac output
   c. Transfusion reaction
10. Systemic emboli
    a. Microemboli
    b. Catheters
11. Postoperative psychosis
    a. ICU environment
    b. Metabolic changes
    c. Pump time

Low cardiac output syndrome. This is the most serious complication of cardiac surgery. In the past, the mortality has been 80%. It is thought to be the result of subendocardial ischemia produced during surgery, it is seen after both coronary artery bypass and valve operations, and it may be a factor in the patient's inability to be weaned off bypass.

A combination of factors alter the heat's oxygen supply-demand balance during surgery. These factors include cross-clamp time, ventricular fibrillation, body temperature, ischemic arrest, intraoperative hypotension, and intraoperative arrhythmias. The symptoms that will result from diminished cardiac output are cardiac index less than 2.0 L/minute/M², signs of decreased peripheral perfusion, decreased urine output, decreased mental sensorium, and decreased mean arterial pressure.

The goal for treatment is to restore the cardiac output to normal values and prevent further ischemia. In order to do this, the clinician must be

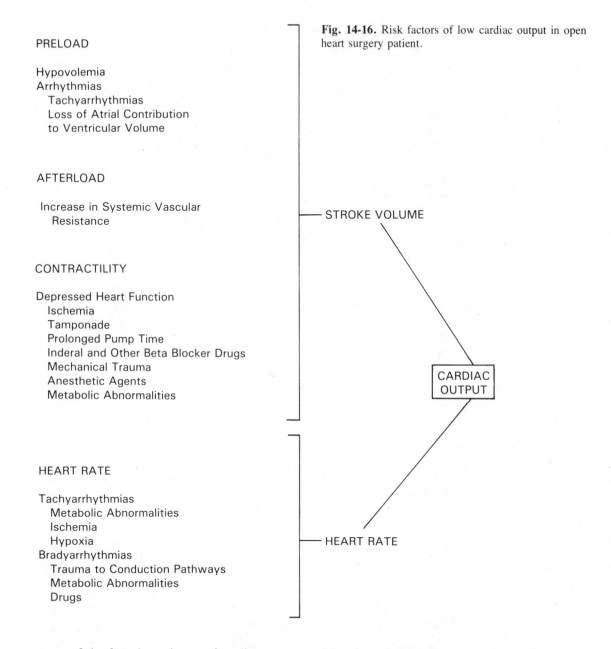

PRELOAD

Hypovolemia
Arrhythmias
   Tachyarrhythmias
   Loss of Atrial Contribution
   to Ventricular Volume

AFTERLOAD

Increase in Systemic Vascular
   Resistance

CONTRACTILITY

Depressed Heart Function
   Ischemia
   Tamponade
   Prolonged Pump Time
   Inderal and Other Beta Blocker Drugs
   Mechanical Trauma
   Anesthetic Agents
   Metabolic Abnormalities

HEART RATE

Tachyarrhythmias
   Metabolic Abnormalities
   Ischemia
   Hypoxia
Bradyarrhythmias
   Trauma to Conduction Pathways
   Metabolic Abnormalities
   Drugs

STROKE VOLUME

CARDIAC OUTPUT

HEART RATE

Fig. 14-16. Risk factors of low cardiac output in open heart surgery patient.

aware of the four determinants of cardiac output and the problems of each that can contribute to a low cardiac output. These four determinants are shown in Fig. 14-16 with the problems that can occur in each. By correcting these problems, one should see improved cardiac output, improved pe-ripheral perfusion, increased urine output, and improved mental status.

Hypovolemia/hemorrhage. Several factors can lead to postoperative bleeding and hypovolemia. Inadequate reversal of heparin, prolonged pump time with destruction of platelets, scar tissue requiring extensive dissection, inadequate or improper suture placement, deficient clotting factors, and failure to provide adequate hemostasis during surgery.

Chest tubes are placed in the anterior and posterior mediastinum to assist in the detection of hemorrhage. Blood loss in excess of 100 ml/hour for 3 or more hours will probably necessitate return to surgery. The hemorrhage may be slow (50 ml/hour for 5 to 6 hours) or very rapid (1000 ml in 20 minutes). If the tubes are patent the first clue will be the chest tube output. If the chest tubes become clotted, the blood will collect in the mediastinum and lead to cardiac tamponade and shock. This seems to be especially common after aortic valve replacement. The first signs of a problem will be a sudden cessation in chest drainage followed by decreased blood pressure, increased right atrial pressure, pulmonary capillary wedge pressure, pulsus paradoxus, a respiratory variation in systolic blood pressure that is greater than 10 mm Hg, narrowing pulse pressure, and distant heart sounds.

Hemorrhage and tamponade require immediate intervention. The goal in treating hemorrhage is to restore an adequate circulating blood volume and control the source of bleeding. For tamponade, the goal is relief of myocardial compression by evacuation of the blood.

Although hemorrhage is a major cause of hypovolemia, the patient may also experience inadequate fluid replacement and overuse of diuretics that can lead to hypovolemia. Indicators that would be seen are decreased blood pressure, decreased right atrial pressure and pulmonary capillary wedge pressure, increased heart rate, decreased cardiac output, and oliguria. Vasodilating drugs (such as nitroprusside) can also produce a relative hypovolemia that can cause a precipitous fall in blood pressure if the patient is already hypovolemic.

Arrhythmias. Studies have found that close to 50% of all cardiac surgery patients exhibit arrhythmias postoperatively.[1] They usually occur in the early postoperative period and are associated with all types of cardiac surgery.

Premature ventricular contractions occur most frequently following aortic valve replacement and coronary artery bypass. The danger is that they often precede ventricular tachycardia or ventricular fibrillation. Also, if they occur frequently, they cause a significant drop in stroke volume and may lead to an overall decrease in cardiac output.

When they are frequent enough to require treatment, they should be treated rapidly and the patient assessed for possible causes. The causes include hypoxia, hyperkalemia, acidosis, alkalosis, infusion of catecholamines, myocardial ischemia, pain, hypotension, and anemia.

Atrial arrhythmias are very common the first 36 hours after surgery because of the pericarditis associated with surgery. They will especially be seen following mitral valve replacement and aortic valve replacement. The danger of premature atrial contractions is that they often precede faster atrial arrhythmias. Atrial tachycardia will cause a decrease in diastolic filling time with a decreased cardiac output. Normally, a heart rate of 80 to 100 beats per minute is maintained in the early postoperative period so that there is adequate cardiac output.

The conduction system may be damaged during aortic valve replacement when calcium deposits are removed or when the new prosthesis is secured. Heart block and junctional rhythms may therefore be seen postoperatively. Physiologically they result in loss of the synchronized atrial kick, which is necessary for adequate cardiac output. Any arrhythmias that decrease cardiac output in the presence of an already compromised ventricle will result in ischemia and further deterioration of left ventricular contraction.

Perioperative myocardial infarction. This is the leading cause of mortality following coronary artery bypass surgery. There is a higher risk of MI in patients who have hypertrophied ventricles, prolonged pump time, preoperative decreased ejection fraction, prolonged arrhythmias, or hypotension during surgery.

MI is diagnosed by the presence of significant new Q waves (greater than 0.04 second), creatine phosphokinase-MB elevation (which may be normally elevated postoperatively and therefore not the best indicator), and pathological thallium scan postoperatively.

Inadequate ventilation/atelectasis. Respiratory complications occur most frequently in the patient with a history of smoking and lung disease. During bypass, the lung tissue becomes stiff and resistant to expansion, leading to increased work of breathing. Adding to this problem is operative pain, which also interferes with the ability to deep breathe. Anesthesia, sedatives, and narcotics further compound the problem by their respiratory depressant effects. The end result is hypoventilation, retained secretions, and the development of atelectasis. The clinical indicators of atelectasis include temperature elevation, normal P_{CO_2}, decreased P_{O_2}, decreased pH and diminished breath sounds over the affected area.

Pulmonary embolism. This may follow coronary artery bypass or valve replacement. It is thought to result from emboli formed while on bypass, problems in coagulation, and mural emboli associated with atrial fibrillation. It is difficult to diagnose because of normal operative chest pain. The clinical manifestations are hemoptysis, tachypnea, decreased P_{O_2}, apprehension, feeling of faintness, hypotension, and cyanosis. A lung scan and/or pulmonary angiogram is done to substantiate the diagnosis.

Respiratory failure. The patient who has an unstable postoperative course with myocardial failure, major fluid shifts, or pulmonary edema and prolonged intubation is prone to the development of respiratory failure and adult respiratory distress syndrome. The patient may not wean readily from the ventilator. He then may require higher and higher oxygen flow rates and the use of positive end-expiratory pressure or constant positive airway pressure. Meanwhile, carbon dioxide levels continue to increase and are persistently high. This complication can become a very serious one in terms of management and associated morbidity and mortality.

Cerebral infarction. Air or particulate emboli during bypass have been a major problem in the past. Now with newer techniques and filters, this does not present as serious a danger to the patient.

Sources of emboli that remain a potential problem are valvular calcium deposits breaking free and lodging in the brain, emboli from an endocardial thrombus in the patient with chronic atrial fibrillation or ventricular aneurysm, plaque in the aorta breaking away with cannulation, and deep vein emboli.

When this occurs, it is manifested by sudden onset of neurological indicators, including shortened attention span, deviation of the head and eyes to one side, paralysis or weakness on one side of the body, aphasia, and a change in the level of consciousness.

Renal failure. Acute tubular necrosis may develop from ischemic injury to the kidneys. Some factors contributing to this are microemboli, intraoperative hypotension, postoperative low cardiac output, and transfusion reaction. The clinical indicators include oliguria (less than 400 ml/24 hours), elevated BUN and creatinine, possible hematuria, and possible proteinuria. The urinary sodium level can be very helpful in differentiating the cause of oliguria. Urinary sodium of less than 10 mEq/L is associated with renal failure resulting from low-output states. A urinary sodium level of greater than 10 mEq/L is usually seen in medullary disease.

Systemic emboli. As discussed previously, emboli may develop from any number of manipulations being done during surgery. In addition, intravenous and intra-arterial catheters are a source of irritation to the vessel wall and may precipitate the development of emboli.

Arterial embolization to the extremities is immediately recognizable by pain, pallor, pulselessness, and paresthesia. Venous embolism or thrombosis is characterized by pain, redness, swelling, and a positive Homans' sign. Both problems require immediate attention. Arterial occlusion, if allowed to go beyond 12 hours, may result in gangrene of the extremity. Venous emboli can migrate to the lungs, causing pulmonary infarction and death.

Postoperative psychosis. Postoperative psychosis, postcardiotomy delirium, and ICU psychosis are all similar phenomena given various titles in the literature. For reasons that are unknown, cardiac surgery patients have a higher than average incidence of this problem. Some of the postulated variables that could contribute to this are pump time, premorbid personality, microemboli, denial of anxiety, preoperative coping, age, ICU environment, prolonged hypotension during surgery, decreased cardiac output, and medications. In assessing this patient, manifestation may include hallucinations; nocturnal disorientation, increased motor activity and restlessness, paranoid delusions; and pulling at lines and tubes. This behavior usually occurs after 2 to 5 days of normal, lucid behavior. The average duration is 2 to 5 days and most patients return to normal upon discharge from the ICU.

Problem in adjustment to valve. The prosthetic valves currently used in patients have the major benefit of durability, which prevents the patient from having to repeat the operation 5 years later. However, noise is one flaw in this artificial device. Not all prosthetic valves are noisy, nor do all patients have problems with the same valve. However, when they are noisy, they may be heard as far away as 12 feet. Initially, most patients find this extremely annoying and disappointing. They may become preoccupied with their heart rate or rhythm. They may also become worried about how they will handle social situations where others hear the clicking.

HEALTH CARE IMPLICATIONS
Preoperative patient problems

The patient with congestive heart failure who is about to undergo cardiac surgery faces four potential problems that may develop in the preoperative period (1) potential for anxiety and fear of the unknown; (2) potential for complicated recovery; (3) potential for patient crisis; and (4) potential for alteration in family process. The nurse must be aware of these potential problems and assess the patient as early as possible so that interventions can be initiated.

Anxiety and fear. All patients experience some anxiety and fear in the preoperative period. This anxiety may be manifested in a variety of behaviors. The patient may be talkative and gregarious or withdrawn and quiet. He may admit to being very frightened or he may tell the nurse he is not frightened at all. The patient may also use denial up to the time of surgery and relate that there is really nothing wrong with his heart. With all these behaviors it is imperative that the nurse sit down and talk with the patient and assess his perceptions of the surgery he is about to have. His anxiety and fear may be the result of (1) a previous experience with surgery, (2) fear of death, (3) fear of pain, (4) fear of the unknown, (5) lack of knowledge about the surgery, (6) fear of mutilation, (7) feelings of loss of control, or (8) other personal experiences.

Once the assessment is made, the nursing diagnosis can be formulated and focus on the patient's lack of knowledge or on his behaviors demonstrating anxiety.

The major intervention for a lack of knowledge would be preoperative teaching. The expected outcome for the patient would be his ability to discuss the preparations for surgery, the surgical procedure, and the expectations for the ICU phase. In addition, the nurse would expect to see a decrease in anxiety and fear with the patient verbally confirming this.

Potential for complicated recovery. Atelectasis, pneumonia, and peripheral thrombosis can complicate a smooth postoperative recovery and are problems that can be prevented by the preoperative intervention of teaching. The patient is instructed in the proper methods for deep breathing, coughing, leg exercises, and the use of the incentive spirometer. The proper procedure for deep breathing and coughing is discussed in the section on ICU patient problems.

Potential for patient crisis. The potential for patient crisis and the potential for physiological alterations are related to the problem of preoperative anxiety and fear. If preoperative anxiety is allowed to build out of control, the patient may go into crisis that could result in hysterical crying, severe depression, feelings of loss of control and helplessness, and a "flight response"—the patient refuses surgery or leaves the hospital. In addition, physiological changes of tachycardia, tachypnea, hypertension, and tremors appear and may exacerbate heart failure. It is rare that this will occur in the setting of supportive health care personnel, but it is important to be cognizant of it and to take measures to prevent it.

Potential for alteration in family process. The final potential problem for the preoperative period is family disintegration. At this time, the family members also experience feelings of helplessness and anxiety that can be manifested by repeated summoning of the nurse to the bedside, repeated questions related to the surgery, treatment of the patient as helpless, indecisiveness, rapid speech, insomnia, and anorexia. If two or more of these behaviors are present in a key family member there is the potential for family conflict and the development of family crisis.

Nurses are in the position to identify these behaviors and intervene before a crisis situation develops. They can intervene in this situation in the following manner.

1. Clarify misconceptions about surgery and explain what to expect in the postoperative period.
2. Have the surgeon talk with the family if further reassurance is needed.
3. Encourage family members to rely on methods of coping that have been beneficial in the past.
4. Assist family members with problem-solving by having them examine all options and prioritize steps to be taken.
5. Establish a means of communication with family members while the patient is in surgery.

6. Call in support persons (friends, relatives) as needed to be with family members.
7. Have a social worker see the family and serve as a support and resource person.

The expected outcome for these interventions is that the family will be able to verbalize feelings of less anxiety and diminished feelings of helplessness.

Intensive care unit patient problems

During the ICU phase of hospitalization the health care plan will focus on the recognition and prevention of the complications of cardiac surgery and the psychological responses of the early postoperative period. The major potential problems of this phase include:

1. Myocardial failure and shock state
2. Hypovolemic shock
3. Respiratory failure
4. Renal failure
5. Cerebrovascular accident (stroke)
6. Potential for complications of immobility
7. Postoperative psychosis
8. Postoperative depression
9. Death from arrhythmias
10. Protracted postoperative progression

Because many of these problems are physiological in nature, interventions will focus on physical assessment of the patient for signs and symptoms of these problems.

Myocardial failure and shock state. This potential problem may be the result of low cardiac output syndrome, intraoperative MI, or cardiac tamponade. The nursing diagnosis, based on the clinical signs of the problem, is inadequate peripheral perfusion related to changes in preload, afterload, contractility or heart rate (depending upon the primary problem). Therefore the outcome criteria would be: the patient will have adequate peripheral perfusion as evidenced by:

1. Cardiac index >2.2 L/minute/M^2
2. Warm extremities
3. Strong peripheral pulses
4. Urinary output of at least 20 ml/hour
5. Heart rate of 80 to 100

6. Systolic blood pressure >90 mm Hg
7. Awake and alert mentally

The first step toward intervention is to check all vital signs and hemodynamic values to assure that they are accurate. A change in patient positioning or the introduction of air into a pressure line can significantly alter pulmonary artery and arterial pressures. If the cardiac output is low and if the patient is warm with adequate peripheral pulses then a test of arterial-venous oxygen saturation difference is indicated. If this difference is greater than 30%, then the patient most likely has an actual decrease in cardiac output.

A second intervention is to provide supportive health care, as in turning every 2 hours, passive range of motion, skin care, and application of anti-embolism stockings. All of these measures contribute to improved peripheral circulation.

The third intervention is to consult with the physician regarding treatment modalities. This includes increasing preload by administering crystalloids, colloids, or blood products to maintain pulmonary capillary wedge pressure >6 mm Hg, increasing contractility by administering inotropic drugs such as dopamine, dobutamine, isoproterenol, or epinephrine, decreasing afterload by administering nitroprusside, nitroglycerin, or hydralazine to maintain systemic vascular resistance <1500 dynes. Assisting with insertion of IABP if indicated, and controlling heart rate with antiarrhythmics or pacemaker as indicated.

The fourth intervention for inadequate peripheral perfusion related to myocardial failure is to continually evaluate the patient's response to therapy and monitor his clinical status.

Hypovolemic shock. The clinical indicators and causes of hypovolemic shock have been discussed in the section of this chapter on "Clinical findings." Regardless of the problem's cause, the outcome criteria will be the same. The patient will have normovolemia as evidenced by:

1. Normal blood pressure
2. Heart rate of 80 to 100
3. Urine specific gravity 1.005 to 1.025

4. Urine sodium 10 to 20 mEq/L
5. Chest tube output <50 ml/hour
6. PCWP 6 to 12 mm Hg
7. Normal skin turgor
8. Warm, well-perfused extremities

Monitoring of the patient's vital signs takes first priority for nursing interventions. Hemodynamic parameters, blood pressure, urine output, and chest tube output are evaluated every hour. Hemoglobin, hematocrit, and clotting studies are followed carefully for any changes.

If the systolic blood pressure drops below 80 mm Hg, or if chest tube output exceeds 100 ml/hour for 3 consecutive hours, then urgent measures of volume replacement and the Trendelenburg position are initiated. One word of caution: Trendelenburg position should not be used on the patient with respiratory distress or heart failure. This position may aggravate these conditions by increasing venous return to the heart.

Vasoconstricting drugs are contraindicated until there has been adequate volume replacement. Vasoconstrictors cannot increase the venous return to the heart if there is no volume in venous or arterial vessels, and in the presence of heart failure they may increase afterload and the work of the heart. Finally, supportive health care measures will also prove beneficial in improving circulation and peripheral perfusion.

Respiratory failure. In the postoperative cardiac surgery patient, inadequate respiratory ventilation may be related to atelectasis, anemia, retained secretions, narcotics/sedation/anesthesia, or chronic obstructive pulmonary disease. If inadequate ventilation is allowed to continue, the patient may develop respiratory failure. The goal in prevention of this problem is that the patient will exhibit the clinical signs of adequate ventilation. Lungs will be clear to auscultation and the chest roentgenogram will demonstrate clear lung fields without pleural effusion or atelectasis. The patient will have a normal respiratory rate and verbalize that he is breathing easily. If he is on the mechanical ventilator, he will have normal lung compliance and normal inspiratory pressures.

Interventions to prevent respiratory failure include the following:

1. Check mechanical ventilator to ensure that the patient is receiving an adequate tidal volume (10 to 15 ml/kg of ideal body weight). Ensure that he is receiving 6 sighs/hour, minimally.
2. Suction secretions every 2 hours and whenever necessary while the patient is intubated.
3. Keep the head of the bed elevated to encourage gas exchange in lower lobes.
4. Have the patient who has been extubated breath deeply and cough every 2 hours.
5. Auscultate breath sounds every 2 hours and report any new pathological findings.
6. Obtain blood gases with each ventilator change and whenever the patient has signs of respiratory distress.
7. Correct anemia as rapidly as possible.

Renal failure. There is always the potential for the development of acute renal failure in the patient who has undergone cardiac surgery. The first and second postoperative days, the patient may normally experience diminished urinary output that is related to the secretion of antidiuretic hormone. However, if the urinary output falls below 20 ml/hour, an immediate assessment should be done to determine the cause.

The nursing diagnosis for this problem can be stated as potential for fluid volume imbalance manifested by diminished urinary output of ___ ml/hour. The goal or expected outcome for interventions is that the patient will have an adequate urinary output of at least 20 ml/hour.

The most common cause of diminished urinary output in postoperative cardiac surgery is hypovolemia. Therefore the first intervention will be the administration of fluids and possibly a fluid challenge. If the patient does not respond to the infusion of fluids, then a test dose of furosemide is administered intravenously. If the patient again fails to respond, then acute renal failure is suspected and appropriate laboratory tests are done to confirm the diagnosis. These laboratory tests and the clinical signs of acute renal failure are summarized in the boxed material below.

The nurse has an important role in monitoring the patient with acute renal failure. Electrolyte,

---

LABORATORY VALUES AND CLINICAL SIGNS AND SYMPTOMS OF ACUTE RENAL FAILURE

Oliguria—< 400 ml urine in 24 hours

Rising BUN—greater than 18 mg/dl*

Rising serum creatinine—greater than 1.5 mg/dl†

Elevated urine sodium—greater than 40 mEq/L

Low urine-plasma osmolarity ratio—less than 1.2

No response to fluid challenge or high dose furosemide

Lethargy and nausea

Leukocytosis

---

*An elevated BUN usually indicates prerenal causes of renal failure. Borderline elevations in BUN may be the result of increased intake of protein, or increased protein catabolism as seen in sepsis, fever, or gastrointestinal bleeding.
†Creatinine is elevated in all diseases of the kidney where 50% or more of nephrons are destroyed.

BUN, and creatinine levels must be measured at least daily. Hyperkalemia must be guarded against and potassium removed from all intravenous fluids and from the patient's diet. A rising serum sodium may indicate dehydration and therefore must be reported immediately. Strict intake and output records must be maintained while the patient is fluid restricted. Daily weights are obtained in order to document the state of hydration.

Special attention must be given to the medications the patient is receiving. Drugs such as digitalis, quinidine, and procainamide, which are normally excreted by the kidneys, may require reduced dosages.

Finally, the nurse may be asked to assist with the initiation of peritoneal dialysis. Peritoneal dialysis is often preferred over hemodialysis in the cardiac surgery patient because there is less hemodynamic instability produced. In addition, the dialysate for peritoneal dialysis does not require the use of heparin or other anticoagulants that could result in a cardiac bleed and tamponade.

Cerebrovascular accident (stroke). This is one potential problem the nurse can do little to prevent. Often the first sign of a cerebral insult is the failure of the patient to awaken from surgery. The cause may be unclear. Interventions are therefore directed toward the prevention of cerebral edema and the prevention of complications of immobility. These interventions include:

1. Provision of adequate ventilation to prevent hypercapnia and maintain adequate oxygenation
2. Administration of urea, mannitol, steroids, and anticoagulants as ordered by the physician
3. Quick treatment of premature atrial contractions and atrial fibrillation that can encourage the development of endocardial emboli
4. Monitoring of acid-base and electrolyte values
5. Provision of supportive health care, to include skin care, use of an egg crate mattress, passive range of motion exercises, and Clinitron therapy

6. Provision of emotional support to the family

Potential for complications of immobility. The complications of immobility that the patient can develop include pneumonia, decubitus, muscle atrophy, peripheral emboli, and diminished peripheral circulation. The cardiac surgery patient is particularly prone to these problems if he is hemodynamically unstable or if he is on the IABP. The goal for health care is that the patient will not develop these complications of immobility.

The first intervention is the repositioning of the patient every 2 hours. There is rarely a contraindication to turning the postoperative cardiac surgery patient. If any major changes in vital signs are observed, such as a decrease in blood pressure, the physician should be notified for this may indicate hypovolemia. Some change in pulmonary artery pressure may also be observed that may require leveling of the transducer. If an IABP is present, one must prevent flexion of the affected leg and position the legs of the coronary artery bypass patient in a way that will facilitate blood flow in the affected extremity.

The second intervention is to have the patient deep breath and cough every 2 hours. This is an important intervention in all immobile patients, but it is especially important for the cardiac surgery patient who is prone to pulmonary atelectasis and pleural effusion.

The patient should be positioned supine with the head of the bed elevated as high as he will tolerate or preferably sitting on the edge of the bed. A pillow should be used for splinting of the incision. The patient takes three deep diaphragmatic breaths through the nose and exhales out of the mouth. He wraps his arms around the pillow and on exhalation of the third breath he hugs the pillow tightly and coughs. The patient should concentrate on tightening his diaphragm and forcing all of the air out. This procedure should be repeated at least once. If the patient is having difficulty in generating one large cough, a series of six small coughs in a row has been recommended. In addition, it may be helpful to administer pain medication before vigorous deep breathing and coughing.

The third intervention is the use of active and passive range of motion to extremities, which should be performed at least three times a day. In 24 hours following surgery, the patient will most likely need assistance with these exercises. Thereafter, he should be encouraged to exercise on his own. The nursing photobook, *Providing Early Mobility*, has excellent illustrations of exercises that can be done.

The provision of skin care is the fourth intervention for preventing complications of immobility. All skin surfaces should be observed for breakdown, pressure, or irritation.

Skin should be kept clean and dry, especially around the chest and leg incisions. Egg crate or similar pressure relieving mattresses should be used on all cardiac surgery patients who (1) are on the IABP, (2) are intubated for more than 24 hours postoperatively, (3) have impaired peripheral circulation or venous disease, and (4) who are elderly or have thin friable skin.

The skin surrounding a pressure area should be massaged gently every 2 hours. One must never massage directly on the pressure point. The nurse should use a draw sheet to reposition the patient. When chest x-ray plates are positioned, the nurse must be sure they are separated from the patient's skin with a pillowcase so that shearing of the skin does not occur. All of these measures will deter the development of skin breakdown.

Postoperative psychosis. The cause of postoperative psychosis is usually unknown and therefore the nursing diagnosis may be stated as a "change in mental alertness and personality related to cardiac surgery." The expected outcome for interventions is that the patient will exhibit a normal mentation and return to his preoperative behavioral state. Nursing interventions are:

1. Have the patient visit the ICU before surgery and point out landmarks such as the clock, calendar, nursing station, window.
2. Encourage family members to visit the patient as frequently as possible and bring familiar objects from home.
3. Orient the patient to his environment, time, and day every 2 hours.
4. If the patient exhibits psychotic behavior, do not argue with him. Do not support or refute delusions or hallucinations. Simply tell the patient that you do not see what he sees. Use a supportive, friendly approach.
5. Minimize noise and external stimuli at the patient's bedside.
6. Nighttime sedation may be needed if the patient is prone to "sundowning." Haloperidol (Haldol) is the drug of choice.
7. Arrange for transfer of the patient from the ICU as early as possible.

Postoperative depression. The patient with congestive heart failure is particularly susceptible to the development of feelings of powerlessness and loss of control. He has been through a life-threatening surgery, he is feeling fatigued and weak, and he is wondering if he will ever lead a normal life again. These feelings may become intensified when the patient is in the ICU and unable to meet his basic needs. If these feelings of powerlessness continue, the patient could develop a severe postoperative depression.

The nursing diagnosis should reflect the powerlessness that the patient feels. The expected outcome for interventions is that the patient will verbalize a feeling of being in control of himself and his environment and that he will participate in decisions regarding his care.

The nurse can begin to assist the patient by listening to him. It is not unusual for the cardiac surgery patient to have feelings of "unreality" in the early postoperative period. In his mind, the time spent in surgery is unaccounted for. There are needles in his arms and tubes in every orifice, and he is experiencing unfamiliar pains and sensations. The patient may need to talk about his perceptions of the experience and receive reassurance that these feelings are normal and temporary.

The patient should be given choices whenever possible. A call light should always be available. While the patient is intubated, a Magic Slate, alphabet board, or flash cards should be available to facilitate communication.

The nurse should encourage the patient to assist with his own care as early as possible. This will give him a feeling of control as well as indicate that his condition is improving.

The nurse should explain all procedures to the patient before performing them. This is especially important when catheters, chest tubes, or needles are being removed. The nurse may know a procedure is painless, but the patient may not and a reassuring explanation will be much appreciated.

Death from arrhythmias. When a patient develops postoperative arrhythmias, the nursing diagnosis will focus on the origin of the arrhythmia (atrial versus ventricular versus other), the heart rate produced, and the patient's clinical response. Interventions are focused on the treatment of the arrhythmia with the goal of returning the patient to normal sinus rhythm or a rhythm that is hemodynamically tolerated.

For atrial arrhythmias, digitalis, propranolol, quinidine, or procainamide may be administered. Frequent premature atrial contractions are treated to prevent atrial fibrillation. Supraventricular tachycardias are treated with carotid massage and then with verapamil if the former is unsuccessful. Serum potassium levels are monitored closely when digitalis is given.

Bradycardias are treated with epinephrine, atropine, isoproterenol, or pacing. Connecting the patient to a temporary pacemaker can be done rapidly and efficiently if the pulse generator is at the bedside.

When sinus tachycardia is present, one must look for possible causes. These include hypovolemia, fever, pain, atelectasis, or anxiety. The danger of tachyarrhythmias is that they result in a decreased diastolic filling time and they increase myocardial oxygen consumption. Therefore measures should be taken to identify and treat the underlying cause.

Premature ventricular contractions (PVCs) are of concern when they are multifocal, number six or more a minute, occur three or more in a row, or land on the preceding T wave. Under these circumstances they are treated immediately with a lidocaine bolus and a continuous lidocaine infusion. Ventricular tachycardia, three or more premature ventricular contractions in a row, is also treated with lidocaine, procainamide, or bretylium, and cardioversion or defibrillation if necessary.

For all arrhythmias, possible underlying causes must be investigated and eliminated. These include hypoxia, electrolyte disturbances, acidosis/alkalosis, catecholamine drug therapy, myocardial ischemia, pain, hypotension, and anemia. Once the arrhythmia has been eliminated, the patient should be monitored for 24 hours for possible recurrence.

Slowed postoperative progression. This is a potential problem that can result when any of the complications of cardiac surgery appear. Postoperative pain is a patient problem that can develop, which requires the nurse to assume a major role in its control and treatment.

Postoperative pain is very individualized for the cardiac surgery patient. Most patients describe the incisional chest pain as a "muscle ache" that inhibits them from taking a deep breath. Their ribs ache much like the ache of a muscle that has been dormant and is suddenly called into use. The patient who has had a bypass may complain of the leg hurting more than the chest. In general then, the pain of cardiac surgery is not a sharp, unbearable pain as one would see in abdominal or other surgeries. At times, though, there is the patient who is very uncomfortable and afraid to move because of pain. This is the patient who is susceptible to a slowed postoperative recovery.

In assessing pain, one needs to gather the following information:
1. Where exactly is the pain located? Does it radiate anywhere?
2. What does it feel like?
3. Is it intermittent or continuous?
4. How intense is the pain?
5. Is there anything that alleviates the pain or

makes it feel better (such as change in position)?

6. What pain medication is the patient receiving? Is he experiencing adequate relief?

This assessment may provide clues to the development of new pains (as in myocardial infarction) and provides clues to pain management.

Comfort measures should always be tried when pain medication is inadequate. The patient should be positioned to his comfort. For the cardiac surgery patient, any position that prevents pull on the incision is comfortable. The nurse should keep the head supported. If allowed to fall in an extended position, the head can cause a significant amount of tension on a midline chest incision. One should always have the patient roll to his side before sitting up and allow the patient to do as much as possible for himself. A backrub is an additional soothing measure to relieve back pains that are present after cardiac surgery.

Narcotic analgesics such as meperidine and morphine are used in the early postoperative period. Side effects that may be observed include respiratory depression, hypotension, bradycardia, convulsions, nausea, vomiting, paralytic ileus, and urinary retention. As postoperative pain lessens, acetaminophen (Tylenol) with codeine, oral meperidine, and oxycodone (Percodan) are prescribed.

Other techniques that have not been well publicized for their use in the cardiac surgery patient include progressive relaxation, distraction techniques, meditation, and biofeedback. (See Chapter 13 for progressive relaxation technique.)

Post-ICU patient problems

The patient usually transfers from the ICU on the second or third postoperative day. The potential problems for this phase of hospitalization include potential late complications, potential nutritional dysfunction, and slowed postoperative progression.

Potential late complications. Potential late complications appear in the following outline with their signs and symptoms.

1. Postpericardiotomy syndrome
   a. Fever
   b. Chest, upper sternum, or shoulder pain
   c. Pericardial friction rub
   d. Possible pleural rub
   e. Leukocytosis
2. Wound infection
   a. Pain, erythema, heat, and swelling along incision
   b. Fever
   c. Drainage from incision
   d. Increased white blood count
3. Pulmonary embolism
   a. Sudden onset of unexplained dyspnea
   b. Possibly pleuritic-type chest pain (rarely occurs)
   c. Confusion
   d. Hypoxia unrelieved by oxygen (because of shunt that is present)
   e. Tachypnea
   f. Diaphoresis
   g. Atrial fibrillation may develop
4. Thromboembolism/phlebitis
   a. Fever
   b. Local swelling, erythema, and pain
   c. Possible edema of extremity
   d. Palpation of a cordlike vein
5. Endocarditis
   a. Persistent fever
   b. Chills
   c. Diaphoresis, anorexia, and malaise
   d. Changing heart murmur, especially with development of a new diastolic murmur
   e. Evidence of emboli to other parts of the body
   f. Splinter hemorrhages in fingernails
   g. Petechiae in mucous membranes, neck area, wrists, or ankles

Many of these complications are treatable with medical therapy and therefore early recognition is vital. The nursing diagnosis will focus on the patient's response to the complication. Interventions for these problems should focus on clinical monitoring of the patient and the administration of needed drugs and treatment.

Potential for nutritional dysfunction. Constipation is not unusual in the cardiac surgery patient. He is immobile for 2 days, taking narcotics, on fluid restrictions, and has had little to eat. Constipation is not only uncomfortable for the patient but can lead to appetite loss and poor absorption of foods. Therefore a potential for nutritional as well as eliminative dysfunction exists.

The patient should be questioned daily for the status of his bowel movements. A laxative may be needed at first, followed by an enema if necessary. The patient's diet should provide a variety of fruits, vegetables, and whole grain breads. Ambulation should be initiated as early as possible. Finally, provisions should be made for privacy during elimination.

Slowed postoperative progression. This is a potential problem for the patient who becomes dysfunctionally dependent. The patient who is dysfunctionally dependent seeks assistance for many of his daily activities such as bathing, dressing, and ambulation. He rarely initiates his own care and he will not progress in his activity level without encouragement and assistance. This behavior is detrimental to the patient's eventual recovery and can result in the patient becoming a "cardiac invalid."

In assessing the patient it is important to evaluate the patient's perceptions of himself and his heart function. Does he feel the surgery was beneficial? Does he anticipate a return to a normal lifestyle? Where will he go when he leaves the hospital? Does he have a reason to get well; someone to get well for? Does he see his body as stronger or weaker after surgery? Does he know what the normal progression is after cardiac surgery? The answers to these questions should provide some indication regarding the patient's perceptions and causes for his dysfunctional dependency.

While a psychosocial assessment is being made, the patient's physical limitations are also assessed. Leg strength and ability to ambulate without help are tested. The nurse then meets with the patient to establish goals for his daily progression in activity. The patient may benefit from a reward or incentive system that encourages him to move a little more each day. Some hospitals have colored lines on hallway floors, and each color represents a differ-

ent distance the patient must walk. He walks one color for 2 days, then moves on to the next, and gradually increases the distance walked. Other hospitals post charts of progress the patient can view and, the patient is rewarded for his daily progress. These and other measures will contribute to the patient's rapid recovery.

Discharge planning

Discharge planning should begin as soon as the patient leaves the ICU. The nurse should begin by doing a discharge assessment to evaluate the following:

1. Does the patient have someone who will be at home with him and be able to drive him to the store and to appointments?
2. What medications will he take at home?
3. What is his exercise prescription for home going to be? Will he be started in a cardiac rehabilitation program? Does he know when and where to go?
4. Does he know how to care for his incisions?
5. What kind of diet is he going home on? Does the dietitian need to see him?
6. What are his cardiac risk factors? Which of them can be changed? How can the nursing staff assist him to begin changing these?
7. How does his family feel about him coming home? Are they frightened about possible arrhythmias or complications? Do they know how to respond in an emergency?

These and other questions should be answered in preparing the patient for discharge. It should be obvious that there is a lot of teaching involved in discharge planning. Topics for teaching should include medications (purpose, dose, toxic effects), diet, care of incisions, activity at home, sleep and rest, sexual relations, risk factor modification, cardiac rehabilitation programs, and special instructions for valve patients (antibiotic prophylaxis for dental work, avoidance of infection).

Follow-up care/cardiac rehabilitation

The patient should have an appointment made with the surgeon or cardiologist for 1 to 2 weeks after discharge. If he is going to be in a rehabilitation program, the program coordinator should visit the patient before discharge to discuss the program goals, costs, and schedule. Cardiac rehabilitation offers the patient a positive and goal-directed program to assist him in developing cardiovascular endurance and control of risk factors. All cardiac surgery patients should be encouraged to participate in such a program for total mental and physical recovery from cardiac surgery.

CASE STUDY

Mr. L was a 68-year-old man admitted to the hospital on August 4 with paroxysmal nocturnal dyspnea, bilateral ankle edema, and acute pulmonary edema. He had a history of anterior myocardial infarction that had occurred 6 years earlier. From the time of his MI up until 1 year ago, he had been asymptomatic. In November of last year, he had a second inferior wall MI associated with bradyarrhythmias and congestive heart failure. He was also diagnosed as having essential hypertension. A permanent AV sequential pacemaker was implanted under the left clavicle at that time and has been functioning without difficulty. He was discharged home taking quinidine, digoxin, and hydralazine. The patient discontinued the hydralazine himself, developed fluid retention, and was readmitted to the hospital in January for moderate heart failure. This was successfully treated and the patient sent home. He did well up until August 4 when he came into the emergency room in acute pulmonary edema.

He was admitted to CCU where he became hypotensive and was subsequently started on nitroprusside and dopamine drips.

Insertion of a flow-directed catheter demonstrated a pulmonary arterial pressure of 48/23, a pulmonary capillary wedge pressure of 25, a cardiac output of 3.0, and a systemic vascular resistance of 1450. A MUGA scan was performed on August 6 and revealed ejection fraction 21%, enlarged left ventricle and anteroapical akinesis. A cardiac catheterization was performed on August 10 and demonstrated markedly enlarged left ventricle, severe mitral regurgitation, diffuse hypokinesis of left ventricle, occlusion of the left anterior descending and right coronary arteries, and severe stenosis of the circumflex coronary artery.

Over the next few days Mr. L's condition was stabilized in preparation for surgery. He experienced one episode of ventricular tachycardia, which was treated with lidocaine intravenously and procainamide orally.

On August 15 Mr. L underwent mitral valve replacement with a Bjork-Shiley prosthesis, a tricuspid annuloplasty, and coronary artery bypass to the left circumflex marginal, the left median ramus, and right coronary arteries. Because of his left ventricular failure, Mr. L could not be weaned from bypass and therefore an intra-aortic balloon pump was inserted and 1:1 counterpulsation initiated.

Mr. L remained on the IABP for 2 days after surgery. He was also receiving low doses of nitroprusside and dopamine. His first postoperative day he experienced a run of ventricular tachycardia that lasted less than a minute and was treated by defibrillation and a lidocaine bolus. He was started on a lidocaine drip and later changed to a procainamide drip in preparation for taking oral procainamide. Once the IABP was discontinued, his cardiac output remained low (3.0) and he continued to require inotropic and vasodilator therapy.

His left foot had been pale, cold, and pulseless the first 48 hours after surgery, but it began to regain color when the balloon was removed. While in the ICU, he began to take oral fluids and food.

Mr. L was transferred back to CCU on his fifth postoperative day because of continued arrhythmias and low cardiac output. He was gradually weaned off of all intravenous medications and began getting up in the chair twice a day.

On his seventh postoperative day he was noted to be very withdrawn and anorexic. He refused to get out of bed or participate in self-care. On his ninth postoperative day he was transferred to the coronary observation unit. His arrhythmias had improved significantly, and he was getting up to the chair three times a day. He remained on three cardiovascular drugs: propranolol, hydralazine, and procainamide, and he had been started on oral warfarin. He continued to progress well and was discharged home on his fourteenth postoperative day. The problem list for Mr. L is as follows:

PREOPERATIVE PROBLEMS

1. Inadequate peripheral perfusion related to decreased myocardial contraction and elevated systemic vascular resistance
2. Inadequate tissue perfusion related to ventricular tachycardia
3. Lack of knowledge about cardiac surgery
4. Inadequate respiratory gas exchange related to left ventricular failure with transudation of fluid into alveoli

ICU PROBLEMS

1. Inadequate tissue perfusion related to ventricular tachycardia
2. Inadequate peripheral perfusion to left leg, related to presence of IABP
3. Inadequate peripheral perfusion related to postoperative low cardiac output syndrome
4. Potential for renal failure related to prolonged bypass time and low cardiac output syndrome

5. Potential for emboli to brain related to presence of valve prosthesis
6. Potential for complications of immobility

POST-ICU PROBLEMS

1. Postoperative depression
2. Lack of knowledge about care of self at home after cardiac surgery

The health care plan for Mr. L is given below.

Text continued on p. 464.

HEALTH CARE PLAN FOR MR. L

Potential problems	Nursing diagnosis	Expected outcome	Nursing activities
PREOPERATIVE PROBLEMS			
1. Shock state with metabolic acidosis and eventual death	Inadequate peripheral perfusion related to decreased myocardial contractility and increased systemic vascular resistance	Mr. L will have adequate peripheral perfusion as evidenced by: CI 2.0 L/min/M²; Warm extremities; Urinary output of at least 30 ml/hr; Heart rate of 80-100; Systolic BP 90 mm Hg; Awake and alert mentally	Obtain accurate measures of CO, SVR, PVR, PAP, PCWP, RAP, heart rate, respiratory rate. If CO is low and patient is warm with good pulses, obtain order to check A-Vo₂ difference (saturations). If 30%, then patient has low CO. Provide supportive care. Turn q2h, suctioning, deep breathing, and coughing q2h, active ROM to extremities t.i.d. Administer medical treatment: Inotropic drugs to increase contractility (epinephrine, dopamine, isoproterenol) Crystalloid, colloids, or blood if hypovolemic to increase preload and maintain PCWP > 8 mm Hg

Continued.

Potential problems	Nursing diagnosis	Expected outcome	Nursing activities
			Afterload reducing agents if SVR, >1500 dynes (nitroprusside, nitroglycerin, IABP)
			Control heart rate with antiarrhythmics or pacing as indicated
			Evaluate response to therapy and clinical status hourly.
2. Shock state with metabolic acidosis and eventual death	Inadequate peripheral perfusion related to ventricular tachycardia	Mr. L will have normal sinus rhythm or a rhythm that is hemodynamically tolerated.	Give lidocaine bolus of 1.0-1.5 mg/kg. Start a lidocaine drip at 2 mg/mm.
			Use cardioversion with 200 watt-seconds of energy, if ventricular tachycardia continues.
			Prepare other IV antiarrhythmics for administration:
			Bretylium tosylate 5 mg/kg IV bolus or 5-10 mg/kg diluted in 50 ml over 10-20 min.
			Amiodarone 5-10 mg/kg IV bolus
			Procainamide 100 mg IVP over 1 min, may repeat in 5 min.
			Monitor vital signs and ECG closely for first 24 hours following arrhythmia.
			Investigate possible correctable causes:
			Hypokalemia or hyperkalemia
			Hypoxia
			Metabolic disorder
			Hypercapnea
			Anemia

Potential problems	Nursing diagnosis	Expected outcome	Nursing activities

3. Patient and family anxiety and fear of the unknown; potential for complicated recovery	Lack of knowledge about cardiac surgery	Mr. L and his family will be able to discuss:
		Preparations for surgery
		Their feelings about the surgery
		Routines the day before surgery
		Expectations the morning of surgery
		Expectations for ICU period
			Assess Mr. L's and his family's understanding of the surgery.
			Teach Mr. L using teaching aids such as heart model, drawings, actual catheters and equipment. Content of teaching to include:
			Preparations for surgery
			  Anatomy and physiology of heart
			  Their disease process
			  Surgical procedure
			Feelings about surgery
			  Informal discussion of their concerns
			Routines the day before surgery:
			  Weights
			  pHisoHex shower
			  Tour of ICU
			  Enema
			  Food and fluid restrictions
			  Sleeping pill for night
			  Visit by anesthesiologist
			Expectations of the morning of surgery
			  Preoperative medication
			  Starting of IV
			Waiting during surgery
			  Where family can wait
			  Length of time for surgery

Continued.

Potential problems	Nursing diagnosis	Expected outcome	Nursing activities
			Expectations for ICU
			Purpose of the ICU
			The ICU environment
			Routine care in the ICU
			Explanation of tubes, lines
			Surgical incision/pain management
			Deep breathing and coughing
			Leg exercises
			Psychological responses in ICU
4. Potential for hypoxemia and exacerbation of left ventricular failure	Inadequate respiratory gas exchange related to left ventricular failure with transudation of fluid into alveoli	Mr. L will exhibit the following signs of improved respiration and gas exchange: Respiratory rate of 12-16 Absence of air hunger, wheezing, and coughing Breath sounds clear to auscultation Decreased restlessness Improved Po_2 blood gas value	Assess breath sounds, respiratory rate, amount and color of secretions hourly. Keep Mr. L in a high Fowler's position. Administer high flow oxygen per physician's order. Assist with other treatment measures for heart failure: Morphine sulfate IM or IV Furosemide IV Rotating tourniquets Unloading therapy; dopamine and nitroprusside Monitor daily chest roentgenograms and b.i.d. blood gases.

ICU PROBLEMS

Potential problems	Nursing diagnosis	Expected outcome	Nursing activities
1. Shock state with metabolic acidosis and eventual death	Inadequate peripheral perfusion related to ventricular tachycardia	See preoperative problem 2.	See preoperative problem 2.

Potential problems	Nursing diagnosis	Expected outcome	Nursing activities
2. Potential for loss of left lower leg or foot to gangrene	Inadequate tissue perfusion to left leg related to presence of IABP	Mr. L will have improved circulation to left leg as indicated by: 　Palpable dorsalis pedis pulses 　Warm foot 　Normal capillary filling time 　Ability to move toes 　Pink coloration of toes and nailbeds	Notify physician of any circulatory changes, especially if sudden pain, pallor, pulselessness, and immobility develop. Give active ROM to left leg and foot; do not flex at hip. Provide protection for skin of left foot by using: 　Heel protector 　Sheepskin 　Lamb's wool between toes 　Foot cradle Keep foot clean and dry; use lukewarm water for bathing.
3. Shock state with metabolic acidosis and eventual death	Inadequate peripheral perfusion related to postoperative low cardiac output syndrome	See preoperative problem 1.	See preoperative problem 1.
4. Acute renal failure	Potential for renal failure related to prolonged bypass time and low cardiac output syndrome	Mr. L will have an adequate urinary output of 20 ml/hour and normal BUN and creatinine.	Prevent hypovolemia by monitoring BP, PCWP, and RAP qlh for a decrease. Monitor daily BUN and creatinine. Report a BUN >20 or a creatinine >1.2 mg/100 ml Monitor hourly intake and output. Daily weights—report a gain or loss of 1 kg. Monitor urine/serum osmolality ratio. A high serum osmolality indicates renal dysfunction. Report any new hematuria to physician. Assist with peritoneal dialysis or renal dialysis if either of these becomes necessary.

Continued.

Potential problems	Nursing diagnosis	Expected outcome	Nursing activities
5. Cerebrovascular accident	Potential for emboli to the brain related to presence of valve prosthesis	Mr. L will have normal neurological functioning; be alert; be oriented to person, place, and time.	Monitor in early postoperative period for signs and symptoms of cerebral complications: Decreased level of consciousness Inability to move extremities Change in response to verbal commands Pupil changes Unilateral weakness Aphasia Changes in respiratory pattern Monitor circulatory status: CO heart rate, BP, SVR, Hgb. and Hct., PT, PTT. Correct atrial fibrillation as quickly as possible. Monitor acid/base and electrolyte status. Maintain adequate oxygenation.
6. Potential for complications of immobility; pneumonia, decubitus, muscle atrophy, decreased peripheral circulation	Immobility associated with early postoperative recovery, presence of IABP, and hemodynamic instability	Mr. L will not develop complications of immobility.	Turn Mr. L q2h. While IABP is present, do not flex leg in which balloon is inserted. There are no contraindications to turning a postoperative cardiac surgery patient. If there are changes in vital signs with turning, the physician should be notified. Deep breathe and cough q2h. Mr. L should be sitting up with pillow splint and breathing from diaphragm. Active range of motion to all extremities while intubated or unstable t.i.d.

Potential problems	Nursing diagnosis	Expected outcome	Nursing activities
			Provide skin care to coccyx, back, perineum, and other skin folds q6-8h.
			Monitor skin and circulation continuously.
			Provide egg crate, air mattress, sheepskin, or Clinitron therapy as needed.
POST-ICU PROBLEMS			
1. Depression	Postoperative depression related to cardiac surgery and life-threatening disease	Mr. L will verbalize that feelings of depression have improved.	Explain to patient that depression or letdown feelings are common the third to sixth day after cardiac surgery.
			Encourage patient to talk about the experience of surgery and the ICU.
			Point out to the patient the progress he is making on a daily basis.
			Get patient involved in his own care.
			Assist patient to begin making plans for when he goes home; what he will do during the day, exercise, and recreation.
2. Potential for complications of recovery at home	Lack of knowledge about care of self at home after cardiac surgery	Mr. L and his family will be able to verbalize the following: Care of incisions Exercise limits The contents of a low-fat, no-added-salt diet. Purpose, dose, and toxic effects of discharge medications The purpose of the cardiac recovery program	Do discharge teaching with patient and his family present. Topics to be covered: Care of incisions: bathing, use of lotions, normal sensations, signs of infection Exercise: how much to do initially, the importance of regular exercise, do's and don't's for exercising

Continued.

HEALTH CARE PLAN FOR MR. L—cont'd

Potential problems	Nursing diagnosis	Expected outcome	Nursing activities
			Diet: Rationale for a low-fat or no-added-salt diet. Provide booklets with menus and sample recipes.
			Sexual relations: when, positions
			Cardiac risk factors and methods for modification
			Cardiac recovery programs
			Valve patients: antibiotic prophylaxis, use of warfarin
			Importance of moderation in all activities and importance of a good sleep and rest periods during the day

SUMMARY

The patient with a viable myocardium and heart failure refractory to all medical interventions usually requires surgery. The goals for surgical intervention are to salvage viable myocardial tissue, to reverse life-threatening situations, and to improve the quality and prolong life. The value of surgical intervention continues to be a controversial issue; however, some physicians have had outstanding results in patients with marginal cardiac function (ejection fractions as low as 15%).

The physiological response to heart surgery is a shock-like response with mobilization of all neuroendocrine mechanisms. Special techniques in heart surgery have been developed—myocardial preservation, hypothermia, hemodynamic monitoring, intra-aortic balloon pumping—that are extremely beneficial in supporting compensatory mechanisms and preventing intraoperative complications.

The nursing assessment of cardiac surgery patients was reviewed with special emphasis on patients with heart failure. It is clear that nurses play a pivotal role in coordinating the care of these patients. Not only must clinicians be adept at physical assessment, but they must provide vital preoperative instruction in a timely and effective manner.

Eleven major complications of cardiac surgery were discussed with the precipitating factors, clinical manifestations, and therapeutic interventions.

Low cardiac output syndrome is the most common complication in the patient with preoperative heart failure.

Major patient problems in the preoperative, intensive care, and postoperative recovery phases were presented. A problem common to all patients in the preoperative phase is anticipatory fear and anxiety. Regardless of what the patient or family relates, they are fearful and anxious, and the most effective means of alleviating this problem is through acceptance, support, and preoperative teaching. This is accomplished by imparting information regarding the events of the intraoperative and postoperative period. In addition, the patient and family are afforded the opportunity to ask all of those ''little'' questions that generate so much concern.

During the intensive care phase, the clinician initially focuses on physiological monitoring of the patient and the prevention of complications. All major body systems are repeatedly assessed during the first 24 hours following surgery. Following this period, when the patient's condition is stabilized, altered perception, sleep deprivation, and intense unfamiliar environmental stimuli may cause the patient to suffer from time disorientation and demonstrate altered mental status characteristic of ICU and/or postcardiotomy psychosis. Postoperative euphoria or depression may also appear 1 to 3 days after surgery.

As the patient returns to floor care, he focuses on regaining a sense of well-being and feeling good again. He is body-oriented and may experience unfamiliar aches, pains, or annoying sensations. The nurse assists the patient through this phase with patience, understanding, and explanations, and encourages the patient to gradually increase self-care and daily physical activity.

Discharge planning is the final step in the patient's hospitalization. The patient should have knowledge of wound care, activity level, diet, medications, and risk factor modification. The cardiac rehabilitation coordinator should consult with the patient before discharge to discuss the purpose and benefits of the program.

Cardiac surgery performed on the patient in heart failure presents many challenges to the health care team. With the new techniques in heart surgery, heart transplants, and development of artificial implants, what was considered intractable heart failure is now treatable. Care of these patients by a sophisticated collegial team is as equally important to patient survival as technical advances. Furthermore, the role of the skilled nurse clinician is vital to the functioning of the health care team and to the delivery of quality health care.

REFERENCES

1. Behrendt, D.M.: Patient care in cardiac surgery, Boston, 1980, Little, Brown, & Co.
2. Braunwald, E.: Heart disease: a textbook of cardiovascular medicine, Philadelphia, 1980, W.B. Saunders Co., p. 557.
3. Bregman, D.: Clinical experience with intra-aortic balloon pumping and the pulsatile assist device. In Unger, F., editor: Assisted circulation, New York, 1979, Springer-Verlag New York, Inc.
4. Buckberg, G.D.: Left ventricular subendocardial necrosis, Ann. Thorac. Surg. **24:**379, 1977.
5. Carabello, B.A., and others: Hemodynamic determinants of prognosis of aortic valve replacement in critical aortic stenosis and advanced congestive heart failure, Circulation **62:**42, 1980.
6. Cooley, D.A., and Norman, J.C.: Techniques in cardiac surgery, ed. 1, Houston, 1975, Texas Medical Press, Inc.
7. Davila, J.C.: Second Henry Ford hospital international symposium on cardiac surgery, New York, 1977, Appleton-Century-Crofts.
8. DeLong, D.R.: Individual differences in patterns of anxiety arousal, stress-relevant information and recovery from surgery, University of California, Los Angeles, 1970, unpublished doctoral dissertation.
9. Gazes, P.C.: The management of congestive heart failure, Curr. Probl. Cardiol., p. 6, May 1980.
10. Hellman, C., and others: Bypass graft surgery in severe left ventricular dysfunction, Circulation (Suppl.) **62:**I-103, 1980.
11. Hung, J., and others: Aortocoronary bypass grafting in patients with severe left ventricular dysfunction, J. Thorac. Cardiovasc. Surg. **79:**718, 1980.
12. Keon, W.J., and others: Experience with emergency aortocoronary bypass grafts in the presence of acute myocardial infarction, Circulation (Suppl.) **47** and **48:**III-151, 1973.
13. King, S.B., and Hurst, J.W.: Indications for bypass in atherosclerotic heart disease, Res. Staff Phys. **25:**21s, 1979.
14. Norman, J.C.: Cardiac surgery, ed. 2, New York, 1972, Meredith Corp.

15. Ochsner, J.L., and Mills, N.L.: Coronary artery surgery, ed. 1, Philadelphia, 1978, Lea & Febiger.
16. Rose, S.D., and others: Cardiac risk factors in patients undergoing noncardiac surgery, Med. Clin. North Am., **63:**1271, 1979.
17. Russell, R.O., and others: Who should have coronary bypass? Consultant p. 121, Jan 1981.
18. Stiles, Q.R., and others: Myocardial revascularization: a surgical atlas, ed. 1, Boston, 1976, Little, Brown & Co.
19. Thorn, G.W., and others: Harrison's principles of internal medicine, ed. 8, New York, 1977, McGraw-Hill Book Co.
20. Wolfgang, T.C., and others: Heart transplants: how far have we come? J. Cardiovasc. Med. **12:**1225, 1981.

ADDITIONAL READINGS

Bourne, G.H.: Hearts and heart-like organs, vols. I-IV, New York, 1980, Academic Press Inc.
DeBakey, M., and Grotto, A.: The living heart, New York, 1977, Grosset & Dunlap, Inc.
Derrick, H.F.: How open heart surgery feels, Am. J. Nurs. **79:**277, 1979.
Dubin, W.R., and others: Postcardiotomy delirium: a critical review, J. Thorac. Cardiovasc. Surg. **77:**586, 1979.
Johanson, B.C., and others: Standards for critical care, St. Louis, 1981, The C.V. Mosby Co.
Sade, R.M., and others: Infant and child care in heart surgery, Chicago, 1977, Year Book Medical Publishers, Inc.
Stuart, E.M., and others: Nursing rounds: care of the patient with a mitral commissurotomy, Am. J. Nurs. **80:**1611, 1980.
Thorpe, C.J.: A nursing care plan: the adult cardiac surgery patient, Heart Lung **8:**690, 1979.
Urosevich, P.R.: Providing early mobility, Horsham, Pa., 1980, Intermed Communications, Inc.

PATIENT EDUCATION RESOURCES
American Heart Association

Coronary Heart Bypass Graft Surgery, AHA #50-047A
Smoking and Heart Disease, AHA #51-091A
E is for Exercise, AHA #51-027A
How can high blood pressure hurt you? AHA #50-011A
Living with your pacemaker, AHA #50-016B
High blood pressure, AHA #51-022A
Your [500 mg, 1000 mg, 2000 mg] sodium diet, AHA #50-031A
Bacterial Endocarditis Antibiotic Prophylaxis Identification Card, AHA #78-004C
Active Partnership for the Health of Your Heart After Your Coronary Bypass Surgery, AHA #64-006D

American Lung Association

Cigarette Smoking: The Facts about your Lungs, #0171

American Society of Hospital Pharmacists

Understanding your Prescription

Miles Grocery Products Division (maker of Morningstar Products)

Living Comfortably with a Low Cholesterol Diet
Cholesterol Counter, Menu Planner

Other Booklets, Books

Moving Right Along . . . After Open Heart Surgery published by Pritchett and Hull Associates, Inc., Suite 110, 3440 Oakcliff Road N.E., Atlanta, Ga., 30340. (In English and Spanish.)
The Living Heart by Michael DeBakey, New York, 1977, Grosset & Dunlap Publishers. A book for laymen with in-depth information on all cardiovascular diseases. Available in most bookstores.
The American Heart Association Heartbook, published by E.P. Dutton, New York. A book for the laymen that has in-depth information on the cause, treatment, and prevention of cardiac disease. Available in most bookstores.

Films, Movies

"Living Proof," is a preoperative teaching film that follows a patient through his hospitalization for cardiac surgery. Past patients are interviewed for their perceptions of what it was like to go through cadiac surgery. A reassurance-oriented film. Purchase from: Stacy Keach Productions, 5216 Laurel Canyon Blvd., North Hollywood, Ca., 91607, (213) 877-0472
"Your Heart Surgery," is an American Heart Association slide-tape program for preoperative teaching.
"Open-Heart Surgery," is a preoperative teaching slide-tape program produced by Trainex Corporation, P.O. Box 116, Garden Grove, Ca, 92642.

COMMUNITY RESOURCES

American Heart Association
National Center
7320 Greenville Avenue
Dallas, Texas 75231

American Society of Hospital Pharmacists
4630 Montgomery Avenue
Washington, D.C. 20014

Miles Laboratories, Inc.
7123 West 65th Street
Chicago, Illinois 60630

The Mended Hearts, Inc.
(See local phone directory.)

CHAPTER 15

Heart failure in infants and children

MADELEINE DISTASO BRUNING
JANET UZANE SCHNEIDERMAN

Congestive heart failure is a common complication of heart disease in pediatric patients. Children with congestive heart failure are usually under 1 year of age with diagnostic evidence of a congenital cardiac anomaly. The incidence of congenital heart disease in children is approximately 8 to 10 per 1000 live births.[8] Ninety percent of children with cardiac lesions causing heart failure will develop the symptoms either in the first year of life or not until adulthood. Ten percent occur between 1 and 5 years of age. Heart failure occurring between the ages 5 and 15 years is usually caused by acquired lesions, such as those that result from acute rheumatic fever.[4]

Congestive heart failure is a serious, potentially fatal complication of heart disease in children. The pathophysiology is similar to that of adults, although the causes, clinical indicators, health care interventions, and psychosocial implications are unique to the child. This chapter elaborates upon these pediatric differences with special emphasis placed on the nurse's role with both the child and the family. Aggressive case finding is instrumental to therapeutic intervention, which frequently necessitates surgical correction of the underlying cardiac defect. The nurse has an important role in identifying the infant with congestive heart failure and suspected congenital heart defects. The material presented in this text is designed to facilitate that role.

This chapter accomplishes the following: reviews the major causes of heart failure in infants and children; identifies the major clinical indicators of heart failure in a pediatric population; delineates the diagnostic studies and relates the psychological implications of these tests on children; discusses the effect of the disease process on the child's developmental status; presents the major psychological implications of heart disease and failure on the parent-child-family relationship; and puts into operation the major concepts in a case study and care plan for children in heart failure.

CAUSES OF CONGESTIVE HEART FAILURE AND MEDICAL INTERVENTIONS
Embryological development

The primary cause of congestive heart failure in infants and children is directly related to the structure and function of fetal circulation and early postnatal circulatory changes; therefore it is necessary to have an understanding of the embryological development of the cardiovascular system.

By the third week of gestation, the fetal heart is a simple tube composed of mesenchymal cells that proliferate into a primitive vascular system.[5] A two-layered tube gradually forms during the third week. The inner lining will develop into the endocardium of the heart and the myocardium and epicardium will develop from the fetal epicardial tissue. Rapid differentiation and identification occurs during the first 4 weeks. A four-chambered heart develops during the fourth to eighth week of intrauterine growth.[5] Endocardial cushions or tissue bundles are located on the dorsal and ventral aspects of the atrioventricular canal and differentiate

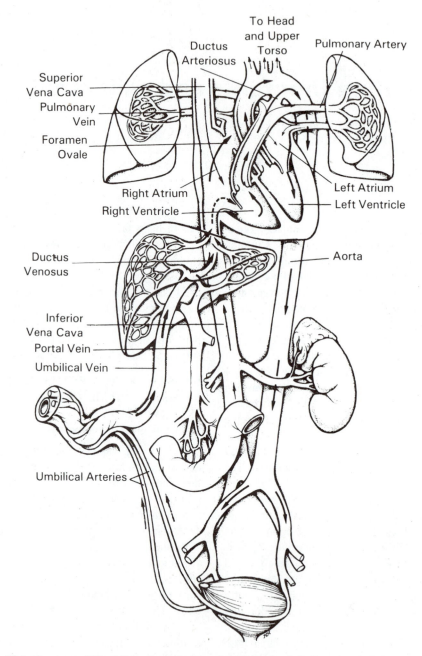

Fig. 15-1. Oxygenated blood flows from placenta via umbilical vein to liver; into inferior vena cava, where it combines with some unoxygenated blood; on to right atrium; through the foramen ovale to left atrium, left ventricle, and aorta. This blood perfuses the brain, coronary arteries, and upper torso. Venous blood returning to right atrium from superior vena cava mixes with some oxygenated blood entering from inferior vena cava and flows into right ventricle and out through pulmonary artery. Some blood continues to lungs, but most is shunted through ductus arteriosus into descending aorta and eventually reaches placenta through umbilical arteries. (From Sacksteder, S., Congenital cardiac defects: embryology and fetal circulation, Am. J. Nurs. **78:**264, Feb. 1978.)

into the right and left circulatory pathways.

Anatomical structure (Fig. 15-1). There are three anatomical structures unique to the fetal circulatory pattern: the patent ductus arteriosus, the patent foramen ovale, and the ductus venosus. The structure utilized for gaseous exchange in utero is the placenta. The placenta serves as the organ that transports nutrients, eliminates metabolic waste products, and acts as a respiratory organ for the fetus. The distribution and pattern of fetal blood flow are greatly influenced by elevated fetal pulmonary vascular resistance. This increased resistance is accentuated by the relatively hypoxic intrauterine environment. This hypoxic state is adaptive for the fetus because hypoxia is a stimulus for pulmonary vasoconstriction. Conversely, the fetal systemic vascular resistance is relatively low. Because of these hemodynamic principles, the unexpanded fetal lungs receive approximately 25%[8] of the total blood volume circulating throughout the fetal cardiovascular system.

Fetal blood flow. Oxygenated blood enters the fetal right side of the heart from the placenta via the umbilical vein. The umbilical vein directs blood to the liver where the circulation divides. The majority of the volume is shunted through the ductus venosus to the inferior vena cava, while the remainder is diverted through the hepatic circulation. Most of the blood entering the right atrium is shunted through the foramen ovale into the left atrium. As a result of this right-to-left shunting, the right ventricle and lungs are bypassed. The left atrium receives blood through the foramen ovale and mixes with small amounts of blood from the pulmonary veins. The blood then circulates to the left atrium and the left ventricle and through the aorta. Fetal brain and cardiac structures require highly oxygenated blood; therefore blood from the aorta is distributed to the coronary and cerebral arteries. Blood returning from the inferior vena cava enters the right ventricle. From the right ventricle blood will enter the pulmonary artery, where bidirectional circulation occurs. Most of the blood returns to the heart from the aorta while a small portion enters the pulmonary vasculature. The patent ductus arteriosus allows this bidirectional circulation. Deoxygenated blood is returned to the placenta from the descending aorta through two umbilical arteries.

Circulatory transition at birth (Fig. 15-2). At birth there are major cardiopulmonary changes. The infant must be able to initiate respirations. Respirations provide alveolar expansion and redirect blood flow to the lungs. There is an increase in pulmonary blood flow and left atrial pressure, whereas there is a decrease in pulmonary vascular resistance and right atrial pressure. The patent ductus arteriosus closes as a result of this hemodynamic transition and increase in partial pressure of oxygen (Po_2). The ductus venosus, umbilical vein, and umbilical arteries degenerate with the clamping of the umbilical cord. With the deletion of the placenta and clamping of the umbilical cord, the infant must adapt to an extrauterine existence.

Causes of congestive heart failure and medical management

Congestive heart failure in infants and children most often results from congenital heart defects and is usually the sequela to congenital heart disease rather than a primary disease entity. The causes for many congenital heart lesions are not identified. However, there are several contributing factors. The first trimester of pregnancy is a critical period for cardiac growth and differentiation. Maternal factors that may alter fetal development include viruses such as rubella (German measles) and coxsackie virus, poor maternal nutrition, maternal age and parity, and maternal drug or alcohol ingestion. There is an increased incidence of congenital heart disease in infants of diabetic mothers, although the relationship is not clearly understood.[8] Other predisposing factors are genetic aberrations such as Down's syndrome (trisomy 21), parents who have congenital heart disease, and siblings with heart lesions. Infants born with noncardiac congenital anomalies should also be assessed for clinical indicators of congestive heart failure that may be secondary to the presence of other anomalies (for example, hypoplastic lungs, diaphragmatic hernia).

Congenital heart defects are classified as acya-

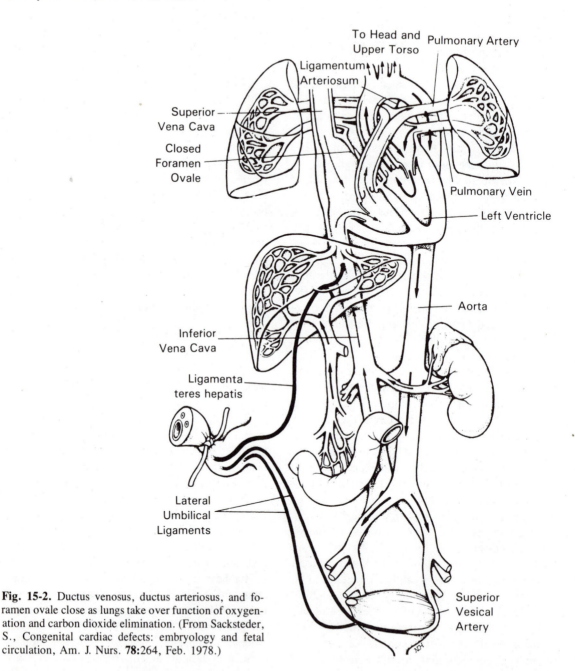

To Head and Upper Torso

Pulmonary Artery

Ligamentum Arteriosum

Superior Vena Cava

Closed Foramen Ovale

Pulmonary Vein

Left Ventricle

Aorta

Inferior Vena Cava

Ligamenta teres hepatis

Lateral Umbilical Ligaments

Superior Vesical Artery

Fig. 15-2. Ductus venosus, ductus arteriosus, and foramen ovale close as lungs take over function of oxygenation and carbon dioxide elimination. (From Sacksteder, S., Congenital cardiac defects: embryology and fetal circulation, Am. J. Nurs. **78:**264, Feb. 1978.)

notic and cyanotic. Differential diagnosis is based on the hemodynamic alterations, clinical manifestations, and diagnostic tests. In acyanotic lesions deoxygenated blood does not mix with oxygenated blood in the systemic circulation. Conversely, in the presence of cyanotic lesions unoxygenated blood circulates systemically. Clinical manifestations correlate with the severity of the defect and the degree of cyanosis. The patient may be asymptomatic if the defect does not alter the workload of

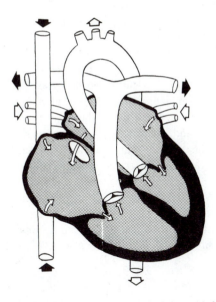

Fig. 15-3. Atrial septal defect is abnormal opening between right and left atria. Basically three types of abnormalities result from incorrect development of atrial septum. Incompetent foramen ovale is most common defect. High ostium secundum defect results from abnormal development of septum secundum. Improper development of septum primum produces a basal opening known as an ostium primum defect, frequently involving atrioventricular valves. In general, left-to-right shunting of blood occurs in all atrial septal defects. (From Congenital heart abnormalities, Clinical Education Aid No. 7. Courtesy Ross Laboratories, Columbus, Ohio, 1968.)

the heart (that is, cardiac output, heart rate, and respiratory rate may be within normal limits). Changes in pulmonary and systemic vascular resistance, cardiac compensation, and the amount of blood shunting through a defect influence the severity of an acyanotic lesion. Severe acyanotic defects are potentially cyanotic contingent upon hemodynamic alterations.

Acyanotic lesions as stimuli for congestive heart failure

Atrial septal defect (ASD) (Fig. 15-3). An atrial septal defect is an abnormal communication between the two atrial chambers. There are several sites where the lesion may occur, and the lesion is identified by its location. Generally, there are three types of atrial defects that may occur during the embryologic development of the heart: sinus venosus defects, located at the superior vena cava and the right atrium; ostium secundum defects, found at the center of the cardiac septum; and ostium

primum defects, found at the inferior aspect of the septum. Hemodynamically, left atrial pressure exceeds the pressure of the right atrium and blood is shunted through the defect from the left to right. Since the blood shunted from left to right is oxygenated blood, systemic cyanosis is absent. However, there is an increase in the pulmonary circulatory volume. The infant may be asymptomatic or manifest signs and symptoms of respiratory distress and congestive heart failure. The presence and severity of symptoms are related to the size of the atrial septal defect and atrial pressures. Surgical correction of the defect consists of direct closure by cardiopulmonary bypass, or a patch graft if the lesion is large. Operative intervention is rarely needed during infancy.

Ventricular septal defect (VSD) (Fig. 15-4). A ventricular septal defect allows shunting of blood through an abnormal orifice between the ventricles. The defect varies greatly in its size and therefore the severity of symptoms. The lesion may be found at the muscular, interventricular, or membranous aspects of the septum and can be combined with other congenital heart defects such as tetralogy of Fallot, patent ductus arteriosus, transposition of the great vessels, coarctation of the aorta, and pulmonic stenosis. Hemodynamic alterations occur because left ventricular pressure exceeds right ventricular pressure and blood is shunted from left to right through the defect. Right ventricular overload may cause right atrial hypertrophy. Spontaneous closure frequently occurs within the first 3 years of life.[8] Medical management is initiated if patients present clinical manifestations of congestive heart failure. If medical management is unsuccessful, then surgical inter-

vention is implemented by direct closure or patch graft.

Aortic stenosis (Fig. 15-5). Aortic stenosis is an obstructive lesion caused by the stricture of the aortic valve. The narrowing may be at the valvular level but may also be subaortic or supra-aortic. The severity of symptoms will vary with the degree of constriction. Left ventricular pressure will increase to maintain normal aortic pressures. Left ventricular hypertrophy may develop secondary to the increased left ventricular pressure. Congestive heart failure may be present at birth if the obstruction is severe. Surgical intervention consists of a valvotomy or commissurotomy if the stricture is located at the valvular level. Excision of the ob-

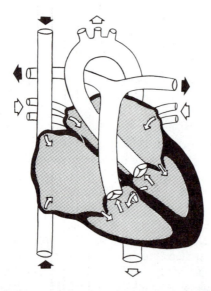

Fig. 15-4. Ventricular septal defect is an abnormal opening between right and left ventricle. Ventricular septal defects vary in size and may occur in either membranous or muscular portion of ventricular septum. Because of higher pressure in left ventricle, a shunting of blood from left to right ventricle occurs during systole. If pulmonary vascular resistance produces pulmonary hypertension, shunt of blood is then reversed from right to left ventricle, with cyanosis resulting. (From Congenital heart abnormalities, Clinical Education Aid No. 7. Courtesy Ross Laboratories, Columbus, Ohio, 1968.)

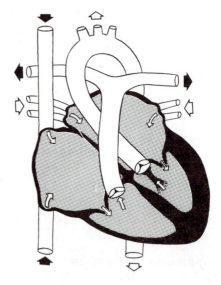

Fig. 15-5. In many instances, stenosis is valvular with thickening and fusion of cusps. Subaortic stenosis is caused by a fibrous ring below aortic valve in outflow tract of left ventricle. At times, both valvular and subaortic stenosis exist in combination. Obstruction causes increased workload for normal output of left ventricular blood and results in left ventricular enlargement. (From Congenital heart abnormalities, Clinical Education Aid No. 7. Courtesy Ross Laboratories, Columbus, Ohio, 1968.)

structive tissue is indicated if the lesion is at the supravalvular or subaortic level.

Coarctation of the aorta (Fig. 15-6). Coarctation of the aorta is a narrowing of the aorta. The narrowing may be preductal (proximal to ductus arteriosus), postductal (distal to the insertion of ductus arteriosus), or juxtaductal (close to the aorta). This lesion may be found in conjunction with other cardiac defects such as hypoplastic left heart. Hemodynamically, there is left ventricular hypertension and increased pressure in the ascending aorta that can lead to congestive heart failure. With a postductal lesion, the blood pressure is increased in the upper extremities and pulses are full. Blood pressure will be decreased in the lower ex-

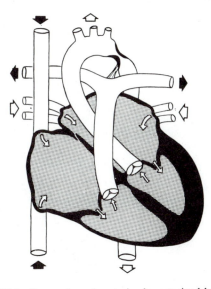

Fig. 15-6. Coarctation of aorta is characterized by narrowed aortic lumen. It exists as preductal or postductal obstruction, depending on position of obstruction in relation to ductus arteriosus. Coarctations exist with great variation in anatomical features. Lesion produces an obstruction to flow of blood through aorta, causing an increased left ventricular pressure and workload. (From Congenital heart abnormalities, Clinical Education Aid No. 7. Courtesy Ross Laboratories, Columbus, Ohio, 1968.)

tremities and pulses may be weak, diminished, or absent. Medical management is indicated for clinical indicators of congestive heart failure. Surgical intervention consists of aortic resection with end-to-end anastomosis or transplanted graft resection. Thoracic entrance will facilitate these surgical corrections because the defect is exterior to the cardiac chambers. For asymptomatic children, surgery is usually performed between the ages of 3 and 10.

Endocardial cushion defect (Figs. 15-7 and 15-8). The endocardial cushions divide the heart into a four-chambered organ. Failure of this development results in a large opening that allows blood to circulate between the four chambers. Communication exists at the upper interventricular septum, at the interatrial septum, and at the mitral and tricuspid valves. The degree of shunting depends on ventricular pressures, chamber compliance, and the level of pulmonary and systemic vascular resistance. Pulmonary hypertension with resultant congestive heart failure and cardiomegaly are common sequelae of an endocardial cushion defect. Surgical corrections include closure of the septal defects and mitral/tricuspid valve repair. Mitral insufficiency may exist after surgery, which necessitates valvular replacement. Because of extensive malformation an increased mortality is associated with this defect.

Pulmonic stenosis. Pulmonary stenosis is a stricture of the pulmonary valve or the pulmonary artery. It is an obstructive lesion that impedes right ventricular outflow. The right ventricle must then pump against the obstruction. Right ventricular pressure increases with resultant right ventricular hypertrophy. Right atrial hypertrophy may develop as a consequence of the elevated right ventricular pressure. If the lesion is severe, right-sided heart failure may occur soon after birth. Cyanosis may be present because of right-left shunting through a patent foramen ovale. Children with moderate defects experience fatigue or dyspnea on exertion and those with mild defects may be asymptomatic until late childhood. A valvotomy is performed for pulmonary valvular lesions. Open-heart technique is utilized to permit entrance to the stenotic area via the right ventricle.

Cyanotic lesions as stimuli for congestive heart failure

Transposition of the great vessels (Fig. 15-9). In transposition of the great vessels, systemic and pulmonary systems function independently and simultaneously. Separate circulations exist because the aorta arises from the right ventricle while the pulmonary artery exits from the left ventricle. If a septal defect or patent ductus arteriosus is found in conjunction with the transposition, shunting will allow unoxygenated systemic and oxygenated pulmonary blood to mix.

Oxygenated blood from the lungs enters the left atrium, flows into the left ventricle, and returns to the lungs through the pulmonary artery. Concurrently, unoxygenated blood enters the right atrium

to the ventricle, flows into the aorta, and then flows through the systemic circulation. The degree of cyanosis is related to the amount of interarterial mixing from a coexisting septal defect. Children with large communications may be in congestive heart failure and will have mild cyanosis. Without lesions such as ventricular septal defect or patent ductus arteriosus, this defect is incompatible with life. To provide interarterial mixing, two palliative surgeries may be performed. An atrial septal defect can be created by the Blalock-Hanlon operation or an existing atrial communication can be enlarged through the balloon septostomy technique (Rashkind procedure).

The Mustard procedure is commonly used for corrective surgery. The therapeutic results from this surgery are (1) a new atrial septum is created from the pericardium, (2) systemic (venous) blood is diverted through the mitral valve, (3) oxygen-

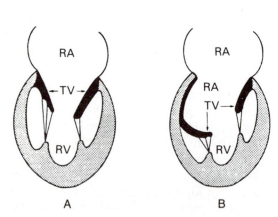

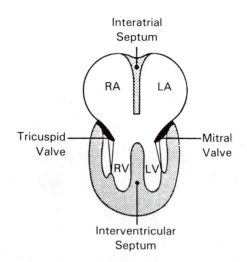

Fig. 15-7. Endocardial cushion defect. Diagrammatic representation of anatomic appearance of tricuspid valve in Ebstein's anomaly. **A,** Normal insertion of the tricuspid valve. **B,** Displacement of one leaflet of tricuspid valve. There is a very small right ventricle and a very large right atrium. *RA,* Right atrium; *TV,* tricuspid valve; *RV,* right ventricle. (Reproduced with permission from Fink, B.W.: Congenital heart disease: a deductive approach to its diagnosis. Copyright © 1975 by Year Book Medical Publishers, Inc., Chicago.)

Fig. 15-8. Endocardial cushion defect. Schematic representation of anatomy in complete endocardial cushion defect. Salient feature is large central hole. *RA,* right atrium; *RV,* right ventricle; *LA,* left atrium; *LV,* left ventricle. (Reproduced with permission from Fink, B.W.: Congenital heart disease: a deductive approach to its diagnosis. Copyright © 1975 by Year Book Medical Publishers, Inc., Chicago.)

ated blood from the pulmonary veins is directed to the tricuspid valve, and (4) oxygenated blood enters the right ventricle, aorta, and systemic circulation.

Tetralogy of Fallot (Fig. 15-10). In tetralogy of Fallot, there are four coexisting lesions: (1) ventricular septal defect, (2) pulmonic stenosis, (3) right ventricular hypertrophy, and (4) overriding or dextroposition of the aorta. Hemodynamically, the pulmonic stenosis hinders blood flow to the lungs, causes right ventricular hypertension, and creates right-to-left shunting of unoxygenated blood through the ventricular septal defect. The right ventricular hypertrophy results from the increased workload on the right ventricle secondary to pulmonic stenosis. The overriding aorta receives unoxygenated blood from the right ventricle, which contributes to generalized cyanosis. Polycythemia may develop to compensate for the

anoxia; however, the increased blood viscosity may impede systemic circulation and cause systemic hypertension. Other complications include thrombophlebitis, embolism, and cerebrovascular disease. The child learns to limit play and may assume the ''squatting position'' in an attempt to relieve hypoxia. In addition to cyanosis, clubbing of the nail beds may be observed. Congestive heart failure is not typical with tetralogy of Fallot because blood pumped from the right ventricle enters the overriding aorta from the ventricular septal defect. Blood flows from the aorta into the systemic circulation. Palliative surgery in neonates[8] consists of a side-to-side anastomosis of the ascending aorta to the right pulmonary artery (Waterston-Cooley procedure). In older children the procedure involves anastomosis of the right subclavian artery to the right pulmonary artery (Blalock-Taussig operation). The Pott's operation,

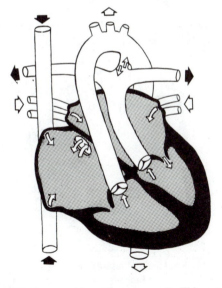

Fig. 15-9. Transposition of great vessels. This anomaly is an embryological defect caused by straight division of bulbar trunk without normal spiraling. As a result, aorta originates from right ventricle and pulmonary artery from left ventricle. Abnormal communication between two circulations must be present to sustain life. (From Congenital heart abnormalities, Clinical Education Aid No. 7. Courtesy Ross Laboratories, Columbus, Ohio, 1968.)

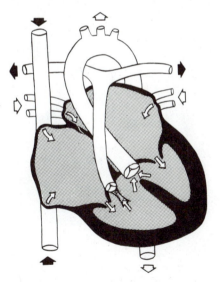

Fig. 15-10. Tetralogy of Fallot is characterized by combination of four defects: (1) pulmonary stenosis, (2) ventricular septal defect, (3) overriding aorta, and (4) hypertrophy of right ventricle. It is most common defect causing cyanosis in patients surviving beyond 2 years of age. Severity of symptoms depends on degree of pulmonary stenosis, size of ventricular septal defect, and degree to which aorta overrides septal defect. (From Congenital heart abnormalities, Clinical Education Aid No. 7. Courtesy Ross Laboratories, Columbus, Ohio, 1968.)

anastomosis of the descending aorta to the left pulmonary artery, is another surgical procedure that may be used. Complete surgical intervention includes closure of the ventricular septal defect, correction of the overriding aorta, and pulmonic valvotomy.

Truncus arteriosus (Fig. 15-11.) With truncus arteriosus a single large vessel overrides both ventricles. In embryological development the bulbar trunk does not divide into the aorta and pulmonary artery. Therefore blood from both ventricles enters the common artery and circulates to the lungs or to the aortic arch and systemic circulation. Pulmonary vascular congestion develops from an increased blood flow to the lungs from the ventricles.

Clinical indicators of congestive heart failure appear in early infancy. Cyanosis develops with progressive pulmonary and cardiac congestion.

The Rastelli procedure may be used to close the ventricular septal defect and allow the truncus to originate from the left ventricle. The pulmonary arteries are excised from the aorta and connected to the right ventricle with a prosthetic valved conduit.

Total anomalous venous return (Fig. 15-12). Total anomalous venous return is a rare lesion in which the pulmonary veins join to the right atrium or to other veins directing blood to the right atrium (for example, coronary sinus, ductus venosus, innominate vein, superior vena cava). Classification is based on the location of the attachment. In a

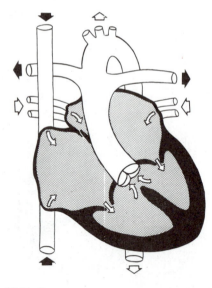

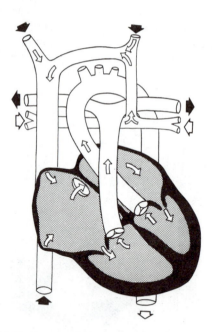

Fig. 15-11. Truncus arteriosus is retention of embryological bulbar trunk. It results from failure of normal septation and division of this trunk into aorta and pulmonary artery. This single arterial trunk overrides ventricles and receives blood from them through ventricular septal defect. Entire pulmonary and systemic circulation is supplied from this common arterial trunk. (From Congenital heart abnormalities, Clinical Education Aid No. 7. Courtesy Ross Laboratories, Columbus, Ohio, 1968.)

Fig. 15-12. Total anomalous venous return. Oxygenated blood returning from lungs is carried abnormally to right side of heart by one or more pulmonary veins emptying directly, or indirectly, through venous channels into right atrium. Partial anomalous return of pulmonary veins to right atrium functions same as atrial septal defect. In complete anomalous return of pulmonary veins, interatrial communication is necessary for survival. (From Congenital heart abnormalities, Clinical Education Aid No. 7. Courtesy Ross Laboratories, Columbus, Ohio, 1968.)

"cardiac" lesion the pulmonary veins are joined to the right atrium or coronary sinus. The other types include "infracardiac"[8] (below the diaphragm), for example, at the inferior vena cava, and "supracardiac" (above the diaphragm), for example, at the superior vena cava. Congestive heart failure develops in infancy. The outcome of surgery depends on the location of the lesion. There is a greater surgical risk with infracardiac lesions, whereas cardiac types are the most successful.

Tricuspid atresia (Fig. 15-13). Absence of the tricuspid valve is the chief characteristic of tricuspid atresia. Because there is no communication between the right atrium and right ventricle, a coexisting defect allows for some shunting of blood to the lungs. A ventricular septal defect allows blood to enter the right ventricle and pulmonary artery to be oxygenated by the lungs. When the ductus arteriosus begins to close, blood flow to the lungs is diminished and right-sided heart failure may appear. The objective of surgical intervention is to increase blood flow to the lungs for oxygenation. The techniques are the same as those used for tetralogy of Fallot. An atrial septostomy can be done during cardiac catheterization to enlarge an existing atrial septal defect.

Patent ductus arteriosus (Fig. 15-14). Contraction of the ductus arteriosus usually occurs within the first 3 days of life. Failure of this closure results in the shunting of blood from left to right,

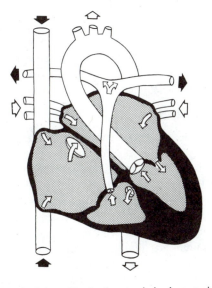

Fig. 15-13. Tricuspid valvular atresia is characterized by small right ventricle, large left ventricle, and usually diminished pulmonary circulation. Blood from right atrium passes through atrial septal defect into left atrium, mixes with oxygenated blood returning from lungs, flows into left ventricle, and is propelled into systemic circulation. Lungs may receive blood through one of three routes: (1) a small ventricular septal defect, (2) patent ductus arteriosus, and (3) bronchial vessels. (From Congenital heart abnormalities, Clinical Education Aid No. 7. Courtesy Ross Laboratories, Columbus, Ohio, 1968.)

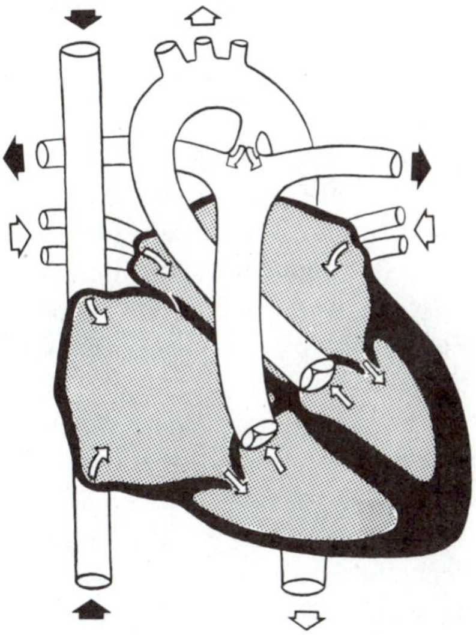

Fig. 15-14. Patent ductus arteriosus is vascular connection that, during fetal life, short circuits pulmonary vascular bed and directs blood from pulmonary artery to aorta. Functional closure of ductus normally occurs soon after birth. If ductus remains patent after birth, direction of blood flow in ductus is reversed by higher pressure of aorta. (From Congenital heart abnormalities, Clinical Education Aid No. 7. Courtesy Ross Laboratories, Columbus, Ohio, 1968.)

that is, blood is pumped from the aorta through the patent ductus arteriosus to the lungs. This increased blood volume to the lungs causes an excessive workload for the left side of the heart. Clinical indicators correlate with the size of the defect and degree of shunting. There is a higher incidence of patent ductus arteriosus with premature infants and respiratory distress syndrome (hyaline membrane disease).

Enteral indomethacin has been utilized for medical closure of the patent ductus arteriosus. Indomethacin is a nonsteroidal, antiinflammatory agent that interferes with or inhibits prostaglandin synthesis.[9] Surgical correction involves ligation of the patent ductus.

Acquired heart disease as cause for congestive heart failure

Acute rheumatic fever. Acute rheumatic fever is a systemic, inflammatory collagen disease that usually occurs after a group A beta-hemolytic streptococcal infection. Acute rheumatic fever frequently occurs in school-age children. Clinical indicators are vague and generalized. Pallor, anorexia, weight loss, and malaise may be apparent during a routine physical examination. The formation of lesions, or Aschoff bodies, is present with the inflammatory process. Aschoff bodies cause swelling and fragmentation in the connective tissue of the heart. These vegetations produce fibrous scar tissue when healed. The scar tissue may cause valvular stenosis; stenotic valves are unable to completely close and regurgitation or backflow may occur. Valvular insufficiency inhibits forward blood flow with subsequent congestive heart failure.

Bacterial endocarditis. Bacterial endocarditis is usually caused by *Streptococcus viridans (S. viridans)* but can also develop from infectious organisms such as enterococci, staphylococci, and to a lesser degree, *Candida albicans* and *Rickettsia*. This infection of the endocardium and cardiac valves usually follows invasive procedures, that is, oral surgery, bronchoscopy, urinary bladder catheterization, or gastrointestinal invasive manipulation.

The virulent agents enter the heart via the systemic circulation (bacteremia) from any localized portal of entry or infection. The child may experience a number of generalized symptoms including fatigue, malaise, loss of appetite, low-grade fever, and weight loss. Splenomegaly may be assessed during abdominal palpation. Petechiae, Janeway's lesion, and Osler's nodes may also be observed during the physical examination. A murmur may be heard on auscultation if the infection has produced valvular damage. Intravenous antibiotics are introduced and maintained for approximately 4 to 6 weeks. The antibiotic should be agent-specific based on accurate blood culture results. Antibiotics such as ampicillin, methicillin, and penicillin may be administered when blood culture results are pending. Bacterial endocarditis can occur at any age but is more prevalent with children than young infants. Coronary emboli are complications that can lead to myocardial infarction. The emboli cause occlusions in the coronary vessels, which lead to coronary tisue ischemia. Congestive heart failure remains a risk from cardiac valvular damage.

ASSESSMENT

The onset of congestive heart failure in infants and children is most often insidious and requires prompt action. The clinical indicators develop when the infant's growth and energy needs exceed the heart's ability to function adequately to meet oxygen demands of the body tissues. Since the majority of children who experience congestive heart failure are infants, we will primarily discuss the assessment of the infant. Newborns' reaction to illness is generalized; therefore it is difficult to identify specific indicators that reflect congestive heart failure versus other diseases or conditions. The slightest change in a child's usual behavior—for example, eating, activity, or disposition—may reflect illness and a complete subjective and objective assessment should be performed.

Subjective data

History. Since the onset of congestive heart failure is insidious, the nurse's role in identifying children with early signs of heart failure is very important. Often the symptoms do not appear during the physical examination but have occurred at home. The history is an essential tool in assessing the child's level of wellness and potential problems. Components of a nursing history for congestive heart failure include maternal-antepartum history, comparison to siblings, feeding problems, activity-sleep patterns, respiratory difficulties or infections, and evidence of cyanosis.

Maternal-antepartum history can provide clues regarding the possibility of congestive heart failure. Prematurity, diabetes in the mother, and/or birth by cesarean section can be warning signs of potential problems. It often is helpful to ask the mother to compare the child to siblings. A mother may express that something is different about this baby compared to her others. The nurse can offer clues as to the possible differences. The mother's comparison will often include developmental delays, more irritability, smaller physical size, and a decreased exercise tolerance.

Feeding difficulties are one of the most frequent complaints by parents of children with congestive heart failure. The feeding problems are often caused by the tachypnea and dyspnea. An infant expends most of his energy during eating; therefore this may be the only time when the heart cannot provide adequate systemic oxygenation. The feeding difficulties range from refusal to suck, vomiting, prolonged feeding time, difficulty swallowing, or inadequate sucking ability. Women who are breastfeeding may blame their child's disinterest in feeding on their lack of milk production. The infant usually sucks vigorously at first and then slows down and appears fatigued. The child appears dusky and closes his eyes. After a few minutes, the infant will take the nipple and suck again, and the cycle repeats itself. Older children may have difficulty eating solids.

The child's activity-sleep pattern includes easy fatigability. The child may go to sleep for short periods and wake irritable and pale as a result of orthopnea. Even while the child sleeps, he may grimace and squirm. The infant often has decreased muscle tone and a faint, weak cry. The

parent may identify that the child assumes the knee chest position or squats when playing or the infant prefers being held upright or sitting up.

Respiratory difficulties include recurrent respiratory infections, congestion, dyspnea, anoxic spells, stridor, paroxysmal hyperpnea, wheezing, or grunting. The parent may notice cyanosis after exertion described as a pasty, grayish coloring of the skin.

Family assessment. The family is an integral part of the child's disease and totally influences the child's reaction to congestive heart failure, adjustment to the disease process, and recovery. Parental acceptance of a child's illness is a process. One needs to assess the parents' orientation to their ill child to provide appropriate support and intervention. "Parents initial response is shock and disbelief. Accompanying and following the disbelief are feelings of anger, sadness, helplessness, guilt, fear, and anxiety."[12]

The parents' concept of their child's disease is influenced by information acquired from health team members, accessible literature, significant others, and their past experiences with illness. The nurse needs to assess the parents' understanding of the disease process and prognosis. Chronic congestive heart failure creates prolonged stress for the family. The peaks and valleys of the disease relate directly to the parents' understanding and coping ability. The disease may also affect the parents' attachment to the child.

The relationship between the parents is also important in assessing the family. Who is the caregiver to the ill child? Does one parent protect the other from difficulties and from knowing about the child's disease and prognosis? Is the child in a single-parent family?

The ill child's position within the family may influence the parents' and siblings' reaction as well as the child's own view of his illness. The oldest sibling is supposed to be the strongest, whereas the youngest is the weakest, the baby. The child can use his disease to his own advantage by encouraging overprotection and eliciting symptoms (for example, dyspnea) when needed.

The siblings' view of their sick brother or sister

is influenced mostly by the parents' reaction. Young children find it difficult to understand why parents must go to the hospital. The siblings and sometimes the father can feel neglected and resentful of the child with congestive heart failure.

All members of the family are affected when a child has congestive heart failure. There may be financial burdens, anxiety over prognosis, guilt, and resentment. Each family reacts differently to the stress of chronic illness in a child. It is essential to assess the families' coping mechanisms and adaptation to properly care for the child.

Objective data

Performing a physical examination on an infant or child. When approaching an infant or child, one should move slowly into the room and speak to the parent or significant other first. The parent's acceptance of the clinician may help allay the child's fears. The parents should be encouraged to stay during the examination and incorporate them into the activities. Often the child will tolerate the examination better if held by the par-

ent. The parent should be asked to undress the infant. The clinician should count the child's respirations before touching the child. Since the infant or child is attached to the parent, any separation may cause anxiety. Especially during a trying situation such as a physical examination, this attachment and trust are helpful.

A small child learns and accepts new objects and situations best by touching and exploring with his hands; therefore it is helpful when possible to let the child feel the equipment before using it. The examiner should offer the child the stethoscope to play with before auscultation. Also children are sensitive to environmental extremes, for example, cold or loud noises. These distractions should be minimalized. For instance, hands and equipment should be warm before touching the child.

Physical assessment (Figs. 15-15 to 15-17, Tables 15-1 and 15-2)

Cardiac indicators. The principal clinical manifestation of congestive heart failure is rapid heart rate (in infants tachycardia is above 160 beats per minute auscultated apically). The infant's heart rate at rest should be assessed. Any exertion,

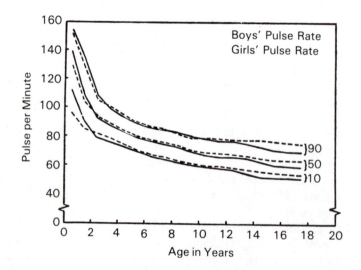

Fig. 15-15. Pulse rates in infants and children. (From Vaughan, V., McKay, R., and Behrman, R., editors: Nelson's textbook of pediatrics, ed. 11, Philadelphia, 1979, W.B. Saunders Co.)

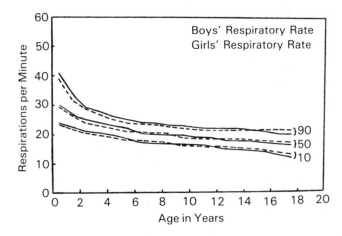

Fig. 15-16. Respiratory rates in infants and children. (From Vaughan, V., McKay, R., and Behrman, R., editors: Nelson's textbook of pediatrics, ed. 11, Philadelphia, 1979, W.B. Saunders Co.)

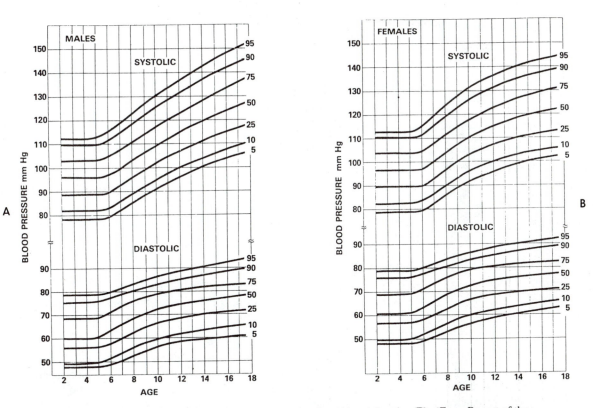

Fig. 15-17. Percentiles of blood pressure in seated males (**A**) and females (**B**). (From Report of the Task Force on Blood Pressure Control in Children. National Heart, Lung, and Blood Institute, Pediatrics [suppl.] **59**[5]:803, Part 2, May 1977.)

Table 15-1. Physical assessment: average pulse rates at rest

Age	Lower limits of normal		Average		Upper limits of normal	
Newborn	70		125		190	
1-11 months	80		120		160	
2 years	80		110		130	
4 years	80		100		120	
6 years	75		100		115	
8 years	70		90		110	
10 years	70		90		110	
	Girls	Boys	Girls	Boys	Girls	Boys
12 years	70	65	90	85	110	105
14 years	65	60	85	80	105	100
16 years	60	55	80	75	100	95
18 years	55	50	75	70	95	90

From Vaughan, V., McKay, R., and Behrman, R.: Nelson's textbook of pediatrics, Philadelphia, 1979, W.B. Saunders Co., p. 1252.

Table 15-2. Summary of clinical indicators of congestive heart failure in infants and children

Clinical indicators	Physiological causes
CARDIAC	
Tachycardia	Compensatory mechanism to increase cardiac output
Murmurs	Intracardiac shunts and high flow rates across normal or narrow valves
Decreased systemic arterial pulses	Peripheral vasoconstriction
Cardiomegaly	Dilation resulting from increased end-diastolic volume
PULMONARY	
Tachypnea	Pulmonary congestion
Cyanosis	Hypoxemia and arterial desaturation
Orthopnea in walking children	Pulmonary congestion—need for increased thoracic space
Rales, rhonchi	Pulmonary edema and obstruction
SYSTEMIC	
Edema/weight gain	Systemic congestion and decreased urinary output
Hepatomegaly	Liver congestion resulting from congested systemic circulation

which will often increase the heart rate dramatically, should be noted. The absence of tachycardia does not necessarily rule out heart failure because myocardial hypoxia can decrease the heart rate. Auscultation of an infant's heart sounds requires patience and much practice. Infants have innocent murmurs more frequently than adults. Therefore the presence or absence of a murmur is not a definitive sign of heart disease.

Many children also have "innocent," or "functional," murmurs and no cardiac disease, whereas others may have no murmur with severe cardiac

Table 15-3. Typical murmurs associated with congenital heart defects*

Sounds heard		Characteristics and location	May indicate
Pansystolic murmur		Maximum in the 4th, 5th, and 6th intercostal spaces at left sternal border; high, harsh murmur heard throughout systole; may be associated with palpable thrill	Ventricular septal defect
		Heard in the apical area	Endocardial cushion defect
Split S_2 on expiration; Systolic ejection murmur		Split is heard in 2nd, 3rd, or 4th intercostal space; murmur maximum in 2nd and 3rd left intercostal spaces	Atrial septal defect
Loud aortic closure sound; Systolic murmur		Aortic sound heard at 2nd left intercostal space; murmur heard if ventricular septal defect is present	Transposition of the great arteries
Single S_2; Systolic murmur		Murmur maximal in 2nd and 3rd intercostal spaces at left sternal border	Tetralogy of Fallot
Continuous murmur		Maximum in 2nd left intercostal space; envelops S_2 with late systolic accentuation; terminates in late or middiastole; radiates to 1st intercostal space and beneath left clavicle	Patent ductus arteriosus
Systolic ejection click		Loudest to left of sternum; sometimes heard at apex	Aortic stenosis
		Loudest during expiration; heard at base of the heart	Pulmonary stenosis
		Heard at both base and apex of the heart; associated with systolic or continuous murmur between scapulae	Coarctation of the aorta

From Shor, V.Z.: Congenital cardiac defects assessment and case finding, Am. J. Nurs. **78:**259, Feb. 1978.

*The preceding murmurs and abnormal heart sounds are generally, but not always, associated with the identified congenital defects. In the presence of multiple defects, various combinations of these sounds may be heard.

disease. A murmur is an audible vibration caused by turbulent blood flow. Turbulence is caused by some intracardiac shunts and high flow rates across normal or narrow valves. S_1, the first heart sound, is associated with closure of the mitral and tricuspid valves. It is heard at the beginning of systole and is synchronous with the apical impulse. S_2, the second heart sound, is produced by closure of the aortic and pulmonic valves and marks the beginning of diastole. Splitting of this sound is usual during inspiration as the aortic valve closes before the pulmonic valve (Table 15-3).

Decreased systemic arterial pulses are a sign of severe congestive heart failure. Decreased or absent pulses can be an important diagnostic tool to identify cardiac lesions.

Respiratory indicators. Tachypnea is usually the first sign and may be the only sign of cardiac failure. Normally, a newborn's respiratory rate is less than 50 breaths per minute with shallow, irregular respirations. The neonate's chest and abdomen rise in unison with each breath. Tachypnea occurs when the respiratory rate is greater than 60 breaths per minute at rest existing for several hours. Dyspnea also is a significant indication of pulmonary congestion and is usually accompanied by costal retractions, expiratory grunting (especially in neonates), and nasal flaring. Retractions in infants are seen laterally rather than in the lower sternum as with primary pulmonary disease.[6] Dyspnea may become evident upon an increase in activity, crying, or feeding but can progress to existing at rest. Paroxysmal nocturnal dyspnea may also occur in children who are walking. During late failure the infant's head bobs as the child appears to be gasping for air when the ancillary chest muscles work to aid respiration.

Cyanosis, a sign of progressive congestive heart failure, indicates hypoxemia and arterial desaturation. It is first seen in nail beds, mucous membranes, and conjunctiva. In black or dark-skinned infants, cyanosis is primarily observed in the mucous membranes. On exertion, the infant's skin may appear mottled or dusky.

Rales and rhonchi are present when pulmonary edema and obstruction occur. Frequent coughing is a result of mucosal swelling and irritation. As pulmonary edema increases, the cough becomes more productive.

Orthopnea may be seen as the child becomes intolerant of the supine position. The child may prefer to be held upright or assume a sitting position.

Systemic indicators. Distended neck, peripheral veins, and anasarca are more commonly seen in older children than in infants. The earliest signs of edema in infants and toddlers are weight gain and facial or sacral edema. Dependent edema occurs in children who are walking. Ascites and pleural effusion can occur when heart failure becomes severe.

Hepatomegaly in infants occurs early after the onset of heart failure. A soft liver 1 to 2 cm beneath the anterior costal margin is normal in infants. Hepatomegaly is diagnosed as a tense liver felt 2 cm below the rib cage.

Generalized objective indicators. The overall appearance of a child with congestive heart failure is one of anxiety, irritability, and lethargy. The infant may have a tense facial expression as if he is "worrying" about where he will get his next breath. The child who has suffered from congestive heart failure has poor weight gain, failure to thrive, and retarded development. Excessive sweating is also a sign of congestive heart failure but rarely occurs in the neonate.

Diagnostic findings

Laboratory tests. Increases in erythrocyte, hemoglobin, and hematocrit levels result from the alteration in cardiac function. Polycythemia is a compensatory mechanism for decreased tissue oxygenation. The increase in red blood cells allows greater oxygen-binding capacity and therefore more oxygen is carried to the body's tissues. Thrombocytopenia is frequently associated with cyanotic cardiac defects and results from the polycythemia accompanied by the lack of subsequent blood volume expansion.

Arterial blood gases usually show a normal or

increased Pco_2 and a decreased Po_2. Urinary output is low, resulting in a high specific gravity and mild proteinuria.

Electrocardiography. An ECG is done essentially to rule out arrhythmias as a cause of congestive heart failure, but the test does not aid in the diagnosis of a congenital cardiac lesion. The ECG can provide information about muscular damage, ventricular hypertrophy, and the effect of various drugs. The vectorcardiograph reflects both direction and amplitude of electrical impulses and is more useful in diagnosing congenital heart defects.[8] The echocardiograph produces the image of sound waves on paper and is helpful in determining the exact location of the defect. Chapter 5 describes echocardiogram technique.

Chest radiogram. The chest radiogram is useful in identifying position of the heart, cardiac size, individual chamber enlargement, and pulmonary congestion.

Cardiac catheterization. This invasive diagnostic tool is essentially the same as in adults, although the catheter size and length are commensurate with the child's anatomical structures. A detailed discussion of this procedure is beyond the scope of this text.

HEALTH CARE PROBLEMS AND INTERVENTIONS

In caring for pediatric patients, it is imperative to consider the developmental stage and chronological age of the individual patient. It is a primary nursing objective to evaluate the rest and activity patterns of the child. A preliminary or admission interview with the parents or primary caregivers can reveal useful information about the child's daily routine.

PROBLEM: Alteration in cardiac output

INTERVENTION: Decreasing cardiac demands

Rest. The child should be provided with prolonged rest periods throughout the day. Health care procedures should be implemented based on an assessment of the child's tolerance (that is, vital signs, bathing, and feeding can be done at one time so the child does not have to be disturbed con-

tinuously, or procedures can be implemented throughout the day if the child becomes fatigued with routine care). Organization in providing care will allow the child to rest between procedures.

Crying increases caloric demands, oxygen consumption, and cardiac workload. Children should be comforted to allay crying episodes and decrease energy expenditure. Children are usually placed on bedrest. Minimizing boredom and providing age-appropriate activities will help the child comply with this restriction. For hospitalized children with acute congestive heart failure, morphine sulfate may be administered as sedation for excessive irritability, agitation, or discomfort.

Feeding. Demand feedings for infants may be more beneficial than strict adherence to a feeding schedule. Because the infant must coordinate breathing, sucking, and swallowing, feeding time is exhausting in the presence of congestive heart failure. Caloric expenditure should not exceed the amount of calories consumed. Frequent, small feedings may be ordered to meet the caloric requirements. Feeding time should not exceed 30 minutes, because the infant will tire easily past this point. Tachypneic infants may be gavage-fed to decrease the risk of aspiration and to provide rest during the feeding. Allowing the infant to suck on a pacifier during "fussy" episodes will be comforting.

Digitalis. Digitalis remains the drug of choice in therapeutic management for children in congestive heart failure. Digoxin levels are obtained and monitored closely in children as dosages are calculated according to the child's weight (μg/kg/day). The pharmacokinetics of the drug must be considered in calculating dosages for neonates and infants. Because of the infant's distribution of body water (that is, the full-term newborn is approximately 70% to 75% water and adults are 57% to 60% water),[1] there may be variable distribution of the drug systemically. Immature or impaired hepatic and renal function may impede absorption, detoxification, and excretion of the therapeutic agent. The half-life of digitalis may accentuate the

Table 15-4. Comparison of digitalis preparations

Variable	Digoxin	Digitoxin
Onset		
Oral	1 hour	2-4 hours
Intravenous	5-10 minutes	½-2 hours
Peak action		
Oral	6-7 hours	12-24 hours
Intravenous	1-2 hours	8-9 hours
Half-life	28-48 hours	8 days
Absorption and excretion	80%-90%	Complete
	Minimally recycled through liver or bowel	Extensively recycled through liver and bowel
	Poorly bound to serum albumin	Closely bound to serum albumin
	Excreted unchanged in urine	Excreted as cardioinactive metabolites in urine

From Whaley, L.F., and Wong, D.L.: Nursing care of infants and children, ed. 2, St. Louis, 1983, The C.V. Mosby Co.

Table 15-5. Total digitalizing doses (TDD) (Lanoxin)

Premature	0.03 mg/kg = 30 μg/kg to 0.04 mg/kg = 40 μg/kg
Full term	0.05 mg/kg = 50 μg/kg
2 weeks	0.06 mg/kg = 60 μg/kg
Over 2 years	0.03 mg/kg = 30 μg/kg to 0.05 mg/kg = 50 μg/kg

Maximum TDD = 1 mg

Give ½ TDD at time 0, wait 6-8 hours to give additional ¼ TDD, wait further 6-8 hours to give final ¼ TDD (obtain rhythm strip first).

If giving IV, reduce TDD by 25%. Also, if giving IV, digitalize by ⅓, ⅓, ⅓.

After digitalization, daily maintenance is ¼ TDD per day, in two divided doses.

How supplied: *Parenteral:* 100 μg/ml and 250 μg/ml; *Oral:* 50 μg/ml elixir.

accumulation of the drug, resulting in toxic serum levels (Tables 15-4 and 15-5).

The onset of symptoms with digitalis toxicity is insidious in infants and children. Abdominal distention and feeding intolerance (vomiting or gastric residuals) may be the first sign of digitalis toxicity. These gastrointestinal signs may be accompanied by a loss of appetite. Other symptoms include insomnia, drowsiness, visual disturbances, and changes in sensorium. On ECG, prolonged atrioventricular conduction, and premature ventricular contractions may be evident. Bradycardia is a significant finding. As a rule of thumb, digoxin is usually withheld for infants with an apical pulse of 100 beats per minute or below and for young children with an apical pulse of 70 beats per minute. The baseline apical pulse should be determined upon admission. One should document and communicate any aberrations from the baseline data.

Digoxin may be given by parenteral, intramuscular, or oral route (Figs. 15-18 and 15-19). Intravenous administration is the most accurate during digitalization. Intramuscular (IM) absorption may be poor because of diminished peripheral circulation and small muscle mass (IM injections are usually given in the vastas lateralis until the child is 3 to 5 years old). Feeding difficulties and vomiting hinder the effectiveness of digitalis elixirs.

ECG monitoring. Continuous cardiac monitoring and a 12-lead ECG should be initiated to determine factors such as baseline PR intervals, QRS duration, QT segments, and atrial and ventricular rates. The skin should be gently prepared before placing the prelubricated electrodes. This will minimize artifact that appears when there is inadequate conductive gel or skin adherence. Lead

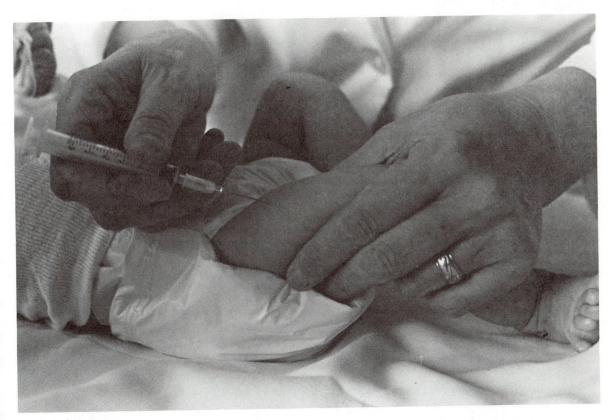

Fig. 15-18. Infant's leg stabilized for intramuscular injection. (From Whaley, L., and Wong, D.: Nursing care of infants and children, ed. 2, St. Louis, 1983, The C.V. Mosby Co.)

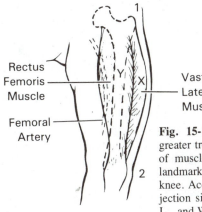

Rectus Femoris Muscle

Femoral Artery

Vastus Lateralis Muscle

Fig. 15-19. Vastus lateralis muscle. Landmarks: *1,* greater trochanter; *2,* knee. Injection site: lateral aspect of muscle mass in middle third of distance between landmarks; injected at 45-degree angle in direction of knee. Acceptable intramuscular sites for children: *X,* injection site; *Y,* alternate injection site. (From Whaley, L., and Wong, D.: Nursing care of infants and children, ed. 2, St. Louis, 1983, The C.V. Mosby Co.)

wires should remain untangled. Monitoring limits are set according to the child's baseline heart rate. Infants and children frequently have bradyarrhythmias or tachyarrhythmias, so careful determination of low and high settings is essential.

PROBLEM: Ineffective oxygenation

INTERVENTION: Reducing oxygen demand

A cardiac chair (or infant seat) may be used with infants and a head elevation position of 30 to 45 degrees may be used with older children. This position will minimize respiratory effort by decreasing venous return and consequent volume overload to the heart. Clothing should be nonconstricting, especially around the chest and abdomen. The knee-chest position may be naturally assumed by children with congestive heart failure. Infants can be maintained in this position by placing them on their sides with knees bent toward the chest and propped up by blankets. The nurse should encourage turning, coughing, and deep breathing for the older child.

The child or infant may be placed in a humidifying tent to liquefy secretions. Oxygen must be humidified. Conscientious monitoring of respiratory rates and blood gases is necessary. Any evidence of Cheyne-Stokes respirations should be reported to the physician immediately, since this is a sign of progressive congestive heart failure. Ventilatory support may be needed for severe pulmonary edema.

PROBLEM: Alteration in nutrition: less than body requirements

INTERVENTION: Provide adequate nutrition

When the infant should consume solids, they can be slightly pureed and fed with the formula or juice through the bottle.

The diet of older children should be highly nutritious, appealing, and easy to consume. Most children have a favorite food or dish that can be used to encourage eating. They usually enjoy milkshakes or commercially available food preparations.[8]

The nursing staff should encourage the family to bring food from home that complies with dietary restrictions, for example, foods for a low-sodium diet or for a diet with fluid restrictions. The dietitian should speak with the family if necessary to explain the food requirements. Also, the family should be helped to interpret these restrictions to fit with their cultural food habits. It is also helpful to have members of the child's family eat with the child in the hospital.

PROBLEM: Alterations in normal body temperature

INTERVENTION: Thermoregulation

Hyperthermic states increase the metabolic rate and therefore oxygen consumption and caloric expenditure. Neonates and infants are sensitive to ambient temperatures, and hypothermia is a risk. Axillary temperatures should be taken on neonates and young infants. Rectal temperatures are avoided because of the risk of anal sphincter perforation. Vagal stimulation may also occur during rectal thermometer manipulation. Rectal temperatures are usually taken on children until 5 years of age. Children under 5 years are unable to safely secure an oral thermometer. When axillary temperatures are taken, the thermometer should be held in place for at least 3 minutes. The infant or child should always be attended during this time to reduce hazardous accidents with the thermometer.

The neonate and young infant will attempt to increase their core temperatures by utilizing calories. Catabolism in hypoxic states will lead to anaerobic processes resulting in a metabolic acidosis, which may complicate an already compromised circulation. After glycogen stores are depleted, the breakdown of fats and resultant ketone accumulation will accentuate an existing metabolic acidosis. Profound and sustained hypothermia may cause apnea and respiratory arrest. Older infants and children are less sensitive to ambient air changes and will usually respond to systemic infections with a febrile state. Febrile seizures or convulsions can occur.

All health care interventions should be initiated to avoid the complications of nonnormothermic states. Providing a neutral thermal environment will decrease needless utilization of calories and oxygen. Clinicians should keep the child warm and dry, control the ambient room temperature and humidity, and administer warmed, humidified oxygen as ordered.

Table 15-6. Comparison of average serum electrolyte concentrations of infants and adults

Electrolyte	Average serum concentrations, mEq/L		
	Newborn*	Infants	Adults
Sodium	149 (139-162)	140 (143-150)	140 (136-145)
Potassium	5.9 (5.0-7.7)	5.0 (4.1-5.6)	4.2 (3.5-5.0)
Calcium	≤4.0 (3.5-4.0)	5 (5.0-6.0)	5 (4.5-5.5)
Magnesium	≤1.8 (1.2-1.8)	2 (1.65-2.5)	2 (1.5-2.5)
Chloride	103 (93-112)	105 (98-106)	104 (96-106)
Bicarbonate	21	20 (19-20)	24 (22-26)
Phosphate	up to 5.0	2 (2.3-3.8)	2 (1.7-2.6)
Sulfate	†	1 (0.5-1.0)	1 (0.4-1.3)
Organic acids	13.5 mg/100 ml	5	3
Protein	†	20	13

Adapted from Bonica, J.J.: Principles and practice of obstetric analgesia and anesthesia, vols. 1 & 2, Philadelphia, 1972, F.A. Davis Co.; Conn, R.B.: Normal laboratory values of clinical importance. In Sabiston, D.C., editor: Davis-Christopher textbook of surgery, ed. 10, Philadelphia, 1972, W.B. Saunders Co.; Robinson, H.: Laboratory values. In Nelson, W.E., Vaughan, V.C., III, and McKay, R.J., editors: Textbook of pediatrics, Philadelphia, 1969, W.B. Saunders Co.; Sodeman, W.A., and Sodeman, W.A., Jr., editors: Pathologic physiology: mechanisms of disease, ed. 4, Philadelphia, 1967, W.B. Saunders Co.; Wasserman, E., and Slobody, L.B.: Survey of clinical pediatrics, ed. 6, New York, 1974, McGraw-Hill Book Co.; from A nurse's guide to fluid and electrolyte balance by Audrey Burgess. Copyright © 1979 by Audrey Burgess. Used with the permission of McGraw-Hill Book Company.
*Term infant 72 h old.
†No comparative data.

PROBLEM: Alteration in fluid volume, excess: potential for electrolyte imbalances

INTERVENTION: Maintenance of normal fluids and electrolytes (Table 15-6)

Febrile states as well as diarrhea and vomiting precipitate dehydration. Potassium loss from diarrhea may result in hypokalemia. Decreased myocardial contractility and cardiac output may result from this electrolyte imbalance. Loss of fluid may result in hypernatremic states. Hyponatremic dehydration develops when fluid loss is replaced with hypotonic, electrolyte-free solutions (that is, the child refuses formula or juice and consumes only tap water). Volume loss is evidenced by sunken eyes, depressed fontanelles, diminished tissue turgor, dry mucous membranes, and oliguria.

Intake and output. The child's weight is taken on admission and daily weights are monitored throughout hospitalization. Weights taken at a consistent time with the same scale will ensure accuracy. Oliguria may occur from vasoconstriction of the renal vasculature. Strict intake and output should be maintained with urine protein and specific gravity determinations. As cardiac output and tissue perfusion improves, urinary output will increase with a lower specific gravity.

Diuretics (Table 15-7). Administration of diuretic therapy is indicated to decrease circulating volume and cardiac workload; however, dehydration and electrolyte imbalances are possible complications. Clinical indicators of dehydration include dry mucous membranes, depressed fontanelles, sunken eyes, and poor tissue turgor. An electrolyte panel including potassium, sodium, bicarbonate, and chloride should be closely monitored. When potassium-depleting diuretics are given, hypokalemia may develop. Hypokalemia can potentiate the effects of digitalis. Supplemental potassium by parenteral route may be ordered. Parenteral potassium may be irritating to a peripheral vein and subsequently cause pain at the intravenous site. The school-age child should be informed of this discomfort before the administration. When possible concentrated doses of par-

Table 15-7. Diuretics used in congestive heart failure

Drug	Route	Onset	Peak	Duration	Action	Comments	Nursing considerations
Furosemide (Lasix)	Oral IV	20-30 minutes 5 minutes	2-4 hours ½ hour	6-8 hours 2-4 hours	Blocks reabsorption of sodium and water in proximal renal tubule and interferes with reabsorption of sodium in Henle's loop and in the most proximal portion of distal tubule	Drug of choice in severe congestive heart failure Causes excretion of chloride and potassium (hypokalemia may precipitate digitalis toxicity)	Begin to record output as soon as drug is given Observe for dehydration caused by profound diuresis Observe for side effects (nausea and vomiting, diarrhea, ototoxicity, hypokalemia, dermatitis, postural hypotension) Encourage foods high in potassium and/or give potassium supplements Observe for signs of digitalis toxicity
Chlorothiazide (Diuril)	Oral	2 hours	4 hours	6-12 hours	Acts directly on distal tubules and possibly proximal tubules to decrease sodium, water, potassium, chloride, and bicarbonate absorption Decreases urinary diluting capacity	Most commonly used drugs, inexpensive Causes hypokalemia, acidosis from large doses May be given on alternate days or for 4-5 days and stopped for 2 days to allow for reabsorption of potassium	Observe for side effects (nausea, weakness, dizziness, paresthesia, muscle cramps, skin eruptions, hypokalemia, acidosis) Encourage foods high in potassium and/or give potassium supplements
Hydrochlorothiazide (Hydrodiuril)	Same	Same	Same	Same	Same	Effect is ten times more potent than chlorothiazide; therefore, dose is decreased by one tenth	Same
Spironolactone (Aldactone)	Oral	Gradual	72 hours	48-72 hours	Blocks the action of aldosterone, which promotes retention of sodium and excretion of potassium	Has potassium-sparing effect, frequently used with thiazides Poorly absorbed from gastrointestinal tract, expensive Beneficial for children who are resistant to other diuretics	Observe for side effects (skin rash, drowsiness, ataxia, hyperkalemia) Do not administer potassium supplements
Triamterene (Dyrenium)	Oral	2 hours	4-8 hours	12-24 hours	Appears to interfere with exchange of sodium, potassium, and hydrogen in distal tubule	Has a potassium-sparing effect, frequently used with thiazides	Observe for side effects (diarrhea, nausea and vomiting, weakness, headache, dry mouth, rash, hyperkalemia) Do not administer potassium supplements

From Whaley, L.F., and Wong, D.L.: Nursing care of infants and children, ed. 2, St. Louis, 1983, The C.V. Mosby Co.

enteral potassium should be administered through a central line. If oral preparations are given, they should be mixed with a small amount of juice to conceal the taste and minimize gastrointestinal irritation. The dose should not be mixed into the entire feeding (liquid or solid) because the child may not complete the meal. This leads to inaccurate administration of the drug and variable therapeutic levels.

Fluid restriction. Edema is a common manifestation of fluid retention due to congestive heart failure. The Frank-Starling law states the following: "The force of cardiac contraction is related to the degree of filling of the ventricles; the more the ventricles fill, the greater the subsequent contraction." If the heart is not able to pump adequately, there is diminished renal perfusion. Water and so-

dium retention results from aldosterone secretion. Concurrently, it is postulated there is an increase in the secretion of antidiuretic hormone (ADH). This relative increase in fluid volume causes a greater cardiac workload. Plasma sodium levels are lowered because of water retention. Therefore the retained hypotonic plasma allows fluid to shift from the blood into the interstitial spaces. Edema and weight gain result, and fluid restrictions may be required (Table 15-8).

Oral fluid restrictions may be difficult for toddlers and older children. The clinician may ask the older child to help with monitoring their fluid intake, which provides a sense of control over the situation. Fluids should not be left at the bedside. It is advantageous to use small cups when giving fluids because young children associate the

Table 15-8. Dynamic equilibrium of fluid and its constituents, (adequate daily fluid intake in relation to age and weight in children with normal body temperature)

Age	Weight, kg	ml/kg body weight	ml/24 h
NEWBORN			
0-12 hours	2.5-4.0 (5.5-8.8)*	0	—
12 hours-15 days	Same as above	60-120	150-480
INFANTS			
16 days-5 months	3.0-7.7 (6.6-17.0)	150	450-1156
6-12 months	8.0-12.0 (17.6-26.4)	120-75†	960-900
12-24 months	10.0-15.0 (22.0-33.0)	75	750-1125
CHILDREN			
2-5 years	13.6-20 (30.0-44.0)	45	612-900
6-10 years	22.6-34.0 (50.0-75.0)	30	678-1023

Adapted from Wasserman, E., and Slobody, L.: Survey of clinical pediatrics, ed. 6, New York, 1974, McGraw-Hill Book Co.; from A nurse's guide to fluid and electrolyte balance by Audrey Burgess. Copyright © 1979 by Audrey Burgess. Used with the permission of McGraw-Hill Book Company.

*Weight in pounds is given in parentheses.

†As solid foods are introduced, fluid intake decreases in relation to body weight.

FOODS HIGH IN POTASSIUM AND LOW IN SODIUM

Dried fruit (prunes, apricots, peaches, raisins)
Molasses
Bananas
Bitter chocolate
Citrus fruit juices

FOODS HIGH IN POTASSIUM

Protein rich foods
Nonstarchy vegetables
Most whole fruits (dried or fresh)
Fresh fruit juices (excluding apple and cranberry)
Nuts
Milk solids

From A nurse's guide to fluid and electrolyte balance by Audrey Burgess. Copyright © 1979 by Audrey Burgess. Used with the permission of McGraw-Hill Book Company.

size of the container with the volume of fluid. There will be greater satisfaction if the child is able to drink from a full small cup rather than a partially filled large cup.

Sodium restriction. Loss of fluids may result in hypernatremic states. Discussing sodium restriction with parents will increase compliance to the dietary regimen. The clinician and dietitian can devise meal plans for the child and family that not only meet the daily caloric and fluid requirements but also consider the family's cultural and economic needs. The box above lists foods low in sodium and high in potassium.

Hemoglobin and hematocrit. An elevated hemoglobin and hematocrit may be present because of compensatory polycythemia. In the presence of dehydration, this state of hemoconcentration potentiates thromboembolitic disorders. Component blood therapy (that is, therapy using packed red blood cells) is used to correct anemia without causing circulatory overload.

PROBLEM: Altered gas exchange

INTERVENTION: Monitoring blood gas determinations

Metabolic acidosis is the product of decreased blood flow, tissue perfusion, and systemic oxygenation that may result from congestive heart failure. Ischemic tissues must metabolize in an anaerobic or hypoxic environment. Pulmonary edema or ineffective respiratory patterns result in hypercapnia. As the Pco_2 content increases in the blood, the respiratory centers in the brain are depressed. Tachypnea is then replaced by a slow, irregular, and shallow respiratory pattern. Initially, tachypnea develops as the body attempts to remove ("blow off") the excess carbon dioxide. Slow, shallow, irregular respirations manifest the depressed neurological status. Neonates usually present a mixed or combined acidosis. The primary causes are hypoxia and the inability to effectively remove CO_2 (Table 15-9).

Blood gas analysis reveals the acid-base balance and oxygenation of the patient with congestive heart disease. Samples may be obtained from central indwelling arterial catheters (umbilical arterial lines in neonates) or arterial "stick" methods. In newborns a heelstick sample can be drawn for capillary specimens. Warming the heel of the foot

Table 15-9. Acid-base assessment guide for neonates

Parameter	Birth normals	Postbirth abnormals
Heart rate	120-160 beats/min	From birth: <102 beats/min >160 beats/min

Respirations	40-50 breaths/min
	Slight irregularity
	Nose breathing
		After 20 min:
		  Periods of apnea
		  Flaring alae nasi
		  Substernal retraction
		  Grunting
		  Nasal stuffiness

Blood pressure	30-60 mm Hg mean
	  pressure between
	  systolic and diastolic;
	  same pressure in arm
	  and leg
		<30 arm and leg
		<30 leg and normal in the
		  arm

Temperature	95-97° F (axillary at
	  room temperature of
	  75° F)
		From birth:
		  Drop >2.5° F during first
		    10-15 min
		  Drop >2° F after 1 h

Blood pH	7.2-7.3	<7.3 after 6 h
Blood O_2 sat	0-20%	<65% after 1 h
P_{CO_2}	50-60 mm Hg	>45 mm Hg after 12 h
Serum HCO_3^-	12 meq/liter	<17 meq/liter after 1 h
Hemoglobin	16.8 g/100 ml	<12.5 g/100 ml after few hours
Hematocrit	58-62%	<40-50% after 1 h

From A nurse's guide to fluid and electrolyte balance by Audrey Burgess. Copyright © 1979 by Audrey Burgess. Used with the permission of McGraw-Hill Book Company.

for approximately 15 minutes before the blood is withdrawn will provide an arterialized capillary specimen. The finger stick method is utilized when the child is of walking age.

Blood gases are obtained during the admission examination to establish baseline parameters. PO_2, P_{CO_2}, pH, and bicarbonate values should be evaluated on a timely basis, especially if the patient is receiving oxygen therapy or requires ventilatory assistance. Metabolic acidosis is corrected with sodium bicarbonate. However, in the setting of congestive heart failure this must be judiciously administered.

PROBLEM: Increased risk of infection
INTERVENTION: Infection control

Since the child with congestive heart failure is susceptible to infections in general, and respiratory in particular, good infection control practices are necessary at home and at the hospital. A respiratory infection—for example, bronchopneumonia—can precipitate heart failure in a compensated child. Hospital personnel who have infections themselves or are caring for children with active infections should not care for the infant in heart failure. Clinicians should structure the child's environment to prevent contact with infectious patients (for example, restricted play times, room selection). Hand washing is the single most effective tool in preventing infections. Antibiotics are sometimes ordered prophylactically to decrease the risk of infection. The child's temperature is monitored closely and any elevation reported.

Infection control at home is more difficult than in the hospital. The family needs to weigh the benefits of isolating their child from all sources of infections and of treating their child as normally as possible. In infancy it is easier to keep the child isolated. But when there are siblings in the household or when the child with congestive heart failure is a toddler, life should proceed as normally as possible. The parent should take the usual precautions of dressing the child for the weather and not exposing the child in close quarters to someone with an active upper respiratory infection.

PROBLEM: Knowledge deficit: caring for the child with congestive heart failure

INTERVENTION: Parent education; teaching home care

Parents need help and reassurance when their infant is sent home with congestive heart failure. This happens often when the neonate is diagnosed after birth with a congenital heart lesion—for example, ventricular septal defect—and the surgeon prefers to wait until the child grows before surgical correction can occur. The easiest and most useful preparation for home care is involvement of the parent(s) in hospital care. If the family has a sound knowledge of the medical problem and hospital care, the teaching required is most successfully accomplished.

The most important content to teach the parents is to identify when their child is becoming decompensated, due to progressive congestive heart failure; at this time they should immediately notify the physician. Each child's level of tolerance is different and the parents need specific guidelines for their own child. If the parents or primary caretakers have been actively involved in hospital care, they have seen the infant in acute failure and will be able to identify this condition at home.

Many of the interventions discussed are applicable to home care. Those interventions that worked best in the hospital should be conveyed to the parents so they can be used at home. For example, if a humidifying tent helped the child's pulmonary congestion, the parents can achieve the same effects by turning on the shower and playing with their child in the bathroom. Children are usually discharged without fluid or activity restrictions. It is almost impossible to enforce these restrictions with any child older than 1 year, so it would be frustrating to try. Children tend to regulate themselves; for example, they will sit or lie down when they are tired.

Teaching parents how to give any medication, especially digoxin, includes much more than the skill of administering the drug. The parent must be given information that will enable safe and competent decision-making in various situations. Parents should be instructed to give the medication when the child is not irritable. It is to be given separately from other medications. Digoxin should not be mixed with meals because the child may not finish the food. If a dose is forgotten, the next dose should be given at the regular time. Parents should be informed that digoxin is slowly excreted and that a missed dose will not endanger the child. Likewise, if the child should vomit, the drug should not be repeated if it has been more than 15 minutes since administration. Digoxin elixir is usually absorbed within 15 minutes of administration, so repeating the dose is not necessary.[3] Digoxin should be given at least 1 to 2 hours before or after meals to decrease the risk of vomiting the drug, and the physician should be notified about continued vomiting. The digoxin should be placed in a safe place, out of the reach of all children. If accidental swallowing occurs, the child should be taken to the nearest emergency room. Parents should be instructed to bring the labeled digoxin bottle to the emergency room, so the dosage and concentration can be ascertained by medical personnel.

Parents or primary caregivers will need to practice digoxin administration (that is, drawing up the dosage, checking radial pulse, giving it to the child). Practice sessions should occur before discharge, enabling the parent to seek support from nursing staff. The health care team will have frequent opportunities for feedback, assessment, and evaluation. Repeated practice of digoxin administration in a supportive environment will give the parent a sense of control and competency before implementing the therapeutic routine at home.

PROBLEM: Parental grief over the loss of a "well child"

INTERVENTION: Help parents adjust to diagnosis of congestive heart failure

The health care team must give the family time to adjust to the diagnosis of heart disease. The family's reaction to the illness, hospitalization, child's clinical indicators, and prognosis are individual. Denial most often is the least accepted reaction by nursing staff but may be the most helpful for the parents. Denial allows the parents to cope with the initial trauma, but if it persists, it can impede their ability to meet the day-to-day needs of their child. The family suffers an important loss—that of a prospective healthy child and the joys of child-rearing. The parents' acceptance of their child as "sick" is a process that is continuous.

The nurse can be instrumental in helping the family adjust to their child's illness by supporting the parents, accepting their coping mode, answering questions, and assessing their level of understanding. Since most of the children with congestive heart failure are infants, the attachment process is a vital part of the parent-child relationship. With hospitalized infants the health team must foster attachment by encouraging the parent to care for the child and by providing liberal visiting hours and/or rooming-in.

PROBLEM: Parent/child inability to understand diagnosis/treatment

INTERVENTION: Provide knowledge based on entering behavior and ability to understand

In preparing the family for procedures, the nurse is often the central member of the health team to teach the child and parents about the disease and their role in treatment. It is essential that the explanations are clear and based on the learner's level of understanding. The child's developmental stage is reflected in his understanding of the heart:

4 to 6 year old child:
Describes it as valentine shaped
Knows approximate anatomic location
Characterizes it by sounds

7 to 10 year old child:
Classifies it as vital organ
Has beginning concept of function

Child over 10 years:
Has more involved and correct concept of function
Relates stopping of heart to death[8]

(Childrens' drawings on pp. 496 and 497)

All teaching should focus on the familiar. The technical information should be simple and should convey the same information (using the same words) as the other health team members. It is especially important not to explain a procedure too far ahead of time to children but rather explain it a short time before it happens. The child will indicate how much he wants to know. Play therapy is an excellent way to help the child learn as well as encourage expression of his feelings. Parents will often understand visual explanations of the heart defect better; they should receive complementary written information also.

Preparation for cardiac catheterization or cardiac surgery is imperative for the child and family. The parents' attitude and knowledge are important factors when the child must undergo invasive procedures. The nurse should prepare the parents by giving information about the mechanics of the procedure, what the child will feel, time sequence (that is, when the child will leave, the time of procedure, and when the parents can see the child after the procedure), risks, and benefits. The child's preparation depends on the cognitive level. Under 3 years old, the child needs little prepara-

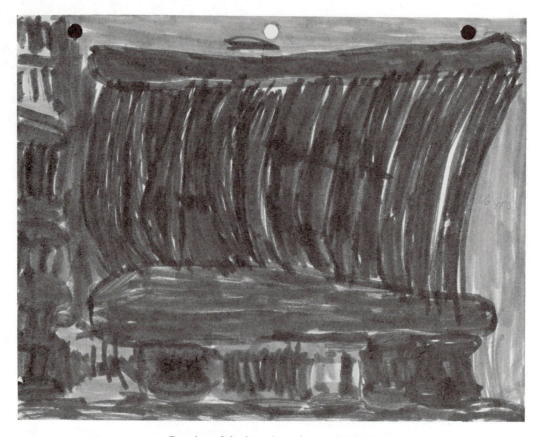

Drawing of the heart by a 6-year-old child.

tion, although a favorite toy or blanket will be helpful. From ages 3 to 7 years (Piaget's preoperational stage), there is a lag between cognition and language. The child reasons from particular to particular and cannot generalize. After 7 years old, the child's thinking is more mature and he can understand more information.[7]

PROBLEM: Parental inability to care for the child at home

INTERVENTION: Help the child/parent cope with understanding symptoms of congestive heart failure

Many children have chronic congestive heart failure that fluctuates in severity. The family needs to know how to care for the child at home and when to call the physician. The parents' thorough understanding of the disease will help them care for their child effectively. Most of the interventions listed in the previous section are applicable to home care. It is important for the parents to realize that their reactions to the symptoms (for example, dyspnea or cyanotic spells) will affect their child's ability to cope. An anxious parent leads to an anxious child. The parents should be taught preventive care (for example, keeping their child away from other children with colds) and emergency care (for example, placing their child in a side-lying, knee-chest position with head and chest elevated during a dyspneic episode). Parents should be encouraged to include others in their

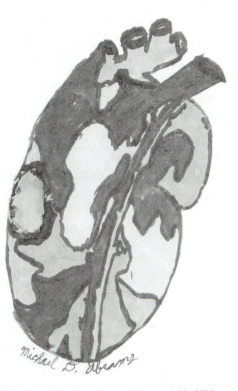

Michael D. Abrams

Drawing of the heart by an 11-year-old child.

child's care to prevent their own exhaustion and resentment.

CASE STUDY

A term infant was born to a 23-year-old primipara. The antepartum, intrapartum, and immediate postpartum periods were uneventful. A murmur was heard on physical examination but was determined to be innocent. The mother and infant were discharged on the third day of hospitalization. She was having difficulty with breastfeeding, because her son would tire easily and cry as if he were hungry. The mother consulted with the pediatri-

cian and was reassured that this was "normal." Over the next week, the infant lost weight and began breathing rapidly, especially during crying and feeding. At 2 weeks of age the infant became congested. The infant was brought to the pediatrician's office because of a "cold." Upon examination, the pediatrician noted the central cyanosis, tachypnea, and tachycardia. The baby was transferred to the neonatal intensive care unit for diagnostic tests and observation.

The admitting diagnosis was congestive heart failure; rule out congenital heart disease. The following diagnostic tests were performed: 12-lead ECG, chest radiogram (anteroposterior and lateral), echocardiogram, and subsequently, a cardiac catheterization. A ventricular septal defect was diagnosed and medical treatment was initiated. The baby was positioned in a cardiac chair with warm, humidified oxygen as needed. The mother was able to provide breast milk by pumping her breasts. Small frequent feedings were offered with a "premie nipple" to diminish exertion during the feedings. Strict intake and output and urine-specific gravities were ordered to assess adequate hydration without circulatory overload. Vital signs were taken with axillary temperatures.

The baby's physicians determined that the heart failure could be managed by palliative medical treatment rather than surgical correction at this time. The infant was digitalized in the hospital with good results. The parents were involved in all realms of the health care treatment. The actions, side effects, and toxicity of digitalis were discussed with the parents. Teaching was initiated and the parents were able to administer the medication under the supervision of the primary nurse. The primary nurse assessed and evaluated the parents' performance and knowledge of the baby's diagnosis, treatment, and prognosis. The nurse provided knowledge, answered questions, and encouraged their participation in giving direct care. Additional emotional support was given to the new parents as they required well baby knowledge and an adjustment to their baby's chronic illness. Surgical correction of the VSD was anticipated when the child reached 6 months of age. The infant was discharged home to his parents and frequent pediatric visits were scheduled.

HEALTH CARE PLAN FOR THE CHILD WITH CONGESTIVE HEART FAILURE

Potential problems	Goal	Interventions

1. Identification of child with congestive heart failure	Prompt, accurate assessment and referral or evaluation as needed	Physical assessment—observe for:
		  Tachypnea
		  Tachycardia
		  Cyanosis
		  Edema
		  Hepatomegaly
		  Failure to thrive
		Subjective history:
		  Feeding difficulties
		  Fatigability
		  Recurrent respiratory infections
		  Parent's perception of child's "difference"

2. Determination of cause of congestive heart failure	Identification of congenital anomaly or acquired heart disease	Diagnostic tests including:
		  ECG
		  Chest radiogram
		  Echocardiogram
		  Cardiac catheterization
		Identification of criteria unique to specific congenital defects
		Frequent physical assessment

HEALTH CARE PLAN FOR THE CHILD WITH
CONGESTIVE HEART FAILURE—cont'd

Potential problems	Goal	Interventions

3. Increased cardiac workload
    Impaired gas exchange
    Alteration in tissue perfusion
    Alteration in nutrition patterns—less than body requirements
    Fluid volume excess
    Sleep pattern disturbance
    Alteration in cardiac output
	Decreasing cardiac demands and oxygen consumption	Bed rest or sedation if necessary
		Minimize crying by anticipating child's needs
		Semi- or high Fowler's position; infant seat; knee chest position
		Avoid constricting clothing
		Thermoregulation
		Infection control
		Provide small, frequent feedings
		Warm, humidified oxygen as necessary

4. Inability of heart to meet baby's metabolic demands
    Potential for altered tissue perfusion
    Potential for fluid volume excess
	Improving cardiac function	Administer digitalis; diuretic therapy
		Prevent digitalis toxicity
		Teach proper drug administration to parents
		Fluid and sodium restriction
		Potassium supplements as indicated

5. Potential for alteration in family dynamics and ineffective coping Alterations in parenting	Child-family adjustment to symptoms, treatment, and prognosis	Foster helping relationship between health care team and patient-family Help parents adjust to diagnosis Assess level of understanding Help child-parent cope with symptoms Prepare child-family with hospitalization and procedures
6. Potential knowledge deficit in both parent and child	Child-parent will understand disease process and course of treatment and comply with medical-nursing regimen	Assess baseline knowledge Focus teaching on the familiar Use child-parent's language Anticipate and answer questions Provide positive feedback for parent's participation in caring for child

SUMMARY

Congestive heart failure in children usually occurs before 1 year of age and is a result of congenital heart defects. Clinical indicators are uniquely presented by pediatric patients. In order to care for children with congestive heart failure, the health care team must be aware of the physiological, developmental, and psychological stages of the pediatric patient. Consideration must also be given to the role of the parents and family in caring for the chronically ill child. Community and hospital nurses should liaison to provide continuity of care for the child and family.

REFERENCES

1. Burgess, A.: A nurses' guide to fluid and electrolytes balance, ed. 2, New York, 1979, McGraw-Hill Book Co., p. 335.
2. Holaday, B.J.: Parenting the chronically ill child, Curr. Pract. Pediat. Nurs. **2**:70, 1978.
3. Jackson, P.L.: Digoxin therapy at home: keeping the child safe, Matern. Child Nurs. J. **4**:106, March/April 1979.
4. Oakes, A.R.: Critical care nursing of children and adolescents, Philadelphia, 1981, W.B. Saunders Co., p. 139.
5. Sacksteder, S.: Congenital cardiac defects: embryology and fetal circulation, Am. J. Nurs. **78**:262, Feb. 1978.
6. Smith, K.M.: Recognizing cardiac failure in neonates, Matern. Child Nurs. J. **4**:100, March/April 1979.
7. Uzark, K.: A child's cardiac catheterization—avoiding the potential risks, Matern. Child Nurs. J. **3**:160, May/June 1978.
8. Whaley, L.F., and Wong, D.L.: Nursing care of infants and children, ed. 2, St. Louis, 1983, The C.V. Mosby Co., ch. 15, 35.
9. Yanagi, R.M., and others: Indomethacin treatment for symptomatic patent ductus arteriosus: a double blind control study, Pediatrics, **67**:647, May 1981.

ADDITIONAL READINGS

Argawala, L.R., and others: Congestive heart failure in infants, Heart Lung **5**:62, Jan./Feb. 1976.
Filipek, J.E.: Postoperative care of the pediatric cardiac patient, Crit. Care Q. **3**:45, June 1980.
Fink, B.W.: Congenital heart disease—a deductive approach to its diagnosis, Chicago, 1975, Year Book Medical Publishers, Inc., pp. 37, 129.
Fochtman, D., and others: Principles of nursing care for the Pediatric surgery patient, ed. 2, Boston, 1976, Little, Brown & Co., p. 73.
Frater, R.W.M.: Postoperative care in the pediatric cardiac patient, Heart Lung **3**:903, Nov./Dec. 1974.
Gildea, J.H., and others: Pre- and postoperative nursing care, Am. J. Nurs. **78**:273, Feb. 1978.
Gillon, J.E.: Behavior of newborns with cardiac distress, Am. J. Nurs. **73**:254, Feb. 1973.
Gottesfeld, I.B.: The family of the child with congenital heart disease, Matern. Child Nurs. J. **8**(1):101, March/April 1979.
Herrera, A.J.: Persistent fetal circulation, Perinatol./Neonatal. **3**:50, Sept./Oct. 1979.
Holaday, B.J.: Parenting the chronically ill child, Curr. Pract. Pediatr. Nurs. **2**:68, 1978.
Jackson, P.L.: Digoxin therapy at home: keeping the child safe, Matern. Child Nurs. J. **4**:105, March/April 1979.
James, F.W., and Love, E.: Congestive heart failure in infants and children, Heart Lung **3**:392, May/June 1974.
Joransen, J.A.: Recent advances in pediatric cardiac catheterization, C.V.P. **8**:29, June/July 1980.
Korones, S.B.: High-risk newborn infants—the basis for intensive nursing care, ed. 3, St. Louis, 1981, The C.V. Mosby Co.
Marlow, D.: Textbook of pediatric nursing, ed. 5, Philadelphia, 1977, W.B. Saunders Co., p. 292.
McGuire, M., Shepherd, R., and Greco, A.: Hospitalized children in confinement, Pediatr. Nurs. **4**:31, Nov./Dec. 1978.
Nelson, W.: Nelson textbook of pediatrics, ed. 11, Philadelphia, 1979, W.B. Saunders Co.
Oakes, A.R.: Critical care nursing of children and adolescents, Philadelphia, 1981, W.B. Saunders Co., p. 99.
Peterson, M.C.: Preparation of the cardiac child and family for surgery, Issues Comprehens. Pediatr. Nurs. **31**:61, Dec. 1979.
Pidgeon, V.: The infant with congenital heart disease, Am. J. Nurs. **67**(2):290, Feb. 1967.
Pikl, B.H.: Massachusetts General Hospital manual of pediatric nursing practice, Boston, 1981, Little, Brown & Co., p. 57.
Sacksteder, S., Gildea, J.H., and Dassy, C.: Common congenital cardiac defects, Am. J. Nurs. **78**:271, Feb. 1978.
Saucier, P.H.: Persistent fetal circulation, J. Obstet. Gynecol. Nurs. **9**:50, Jan./Feb. 1980.
Scipien, G.M.: Comprehensive pediatric nursing, New York, 1975, McGraw-Hill Book Co., p. 547.
Shor, V.Z.: Congenital cardiac defects: assessment and case finding, Am. J. Nurs. **78**(2):256, Feb. 1978.
Shor, V.Z.: Long-term implications of cardiovascular disease, Issues Comprehens. Pediatr. Nurs. **2**:36, Jan./Feb. 1978.
Shuler, S.N.: Death during childhood: reactions in parents and children, Curr. Pract. Pediatr. Nurs. **2**:109, 1978.
Smith, K.M.: Recognizing cardiac failure in neonates, Matern. Child Nurs. J.: **4**:98, March/April 1979.
Talner, N.S.: Congestive heart failure in the infant, Pediatr. Clin. North Am. **18**:1011, Nov. 1971.
Tesler, M., and Hardgrove, C.: Cardiac catheterization: preparing the child, Am. J. Nurs. **73**:80, Jan. 1973.
Uzark, K.: A child's cardiac catheterization—avoiding the potential risks, Matern. Child Nurs. J. **3**:158, May/June 1978.

Index